# Glial Physiology and Pathophysiology

# Glial Physiology and Pathophysiology

**Alexei Verkhratsky**
The University of Manchester, UK

and

**Arthur Butt**
University of Portsmouth, UK

**WILEY-BLACKWELL**
A John Wiley & Sons, Ltd., Publication

*Library of Congress Cataloging-in-Publication Data*
Verkhratskii, A. N. (Aleksei Nestorovich)
  Glial physiology and pathophysiology : a handbook / Alexei Verkhratsky and Arthur Butt.
      p. ; cm.
  Includes bibliographical references and index.
  ISBN 978-0-470-97852-8 (cloth) – ISBN 978-0-470-97853-5 (pbk.)
  I. Butt, Arthur. II. Title.
  [DNLM: 1.  Neuroglia–physiology. 2.  Nervous System Diseases–physiopathology. 3.  Neuroglia–pathology.  WL 102]
  612.8'1046–dc23

                                                    2012034773


A catalogue record for this book is available from the British Library.

Wiley also publishes its books in a variety of electronic formats. Some content that appears in print may not be available in electronic books.

Set in 10.5/13pt Times by Thomson Digital, Noida, India.
Printed and bound in Singapore by Markono Print Media Pte Ltd


First Impression 2013

*Dedicated to our families*

# Contents

        10.16.1   Hereditary neuropathies                              499
        10.16.2   Acquired inflammatory neuropathies                   500
        10.16.3   Diabetic neuropathies                                500
        10.16.4   Leprosy                                              501
10.17   Gliomas                                                        501
        10.17.1   Glial complications of glioma therapy                504
10.18   Concluding remarks                                             504
        References                                                     504

        **Author Index**                                               **513**

        **Subject Index**                                              **517**

# Preface

In 2007, we published the first textbook on glial neurobiology, *Glial Neurobiology: A Textbook*. The aim of our first book was to provide an introduction to glial cells, aimed at undergraduates and postgraduates in neuroscience. However, it has become clear to us that there is also the need for a more detailed and comprehensively referenced account of glial neurobiology for researchers and clinicians. This is the aim of our new book, *Glial Physiology and Pathophysiology*. We have deliberately shaped this to be a textbook that is readily accessible to those who want to get a systematic view on neuroglial function in physiology and pathophysiology.

This is meant to be a learning resource, not a reference book. The glial field has a weighty reference book, *Neuroglia*, written by several dozen experts in the different aspects of glial cell biology under the auspices of H. Kettenmann and B. Ransom. However, a substantial gap exists between the reference book *Neuroglia* and our first book *Glial Neurobiology: A Textbook*, both in the scientific content and complexity. The aim of our new book *Glial Physiology and Pathophysiology* is to fill this gap and to provide an account of glial cell biology that, hopefully, is written in a style that is enjoyable and interesting to read.

Our purpose has been to write a comprehensive, yet concise and readable, account of neuroglia – the class of cells that provide for the housekeeping and defence of the nervous system. Neuroglial functions in health and disease are generally overlooked in contemporary curricula for medics and biologists. Indeed, neuroglia are mentioned only superficially in the absolute majority of university courses. This neglect has been developed over the course of the last century or so, mainly after the discovery of electrical excitability in neurones, the principal signalling cells in the nervous system. The discovery of action potentials and synaptic transmission provided us with a fundamental understanding of nervous system functioning; neuronal networks can be relatively easily reduced to logical units communicating in binary fashion, and electronic summation provides a simple tool to predict how the excitation/inhibition of a given neurone defines output. This has had a mesmerising effect upon the minds of neurophysiologists. We can see the most powerful computers in the world employed to model the brain, based on an assumption of the primary role for action potential-mediated binary encoded signalling between logical elements that can exist in a limited (excited/resting/inhibited) number of states.

Nature, of course, is far more complex than our most ingenious engineering. The nervous system is not a computer, with an output that can be precisely calculated. There are many ways of signalling between neural cells that involve diffusion of many different molecules, each with their own targets, weaving an intricately interconnected canvas for information processing.

This book is not about processing in neural networks, but rather about overall homeostasis in the nervous system. Homeostasis is fundamental for the life of organisms, organs, tissues and cells. The nervous system is not an exception. In the course of the evolution of the nervous system that appeared in the most primitive multicultural organisms, neural cells have divided into the executive branch, represented by neurones (which control reception of sensory input and effect an output to control peripheral organs) and the housekeeping branch, represented by neuroglia. Perfection of fast signalling in neuronal networks required a division of labour, and neurones lost their ability to maintain their own survival adequately; these functions went to neuroglia.

This, then, was our endeavour – to relate the evolutionary history of neuroglia and to demonstrate how these cells assume every conceivable function aimed at maintaining nervous system homeostasis. Indeed, neuroglia oversee the birth and development of neurones, the establishment of inter-neuronal connections (the 'connectome'), the maintenance and removal of these inter-neuronal connections, wiring of the nervous system components, adult neurogenesis, the energetics of nervous tissue, metabolism of neurotransmitters, regulation of ion composition of the interstitial space and many, many more homeostatic functions.

In this book, we start with the history of neuroscience, trying to show the development of ideas and concepts of nervous system organisation. In particular, we emphasise that, from the very beginning of cellular neuroscience, little distinction was made between neural cell types and the great minds of neuroscience regarded glia as an indispensable element of the neural architecture. By doing this, we hope to prime the reader towards the notion that nervous tissue is not divided into 'more important' and 'less important' cells. The nervous tissue functions because of the coherent and concerted action of many different cell types, each contributing to an ultimate output. This reaches its zenith in humans, with the creation of thoughts, underlying acquisition of knowledge, its analysis and synthesis, and contemplating the Universe and our place in it.

Also, we contemplate the role of neuroglia in pathology. All diseases are, fundamentally, failures of the homeostasis that makes organs and organisms incompatible with life. The neurological diseases are, *ipso facto*, failures of homeostasis in the nervous tissue and are, in essence, failures of the homeostatic cells – neuroglia. Indeed, progression and outcome of all neurological diseases are defined by neuroglia, which defends the brain. When this defence system crumbles, the nervous tissue dies.

This book has been shaped by many years of work and discussions with our friends and colleagues, to whom we extend our heartfelt thanks. Also, in writing this book we have relied on many authoritative papers and review articles written by those who are more expert than ourselves in particular aspects of glial cell biology. We hope that we have done a good job in representing their findings. We apologise for any inaccuracies and for any important omissions, which we trust are few.

**Alexei Verkhratsky**
**Arthur Butt**
*June 20, 2012*

# About the Authors

## Alexei Verkhratsky

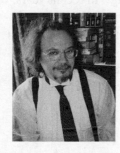 Professor Alexei Verkhratsky, MD, PhD, D.Sc., Member of Academia Europaea, Member of Real Academia Nacional de Farmacia, was born in 1961 in Stanislav, Galicia, Western Ukraine. He graduated from Kiev Medical Institute in 1983 and received his PhD (1986) and D.Sc. (1993) in Physiology from Bogomoletz Institute of Physiology, Kiev, the Ukraine. From 1990 to 1995, he was Head of the Laboratory of Cellular Signalling in Bogomoletz Institute of Physiology.

In the period between 1989 and 1995, Professor Verkhratsky was visiting scientist in Heidelberg and Gottingen, and between 1995 and 1999 he was a research scientist at Max Delbrück Centre of Molecular Medicine in Berlin. He joined the Division of Neuroscience, School of Biological Sciences in Manchester in September 1999, became a Professor of Neurophysiology in 2002 and served as head of the said division from 2002 to 2004. From 2007 to 2010, he was appointed as Visiting Professor/Head of Department of Cellular and Molecular Neurophysiology at the Institute of Experimental Medicine, Academy of Sciences of Czech Republic. In 2010, he was appointed as a Research Professor of the Ikerbasque (Basque Research Council), and in 2011 as a Visitor Professor at Kyushu University, Fukuoka, Japan.

Professor Verkhratsky was elected to membership of Academia Europaea in 2003, and since 2006 he has been Chairman of the Physiology and Medicine section. In 2011, he was elected a foreign member of Real Academia Nacional de Farmacia, Spain. He is editor-in-chief of *Cell Calcium* (2000) and *Membrane Transport & Signalling – Wiley Interdisciplinary Reviews* (2009), Receiving Editor (neuroscience) of *Cell Death & Disease* (2009) and a member of the editorial boards of *Pflugers Archiv European Journal of Physiology, Journal of Molecular & Cellular Medicine, Acta Physiologica (Oxford), Acta Pharmacologica Sinica* (2005), *Glia* (2008), *Frontiers in Neuropharmacology, Frontiers in Aging Neuroscience,* (2009), *Purinergic Signalling, ASN Neuro* (2010), *Neuroscience Bulletin* (2011). He has delivered more than 180 international invited lectures and seminars.

Professor Verkhratsky is an internationally recognised scholar in the field of cellular neurophysiology. His research is concentrated on the mechanisms of inter- and intracellular signalling in the central nervous system, being especially focused on two main types of neural cells, on neurones and neuroglia. He has made important contributions to understanding the chemical and electrical transmission in reciprocal neuronal-glial communications and on the role of intracellular calcium ion signals in the integrative processes in the nervous system. Many of his studies are dedicated to investigations of cellular mechanisms of neurodegeneration.

In collaboration with Dr. P. Fernyhough, Professor Verkhratsky demonstrated that experimental diabetes is associated with disruption of $Ca^{2+}$ homeostasis and mitochondrial function; both of these systems appear to be regulated by insulin-receptor-dependent signalling cascades. He was the first to perform intracellular $Ca^{2+}$ recordings in old neurones in isolation and *in situ*, which provided direct experimental support for the '$Ca^{2+}$ hypothesis of neuronal ageing'. In recent years, in collaboration with Professor J. J. Rodriguez, he has been studying glial pathology in Alzheimer's disease. He is the author of a pioneering hypothesis of astroglial atrophy as a mechanism of neurodegeneration.

Professor Verkhratsky has authored and edited ten books, edited 19 special issues and published approximately 300 papers and chapters. His papers have been cited more than 8,500 times (H-index 53).

# Arthur Butt

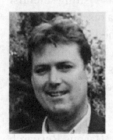 Professor Arthur Butt has worked on glial cells for over 25 years, using multiple cell biological, molecular, anatomical and physiological techniques. He received his PhD from King's College, London in 1986, working with Joan Abbott, a leader in blood-brain barrier research. After a postdoctoral position in the lab of Ed Liebermann (North Carolina, USA) and a Grass Fellowship at the Wood's Hole Marine Laboratories, he joined the lab of Bruce Ransom (Yale University, USA). Here, he began his work on glial cells in the optic nerve, and he has pursued this line of research ever since.

Professor Butt obtained his first position in Guy's and St Thomas's Hospitals Medical Schools in 1990, where he worked closely with Martin Berry, a leader in CNS regeneration studies. After gaining a personal chair in King's College London in 2000, Professor Butt moved to the University of Portsmouth in 2005, where he is currently Director of the Institute of Biomedical and Biomolecular Sciences. Professor Butt is closely associated with the Anatomical Society, in which he sat on the management committee and served as programme secretary for many years. He is on the editorial board of *Glia*, has acted as guest editor for a number of special issues for the *Journal of Anatomy*, and edited the first special issue on novel NG2-glial cells for the *Journal of Neurocytology* in 2000.

Much of Professor Butt's work has focused on oligodendrocytes, using the model tissue of the rodent optic nerve, on which he has published a number of reviews and book chapters. He has focused on the fundamental biology of glial cells, with a particular relevance to multiple sclerosis and neurodegeneration. In this regard, Professor Butt would like to thank especially the Multiple Sclerosis Society, the Anatomical Society and The International Spinal Research Trust, for their support over the years. He is also part of the European consortium Edu-Glia (2009–2013), which provided for the establishment of a European school for glial research training.

# Abbreviations

| | |
|---|---|
| AA | arachidonic acid |
| Aβ | β-amyloid protein |
| α-AR | α adrenergic receptor |
| β-AR | β adrenergic receptor |
| $A_{1-3}$ | adenosine receptor type 1–3 |
| ABC | ATP-binding cassette |
| AC | adenylate cyclise |
| ACh | acetyl choline |
| AChBP | acetylcholine binding protein |
| AD | Alzheimer's disease |
| ADNF | activity-dependent neurotrophic factor |
| ADP | adenosine diphosphate |
| AEP | anterior entopeduncular area |
| AIDP | acute inflammatory demyelinating neuropathy |
| AIDS | acquired immunodeficiency syndrome |
| ALS | amyotrophic lateral sclerosis ("Lou Gehrig's disease" in USA) |
| AMPA | α-amino-3-hydroxy-5-methyl-4-isoxazolepropionate |
| ankG | ankyrinG |
| ANLS | astrocyte–neurone lactate shuttle |
| ANP | atrial natriuretic peptide |
| 4-AP | 4-amynopyridine |
| AQP | aquaporin |
| AR | adrenergic receptor |
| ASIC | Acid Sensing Ion Channel |
| $AT_{1/2}$ | angiotensin receptor type 1/2 |
| ATP | adenosine triphosphate |
| AxD | Alexander disease |
| BACE 1 | β-site APP-cleaving enzyme 1 |
| BBB | blood-brain barrier |
| BC | boundary cap |
| bHLH | basic helix-loop-helix |
| BDNF | brain-derived neurotrophic factor |
| BMP | bone morphogenetic protein |
| BP | binding protein |
| BzATP | 2′,3′-(benzoyl-4-benzoyl)-ATP |

| | |
|---|---|
| cAMP | cyclic adenosine $3',5'$-monophosphate |
| cGMP | cyclic guanosine $3'5'$-monophosphate |
| CAII | carbonic anhydrase II |
| $Ca^{2+}$ | Calcium ion |
| CaM | calmodulin |
| CaM kinase | calcium-calmodulin-dependent protein kinase |
| CaM AC | calcium-calmodulin-dependent-adenylate cyclase |
| CaM-phosphatase | calcium-calmodulin-dependent-protein phosphatase |
| Casp | caspase |
| $Ca_V$ | voltage operated $Ca^{2+}$ channel |
| CB | cannabinoid receptor |
| CBP | $Ca^{2+}$ binding proteins |
| CCR | chemokine receptor |
| Cdk | cyclin-dependent kinase |
| CFTR | cystic fibrosis transmembrane conductance regulator channel |
| CGE | caudal ganglionic eminence |
| CGT | ceramide galactosyltransferase |
| CHN | congenital hypomyelinating neuropathy |
| CICR | calcium-induced calcium release |
| CIPD | chronic inflammatory demyelinating neuropathy |
| CLC | chloride channel |
| CLIC | chloride intracellular channel |
| CMT | Charcot Marie Tooth disease |
| CMT1X | X-linked Charcot Marie Tooth disease |
| CNTF | ciliary neurotrophic factor |
| CNQX | 6-cyano-7-nitroquinoxaline-2,3-dione (AMPA receptor antagonist) |
| CNPase | $2',3'$-cyclic nucleotide-$3'$-phosphodiesterase |
| CNS | central nervous system |
| COX | cyclo-oxygenase |
| CRAC | $Ca^{2+}$-release activated $Ca^{2+}$ channel |
| CREB | cyclic element-binding protein |
| CSF | cerebrospinal fluid |
| CSPG | chondroitin sulphate proteoglycan |
| CST | cerebroside sulfotransferase |
| Cx | connexin |
| CXCR | chemokine receptor |
| CysLT | cysteinyl leukotrienes |
| Da | Dalton |
| DAG | diacylglycerol |
| D-AP5 | D-2-amino-phosphonopentanoic acid (NMDA receptor antagonist) |
| DM20 | isoform of PLP |
| DOPA | dopamine |
| DRG | dorsal root ganglion |
| DRP2 | dystroglycan-related protein 2 |
| EAAT | excitatory amino acid transporter |
| EAE | experimental autoimmune encephalomyelitis |
| ECM | extracellular matrix |
| ECS | extracellular space |
| EGC | enteric glial cell |
| eGFP | enhanced green fluorescent protein |

| | |
|---|---|
| EGFR | epidermal growth factor receptor |
| $E_K$ | equilibrium potential for potassium |
| EM | electron microscopy |
| ENAC | Epithelial Sodium Channel |
| ENCC | Enteric Neural Crest Cell |
| ENS | enteric nervous system |
| Eph | ephrin |
| EPSC | excitatory postsynaptic current |
| ERK | extracellular signal-regulated protein kinase |
| ET | endothelin |
| FDG | Fluorodeoxyglucose |
| FGF2 | fibroblast growth factor 2 |
| FGFR | FGF receptor |
| fMRI | functional magnetic resonance imaging |
| GABA | γ-aminobutyric acid |
| GABA-T | GABA transaminase |
| GAD | glutamate decarboxylase |
| GalC | galactocerebroside |
| GAT | GABA transporter |
| GC | guanylate cyclise |
| GPCR | G-protein coupled receptor |
| GDAP | ganglioside-induced differentiation-associated protein |
| GDNF | glial derived neurotrophic factor |
| GFAP | glial fibrillary acidic protein |
| GFP | green fluorescent protein |
| GI | gastrointestinal |
| GJ | gap junction |
| GLAST | glutamate/aspartate transporter |
| GLT-1 | glutamate transporter-1 |
| GluA1-4 | AMPA receptor subunits |
| GluK1-3 | kainite receptor subunits |
| GluN1-3 | NMDA receptor subunits |
| GluR | glutamate receptor |
| GlyT | glycine transporter |
| GnRH | gonadotropin-releasing hormone |
| GRP | glial restricted precursor |
| GSNO | S-nitrosoglutathione |
| GSK3β | Glycogen synthase kinase 3β |
| 2-HETE | 2-hydroxyeicosatetraenois acid |
| 5-HT | 5 hydroxy tryptamine (serotonin) |
| $H_{1-3}$ | histamine receptor type 1–3 |
| HAD | HIV-1 associated dementia |
| HD | Huntington's disease |
| HDAC | HDAC |
| HIPK | homeodomain interacting protein kinase |
| HIV | immunodeficiency virus |
| HIVE | HIV-encephalitis |
| HNPP | hereditary neuropathy with liability to pressure palsies |
| HTLV-1 | Human T-lymphotropic virus type-1 |
| IFN | interferon |

| | |
|---|---|
| IGF | insulin-like growth factor |
| IGIF | interferon inducing factor |
| iGluR | ionotropic glutamate receptor |
| IL | interleukin |
| InsP$_3$ | inositol-trisphosphate |
| InsP$_3$R | inositol-trisphosphate receptors |
| IPC | intermediate progenitor cell |
| JAK | Janus kinase |
| JAM | junctional adhesion molecule |
| JNK | c-Jun N terminal kinase |
| KA | kainate |
| kDa | kilo Dalton |
| K$_A$ | rapidly inactivating A-type K$^+$ channel |
| K$_D$ | delayed rectifier K$^+$ channel |
| K$_{Ca}$ | calcium-activated K$^+$ channel |
| K$_{ir}$ | inward rectifier K$^+$ channel |
| [K$^+$]$_i$ | intracellular K$^+$ concentration |
| [K$^+$]$_o$ | extracellular K$^+$ concentration |
| LDH | lactate dehydrogenase |
| LEF | lymphoid enhancing factor |
| Les/Ls | late endosomes/lysosomes |
| LGE | lateral ganglionic eminence |
| LIF | leukaemia-inhibitory factor |
| L-MAG | large isoform of myelin associated glycoprotein |
| LN2 | Laminin 2 |
| LPS | lypopolysaccharide |
| LTP | long-term potentiation |
| mChR | muscarinic cholinoreceptor |
| MAG | myelin associated glycoprotein |
| MAP | microtubule associated protein |
| MAPK | mitogen-activated protein kinase |
| MBP | myelin basic protein |
| M-CSFR | macrophage colony-stimulating factor receptor |
| MCT | monocarboxylase transporter |
| MEK | mitogen-activated/extracellular regulated kinase |
| MGE | medial ganglionic eminence |
| mGluR | metabotropic glutamate receptor |
| miRNA | microRNA |
| MLC | Megalencephalic leukoencephalopathy with subcortical cysts |
| MOBP | myelin-associated/oligodendrocyte basic protein |
| MOG | myelin oligodendrocyte protein |
| MOSP | myelin/oligodendrocyte specific protein |
| MPN | medial preoptic nucleus |
| MPTP | mitochondrial transition permeability pore |
| MRF | Myelin gene regulatory factor |
| MRI | magnetic resonance imaging |
| MRS | magnetic resonance spectroscopy |
| MS | multiple sclerosis |
| MSA | multiple system atrophy |
| mTOR | mammalian target of rapamycin |

| | |
|---|---|
| NAADP | Nicotinic acid adenine dinucleotide phosphate |
| NADPH | Nicotinamide adenine dinucleotide phosphate |
| $[Na^+]_i$ | intracellular $Na^+$ concentration |
| $Na_V$ | voltage-gated $Na^+$ channel |
| nAChR | nicotinic cholinoreceptor |
| NBC | sodium-bicarbonate transporter |
| NCAM | neural cell adhesion molecule |
| NCC | neural crest cell |
| NCSC | neural crest stem cell |
| NCX | sodium-calcium exchanger |
| NDPase | nucleoside diphosphatase |
| NF | neurofascin |
| NF-$\kappa$B | nuclear factor $\kappa$B |
| NGF | nerve growth factor |
| NgR | Nogo receptor |
| NHE | sodium-hydrogen exchanger |
| NK-1 | neurokinin-1 receptor (substance P receptor) |
| NKA | sodium-potassium pump ($Na^+/K^+$ ATPase) |
| NKCC | sodium-potassium-chloride cotransporter |
| NMDA | N-methyl-D-aspartate |
| NMO | Neuromyelitis optica (Devic's disease) |
| NO | Nitric oxide |
| NOS | nitric oxide synthase |
| NP | neural precursor |
| NRG | neuregulin |
| NSC | neural stem cell |
| NT | neurotrophin |
| NTDPase | nucleoside triphosphate diphosphohydrolase |
| OEC | olfactory ensheathing cell |
| Olig1/2 | oligodendrocyte lineage transcription factor 1/2 |
| OMgp | oligodendrocyte-myelin glycoprotein |
| OPC | oligodendrocyte progenitor cell |
| OSP/claudin-11 | oligodendrocyte specific protein |
| OVLT | organum vasculosum of the lamina terminalis |
| P0 | peripheral myelin protein zero |
| P2 | peripheral myelin protein 2 |
| PAF | platelet-activating factor |
| PAR | protease-activated receptors |
| PD | Parkinson's disease |
| PDGF | platelet-derived growth factor |
| PDGFR$\alpha$ | platelet-derived growth factor receptor alpha |
| PDGFR$\beta$ | platelet-derived growth factor receptor beta |
| PDS | paroxysmal depolarization shift |
| PET | positron emission tomography |
| PGE2 | prostaglandin E2 |
| PGK | phosphoglycerate kinase |
| $PIP_2$ | phosphatidylinositol (4,5)-biphosphate |
| PIP3 | phosphatidlyinositol (3,4,5)-triphosphate |
| PKA | protein kinase A |
| PKC | protein kinase C |

| | |
|---|---|
| PLC | phospholipase C |
| PLP | proteolipid protein |
| PMCA | plasmalemmal $Ca^{2+}$ ATP-ase |
| PMP22 | peripheral myelin protein 22 |
| PNPase | purine nucleoside phosphorylase |
| PNS | peripheral nervous system |
| POA | pro-oligodendroblast antigen |
| PSD | post-stroke dementia |
| PTEN | Phosphatase and tensin homologue |
| PTP | permeability transition pore |
| RMP | resting membrane potential |
| RMS | rostral migratory stream |
| ROS | reactive oxygen species |
| RTK | receptor tyrosine kinase |
| RyR | Ryanodine receptor |
| RVD | regulatory volume decrease |
| SCI | spinal cord injury |
| SCN | Suprachiasmatic Nuclei |
| SCP | Schwann cell precursor |
| SD | Sleep deprivation |
| SERCA | Sarco(Endo)plasmic Reticulum $Ca^{2+}$ ATP-ases |
| SGC | satellite glial cell |
| Shh | sonic hedgehog |
| αSMA | α-smooth muscle actin |
| S-MAG | small isoform of myelin associated glycoprotein |
| SNAP | synaptosome-associated protein (e.g. 25 kDa SNAP25) |
| SNARE | soluble N-ethyl maleimide-sensitive fusion protein attachment protein receptor |
| SNAT | sodium-coupled neutral amino acid transporter |
| SOCC | store-operated $Ca^{2+}$ channels |
| SOCE | store-operated $Ca^{2+}$ entry |
| STAT | Signal Transducers and Activators of Transcription |
| SUCNR | succinate receptor |
| SVZ | subventricular zone |
| TCA | tricarboxylic acid |
| TEA | tetraethylammonium |
| Tf | transferrin |
| TGF | transforming growth factor |
| TJ | tight junction |
| 7-TM | 7 transmembrane receptor |
| TCF | T-cell factor |
| TLR | Toll-like receptor |
| TNF | tumour necrosis factor |
| TNFR | TNF receptor |
| TRP channel | Transient receptor potential channel |
| TSP-1 | thrombospondin |
| TZ | transition zone |
| TTX | tetrodotoxin |
| VAMP2 | vesicle-associated membrane protein 2 (synaptobrevin 2) |
| V-ATPase | vacuolar V-type proton ATPase |

| | |
|---|---|
| VEGF | vascular endothelial growth factor |
| VGlutT | vesicular glutamate transporter |
| VIP | vasoactive intestinal peptide |
| VPAC | VIP/pituitary adenylate cyclase-activating peptide receptor |
| $V_m$ | membrane potential |
| VNUT | vesicular nucleotide transporter |
| VOCC | voltage-operated $Ca^{2+}$ channel |
| VRAC | volume-regulated anion channel |
| VSOAC | volume-sensitive organic anion channel |
| VSOR | volume-sensitive outwardly rectifying channel |
| VT | Volume Transmission (used only in Chap 1 – so omit?) |
| VWM | Vanishing white matter disease |
| VZ | ventricular zone |
| WT | wiring transmission (used only in Chap 1 – so omit?) |
| YY1 | Yin Yang 1 |
| ZnT | plasmalemmal $Zn^{2+}$ transporter |

# About the Companion Website

This book is accompanied by a companion website:

www.wiley.com/go/verkhratsky/glialphysiology

The website includes:
- Powerpoints of all figures from the book for downloading
- PDFs of tables from the book

# 1
# History of Neuroscience and the Dawn of Research in Neuroglia

## 1.1   The miraculous human brain: localising the brain functions

*'Many things seem miraculous until you understand them and some are so marvellous you could call them miracles.'*

Merlin to young Arthur (Crossley-Holland, 2009)

Human brain and human intellect – these are still miraculous for us. The scientific endeavours driven by human curiosity have deciphered many miracles of nature. Yet our understanding of how we think, and where lies the fundamental mechanism that distinguishes a man from a beast, remains obscure and hazy.

The general concept that brain functions are produced by immensely complex structures localised in the brain parenchyma evolved slowly over history. In the most

*Glial Physiology and Pathophysiology*, First Edition. Alexei Verkhratsky and Arthur Butt.
© 2013 by John Wiley & Sons, Ltd. Published 2013 by John Wiley & Sons, Ltd.

ancient times, the place for sprit, thoughts and cognition was believed to be associated with the heart, and this was considered to be the hegemonic organ by the Hebrews, the Mesopotamians, the Indians, the Egyptians and possibly the Chinese (Gross, 1995). The 'cardiocentric' doctrine was contemplated by ancient Greeks, who were the first to apply logic, scepticism and experimentation to understand the forces that drive the world and life. Possibly, it all began in about the 7th century BC, when Thales of Miletus made the fundamental discovery that our world is mostly made of water, a statement which, at least as far as life is concerned, remains undisputable. Slightly later, Empedocles broadened the list of basic elements of nature to earth, air, fire and water, and Democritus (460–370 BC) introduced the atomic theory, in which all differences between substances was determined by their atoms and inter-atomic relations. More or less at the same time, the idea of a special substance composed of air and vapours, the *thymós* or *pneuma*, which represents the substance of life, came into existence.

The concept of pneuma as the material substance of life, which acts as a vehicle driving all reactions of the body, was formalised by Aristotle (384–322 BC). The pneuma was a sort of 'air' substance that was diffusely present in living organisms; the mind was pneuma and had no specific localisation. According to Aristotle, the pneuma originated from the heart, and the heart was considered to be the primary organ controlling production of pneuma and also the central seat for sensory integration and initiation of movements. The heart was connected to the periphery by vessels and nerves (between which Aristotle made no distinction). The brain, which Aristotle almost certainly dissected, was of a secondary importance. The brain was a cold and bloodless organ; senseless, indifferent to touch, or even to cutting, and disconnected from the body. Most importantly, a brain was absent in many organisms that were able to move and react to the environment. The primary brain function, according to Aristotle, was to cool the pneuma emerging form the heart and thus temper the passions (Aristotle, 1992; Clarke, 1963).

An alternative concept which identified the brain as an organ of cognition was developed in parallel, being initially suggested by Alcmaeon of Croton (6th century BC), who practised dissections; he described the optic nerves and considered them as light guides connecting the eyes with the brain. Democritus suggested the first mechanism of signalling in the body. He thought about the psyche (the substance of soul and mind) as being made from the lightest atoms, which concentrated in the brain and conveyed messages to the periphery. Heavier atoms concentrated in the heart, making it the organ of emotions, and the heaviest in the liver, which therefore was the organ of appetite, gluttony and lust (Gross, 1995).

Plato was very much influenced by the ideas of Democritus and similarly considered the brain as a cognitive organ. The Hippocratic corpus (the assembly of approximately 60 texts on various aspects of medicine likely written by the members of Hippocrates' school in the 5th and 4th centuries BC) contains the treatise *On the Sacred Disease*, which directly identifies the brain as an organ of cognition: '*It ought to be generally known that the source of our pleasure, merriment, laughter, and amusement, as of our grief, pain, anxiety, and tears, is none other than the brain. It is specially the organ which enables us to think, see, and hear, and to distinguish the ugly and the beautiful, the bad and the good, pleasant and unpleasant . . . '* (Hippocrates, 1950).

Systematic studies of the brain developed in the first research institute known to humanity – the Museum at Alexandria, organised and funded by Ptolemaeus I Soter (who in this enterprise consulted Aristotle), and further developed under the reign of the Soter's son Ptolemaeus Philadelphus. The Museum employed, on a tenure basis, about 100 professors, who were provided with laboratories for anatomy and dissection, with an astronomical observatory, zoological and botanical gardens and, above all, with a grand library containing hundreds of thousands of manuscripts.

Two leading neuroanatomists of the Museum were Herophilus (335–280 BC) and Erasistratus (304–250 BC) (Von Staden, 1989; Wills, 1999), who performed numerous dissections of the brains of animals and humans, including vivisections on live human subjects – criminals supplied by royal prisons. Herophilus and Erasistratus were the first to describe macroanatomy of the brain and to discover the brain ventricles. Importantly, Herophilus made a distinction (previously unknown) between nerves and blood vessels and classified the nerves as sensory and motor (Longrigg, 1993). Herophilus and Erasistratus were most likely the first to combine Aristotle pneuma with new anatomical findings, and they proposed the cephalocentric ventricular-pneumatic doctrine (although their works did not survive, and we can judge their ideas only after later texts referring to them). For many other aspects of the history of neuroscience and our understanding of the brain, the reader may consult several comprehensive essays (Clarke and O'Malley, 1996; Longrigg, 1993; Manzoni, 1998; Swanson, 2007).

The ventricular-pneumatic doctrine became widespread and was further developed by Claudius Galen of Pergamon (129–200 AD). According to Galen, the substance of intellect and sensations was the 'psychic pneuma', an extremely light (lighter than the air) substance, which acted as a producer and conveyer of thoughts, afferent and efferent signals. The pneuma was not a gas, however, but rather a fluid which filled the ventricles and hollow nerves. In this scenario, the brain acted as a pneuma producer and as a pump maintaining movement of pneuma through the motor nerves and aspiration of pneuma from sensory nerves. At the same time, the nerves, being rigid, provided for a very rapid signal transduction, much as the pulse wave in the blood vessels. The signal transfer between sensory organs and nerves and nerves and effector organs was made possible by the virtue of microscopic pores that allow free exchange of pneuma between the nerves and peripheral tissues (Galen, 1821–1833; Manzoni, 1998). All these flows of pneuma, according to Galen, had specific anatomic routes; for example, the sensory information were delivered to the anterior ventricles, whereas the afferent signals to the muscles originated from the posterior ventricle.

Thus, the psychic pneuma was assigned the central role in neural processes, from sensation to cognition and memory. The process of pneuma formation was, according to Galen, complex; it went through several stages that involved a specific processing which transferred the inhaled air into the vital spirit. This vital spirit then entered the choroids plexus, through which it eventually reached the ventricles, where the final refinement took place. The brain parenchyma therefore had a purely supportive role, being involved in the production of pneuma, whereas the latter was the true origin of thoughts, sensations, emotions and voluntary movements. These conclusions were experimentally corroborated in experiments on live animals, in which Galen ligated the nerves and selectively compressed different parts of the brain (he believed that by doing so, he affected only the ventricles). The ligation of

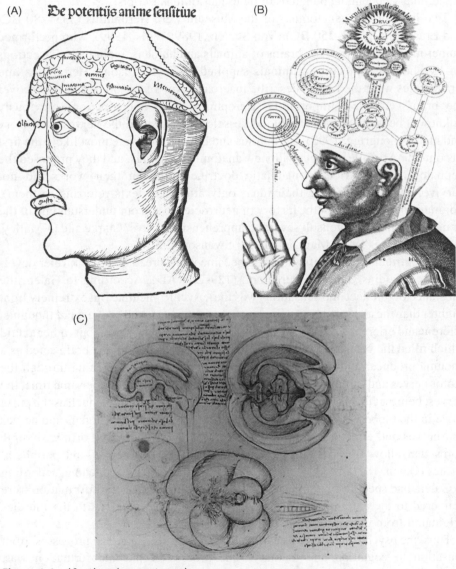

(A)  De potentijs anime sensitiue    (B)

(C)

**Figure 1.1**  (*Continued on next page*)

the nerve, as Galen discovered, led to muscle paralysis; moreover, this process was reversible and removal of the ligature restored muscle contraction. These data were perfectly compatible with an idea of fluid which needed to propagate through the nerve to initiate contraction.

In his experiments on the brain, Galen further found that compression of anterior ventricle caused blindness, whereas compression of the posterior ventricle resulted in paralysis (*De anatomics administrationibus* – cited from Manzoni, 1998). Moreover, he discovered that surgical lesions of the *pia mater* or brain parenchyma did not cause immediate effects unless the ventricle was opened. The damage to the ventricles resulted either in serious sensory deficits (anterior ventricle) or in collapse and death (middle and posterior ventricles). According to Galen, the mechanism concerned was simple – opening of the ventricles led to the escape of psychic pneuma that rendered the brain incapable of performing its functions.

The ventricular-pneumatic doctrine became generally accepted and, with many modifications accumulated during centuries (for a comprehensive account see Manzoni, 1998), it dominated brain physiology through Middle Ages and the Renaissance (Figure 1.1). The main modifications of Galenic neurophysiology were represented by further attempts to localise brain function. In the Middle ages, Arabic (e.g. Avicenna and Averroes), and European (e.g. Albertus Magnus, Tomas Aquinas and Roger Bacon) anatomists and medics associated different faculties of the nervous system with distinct ventricles. Most often, the anterior ventricle was described as a place for sensory inputs and the middle ventricle provided for creative

**Figure 1.1**   Localisation of brain functions in the framework of pneumatic-ventricular doctrine.

A–C. The three-cell concept that divided localisation of functions between different ventricles and assumed sequential information processing from the first ventricle, which receives the sensory input, to the third, which commands the behaviour.

A.  The conceptual scheme of Albertus Magnus in the later version from the 16th century, made by Gregorius Reisch, who was the Prior of House of Carthusians at Freiburg and confessor to the Emperor Maximilian, and who published a concise encyclopaedia of knowledge in 1503 (Reisch, 1503).

B.  The much-elaborated scheme from another encyclopaedic book (from the chapter 'The Art of Memory') by English Paracelcian physician Robert Fludd (Fludd, 1617–1621).

C.  Cerebral ventricles (ox brain), as seen by Leonardo da Vinci in about 1508. In the small drawing on the right, the syringe can be seen inserted into the floor of the third ventricle, which has expanded somewhat with the pressure. The foramen of Monro, linking the lateral ventricles to the third ventricles, can be seen, as can the aqueduct of Sylvius and the two lateral and the fourth ventricles. In the upper left figure, Leonardo expands the drawing and adds the words '*imprensiva*' in the lateral ventricles, '*senso comune*' in the third ventricle, and '*memoria*' in the fourth. The upper right drawing shows the ventricles from below and the lower left drawing shows the base of the brain, demonstrating the arterial network called the '*rete mirabile*'. (da Vinci, 1978–1980).

imagination, cognition and intellect, whereas the posterior ventricle was a seat for memory (see a comprehensive account written by Manzoni, 1998).

A multitude of scholars throughout Europe (e.g. Petrus Montagnana, Lodovico Dolce, Ghiradelli of Bologna and Theodor Gull of Antwerp) produced their own mapping of brain functions within the ventricles. Leonardo da Vinci, for example, believed in the central role of the middle ventricle, where both soul and judgement dwell (Figure 1.1): '*The soul seems to reside in the judgment, and the judgment would seem to be seated in that part where all the senses meet; and this is called the* senso commune.' (cited from Pevsner, 2002).

Leonardo placed the memory into the posterior ventricle, and the anterior ventricles were responsible for interfacing the sensory inputs with *senso commune*, the function defined as '*imprensiva*' (Pevsner, 2002). Leonardo was the first to make an accurate image of the brain ventricles (Figure 1.1), by filling them with melted wax, thus obtaining their precise cast (da Vinci, 1978–1980): '*Make two vent-holes in the horns of the greater ventricles, and insert melted wax with a syringe, making a hole in the ventricle of memory; and through such a hole fill the three ventricles of the brain. Then when the wax has set, take apart the brain, and you will see the shape of the ventricles exactly.*' (cited from Pevsner, 2002; see also Del Maestro, 1998; Woolam, 1952).

Andreas Vesalius placed the *senso commune* in the anterior ventricle, whereas middle and posterior ventricles were respectively associated with intellect and memory (Vesalius 1543). It was Vesalius who made the most detailed drawings of the peripheral nervous system (Figure 1.2).

Final tuning of the ventricular-pneumatic doctrine was made by René Descartes (1596–1650), who regarded the body as a machine and proposed a mechanical theory of nerve propagation, according to which peripheral stimulation triggered mechanical displacement of nerves that almost immediately caused the central end of the nerve to twitch, resulting in the release of 'animal spirit' or 'a very fine flame' (Descartes, 1664). He also introduced the concept of automatic reflexes, which highlighted the rapidity of signal propagation through the nervous system.

Probably the first neuroanatomists who realised that brain functions are associated with the organ parenchyma, and even more specifically with the grey matter, were Marcello Malpighi (*Epist. de cerebro et cort. Cereb. ad Fracassatum* – Malpighi, 1687) and Thomas Willis (Willis, 1672). This conceptual change induced further interest in localising the brain functions. Starting from the 1780s, the works of Georg Prochaska (Prochaska, 1784), followed by prolific writings of Franz Joseph Gall, Johann Gaspard Spurzeim and George Combe (Combe, 1847; Gall, 1835; Gall and Spurzheim, 1810–1819; Spurzheim, 1826), gave birth to phrenology (literally the 'science of mind'). The term 'phrenology' was introduced by Thomas Ignatius Forster; initially this theory was called 'organology' and was also known as 'craniology' or 'physiognomy' – Macalister, 1911).

Phrenology developed rapidly and gained amazing popularity, especially in America, because of the efforts of the Fowler brothers and Samuel Wells

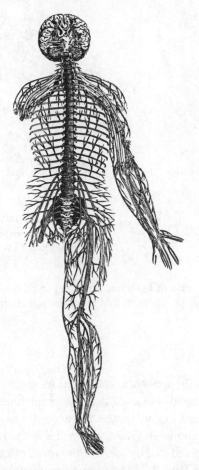

**Figure 1.2** The adult human nervous system as seen from the front, with the brain tilted upward to expose the cranial nerve roots emerging from the base, drawn by Andreas Vesalius in the mid-16th century (Vesalius, 1543).

(Fowler & Fowler, 1875; Wells, 1894). Phrenology assigned a multitude of functions to various regions of the brain, which (it was assumed) were mirrored by the surface of the skull (Figure 1.3). This assignment, however, was based on purely empirical observations of the behaviour of different people. Nonetheless, phrenology introduced a fundamental notion that specific functions may be associated with specific regions of the brain, which initiated a further quest for anatomical correlates of these different functions. Ideas of morphological and functional segregations of the brain regions were developed by Luigui Rolando, who was the first to make direct electrical stimulation of brain structures in search for primary motor areas (Caputi *et al.*, 1995).

The idea of functional sub-divisions of the brain was not generally accepted at the time and much opposition was mounted by the most respected neurophysiologists,

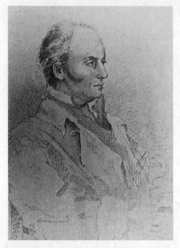

Franz Joseph Gall (1758 - 1828)

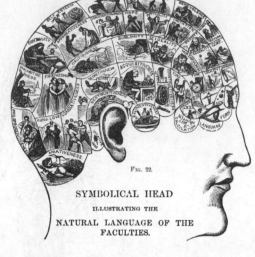

Fig. 22.

SYMBOLICAL HEAD
ILLUSTRATING THE
NATURAL LANGUAGE OF THE
FACULTIES.

**Figure 1.3**  Cortical localization of functions according to phrenology.
Portrait of Franz Joseph Gall (1758–1828) and phrenological chart according to Samuel Wells
(Wells, 1894).

such as Pierre Frourens, François Magendie and Johannes Müller (Frourens, 1846; Müller, 1838–1842), who all believed that the brain functions as a single organ. Even if they were prepared to give some allowances for motor centres (as Johannes Müller did), they believed that the mind and will and thoughts were the product of the entire organ. The heated discussions on the topic of cortical localization were instrumental in inspiring Paul Broca to search for functionally distinct brain areas. This led to the discovery of the Broca area in the posterior-inferior part of the frontal cortex of the dominant hemisphere – the area that controls the exclusive human function of articulate speech (Broca, 1861).

Nine years later, the first electrophysiological mapping of the motor cortex of the dog was performed by Gustav Theodor Fritsch and Edward Hitzig (Fritsch & Hitzig, 1870), who demonstrated that stimulation of certain areas produced specific motor reactions; in all, they found five distinct motor centres. These first experiments were followed by the truly systematic and comprehensive research of David Ferrier, who developed the first advanced map of functional speciality of various brain regions, including motor and sensory (vision, hearing and taste) areas (Ferrier, 1875, 1876, 1878, 1890). Ferrier and many of his contemporaries, including Charles Sherrington, interpreted these findings as a basis for 'scientific phrenology'.

Incidentally, Ferrier's experiments on primates almost led him to jail, when the Victoria Street Society for the Protection of Animals from Vivisection brought charges for 'frightful and shocking' experiments, using as a legal pretext "The

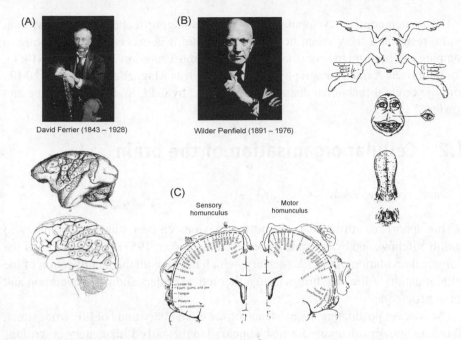

**Figure 1.4**   The sensory motor mapping of the brain.

A.  Cortical mapping of the monkey made by David Ferrier.

B.  The original homunculus, as drawn by Wielder Penfield and Edwin Bouldrey (Penfield & Bouldrey, 1937). In the figure legend, they wrote:

> *'Fig. 28. Sensory and motor homunculus. This was prepared as a visualization of the order and comparative size of the parts of the body as they appear from above down upon the Rolandic cortex. The larynx represents vocalisation, the pharynx swallowing. The comparatively large size of thumb, lips and tongue indicate that these members occupy comparatively long vertical segments of the Rolandic cortex, as shown by measurements in individual cases. Sensation in genitalia and rectum lie above and posterior to the lower extremity but are not figured.'*

C.  The modern view of sensory-motor homunculus as represented in textbooks.

Cruelty to Animals Act of 1876" (Fishman, 1995). The medical community mounted a passionate defence[1] and finally the charges were dropped.

The mapping of the brain continued until Wilder G. Penfield accomplished the task of identifying the sensory and motor cortical representations and introduced the widely accepted 'homunculus' to visualise them graphically (Figure 1.4; Penfield & Bouldrey, 1937; Penfield, 1986).

---

[1] Summons under the Vivisection Act: *British Medical Journal* 1881; **2**, 752. The antivivisection prosecution. *British Medical Journal* 1881; **2**, 785. Dr. Ferrier's localisations; for whose advantage? *British Medical Journal* 1881; **2**, 822–824. Correspondence. Proposed subscription to Dr. Ferrier. *British Medical Journal* 1881; **2**, 834. The Charge against Professor Ferrier under the Vivisection Act: Dismissal of the Summons. *British Medical Journal* 1881; **2**, 836–842.

The contemporary developments of *in vivo* imaging techniques will, without doubt, result in a 'new scientific phrenology', and it is exceedingly interesting to compare the brain maps constructed with Positron Emission Tomography (PET), Computerized Axial Tomography (CAT) or Nuclear Magnetic Resonance (NMR) with the original functional distribution proposed by Gall, Spurzheim, Combe and Fowlers.

## 1.2  Cellular organisation of the brain

*'Omnis cellula e cellula'*

This aphorism, attributed by some to François-Vincent Raspail[2], by many to Rudolf Virchow, and by others to Robert Remak (Baker, 1953), is an epitome of the biological revolution of the 19th century, which begun with the identification of the cellular nature of life, and brings us to a theoretical understanding of evolution and the genetic code.

The concept postulating the existence of the elementary units of life, from which all tissues and organisms are formed, appeared in the early 17th century in writings of several philosophers, most notably Pierre Gassendi and Robert Boyle. The origins of cellular theory are rooted in the discoveries of the first microscopists. The very first microscope is believed to be created by Zacharias Janssen in about 1595 (it is likely that his father, Hans Janssen, was involved, too). According to the general view, Janssen invented both single-lens and compound microscopes.

Microscopes were initially used for microscopic observations of plants, and it was Robert Hooke who, when examining the fine structure of cork, visualised the regular structures that reminded him of the monk's cells in the monastery dormitories, and thus the term 'cell' was born (Hooke, 1665). The first animal cells were discovered, in all likelihood, by Antonius van Leeuwenhoek who, in his many letters to the Royal Society, described bacteria (and named them *animalcules* or little animals) and erythrocytes, observed single muscle fibres, followed the movements of live spermatozoids and was the first to see the regular structure (representing single axons) in sagittal slices of peripheral nerves (Figure 1.5A; Bentivoglio, 1996; Leeuwenhoek, 1673–1696, 1798). Leeuwenhoek reflected on the latter observation made in 1717: *'Often and not without pleasure, I have observed the structure of the nerves to be composed of very slender vessels of*

---

[2] This seems to have become a popular general belief; and is stated in numerous papers, e.g. Tan SY & Brown J. (2006). Rudolph Virchow (1821–1902): 'pope of pathology'. *Singapore Medical Journal* **47**(7), 567–568; Wright NA & Poulsom R. (2012). Omnis cellula e cellula revisited: cell biology as the foundation of pathology. *Journal of Pathology* **226**(2), 145–147; and even in Wikipedia (http://en.wikipedia.org/wiki/François-Vincent_Raspail). The reference to original Raspail writing given in these sources (a paper of Raspail on the development of starch in the grains of wheat – Raspail FV. (1825). Developement de la fecule dans les organes de la fructification des cereales. *Annales Des Sciences Naturelles* **6**, 224) does not contain the sentence in question; we failed to find any original text written by Raspail which contains the phrase.

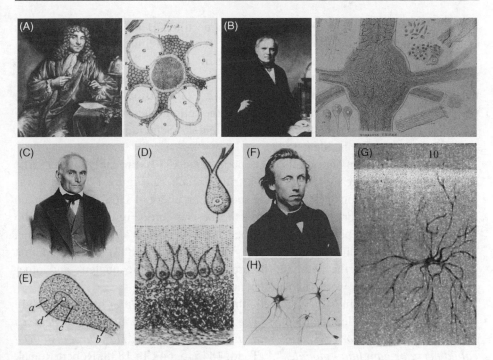

**Figure 1.5**   First images of neural cells.

A. Antonius van Leeuwenhoek (1632–1723) and his drawing of a *'small Nerve (BCDEF)'*,
   composed by many 'vessels' in which *'the lines or strokes denote the cavities or orifices of those*
   *vessels. This Nerve is surrounded, in part, by five other Nerves (GGGGG)'* in which only 'external
   coats' are represented. The image was kindly provided by Prof. Marina Bentivoglio, University
   of Verona.

B. Christian Gottfried Ehrenberg (1795–1876) and his image of the nerve cell of the leech
   (Ehrenberg, 1836) (kindly provided by Professor Helmut Kettenmann, Max Delbruck Center for
   Molecular Medicine, Berlin).

C, D. Johann Evangelista Purkinje (1787–1869) and the first drawings of the Purkinje neurone
   made by him for the Congress of Physicians and Scientists Conference in Prague, in 1837. The
   image was kindly provided by Prof. Helmut Kettenmann.

E. The first published drawing of a neurone, made by Gustav Gabriel Valentin (1810–1883)
   (Valentin, 1836).

F, G, H. Otto Friedrich Karl Deiters (1834–1863) and his drawings (Deiters, 1865) of
   motoneurones and 'connective tissue cells' (astrocytes). The images were kindly provided by
   Prof. Helmut Kettenmann.

*an indescribable fineness, running lengthwise to form the nerve.*' (cited from
Bentivoglio, 1996).

Slightly later, Felice Gaspar Ferdinand Fontana also observed the fine cylindrical
nerve fibres that were mechanically dissected from a nerve and observed at
700× magnification (Bentivoglio, 1996). In 1824, Henri Milne-Edwards identified

the basic life unit as 'globule' and, at the same time, Henri Dutrochet made a statement that cells are morphological and functional units of life, and that 'everything is ultimately derived from the cell' (Harris, 1999). Around 1830, Robert Brown defined the nucleus (Ford, 1992), although the first description of the nucleus was made by Franz Bauer, in 1802. Cell division was discovered (in plants) by Barthelemy Dumortier in 1832, and the cellular theory was formalised by Theodor Schleiden and Matthias Jakob Schleiden (Schleiden, 1838; Schwann, 1839; Schwann and Schleiden, 1847).

Early observations of nerve cells were made in the 1830s. Probably the very first descriptions were made by Christian Gottfried Ehrenberg (Figure 1.5B), who was investigating the nervous system of the leech (Ehrenberg, 1836), and by Johann Evangelista Purkyně (or Purkinje in English transcription) (Figure 1.5C, D), who was studying the cerebellum and described the cell named after him (Purkinje, 1837). Purkinje's pupil, Gustav Gabriel Valentin (1810–1883), made the first published drawing of the neurone (Figure 1.5E), where the nucleus and other intracellular structures were visible (Valentin, 1836).

Purkinje and Valentin named the cells they observed *kugeln* or globules and, in 1845, Robert Todd called them cells: '*The essential elements of the grey nervous matter are "vesicles" or cells, containing nuclei and nucleoli. They have also been called nerve or ganglion "globules".*' (Todd, 1845, p. 64). In 1838, Robert Remak made the description of nerve fibres and visualised the covering sheath around them (Remak, 1838).

Several types of neuroglial cells (see below) were described by Heinrich Müller, Max Schulze and Karl Bergmann. In 1862, the neuro-muscular junction was described by Wilhelm Friedrich Kühne, who named it the '*endplate*' (Kühne, 1862). Slightly later, the very detailed images of both neurones and stellate glial cells (probably astrocytes – Figure 1.5F, G, H) were made by Otto Deiters (Deiters, 1865). Deiters tragically died very young at 29 from typhoid fever.

It has to be kept in mind that these early cellular images were done mostly on unstained preparations, following painstaking isolation of cells by microsurgery. The histological revolution occurred in 1873, when Camillo Golgi developed the silver-chromate staining technique (the famous '*reazione nera*' or black staining – Golgi, 1873, 1903) which, for the first time, allowed neurohistologists to obtain images of neural cells in their entirety (Figure 1.6; for a comprehensive and vividly written account of Golgi's life and research, see Mazzarello, 2010).

The end of the 1880s marked the arrival of the neuronal doctrine, very much driven by the efforts of Santiago Ramón y Cajal. Cajal's first papers dedicated to the fine structure of the nervous system begun to appear in 1888, about one year after he learned the black staining technique. With characteristic determination and originality, Cajal made a special journal for his papers, the *Revista Truimestral de Histologia Normal y Patologica*, of which he naturally became the editor-in-chief, and the first issues of this journal were almost entirely occupied by his papers (Mazzarello, 2010).

Olfactory bulb

Hippocampus

Cerebellum

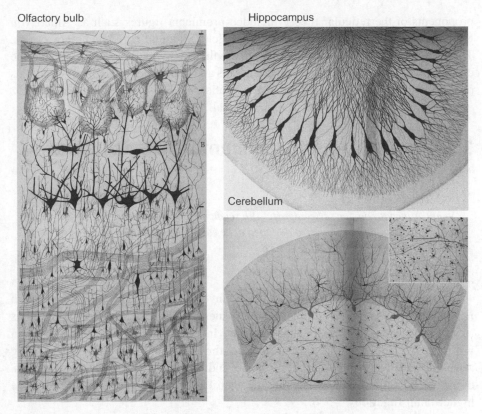

**Figure 1.6** Neural cells stained by Golgi's *reazione nera* or black stain reaction. Reproduced from Golgi, 1875, 1903. Images were kindly provided by professor Paolo Mazzarello, University of Pavia. (Full colour version in plate section.)

In the first paper published in the first issue of his journal, Cajal made the seminal statement that *'each nerve cell is a totally autonomous physiological canton'* (Ramón y Cajal, 1888). One year later, in October, 1889, Cajal attended the German Anatomical Congress, where he demonstrated his numerous microscopic preparations to the delegates; this instantly made his international reputation.

In 1891, Heinrich Wilhelm von Waldeyer, a great admirer and follower of Cajal, coined the term *'neurone'* (von Waldeyer, 1891) and the neuronal doctrine began to conquer the minds of neuroscientists. The neuronal processes received the name of *'dendrites'*, introduced by Wilhelm His in 1889, and the principal process was named *'axon'* by Alfred Kölliker in 1896.

The first general theory about the brain's functional organisation was introduced by Josef von Gerlach (Gerlach, 1871), who proposed that neurofilaments and neural cell processes are internally connected through anastomoses and form a diffuse network that represents the substrate for brain function. This *'reticular'* theory dominated neuroscience for a good 20 years and recruited many supporters, including Camillo Golgi, who was very much convinced of the existence of a *'diffuse neural net'*. Other proponents of the reticular theory included prominent figures such as Albert von Kölliker, Max Schulze, Istvan Apáthy, Hans Held, Sigmund Freud and many others. The history of the neuronism-reticularism conflict was widely popularised, and the curious reader may find all the dramatic details and read about the many participants of the struggle in several comprehensive treatises (Jacobson, 2005; Lopez-Munoz *et al.*, 2006; Mazzarello, 2010; Ramón y Cajal, 1933; Shepherd, 1991).

## 1.3    Mechanisms of communications in neural networks

'Vengo attaccato da due sette opposte – gli scienziati e gli ignoranti. Entrambi ridono di me, chiamandomi "il maestro di danza delle rane". Eppure io so di avere scoperto una delle piùgrandi forze della natura.'

Luigi Galvani (Galvani, 1841)[3]

The notion that there is some substance(s) involved in signal propagation through nerves and between nerves and peripheral tissues, as well as within the brain, has its roots in the ventricular-pneumatic doctrine. Indeed, both Galenic and Cartesian writings describe the 'pneuma' diffusing through the nerves and then being released, either from the peripheral nerve endings to drive muscle contractions, or aspirated from sensory nerves into the ventricles to mediate sensations and drive higher brain functions.

René Descartes introduced a sophisticated mechanistic theory of this 'neurotransmission', contemplating the flow of minuscule particles in the ventricles, from which they diffuse through the multiple pores in the internal surface of the brain and then leave towards the periphery through the nerves. The nerves, in turn, are endowed with a system of valves which allow release of the said particles onto muscles, where they are picked up by a congruent valve system localised in the muscular fibres, thus regulating contraction (Descartes, 1664). The substances for neuronal excitability and communication in the nervous system were found much later and, indeed, they are represented by small molecules – ions and neurotransmitters.

### 1.3.1    Electrical/ionic nature of excitability

The first experimental preparation for use in physiology (and which was to be the most widely used) was introduced in the 1660s, when Dutch microscopist and natural scientist Jan Swammerdam (Cobb, 2002) developed a neuro-muscular preparation (Figure 1.7). Swammerdam used the frog leg, from which '*one of*

---

[3] '*I am attacked by two very opposite sects – the scientists and the know-nothings. Both laugh at me – calling me "the frogs' dancing-master." Yet I know that I have discovered one of the greatest forces in nature*'. English translation Atkinson WW. 1907. The secret of mental magic: A course of seven lessons. Chicago: Authors edition. 1–441 p., p. 20.

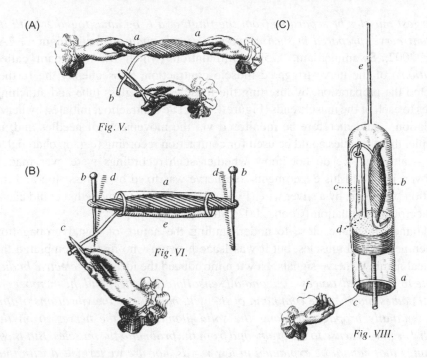

**Figure 1.7** Neuro-muscular preparations of Jan Swammerdam, with his original descriptions (Swammerdam, 1758).

A. *'If [ . . . ] you take hold, aa, of each tendon with your hand, and then irritate b the propending nerve with scissors, or any other instrument, the muscle will recover its former motion, which it had lost. You will see that it is immediately contracted, and draws together, as it were, both the hands, which hold the tendons.'*

B. *'If we have a mind to observe, very exactly, in what degree the muscle thickens in its contraction, and how far its tendons approach towards each other, we must put the muscle into a glass tube, a, and run two fine needles bb through its tendons, where they had been before held by the fingers; and then fix the points of those needles, neither too loose nor too firmly, in a piece of cork. If afterwards you irritate, c, the nerves, you will see the muscle drawing dd the heads of the needles together out of the paces; and that the belly of the muscle itself becomes considerably thicker e in the cavity of the glass tube, and stops up the whole tube, after expelling the air. This continues till the contraction ceases, and the needles then move back into their former places.'*

C. The stimulation of neuro-muscular preparation by silver wire: *'a) The glass tube, or siphon. b) The muscle. c) A silver wire with a ring in it, through which the nerve passes. d) A bras wire . . . through which the silver wire passes. e) A drop of water in glass tube. f) The hand that irritates the nerve, in consequence of which irritation the drop on the muscle, contracting itself, descends a little.'*

Images and quotations were kindly provided by Dr. Mathew Cobb, University of Manchester. see also Cobb, 2002.

*the largest muscles be separated from the thigh of a Frog, and, together with its adherent nerve, prepared in such a manner as to remain unhurt'* (Figure 1.7A; Cobb, 2002; Swammerdam, 1758). Stimulation (which Swammerdam called *'irritation'*) of the nerve triggered muscle contraction. Subsequently, he further perfected the preparation, by inserting the muscle into a glass tube and attaching needles to each of the muscle ends (Figure 1.7B). The contraction, initiated by nerve stimulation, could therefore be monitored via the movements of needles and, in principle, these needles could be used for contraction recording (e.g. on charcoaled paper – although we do not know whether such recordings were ever made). Moreover, in one of his experiments, the nerve was fixed by a brass ring and the 'irritation' was done by a silver wire (Figure 1C) – an arrangement that could cause true electrical stimulation (Cobb, 2002; Stillings, 1975).

Swammerdam came close to understanding the nature of signal propagation between nerves and muscles, but it was Isaac Newton who first contemplated the electrical nature of nerve signals. Newton introduced the idea that: *'electric bodies operate to greater distances . . . and all sensation is excited, and the members of animal bodies move at the command of the will, namely, by the vibrations of this spirit, mutually propagated along the solid filaments of the nerves, from the outward organs of sense to the brain, and from the brain into the muscles. But these are things that cannot be explained in few words, nor are we furnished with that sufficiency of experiments which is required to an accurate determination and demonstration of the laws by which this electric and elastic spirit operates.'* (Newton, 1713). Several other scientists contributed to the elevation of neuro-electrical theories in the 18th century; most prominent was Tommaso Laghi, who surmised the flow of some *'electrified'* substances through the nerve, these latter substances also initiating muscle contraction (Bresadola, 1998).

Experimental support for the electric nature of nerve impulses was furnished in Bologna, and the story of electrophysiology, ion channels and ionic nature of excitability began in 1791, when Luigi Galvani published his fundamental work, *De Viribus Electricitatis in Motu Musculari Commentarius* (Galvani, 1791), on animal electricity. This was the result of 10 years of experimentation on isolated frog nerve-muscle preparations, in which Galvani was assisted by his wife, Lucia Galeazzi and his nephew, Giovanni Aldini.

Initially, Galvani used his version of the nerve muscle preparation (Figure 1.8), which consisted of the inferior limbs with the crural nerves, connecting the spinal cord with the limbs, fully exposed, and a metal wire was inserted across the vertebral canal (Galvani, 1791, 1841; Piccolino, 1997, 1998). Using this preparation, Galvani identified electrical excitation of the nerve-muscle preparation, found the relationship between stimulus intensity and muscle contraction (the latter showed saturation, i.e. increasing the intensity of stimulation above a certain strength did not result in an increased magnitude of contraction), and described the refractory phenomenon by showing that repeated stimulation leads to disappearance of contractions, which can be restored after a period of rest.

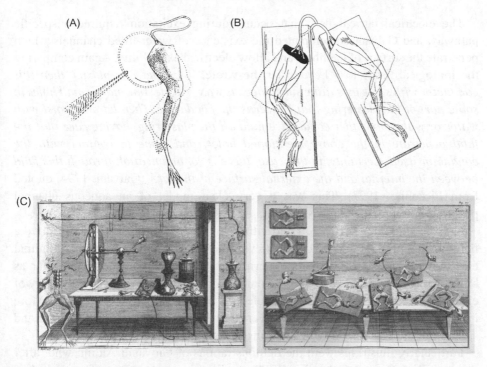

**Figure 1.8** Galvani experiments of muscle contraction without metals (Galvani 1841).

A. The 1794 experiment. When the surface of a section of nerve touches the muscle, the leg contracts.

B. The 1797 experiment. When the surface of a section of the right sciatic nerve touches the intact surface of the left sciatic nerve, both legs contract.

C. Plate I of the *Commentarius* shows the frog preparation and the electric machine; Plate III of the *Commentarius* shows the experiments with metallic arcs (Galvani, 1791).

Images were kindly provided by Professor Marco Piccolino, University of Ferrara.

The crucial experiments, however, were performed in 1794–1797 (Galvani, 1841), when Galvani used two frog legs with long sciatic nerves attached (Figure 1.8). When the nerve of the first preparation was in contact with the nerve or muscle of the second, contraction occurred in both preparations. This was the first demonstration of a propagating action potential. Based on his experimental achievements, Galvani developed the theory of electrical excitation. First, he realized that biological tissues exist in a state of '*disequilibrium*' i.e. at rest the tissue is ready to respond to external stimuli by generating electrical signals. Even more importantly, Galvani postulated that '*animal electricity*' results from accumulation of positive and negative charges on external and internal surfaces of the muscle or nerve fibre, which he compared to the internal and external plates of the Leyden jar (Galvani, 1794; Piccolino, 1997).

The electrical current flow that occurs during excitation required a specific pathway, and Galvani contemplated the existence of water-filled channels which penetrate the surface of the fibres and allow electrical excitability. Again comparing the biological tissue to a Leyden jar, he wrote: ' . . . *let one plaster then this conductor with some insulating substance, as wax . . . let one make small holes in some part of the plastering that concerns the conductor. Then let one moist with water or with some other conductive fluid all the plastering, having care that the fluid penetrate in the above mentioned holes, and come in contact with the conductor itself. Certainly, in this case, there is communication through this fluid between the internal and the external surface of the jar.*' (Galvani, 1794, quoted from Piccolino, 1997). This was a very clear model of an aqueous channel penetrating the membranous structure.

Galvani's findings resonated rapidly throughout the world. First, they inspired a fierce fight with Alessandro Volta, who vehemently opposed the concept of animal electricity (Volta, 1918). Volta's experiments, although proven wrong as far as biology was concerned, resulted in fundamental discoveries in the general theory of electricity and the invention of the electric battery in the 19th century. More importantly, however, the idea of galvanism became a cultural phenomenon and spread throughout Europe with lightning speed.

Particularly illustrious were the demonstrations of Giovanni Aldini, who, after the untimely death of Galvani in 1798, continued investigations of animal electricity. In 1803–1804, Aldini published important books, which combined the ideas of Galvani and Volta and made a coherent theory of electrical excitation of biological tissues (Aldini, 1803, 1804). He also made the most exciting electrical stimulations of body parts of freshly executed criminals, which made a huge impact on the general public. So invigorating was the theory of galvanism that, in 1817, it inspired Mary Shelley to write her novel *Frankenstein, or the Modern Prometheus*, which for the first time addressed the problem of the responsibility of the scientist for the products of his mind and hands.

Besides these demonstrations, Aldini made many other fundamental observations. In particular, he was the first to apply electrical currents to mammalian brains and he found that stimulation of the corpus callosum and cerebellum triggered pronounced motor responses (the experiments were done on the ox brain *in situ*, with the skull opened and all brain-spinal cord connections remaining intact (Aldini, 1803; 1804).

The first instrumental recording of animal electricity (using the frog neuro-muscular preparation), was made by Leopoldo Nobili in 1828, with the aid of an electromagnetic galvanometer (Nobili, 1828), although Nobili interpreted this recording in strictly physical terms, suggesting that he was measuring a thermo-electrical current resulting from unequal cooling of the two ends of the preparation. Several years later, in 1842, Carlo Matteucci repeated this experiment and demonstrated that the galvanometer reading was the exclusive consequence of currents generated by the living tissue (Matteucci, 1842). Furthermore, he succeeded in measuring the resting current between the intact and cut surfaces of the muscle.

The next step was made by Emile du Bois-Reymond, who was able to measure electrical events accompanying the excitation of nerve and muscle, and who realized that excitation greatly decreases the potential difference between the intact surface and the cut portion of the tissue; hence, he called the excitatory electrical response the 'negative Schwankung' (negative fluctuation) (du Bois-Reymond, 1884).

In 1850–1852, another fundamental discovery was made by Hermann von Helmholtz, who, using the nerve-muscle preparation, determined the speed of nerve impulse propagation by measuring the delay between the application of an electrical stimulus and the muscle contraction (Helmholtz, 1850). Furthermore, Helmholtz, for the first time, used a smoked drum to record muscle contractions (Helmholtz, 1852). To measure the velocity of nerve impulse propagation, he used a technique developed by Claude Pouillet, who found that galvanometer excursions induced by brief pulses of current were proportional to the pulse duration (Piccolino, 2003) (incidentally, this technique was successfully used in military practice for determining the speed of cannon balls). By using this method, Helmholtz was able to determine the delay between electrical stimulation of the nerve and muscle contraction, a delay, which he rather poetically defined as 'le temps perdu' (the lost time) (Piccolino, 2003).

The speed of nerve impulse propagation measured by Helmholtz caused some confusion: the values of the propagation velocity were in the range of 25–40 m/s, which was much slower than the propagation of electric current. It was somehow difficult to correlate the Helmholtz data with the excitatory currents of Dubois-Reimond, as the time resolution of the contemporary techniques did not allow measurement of the kinetics of the activity-associated electrical events with any relevant precision. This problem was brilliantly solved by Julius Bernstein, who introduced a truly remarkable piece of scientific machinery – the 'differential rheotome', which allowed adequate recordings of very fast electrical processes. The sampling rate of Bernstein's rheotome was approximately several tens of microseconds (a detailed account of Bernstein's techniques was made by Bernd Nilius (2003).

Using the rheotome, Bernstein made the first true recordings of resting and action potentials (Figure 1.9). He estimated that, at rest, the nerve interior is about 60 mV more negative than the surface, and he showed the kinetics of the action potential (still called 'negative Schwankung'). The action potential measured by Bernstein had a rise time of about 0.3 ms and a duration of ≈0.8–0.9 ms but, most importantly, the potential deflection actually crossed the 'zero potential' line, causing a 'sign reversal' which clearly reflected the action potential overshoot (Bernstein, 1868). Bernstein also estimated the conduction velocity of the nerve, which was very similar (≈25–30 m/s) to the data obtained by Helmholtz.

Bernstein developed several theories of electrical excitability and, in 1896, being prompted by his student Vassily Tschagovetz, he employed the electrolytic theory of Walther Nernst to biological systems and came up with the hypothesis that $K^+$ selectivity of the excitable membrane is responsible for the generation of the resting membrane potential (Bernstein, 1902, 1912). This theory was further developed by Charles Ernst Overton, who demonstrated that $Na^+$ ions are required for producing

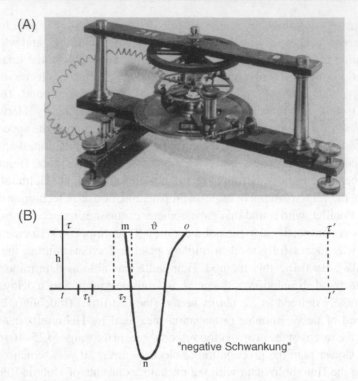

**Figure 1.9** First recording of action potential from the nerve made by Julius Bernstein (Bernstein, 1868).

A. The Bernstein rheotome.

B. The recording of an action potential. The $t_1$ and $t_2$ indicate 'sampling' intervals of the rheotome; the duration $m - o$ is the duration of action potential ('*negative Schwankung*'; and $n$ is the '*sign reversal*' (overshoot).

Images were kindly provided by Professor Bernd Nilius, University of Leuven.

the '*negative Schwankung*', and suggested that the excitation process results from the exchange of $Na^+$ and $K^+$ (Overton, 1902).

Incidentally it was also Overton who, in 1899, proposed a '*lipoidal membrane*' model of the plasmalemma, after discovering that lipid-soluble dyes enter cells substantially easier than the water-soluble ones (Overton, 1899). The bilayer structure of the cellular membranes was confirmed in 1925 by Gorter and Grendel, who found that the amount of lipids extracted from 'chromocytes' (red blood cells) was sufficient to cover the surface of these cells twice (the surface area was determined from microscopic observations of blood cells), which led them to propose the lipid bilayer structure (Gorter & Grendel, 1925). This theory was further developed by Danielli and Davson (Danielli & Davson, 1935), who introduced the concept of the bilayer lipid membrane, which is associated with numerous proteins and is penetrated by narrow water-filled pores that allow the passage of lipid-insoluble molecules, including ions.

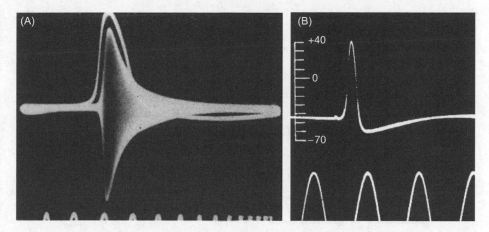

**Figure 1.10** First electrophysiological recordings from squid axons.

A. The increase in conductance of the squid axon during the action potential as seen by Cole and Curtis (Cole & Curtis, 1939). Upper trace: action potential; white-dark band: measure of the membrane impedance obtained with the Wheatstone bridge method by applying a high frequency (20 KHz) sinusoidal signal to two electrodes placed on the opposite site of a giant axon. The time marks at the bottom are 1 millisecond apart.

B. The first published intracellular recording of the action potential in the squid axon. Time mark, 500 Hz (Hodgkin & Huxley, 1939).

Reproduced from Hodgkin and Huxley 1939, Journal of Physiology.

All in all, by the mid-1930s, the structure of the cell membrane was known and the prototypes of ion channels suggested. However, direct physiological data were needed to confirm the electrical theory of excitation. These direct electrophysiological experiments became possible after John Z. Young introduced the squid axon into physiological practice (Young, 1936). In 1939, Kenneth Cole and Howard Curtis performed impedance measurements using extracellular electrodes on axons isolated from the '*Atlantic squid*, Loligo pealii . . . *From early May until late June excellent animals were available, but later they were smaller, not so numerous, and did not live long in the aquarium. Slender animals were preferred because the axons were of nearly uniform diameter over their usable length.*' (Cole & Curtis, 1939).

These experiments directly demonstrated the rapid fall in membrane resistance during the development of the action potential (Figure 1.10A). Slightly later, both Cole and Curtis (Curtis & Cole, 1940) and Alan Hodgkin and Andrew Huxley (Hodgkin & Huxley, 1939) developed intracellular electrodes which could be inserted into the squid axon, and performed the first direct recordings of action potentials (Figure 1.10B). These recordings demonstrated a very clear action potential overshoot and determined the resting potential at approximately –50 mV.

In 1949, the voltage-clamp technique was designed by Cole (Cole, 1949) and Marmont (Marmont, 1949), and it was almost immediately employed by Hodgkin, Huxley and Katz (Figure 1.11) to produce the ionic theory of membrane excitation (Hodgkin & Huxley, 1952). Most importantly, Hodgkin and Huxley clearly

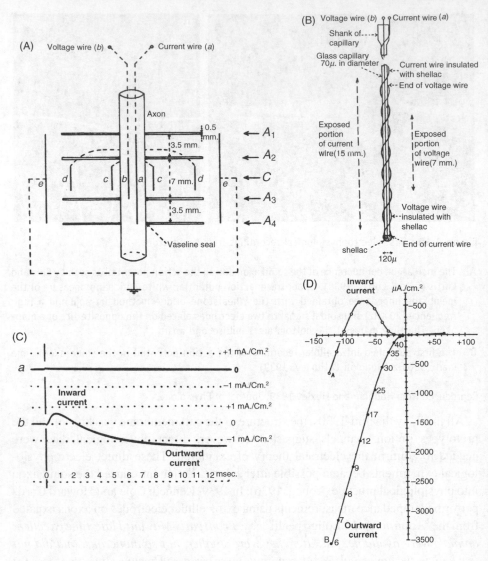

**Figure 1.11**   First recordings of ion currents.

A.   Diagram illustrating arrangement of internal and external electrodes. $A_1$, $A_2$, $A_3$, and $A_4$ and C are Perspex partitions; a, b, c, d and e are electrodes. Insulated wires are shown by dotted lines.

B.   Diagram of internal electrode (not to scale). The pitch of each spiral was 0.5 mm. The exposed portions of the wires are shown by heavy lines.

C.   Records of membrane current under a voltage clamp. At zero time, the membrane potential was increased by 65 mV (record A) or decreased by 65 mV (record B); this level was then maintained constant throughout the record. Inward current is shown as an upward deflexion. Axon 41; diameter 585 μm. Temperature 3.8° C.

D.   The current-voltage relations for inward and outward ion currents.

Reproduced from Hodgkin *et al.* 1952, Journal of Physiology.

demonstrated that membrane excitability is determined by passive ion fluxes according to their electro-chemical gradients, which implied the existence of transmembrane aqueous pathways. Although the ion channels were not directly incorporated into the theory, their existence was suggested. The quest for ion channels occupied the next 30 years.

From the early days of this quest, several technical obstacles had to be sorted. First, further development of the ionic theory of excitation required recordings not only from axons of non-vertebrates but also from mammalian cells, which are generally rather small and difficult to access because of tissue barriers. Second, precise separation of ion currents and dissection of the mechanisms of their regulation required control over both the extra- and intracellular environments. Third, monitoring of single ion channels' currents ultimately required low noise recordings from exceedingly small areas of cellular membranes (i.e. small enough to contain only a few channel molecules, or better still a single ion channel). In fact, the very first evidence for discrete ion currents were obtained in experiments with artificial lipid membranes, introduced by Paul Müller and Donald Rudin (Mueller & Rudin, 1963). When these membranes were exposed to certain antibiotics (e.g. gramicidin A) or to certain proteins, an ionic conductance was induced, which could be recorded as step-like, discrete events of transmembrane currents (Bean et al., 1969).

The problem of connecting recording instruments to single cells was solved with the development of microelectrodes pulled from glass pipettes. These microelectrodes for low-traumatising penetrations of cells were introduced in 1949 by Gilbert Ling and Ralf Gerard (Ling & Gerard, 1949). The microelectrode technique was rapidly adopted by electrophysiological laboratories.

Glass microelectrodes, filled with ion-containing solution, were first employed for extracellular recordings in 1919 by Frederick Pratt and John Eisenberger (Pratt & Eisenberger, 1919), who manufactured a fine-pointed capillary pore electrode with outer diameter $\approx 4$–$8$ $\mu$m and employed these electrodes for focal stimulation of single skeletal muscle fibres. The experiments directly demonstrated that skeletal muscle excitation followed the 'all-or-none' principle.

The first extracellular recordings from cellular membranes of muscle cells were performed by Alfred Strickholm in the early 1960s (Strickholm, 1961, 1962). He used a *smooth tipped, liquid-filled micropipette (several microns tip diameter) . . . placed against a muscle in such a way that the cell surface under it was electrically isolated except for a leakage resistance path between tip and cell*. (Strickholm, 1961). Using these pipettes, Strickholm was able to measure the impedance of frog muscles and obtain recordings of currents flowing through the small membrane patch under the tip of this extracellular pipette. Several years later, Karl Frank and Ladislav Tauc revealed a heterogeneous distribution of $Na^+$ channels in molluscan neurones by voltage-clamping relatively small patches of the plasma membrane with the help of an extracellular glass micropipette (Frank & Tauc, 1963).

In 1969, Erwin Neher and Hans Dieter Lux developed a conceptually similar technique to monitor membrane currents from the somatic membrane of sub-oesophageal ganglion neurones of *Helix pomatia* snails (Neher & Lux, 1969). They pulled micro-pipettes from asymmetrical double-barrelled capillaries to obtain an opening of about 100–150 µm in diameter; the tip of the pipette was subsequently fire-polished. Importantly, gentle suction (2–10 mm Hg) was applied to the pipette interior, which helped approaching the membrane of the neurone located within the ganglia (normally covered by glial cells) and improved the shunt resistance between the pipette wall and the cell membrane.

The problem of controlling intracellular ion concentrations was solved in parallel. The first experiments with complete or partial replacement of the cyto-plasm with artificial salt solution were performed on squid axons in 1961 by Peter Baker, Alan Hodgkin and Trevor Shaw (Baker *et al.*, 1962). About a decade later, the cytoplasm replacement approach was adopted for single cells. The initial version of intracellular perfusion was built around plastic film, which separated two chambers, filled with extra- and intracellular solutions (Kryshtal & Pidoplichko, 1975). A tiny pore, several millimetres in diameter, was made in the film, and the cell soma was placed on top of the pore; a small negative pressure applied to the 'intracellular' chamber helped the cell to invade the pore. After the cell firmly occluded the pore, the membrane facing the intracellular compartment was disrupted and electrical and physical access to the cell interior was gained.

This initial set-up was soon modified and the planar film was replaced by either plastic or glass pipettes (Kostyuk *et al.*, 1981; Lee *et al.*, 1980), which allowed easy hunting for cells and permitted further modification of the method. These modifi-cations included, for example, double perfusion, where the cell was fixed between two pipettes (Kostyuk *et al.*, 1981; Lee *et al.*, 1980), which provided for a very good spatial voltage-clamp and fast and effective exchange of the intracellular milieu. The plastic pipettes were also used for extracellular recordings with the aim of measuring single channel currents (Kryshtal & Pidoplichko, 1977). All of these techniques suffered from a relatively low shunt resistance between the membrane surface and the wall of the recording pipette, which prevented low-noise recordings.

Indeed, in intact cells, the main difficulty is to detect single channel currents in the presence of background electrical noise. A background noise associated with the usage of glass intracellular microelectrodes usually exceeds 100 pA, whereas the current flowing through a single channel is as small as several pA, being therefore only a relatively tiny fraction of this background noise. To overcome this problem, Ervin Neher and Bert Sakmann (Neher & Sakmann, 1976) used an extracellular glass micropipette, the tip of which was pressed against the surface of an isolated skeletal muscle fibre. In this configuration, a patch of a membrane was electrically isolated (Figure 1.12). Intrinsic noise decreases with the area of membrane under voltage-clamp, so when a small area ($1–10 \, \mu m^2$) is isolated, the extraneous noise levels can be made so low that the pico-ampere currents flowing through single ion channels can be recorded (Figure 1.12).

These first recordings (which measured currents through single nicotinic acetyl-choline receptors) were still far from ideal, because the resistance between recording pipette and cell membrane remained relatively low (in a range of tens

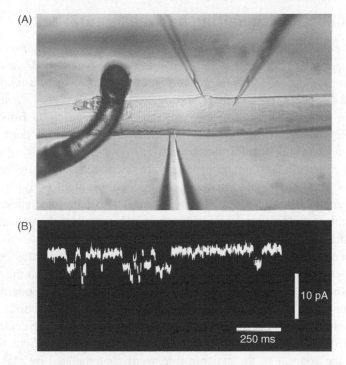

**Figure 1.12**  First recordings of acetylcholine receptor single channel currents from denervated frog *(Rana pipiens)* cutaneous pectoris muscle.

A.   The micro-photograph of the preparation.

B.   Current recordings. The pipette contained 0.2 mM suberyldicholine, an analogue of acetylcholine, which induces long-lived channel openings. Membrane potential –120 mV; temperature 8°C.

Reproduced with permissions from Neher, E. and Sakmann, B. (1976) Single-channel currents recorded from membrane of denervated frog muscle fibres. Nature 260: 5554 © Nature Publishing Group.

of M$\Omega$). The technique was substantially improved in 1980, when the ultra-high resistance (giga-ohm) seal between highly cleaned and very smooth micropipette tips and smooth surface cell membranes (the so-called giga-seal) was achieved (Hamill *et al.*, 1981). This was the patch-clamp technique that revolutionised electrophysiology, allowing entirely new types of experiments to be designed. The astonishing stability and tightness of the giga-seal interaction between micropipette and cell membrane permitted not only electrical isolation but also complete mechanical isolation of a patch of cell membrane in either the inside-out or outside-out configurations. Furthermore, the patch-clamp technique can be used for intracellular perfusion and it can be applied to virtually every cell type in the body, in isolation (cell culture) or in tissues (acutely isolated slices) or, indeed, *in vivo*. The patch-clamp technique was instrumental in the detailed characterisation of ion channels underlying electrical excitability, being one of the very few techniques allowing direct recordings of the functional activity of single protein molecules.

## 1.3.2   Chemical signalling between neural cells

*'Of known natural processes that might pass on excitation, only two are, in my opinion, worth talking about. Either there exists at the boundary of the contractile substance a stimulative secretion in the form of a thin layer of ammonia, lactic acid, or some other powerful stimulatory substance, or the phenomenon is electrical in nature'.* These prophetic words of Emil Heinrich du Bois-Reymond (du Bois-Reymond, 1877) signalled the emergence of the modern theory of molecular mechanisms of information transfer between cells in living organisms. Indeed, all intercellular communications are mediated either by release and reception of transmitter substances, or by direct movement of molecules from one cell to another through intercellular junctions. This latter mechanism provides for direct intercellular electrical and/or chemical signalling by means of inter-cellular diffusion of ions and/or other compounds, respectively.

As has been already mentioned, the notion that cells communicate between each other with some substances that can, for example, be released from the nerves and act upon other cells, has been circulated for a long time. The modern theory of neurotransmission, however, developed entirely in the last 120 years.

The morphological basis for intercellular communications in the central nervous system (CNS) was defined in 1897, when Michael Foster and Charles Scott Sherrington introduced the concept of the synapse (the word contemplated by classic scholar Arthur Woolgar Verrall from Greek roots *syn*, συν meaning together and *haptein* απτειν meaning clasp). The theory of chemical neurotransmission was formulated in 1904 by John Newport Langley and Thomas Renton Elliott, who also suggested adrenaline (epinephrine) as the neurotransmitter in the sympathetic nervous system (Elliott, 1904). A year later, Langley postulated the existence of specific neuro-transmitter receptors (Langley, 1905), which he called the *'receptive substances . . . capable of receiving and transmitting stimuli of target cells'* (Langley, 1906).

Acetylcholine became the first neurotransmitter experimentally discovered by Otto Loewi and Henry Dale (Dale, 1914; Loewi, 1921), and noradrenaline (norepinephrine) followed in 1946 (Von Euler, 1946). Many more neurotransmitters and neuromodulators were discovered in the ensuing decades, including adenosine 5'-triphosphate (ATP), dopamine, serotonin, glutamate, neuropeptides, etc. The theory of chemical transmission in the CNS became fully acknowledged in the mid 1950s, following famous acceptance of this theory by John Carew Eccles, and definition of its cornerstone principles.

The main criteria that allowed a substance to be accepted as a neurotransmitter were formulated by Eccles (Eccles, 1964) as:

1.  The substance and the enzymes necessary for its formation must be present in the neurone.

2.  The substance must be released from the terminal axon when the nerve is activated.

3. The effect of the transmitter released on nerve stimulation must be mimicked by the exogenous application of the substance to the effector.

4. A mechanism for inactivation of the substance must be present, whether it involves enzyme action or uptake or both.

5. Drugs which reduce or potentiate nerve mediated responses should similarly affect the responses to the exogenously applied substance (quoted from Burnstock, 1972).

Another criterion of neurotransmission, the 'Dale principle', was also defined by Eccles (Eccles, 1976). This principle postulates that each neurone produces and releases only one type of neurotransmitter. Based on Eccles interpretation of Henry Dale's Nothamgal lecture in 1934, the principle became a subject of long-standing discussions to date.

Further developments in the field lead to the realisation that these fundamental principles have to be redefined somewhat. Indeed, some neurotransmitters (most notably glutamate) can not be synthesised *de novo* in neurones releasing them; they have to be transported in the form of precursors and then converted into the active substance. Second, it appears that most (if not all) neurones secrete more than one transmitter (the concept of co-transmission was originally formulated by Geoffrey Burnstock (Burnstock, 1976), which greatly adds to the complexity of chemical transmission in the CNS. Third, it became clear that neurotransmitters are released not only by neurones but also by neuroglia.

## 1.4    The concept of neuroglia

*'Ich habe bis jetzt, meine Herren, bei der Betrachtung des Nervenapparatus immer nur der eigentlich nervösen Theile gedacht. Wenn man aber das Nervensystem in seinem wirklichen Verhalten im Körper studiren will, so ist es ausserordentlich wichtig, auch diejenige Masse zu kennen, welche zwischen den eigentlichen Nerventheilen vorhanden ist, welche sie zusammenhäund dem Ganzen mehr oder weniger seine Form gibt.'*
Rudolf Virchow, *Die Cellularpathologie*, p. 246 (Virchow, 1858)[4]

The idea of the coexistence of active (excitable) and passive (non-excitable) elements in the brain was suggested in 1836 by Gabriel Gustav Valentin, who had just been appointed to the Physiology chair in Bern University, in his book *Über den Verlauf und die letzten Enden der Nerven*. The concept and term 'neuroglia' was coined in 1856 by Rudolf Ludwig Karl Virchow (1821–1902; Figure 1.13) in his

---

[4] *'Hitherto, gentlemen, in considering the nervous system, I have only spoken of the really nervous parts of it. But if we would study the nervous system in its real relations in the body, it is extremely important to have a knowledge of that substance also which lies between the proper nervous parts, holds them together and gives the whole its form in a greater or lesser degree.'*

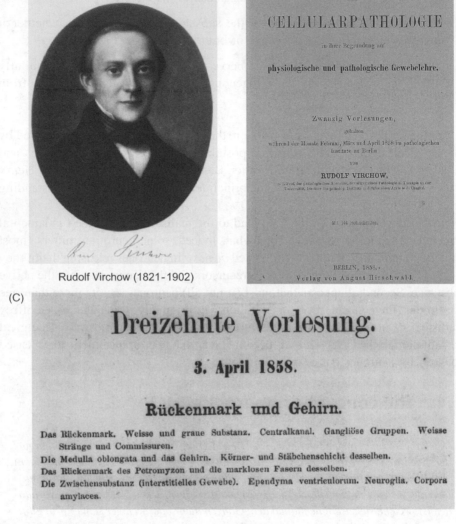

(A)

Rudolf Virchow (1821–1902)

(B)

DIE

CELLULARPATHOLOGIE

in ihrer Begründung auf

physiologische und pathologische Gewebelehre.

Zwanzig Vorlesungen,

gehalten

während der Monate Februar, März und April 1858 im pathologischen
Institute zu Berlin

von

RUDOLF VIRCHOW,

BERLIN, 1858.
Verlag von August Hirschwald

(C)

# Dreizehnte Vorlesung.

## 3. April 1858.

### Rückenmark und Gehirn.

Das Rückenmark. Weisse und graue Substanz. Centralkanal. Gangliöse Gruppen. Weisse
Stränge und Commissuren.
Die Medulla oblongata und das Gehirn. Körner- und Stäbchenschicht desselben.
Das Rückenmark des Petromyzon und die marklosen Fasern desselben.
Die Zwischensubstanz (interstitielles Gewebe). Ependyma ventriculorum. Neuroglia. Corpora
amylacea.

**Figure 1.13**   *(Continued on next page)*

own commentary to the earlier paper 'Über das granulierte Ansehen der Wandungen
der Gehirnventrikel' (published in 1846 in the journal *Allgemeine Zeitshrift fur
Psychiatrie* vol. 3, pp. 242–250). This commentary (Virchow, 1856, p. 890)
indicated the existence of ' . . . *connective substance, which forms in the brain,
in the spinal cord, and in the higher sensory nerves a sort of Nervenkitt (neuroglia),
in which the nervous system elements are embedded*'.

The concept of neuroglia was presented to the public on April 3rd, 1858, when
Virchow delivered the 13th of a series of 20 lectures to medical students of Charite
Hospital in Berlin. These lectures were stenographed and published almost without
any editing in a book, *Die Cellularpathologie in ihrer Begründung auf*

**Figure 1.13**   Rudolf Virchow and the concept of neuroglia.

A.  Portrait of Rudolf Virchow in the 1850s. Rudolf Virchow was born on October 13, 1821, in Schivelbein, which was then under the rule of the Prussian kingdom and now is a city of Swidwin in Poland. He studied medicine in Berlin and worked as a pathologist at the Charité. After the failure of the 1848 revolution, in which he had actively participated, he was forced to leave Berlin and to move to Würzburg, where he became Professor of Pathology. He returned to Berlin in 1856 and occupied the Chair in Pathology for the rest of his life. He had a broad interest in science, ranging from cancer research and neuroscience to anthropology and, as the editor-in-chief of *Virchow's Archiv*, he could oversee it all. Rudolf Virchow was not only a highly influential scientist, but was actively engaged in different aspects of political and cultural life. He initiated laws for meat inspection at slaughterhouses and, as a member of the German parliament, he was instrumental in installing a modern sewage system in the city of Berlin, borne out of the recognition that there is a relationship between infections and hygienic conditions. His interest in anthropology let him to participate in excavations carried out by his friend Heinrich Schliemann in Troy, and it was Virchow who convinced Schliemann to donate the treasures of Priam to the city of Berlin. Virchow assembled a tremendous collection of pathologic specimens and, at the end of his life, he opened a Pathologic Museum, not only for students and medical practitioners, but also for the public. He died in Berlin on September 5, 1902.

B.  The frontispiece of *Cellular Pathology*, published in 1858.

C.  Lecture 13 ('Spinal cord and the brain') from *Cellular Pathology*, where the name neuroglia was first coined.

Reproduced with permission from Kettenmann & Verkhratsky, 2008.

*physiologische und pathologische Gewebelehre* (Virchow, 1858), which became one of the most influential treatises in pathophysiology in the 19th century. Virchow derived the term 'glia' from the Greek 'γλια' for something slimy and of sticky appearance (the root appeared in the form 'γλοιοσ' in writings of the ancient Greek poet Semonides where it referred to 'oily sediment' used for taking baths; in works of Herodotus, for whom it meant 'gum'; and in the plays of Aristophanes, who used it in a sense of 'slippery or knavish'. In modern Greek, the root remains in the word 'γλοιωης', which means filthy and morally debased person[5]).

Virchow did not recognise neuroglia as a specific class of neural cells; the drawings of some round structures (Figure 1.14), which he reproduced in the *Die Cellularpathologie*, show, if anything, activated microglia. This did not matter, because for Virchow neuroglia were a connective tissue, the '*Zwichenmasse* – in between tissue' of mesodermal origin. This misconception of the origin of glia was embraced by many histologists, for example by Andriezen, Robertson and Weigart.

In 1851, Heinrich Müller (Müller, 1851) produced the first images of retinal radial glia, the cells that were subsequently named Müller cells by Rudolf Albert von Kölliker (Kölliker, 1852). In 1858, Max Schulze made a detailed investigation

[5] The linguistic analysis was kindly provided by David Langslow, Professor of Classics at Manchester University.

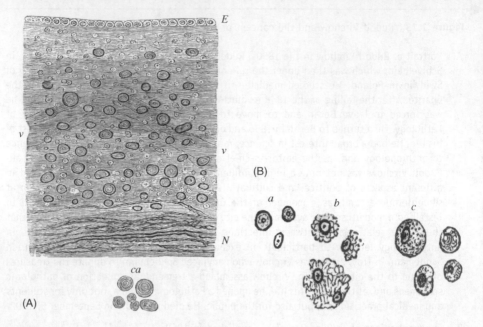

**Figure 1.14**   Neuroglia as seen by Rudolf Virchow.

A.   Ependyma and neuroglia in the floor of the fourth ventricle. Between the ependyma and the nerve fibres is *'the free portion of the neuroglia with numerous connective tissue corpuscles and nuclei'*. Numerous corpora amylacea are also visible, shown enlarged below the main illustration (*ca*). E – ependymal epithelium; N – nerve fibres; v, w – blood vessels.

B.   Elements of neuroglia from white matter of the human cerebral hemispheres. a – free nuclei with nucleoli; b – nuclei with partially destroyed cell bodies; c – complete cells.

Reproduced from Virchow, 1858.

of Müller cells and produced probably the best possible drawings of them in the pre-staining era of histology (Figure 1.15). Simultaneously, Karl Bergmann (Bergmann, 1857) had identified radial glial cells in the cerebellum (the cells now referred to as Bergmann glial cells). At the beginning of 1860, Otto Deiters described stellate cells in white and grey matter, closely resembling what we now know as astrocytes (see Figure 1.5H). Curiously enough, these cells were subsequently named as *Spinnen-zellen*, or spider cells, by Moritz Jastrowitz (Jastrowitz, 1870). Several years later, Jacob Henle and Friedrich Merkel visualised the glial network in the grey matter (Henle & Merkel, 1869).

Further discoveries in the field of the cellular origin of glial cells resulted from the efforts of many prominent histologists (Figures 1.16, 1.17, 1.18), in particular Camillo Golgi (1843–1926), Gustav Retzius (1842–1919), Santiago Ramon y Cajal (1852–1934), and Pio Del Rio Hortega (1882–1945).

Camillo Golgi was born in Brescia on July 7, 1843. He spent most of his life in Pavia, first as a medical student, then as Extraordinary Professor of Histology, and

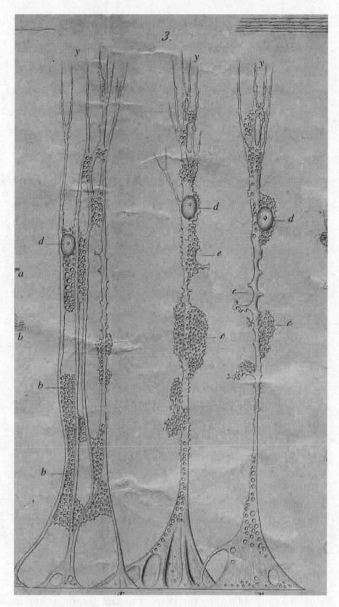

**Figure 1.15**   Müller fibre of the sheep retina, inspected by Max Schulze with a microscope from Amici.

Yyy: brush-like fibrils extending from the outer Müller fibre in the outer granular layer; xx: internal limiting membrane; a: opening in the limiting membrane; b: very delicate network of fenestrated membranes similar in the ganglion cell layer; cc: network in the so-called molecular layer; ddd: nuclei as part of the Müller fibres; ee: cavity in which the nuclei or the cells of the internal granular layer are located.

From Schulze, 1859. Image kindly provided by Professor Helmut Kettenmann, Max Delbrück Center for Molecular Medicine, Berlin.

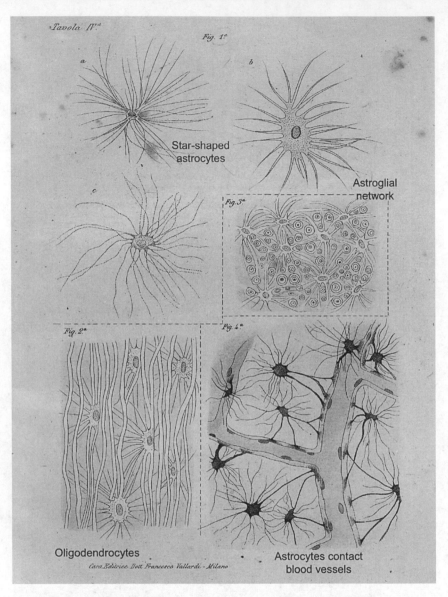

**Figure 1.16**   Neuroglial cells stained by the silver-chromate technique and drawn by Camillo Golgi (Golgi, 1903).

Top panels show individual star-shaped astrocytes and astroglial networks. At the bottom right, astrocytes forming numerous contacts (the end feet) with brain capillaries are demonstrated. The bottom left panel shows the drawing of white matter with numerous cellular processes oriented parallel to axons, which most likely represent oligodendrocytes.

The image was kindly provided by Prof. Paolo Mozzarello.

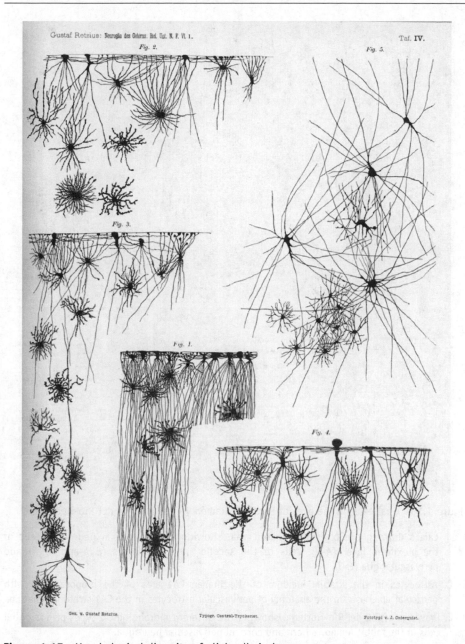

**Figure 1.17** Morphological diversity of glial cells in human cortex.

Plate IV: *Fig. 1*. Glial cells from cerebral cortex of 1 year old kid; *Fig. 2*. Glial cells from cerebral cortex of 5.5 years old kid; *Fig. 3*. Glia in *gyrus occipitalis medius* of 17 year old man; Fig. 4. Glia in *gyrus centralis posterior* of 33 year old man; Fig. 5. Glia in *gyrus centralis posterior* of 42 year old woman.

All images are obtained from Golgi stained preparations.

Reproduced from Retzius, 1894, Plate IV.

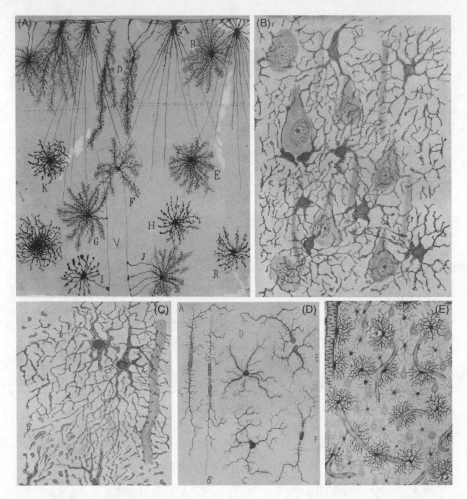

**Figure 1.18**   Glial cells by the eyes of Santiago Ramón y Cajal and Pío del Río-Hortega.

A.   Cajal's drawing of Golgi impregnated glia, showing human cortical neuroglial cells of the plexiform layer (*A-D*), cells of the second and third layers (*E-H* and *K, R*) and perivascular glia (*I, J*).

B, C. Astrocytes in the stratum lucidum of the human CA1 area of the hippocampus, with particular emphasis on the anatomy of perivascular astrocytes in the CA1 stratum radiatum.

D, E. Drawings of Pío del Río-Hortega, showing the different morphological types of microglial cells in the rabbit Ammon's horn and cortical perivascular neuroglia.

Reproduced with permission from Verkhratsky *et al.*, 2011. (Full colour version in plate section.)

from 1881 he occupied the Chair for General Pathology. Camillo Golgi made the first detailed descriptions of glial cells in 1870 (Golgi, 1870), which he observed in thin sections fixed with osmic acid. Already, in this first paper, Golgi identified glia as round cells with many fine processes extended in all directions, many of which were directed towards blood vessels. Using silver nitrate chromate 'black' staining and microscopic techniques, he discovered a huge diversity of glial cells in the brain, and further characterised the contacts (endfeet) formed between glial cells and blood vessels, as well as describing cells located in closely aligned groups between nerve fibres – the first observation of oligodendrocytes (Figure 1.16). Golgi staining was used by many neuroanatomists, who further characterised morphological diversity amongst neuroglia (Figure 1.17). Golgi was the first to demonstrate that glia represent a cellular population distinct from nervous cells, although he also believed that glial cells and neurones may transform into each other.

Santiago Ramon y Cajal was born on May 1, 1852, in Aragon, Spain. In 1883, he was appointed Professor of Descriptive and General Anatomy at Valencia, in 1887 he assumed a Chair in the University of Barcelona, and in 1892 he became Professor of Histology and Pathological Anatomy in Madrid. Cajal was, and remains, one of the most prominent and influential neurohistologists, who described the fine structure of various parts of the nervous system. He was the most important supporter of the neuronal doctrine of brain structure. He won the Nobel Prize in 1906, together with Camillo Golgi.

Cajal was very much interested in neuroglia throughout his career (Figure 1.18). He developed the gold and mercury chloride-sublimate staining method that was specific for both protoplasmic and fibrous astrocytes (Garcia-Marin et al., 2007; Ramón y Cajal, 1913b). We now know that this stain targeted intermediate filaments consisting mainly of glial fibrillary acidic protein (GFAP), a protein used today as an astrocytic marker. Using this technique, Cajal confirmed earlier ideas of the origin of astrocytes from radial glia, and also demonstrated that astrocytes can divide in the adult brain, thus laying the basis for much later discoveries of the stem properties of astroglia (Ramón y Cajal, 1913a, 1916). Cajal contemplated this latter hypothesis about the proliferative capacity of astrocytes after observing pairs of astrocytes joined by their soma; he defined these pairs as twin astrocytes or 'astrocitos gemelos' (see Ramón y Cajal, 1913a, and a comprehensive historic essay by Garcia-Marin et al., 2007).

The term astrocyte (αστρον κψτοσ; astron, star, and kytos, a hollow vessel, later cell, i.e. star-like cell) was introduced by Michael von Lenhossék (Figure 1.19A) to describe stellate glia, which gained universal acceptance within the next two decades. Lenhossék clearly understood the heterogeneity of neuroglia as he wrote: 'I would suggest that all supporting cells be named spongiocytes. And the most common form in vertebrates be named spider cells or astrocytes, and use the term neuroglia only cum grano salis (with a grain of salt), at least until we have a clearer view.' (Lenhossék, 1895).

More or less at the same time astrocytes were further subdivided into protoplasmic and fibrous astrocytes residing in grey and white matter, respectively (Andriezen, 1893; Kölliker, 1893). William Lloyd Andriezen believed that these two types of cells had different origins, the protoplasmic cells being of mesoblastic origin, while the fibrous cell were ectodermal. Interestingly, he also contemplated

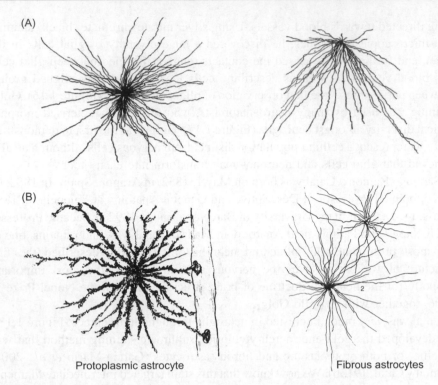

Protoplasmic astrocyte                                    Fibrous astrocytes

**Figure 1.19**   Astrocytes.

A.  Images of astrocytes drawn by Michael von Lenhossék (Lenhossék, 1895).

B.  Protoplasmic and fibrous astrocytes drawn by William Andriezen (Andriezen, 1893).
    Both preparations were stained with Golgi technique.

the complexity of protoplasmic astrocytes processes, indicating that they have '*the shaggy granular contour, as if a fine moss constituted the protoplasmic processes*'. In the same period, Wilhelm His made a fundamental discovery, when in 1889 he found the neuronal origin of neuroglia and directly demonstrated that both nerve cells and neuroglia derive from the neuroectoderm (His, 1889a, 1889b).

Cajal's pupil (and later his adversary) Pío del Río-Hortega identified two other principal classes of glial cells, initially considered by Cajal as the '*third element*' (a group of adendritic cells) which represented, in fact, the oligodendrocytes and the microglia (Figure 1.18D, E). Oligodendrocytes were initially observed and described by the Scottish neuroanatomist William Ford Robertson, who developed for this purpose a specific platinum stain technique. However, Robertson did not realise the myelinating capacity and role of these cells, and he thought them external invaders to the brain, hence identifying them as mesoglia (Robertson, 1899, 1900a). Almost 20 years later, Río-Hortega rediscovered these cells and gave them the name oligodendrocytes (Del Río-Hortega, 1921). He also demonstrated that oligodendrocytes were myelinating cells in the CNS, being thus analogous to the Schwann

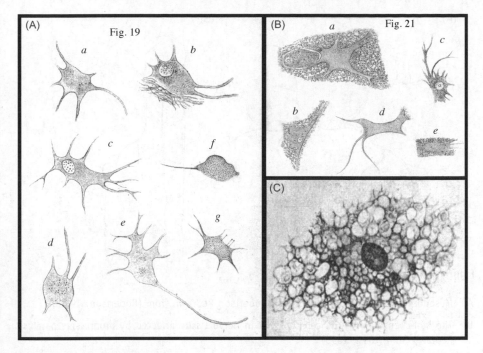

**Figure 1.20**   Neuroglial cells in pathological context as seen by Carl Frommann and Alois Alzheimer.

A, B. Different types of glial cells found in multiple sclerosis plaques of human cortex.

C.   Glial cell close to a 14 days old haemorrhage in human white matter. Axons pass through the network of the cell.

A and B from Frommann, 1878; C from Alzheimer, 1910.

cells in the periphery. It was also Río-Hortega who described microglial cells, the only glial members of non-neuronal origin.

Morphological remodelling of glial cells in neuropathology had already been noted by several neurohistologists by the end of 19th century (Figures 1.20, 1.21). Possibly the first to describe pathology-related remodelling of glia was Carl Frommann, who found, in the brain and in the spinal cord of a patient suffering from multiple sclerosis, glial cells with large somata and small thick processes. He believed these represented their reaction to the disease. Similar pathologically remodelled cells were observed in other pathological contexts, for example *tabes dorsalis* or dementia, by Nissl, Alzheimer and Merzbacher (Alzheimer, 1910; Merzbacher, 1909; Nissl, 1899). These cells received different names, being variously called rod cells (*Stäbchenzellen*), grid cells (*Gitterzellen*) or clearance cells (*Abräumzellen*).

William Ford Robertson introduced the special class of mesoglial cells, which were distinct from parenchymal glia (Figure 1.21A). Robertson found that these

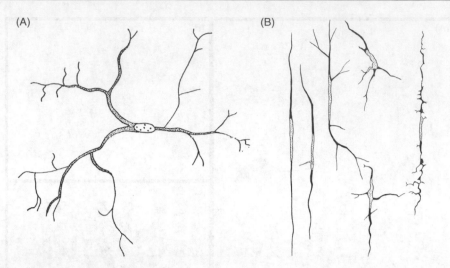

**Figure 1.21**   Early images of microglia.

A.  Mesoglial cells drawn by William Ford Robertson Redrawn from (Robertson, 1900b).

B.  The Stabchenzellen or rod cells of Nissl in nerve tissue affected by progressive paralysis. Redrawn from (Nissl, 1899)

cells did not contact blood vessels and withdraw their processes and transform into granule cells in response to injury (Robertson, 1900b)[6]. At the same time, the possibility of cell exchange between blood and the nervous system was also recorded. First, Campobianco and Fragnito (Campobianco & Fragnito, 1898) and Campobianco (Campobianco, 1901) found that at the early embryonic stages a number of mesoblastic cells migrate into the nervous system and are transformed into neuroglia. Some years later, Hatai (Hatai, 1902) described two types of glial cells in the early postnatal brain of mouse and rat. One form he termed the type 'a' cell, which he considered to be the ectodermal derived glial cells. The second type, the type 'b' cell, was morphologically distinct. Based on his morphologic studies, Hatai concluded that these 'b' type cells separated from the vessel wall, became amoeboid and migrated away from the capillary. He concluded that the brain contains two types of glial cells – one ectodermal, the other of mesodermal origin.

Del Rio-Hortega developed a specific silver carbonate impregnation technique to label the microglial cells (Del Río-Hortega, 1917) and made their detailed description (Del Rio-Hortega, 1919a, 1919b, 1920, 1932). Initially, he called these cells '*garbage collectors*', but subsequently he used the term microglia and called an individual cell a

---

[6] Paul Glees even proposed to call these cells 'Robertson-Hortega cells'. See Glees P. (1955). *Neuroglia morphology and function.* Oxford, Blackwell.

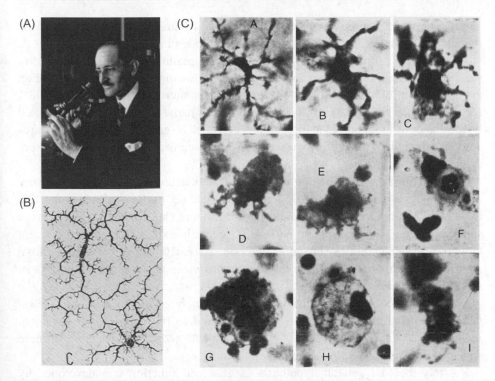

**Figure 1.22**   Microglial cells discovered by Pio del Rio Hortega.

A.   Pio del Rio Hortega (1882–1945).

B.   Images of ramified (resting) microglial cells drawn by Hortega (reproduced from Del Rio-Hortega, 1919a).

C.   Pathology triggers metamorphosis of microglia. a: cell with thick, rough prolongations; b: cells with short prolongations and enlarged cell body; c: hypertrophic cell with pseudopodia; d, e: amoeboid and pseudopodic forms; f: cell with phagocytosed leukocyte; g: cell with numerous phagocytosed erythrocytes; h: fat-granule cell; i: cell in mitotic division. Photomicrographs: reproduction of Fig. 15 from Del Rio-Hortega, 1932.

'*microgliocyte*'. In some of the contemporary publications, these cells were even referred to as '*Hortega cells*' (Metz, 1924). Del Río-Hortega gave microglia a very detailed and comprehensive characterisation (Figure 1.22), which has changed but little up to now (see Chapter 7). He found that microglial precursors invade the brain shortly after birth, disseminate over the brain parenchyma and develop a distinct phenotype. He also found that that these cells reacted to brain damage by morphological and functional modification known as microglial activation, which eventually turns microglial cells in phagocyting macrophages (Del Rio-Hortega, 1932).

The main peripheral glial element, the Schwann cell, was so called by Louis Antoine Ranvier (1871), following earlier discoveries of Robert Remak, who described the myelin sheath around peripheral nerve fibres (Remak, 1838) and Theodor Schwann, who suggested that the myelin sheath was a product of specialised cells (Schwann,

1839). The word myelin was introduced by Rudolf Virchow and means 'marrow' (Greek μυελοσ), because myelin appearance reminded him of bone marrow.

Remarkably, a further glial cell type in the mammalian CNS was discovered in the 1980s by William Stallcup and colleagues, following their development of an antibody to a novel chondroitin sulphate proteoglycan termed NG2 (Stallcup, 1981; see also Chapter 6). These cells have had numerous names, but in general are called NG2-glia or oligodendrocyte progenitor cells. NG2-glia have unique features amongst glia in that they form synapses, previously considered an exclusive feature of neurones.

The functional role of neuroglial cells puzzled neuroscientists from the very beginning. As already mentioned, Virchow regarded neuroglia as a true connective tissue, which provided the structural support for nerve elements in the brain, in the spinal cord and in the peripheral nerves. To a certain extent, this general concept hindered further enquiries into glial function. As early as 1893, William Lloyd Andriezen complained, '*While in the human brain the nerve elements have been largely and extensively studied both in health and in disease, the neuroglia elements have been comparatively neglected, partly owing to a widely-spread belief in a mere passive rôle they were supposed to play, and partly owing to inadequacy of the methods used . . .* ', although '*the growing importance of these elements is becoming daily obvious . . .* ' (Andriezen, 1893).

Possibly the first general hypothesis of glial cell function was developed by Camillo Golgi, who clearly understood that neuroglia are quite distinct from mere connective tissue. He suggested that glial cells are mainly responsible for feeding neurones, by virtue of their processes contacting both blood vessels and nerve cells. In Chapter 8 (dedicated to neuroglia) of his comprehensive treatise, *Sulla fina anatomia degli organi centrali del sistema nervoso* (Golgi, 1885), Golgi wrote: '*Credo conveniente notare che la parola connettivo, da me viene qualche volta usata per indicare il tessuto interstiziale dei centri e quale sinonimo di nevroglia, senza punto voler assimilare il tessuto medesimo col tessuto connettivo ordinario di origine mesodermica o parablastica. Dichiaro anzi che, dopo tutto, la parola nevroglia adoperata nel senso passato in uso, mi sembra abbia titoli di preferenza, valendo ad indicare un tessuto, che sebbene sia connettivo, perchè connette elementi d'altra natura e alla sua volta serve alla* distribuzione del materiale nutritizio, *pure si differenzia dal connettivo comune per caratteri morfologici, chimici, e quasi certamente, come dirò in seguito . . .* '[7].

Golgi, and many other neurohistologists (e.g. Nissl, Striker, Unger and Bauer (Glees, 1955)), being the proponents of the reticular theory of nerve system

---

[7] 'It is convenient to note that I usually use the word "connective tissue" to indicate the interstitial tissue as synonymous with neuroglia, without comparing this particular tissue with the usual connective tissue of mesodermal or parablastical origin. I declare that, however, the word neuroglia, used as in the past, indicates a tissue that although is a connective tissue, because connecting elements of another nature and in turn it serves for *distributing the nutritive material*, it is different from the common connective tissue for morphological and chemical features . . . '.

organisation, considered that astroglial cells were connected into the syncytial structure and were making anastomoses with neurones. In contrast, Carl Weigert believed that glial cells were mere structural elements that filled spaces not occupied by neurones. Weigert actually thought that glial fibres exist independently of glial cell somata, and that these fibres provide for structural scaffolding and filling of the interneuronal spaces (Weigert, 1895). Incidentally, this opinion postulating glial fibres existing independently of cell bodies survived well into 1940s and found many supporters (see Glees, 1955).

Both the nutritional theory of Golgi and the space-filling views of Weigert were opposed by Cajal, who, together with his brother Pedro (see Ramon, 1891), suggested that the main function of neuroglia in the grey matter lies in isolation of neuronal contacts in the CNS, thus controlling information flow. '*In short, as a framework with a thousand beams the neuroglia cells act as a material support and protection of the nerve cells and blood vessels. As an insulator their many branches interpose themselves among the dendritic expansions and nerve fibres which for whatever reason must not be in contact*'. The glial processes in their turn '*provide a medium resistant to the passage of nerve waves*' (Ramón y Cajal, 1909–1911).

Cajal's ideas about the role of glia were, however, in a state of continuous flux and modification. As early as in 1895, he proposed astrocytes as core regulators of functional hyperaemia, suggesting that contraction/relaxation of astroglial

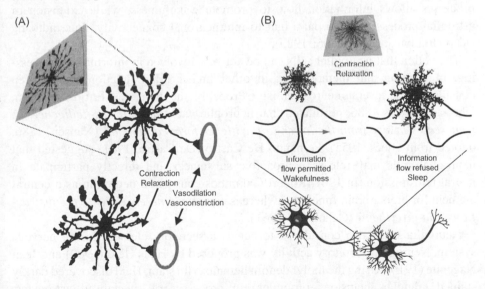

**Figure 1.23**  Integrative functions of astroglia according to Ramon y Cajal (Ramon y Cajal, 1895, 1925).

A.  By contracting and relaxing perivascular processes, astroglia regulate the diameter of brain blood vessels, thus controlling the local blood flow.

B.  Astrocytes, again by contracting or relaxing their processes, may interrupt/permit information flow through neuronal networks, thus regulating transition between sleep and wakefulness.

perivascular processes can increase or decrease the diameter of brain capillaries, thus regulating the blood flow (Figure 1.23A; Ramón y Cajal, 1895).

The idea of active neuronal-glial interactions as a substrate for brain function was first voiced in 1894 by Carl Ludwig Schleich (1859–1922) in his book *Schmerzlose Operationen* (Schleich, 1894; and Figure 1.24). Schleich believed that glia and neurones were equal players and that both acted as active cellular elements of the brain. He also thought that glial cells represent the general inhibitory mechanism of the brain. According to Schleich, neuronal excitation is transmitted from neurone to neurone through intercellular gaps (i.e. synapses), and these interneuronal gaps are filled with glial cells, which are the anatomical substrate for controlling network excitation/inhibition. He postulated that the constantly changing volume of glial cells represents the mechanism for control – swollen glial cells inhibit neuronal communication, while impulse propagation is facilitated when glia shrink. This was also the mechanism for general anaesthesia, which, according to Schleich, led to a maximal increase in glial volume, and therefore in complete inhibition of neuronal transmission.

Similar ideas were developed by Cajal, who suggested that perineuronal glia may actively regulate neuronal transmission, and even considered this as being a mechanism of sleep (Figure 1.23B). Cajal suggested that astrocytes act as a switch between active and passive states of the neuronal networks; retraction of astroglial processes allows information flow to promote wakefulness, while extension of astroglial processes would put a halt to interneuronal connectivity, thus inducing sleep (Ramon y Cajal, 1895; 1925).

The notion that neuroglial cells can be actively involved in information processing, in learning and memory and in other higher brain functions, have been considered by several neuroscientists. Probably the first was Fritjoff Nansen, who, as early as 1886, postulated that neuroglia was '*the seat of intelligence, as it increases in size from the lower to the higher forms of animal*' (Nansen, 1886, quoted from Glees, 1955). Fernando De Castro (De Castro, 1951) suggested that neuroglial cells may release neuroactive substances and directly participate in neural transmission. In 1961, Robert Galambos considered neuroglia as a central element for higher brain functions, whereas neurones '*merely execute the instructions glia give them*' (Galambos, 1961).

Neuroglia were also considered to act as a secretory element in the nervous system. Neuroglial secretory activity was proposed by Hans Held (1909) and Jean Nageotte (1910). Using the molybdenum hematoxylin stain, Held discovered darkly stained granular inclusions (granules) in processes of specialised astrocytes, marginal (subpial) glial cells. This stain also allowed him to determine that glial fibres were actually cellular extensions (not an interstitial mass, as per Virchow), forming an elaborate three-dimensional intercellular (astrocytic) network that interacts with vascular endothelium.

These two findings led him to hypothesize that the granular inclusions he observed, referred to as '*gliosomes*' by Alois Alzheimer (1910), was evidence

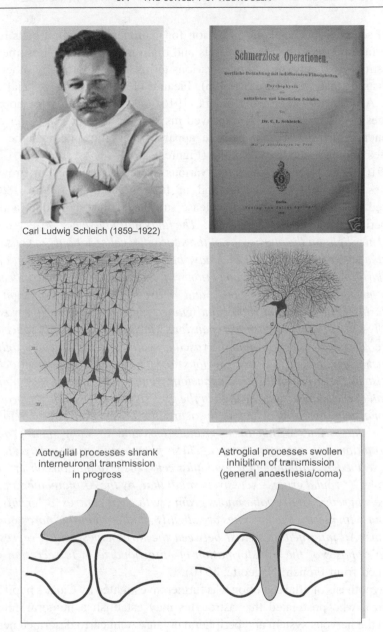

**Figure 1.24** Carl Ludwig Schleich and the neuronal-glial interactions hypothesis.

Schleich was a pupil of Virchow and a surgeon who introduced local anaesthesia into clinical practice. In 1894, he published a book, *Schmerzlose Operationen* (Schleich, 1894), the frontispiece of which is shown here on the right upper panel. Apart from describing the principles of local anaesthesia, this book also contained the first detailed essay on interactions in neuronal-glial networks as a substrate for brain function. Mid panels show original drawings from this book, depicting intimate contacts between glial cells and neurones, and the low panel shows, in a schematic manner, Schleich's theory of neuroglia controlling information flow in neuronal networks.

for glial secretion or metabolic provision for neurones, since glial cells reside at the interface between the blood vessels and brain parenchyma. Gliosomes in the cytoplasm of glial cells were, under various terms, also reported by other micro-anatomists of that era – Eisath (1906), Fieandt (1910), Ramón y Cajal (1913a, 1913b), Achucarro (1915) and Hortega (1916) (see Glees, 1955, for appropriate references). As Penfield (1924) improved his staining methods to better disclose oligodendrocytic processes, it became apparent that gliosomes can be seen in astrocytes and oligodendrocytes alike (Figure 1.25).

In 1910, Jean Nageotte observed various secretory granules in grey matter astrocytes using the Altmann method of fucsin labelling (Figure 1.26), and suggested that astroglial cells may release substances into the blood, acting like an endocrine gland. Nargeotte reported: '*The facts that I have just observed seem to me shed new light on the physiology of the neuroglial cells, not only of cells that are associated with neuronal cells, which have been named satellite cells, but also, and particularly, of cells that are in connection with the vasculature walls. Indeed, I was able to present evidence of robust and active secretion phenomenon in the protoplasm of these cells in rabbit and guinea pig. This observation was visible especially within the protoplasmic expansions which cross the empty space created by the retraction of tissues around the vascular walls, on which the neuroglial cells attach using an enlarged foot. In a previous note, I have described the mitochondria that exist in these protoplasmic expansions, and I have shown that many, and maybe all of the granulations located in the grey substance outside the protoplasm of neuronal cells, in reality belong to the neuroglia. Today, I am poised to follow the evolution that occurs within these granulations and to show their progressive transformation into secretion grains. These phenomena are exactly similar as those described by Altmann in the glandular cells; the granulations observed are of three types: 1° round grains excessively small that, by the Altmann method, colour intensively in red; 2° more voluminous grains, with clear centres; 3° grains that do not colour with fucsin. The last ones are slightly smaller than the more voluminous red grains. All intermediates exist between the three types, which represent the successive phases of the transformation of mitochondria in to secretion grains.*' (Translated from French; Nageotte, 1910).

The hypothesis of glial secretion was further investigated by Cajal's pupil Nicolas Achucarro, who postulated that astrocytes may establish a humoral connection between the nervous system and peripheral organs. Achucarro described neuroglial processes as hollow tubules designed to convey various endocrine factors to the blood vessels (Achucarro, 1915). Similar endocrinological roles of neuroglia were considered by another of Cajal's pupils, Fernando De Castro. Several prophetic ideas about neuroglial function were developed by Ernesto Lugaro (a prominent neurologist who, in particular, introduced the concept of neuronal plasticity), who wrote a comprehensive review on neuroglia (Lugaro, 1907). Lugaro suggested close interactions between astroglial processes and synaptic structures and the critical role

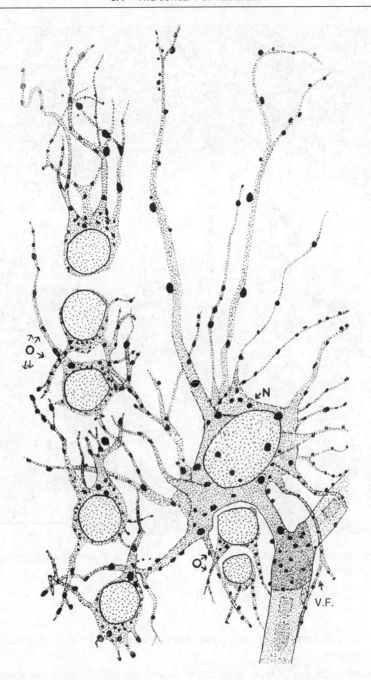

**Figure 1.25**   Gliosomes.

Oligodendroglia of the white matter and one astrocyte with a vascular endfoot, showing the distribution of darkly staining granules (gliosomes) in their processes.

Drawn from Penfield, 1924.

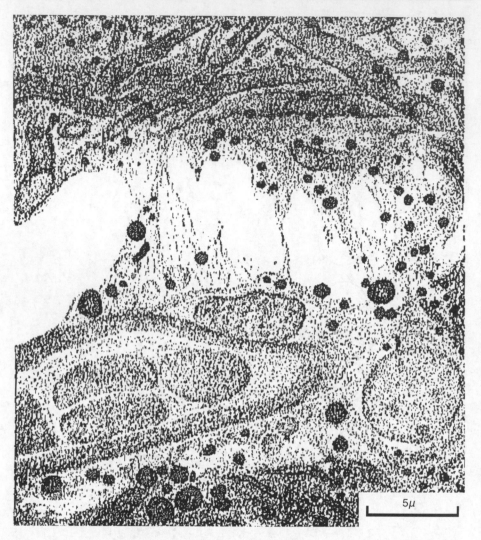

**Figure 1.26**   Neuroglial cells of grey matter in rabbit medulla, most likely astrocytes, contain various secretory granules.

Scale bar, 5 µm. Reproduced from Nageotte, 1910.

of neuroglia in taking up or degrading transmitters employed for interneuronal communications.

Finally, neuroglial cells were implicated in various pathological processes. Nissl and Alzheimer considered the pathological role of neuroglia in a variety of neurological diseases (Alzheimer, 1910). Astrocytes were considered to '*exhibit a morbid hypertrophy in pathological conditions*' (Andriezen, 1893). The role of astrocytes in scar formation was perceived by Cajal, Hortega and Penfield in the early 1920s. The phagocytic activity of glia, which can be instrumental in removal of injured or dying neurones form the lesion site, had already been found in 1896 by Gheorghe Marinesco (Marinesco, 1896).

## 1.5   Beginning of the modern era

The modern era in glial physiology began with two seminal discoveries made in the late 1950s to mid 1960s, when Walter Hild and his colleagues made the first microelectrode recordings from cultured astrocytes (Hild *et al.*, 1958) and Steven Kuffler, John Nicolls and Richard Orkand (Kuffler *et al.*, 1966) demonstrated electrical coupling between glial cells. Slightly later, Milton Brightman and Tom Reese (Brightman & Reese, 1969) identified structures connecting glial networks, which we know now as gap junctions.

Nonetheless, for the following two decades, glial cells were still regarded as passive elements of the CNS, bearing mostly supportive and nutritional roles. The advent of modern physiological techniques, most notably those of the patch-clamp and fluorescent calcium dyes, dramatically changed this image of glia as 'silent' brain cells. Developments in glial cell physiology were also greatly assisted by the introduction of neuroglial cell cultures (Hild *et al.*, 1958; McCarthy & de Vellis, 1980), which allowed the study of these cells in isolation and excluded indirect effects associated with neuronal excitation.

The first breakthrough discovery using these new techniques was made in 1984, when groups led by Helmut Kettenmann and Harold Kimelberg discovered glutamate and GABA receptors in cultured astrocytes and oligodendrocytes (Figure 1.27; Bowman and Kimelberg, 1984; Kettenmann *et al.*, 1984).

Several years later, in 1990, Ann Cornell-Bell and her co-workers (Cornell-Bell *et al.*, 1990) found that astroglial cells are capable of long-distance communication by means of propagating calcium waves (Figure 1.28). These calcium waves can be initiated by stimulation of various neurotransmitter receptors in the astroglial plasma membrane.

Finally, in 1994, two studies carried out by Maiken Nedergaard, Philip Haydon and Vladimir Parpura demonstrated that astrocytes can trigger calcium increases in neurones when growing together in co-cultures (Nedergaard, 1994; Parpura *et al.*, 1994). These discoveries were fundamental in demonstrating that glial cells can mount an active response to brain chemical signalling as well as signal back to neurones, and thus can be involved in information processing in the CNS.

Detailed analysis of the expression of these receptors performed during subsequent decades has demonstrated that glial cells, and especially astrocytes, are capable of expressing virtually every type of neurotransmitter receptor known so far. Moreover, glial cells have been found to possess a multitude of ion channels, which can be activated by various extracellular and intracellular stimuli. Thus, glial cells are endowed with the proper tools to detect the activity of neighbouring neurones. Neurotransmitter receptors and ion channels expressed in glial cells turned out to be truly operational. It has now been shown, in numerous experiments on various regions of the CNS and PNS,

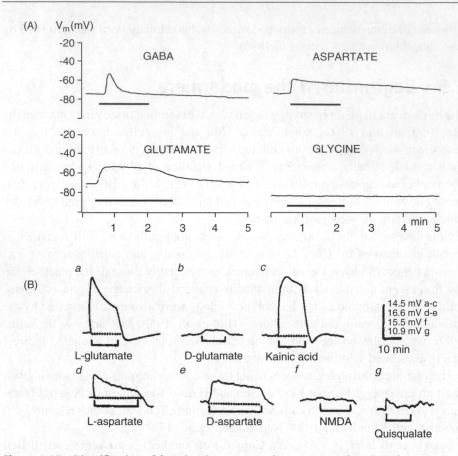

**Figure 1.27**  Identification of functional neurotransmitter receptors in cultured astrocytes.

A. Microelectrode recordings from cultured astrocytes. The traces show effects of γ-amino-butyric acid (GABA), glutamate, aspartate and glycine all applied at a concentration of 1 mM. Reproduced with permission from Kettenmann, H. et al. (1984) Aspartate, glutamate and y-aminobutyric acid depolarize cultured astrocytes. Neuroscience Letters 52:1–2, pp. 25–29 © Elsevier

B. Effects of excitatory amino acids on membrane potential of cultured astrocytes. Amino acids were applied at a concentration of 10 mM. Membrane potentials of the cells shown before addition of the amino acids were: a, –85 mV; b, –87 mV; c, –78 mV; d, –56 mV; e, –70 mV; f, –86 mV; and g, –64 mV. Reproduced with permission from Bowman & Kimelberg, 1984

that neuronal activity triggers membrane currents and/or cytosolic calcium signals in glial cells closely associated with neuronal synaptic contacts.

Finally, glial cells can also feed signals back to neurones, as they are able to secrete neurotransmitters such as glutamate and ATP. This discovery resulted from the efforts of several research groups, and it has led to the concept of much closer

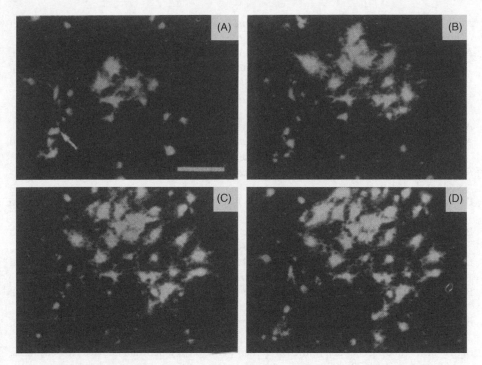

**Figure 1.28** First recordings of $Ca^{2+}$ waves propagating through astroglial syncytium in culture after focal stimulation with glutamate.

Reproduced with permission from Cornell-Bell *et al.*, 1990.

interactions between two circuits – neuronal and glial – which communicate via chemical and electrical synapses.

## 1.6 Concluding remarks

The 150 years of glial research resulted in remarkable changes in concepts and understanding of the role of these cells in the nervous system. Glial cells underwent a long evolutionary history and developed into indispensable homeostatic elements of the brain. Many of the theories of glial cell function originate from the early research of the 19th century, and many of these theories have been forgotten for decades. However, they are now re-emerging, supported by a wealth of newly acquired experimental data.

## References

Achucarro N. (1915). De l'evolution de la nevroglie et specialment de ses relations avec l'appareil vasculaire. *Trab Laboratory Investigation Biol Univ Madrid* **13**, 169–212.

Aldini G. (1803). *An account of the late improvements in galvanism, with a series of curious and interesting experiments performed before the commissioners of the French National Institute, and repeated lately in the anatomical theaters of London, by John Aldini.*

Aldini G. (1804). *Essai théorique et expérimental sur le galvanisme* (2 vol). Paris: Fournier et Fils.

Alzheimer A. (1910). Beiträge zur Kenntnis der pathologischen Neuroglia und ihrer Beziehungen zu den Abbauvorgängen im Nervengewebe. In: Nissl F, Alzheimer A, (eds). *Histologische und Histopathologische Arbeiten über die Grosshirnrinde mit besonderer Berücksichtigung der pathologischen Anatomie der Geisteskrankheiten*, pp. 401–562. Jena: Verlag von Gustav Fischer.

Andriezen WL. (1893). The neuroglia elements of the brain. *British Medical Journal* **2**, 227–230.

Aristotle. (1992). *De partibus animalium I and De Generatione Animalium I*. Edited and translated with notes by D.M. Balme.Oxford: OUP.

Atkinson WW. (1907). *The secret of mental magic: A course of seven lessons*. Chicago: Authors edition. 1–441 p.

Baker Jr, (1953). The cell-theory; a restatement, history, and critique. Part IV. The multiplication of cells. *Quarterly Journal of Microscopical Science* **94**(1), 407–440.

Baker PF, Hodgkin AL, Shaw TI. (1962). Replacement of the axoplasm of giant nerve fibres with artificial solutions. *Journal of Physiology* **164**, 330–54.

Bean RC, Shepherd WC, Chan H, Eichner J. (1969). Discrete conductance fluctuations in lipid bilayer protein membranes. *Journal of General Physiology* **53**(6), 741–57.

Bentivoglio M. (1996). 1896–1996: the centennial of the axon. *Brain Research Bulletin* **41**(6), 319–25.

Bergmann K. (1857). Notiz über einige Strukturverhältnisse des Cerebellums und Rükenmarks. *Z Med* **8**, 360–363.

Bernstein J. (1868). Ueber den zeitlichen Verlauf der negativen Schwankung des Nervenstroms. *Pflugers Archiv* **1**, 173–207.

Bernstein J. (1902). Untersuchingenzurb Thermodynamik der bioelectrischen Strome. *Pflugers Archiv* **92**, 512–562.

Bernstein J. (1912). *Elektrobiologie – Die Lehre von den electrischen Vorgangen im Organismus auf moderner Grundlage dargestellt*. Braunschweig: Vieweg und Sohn.

Bowman CL, Kimelberg HK. (1984). Excitatory amino acids directly depolarize rat brain astrocytes in primary culture. *Nature* **311**(5987), 656–9.

Bresadola M. (1998). Medicine and science in the life of Luigi Galvani (1737–1798). *Brain Research Bulletin* **46**(5), 367–80.

Brightman MW, Reese TS. (1969). Junctions between intimately apposed cell membranes in the vertebrate brain. *Journal of Cell Biology* **40**(3), 648–77.

Broca P. (1861). Perte de la parole, ramolissement chronique et destruction partielle du lobe anterieur gauche du cerveau (Sur la siege de la faculte du langage). *Bulletins de la Societe d'anthropologie de Paris* **2**, 235–238.

Burnstock G. (1972). Purinergic nerves. *Pharmacological Reviews* **24**(3), 509–81.

Burnstock G. (1976). Do some nerve cells release more than one transmitter? *Neuroscience* **1**(4), 239–48.

Campobianco F. (1901). Della participazione mesodermica nella genesi della neuoglia cerebrale. *Archives Italiennes de Biologie* **37**, 152–155.

Campobianco F, Fragnito O. (1898). Nuovo ricerche su la genesi ed i rapporti mutui degli elementi nervosi, e neuroglici. *Anm dei Neuroglia* **12**, 36.

Caputi F, Spaziante R, de Divitiis E, Nashold BS, Jr., (1995). Luigi Rolando and his pioneering efforts to relate structure to function in the nervous system. *Journal of Neurosurgery* **83**(5), 933–7.

Clarke E. (1963). Aristotelian concepts of the form and function of the brain. *Bulletin of The History Of Medicine* **37**, 1–14.

Clarke E, O'Malley CD. (1996). *The Human Brain and Spinal Cord: A Historical Study Illustrated by Writings from Antiquity to the Twentieth Century.* 2nd Edition. San Francisco: Norman.

Cobb M. (2002). Timeline: exorcizing the animal spirits: Jan Swammerdam on nerve function. *Nature Reviews Neuroscience* **3**(5), 395–400.

Cole KS. (1949). Dynamic electrical characteristics of the squid axon membrane. *Archives des Sciences Physiologiques* **3**, 253–258.

Cole KS, Curtis HJ. (1939). Electric impedance of the squid giant axon during activity. *Journal of General Physiology* **22**, 649–670.

Combe G. (1847). *The Constitution of Man considered in relation to External objects*, 8th Edition. Edinburgh, London: MacLahlan Steward & Co.

Cornell-Bell AH, Finkbeiner SM, Cooper MS, Smith SJ. (1990). Glutamate induces calcium waves in cultured astrocytes: long- range glial signaling. *Science* **247**, 470–473.

Crossley-Holland K. (2009). *Arthur. The Seeing Stone.* London: Folio Society.

Curtis HJ, Cole KS. (1940). Membrane action potentials from the squid giant axon. *Journal of Cellular and Comparative Physiology* **15**, 147–157.

da Vinci L. (1978–1980). *Corpus of the Anatomical Studies in the Collection of Her Majesty, the Queen, at Windsor Castle.* Windsor: Harcourt Brace Jovanovich.

Dale HH. (1914). The action of certain esters and ethers of choline, and their relation to muscarine. *Journal of Pharmacology and Experimental Therapeutics* **6**, 147–190.

Danielli JF, Davson H. (1935). A contribution to the theory of permeability of thin Films. *Journal of Cellular and Comparative Physiology* **5**, 495–508.

De Castro F. (1951). Anatomical aspects of the ganglionic synaptic transmission in mammalians. *Archives Internationales de Physiologie* **59**, 479–525.

Deiters O. (1865). *Untersuchungen über Gehirn und Rückenmark des Menschen und der Säugethiere.* Braunschweig: Vieweg.

Del Maestro RF. (1998). Leonardo da Vinci: the search for the soul. *Journal of Neurosurgery* **89**(5), 874–87.

Del Río-Hortega P. (1917). Noticia de un Nuevo y fácil método para la coloración de la neuroglía y del tejido conjuntivo. *Trab Laboratory Investigation Biol Univ Madrid* **15**, 367–378.

Del Rio-Hortega P. (1919a). El tercer elemento de los centros nerviosos. I. La microglia en estado normal. II. Intervencíon de la microglia en los procesos patológicos. III. Naturaleza probable de la microglia. *Bol de la Soc Esp de Biol* **9**, 69–120.

Del Rio-Hortega P. (1919b). Poder fagocitario y movilidad de la microglia. *Bol de la Soc Esp de Biol* **9**, 154.

Del Rio-Hortega P. (1920). La microglia y su transformacíon cn células en bastoncito y cuerpos gránulo-adiposos. *Trab del Lab de invest biol* **18**, 37.

Del Río-Hortega P. (1921). Estudios sobre la neuroglia. *La glia de escasas radiaciones oligodendroglia. Biol Soc Esp Biol* **21**, 64–92.

Del Rio-Hortega P. (1932). *Microglia.* In: Penfield W. (ed). *Cytology and cellular pathology of the nervous system*, pp. 482–534. New York: Hoeber.

Descartes R. (1664). *L'Homme, et un traité de la formation du foetus du mesme autheur. Avec les remarques de Louys de La Forge.* 1st Edition. Paris: Nicolas Le Gras.

du Bois-Reymond E. (1877). *Gesammelte Abhandlungen zur Allgemeinen Muskel-und Nervenphysik.* Leipzig: Veit & Co.

du Bois-Reymond E. (1884). *Untersuchungen über thierische elektricität, 1848–1884 (2 bande)* Berlin: Reimer.

Eccles JC. (1964). *The Physiology of Synapses.* Berlin: Springer-Verlag.

Eccles J. (1976). From electrical to chemical transmission in the central nervous system. *Notes and Records of the Royal Society* **30**(2), 219–30.

Ehrenberg CG. (1836). *Beobachtungeiner auffallenden bisher unerkannten Strukfurdes Seele-norgans bei Menschen und Thieren*. Berlin: Königlichen Akademie der Wissenschchaft.

Elliott TR. (1904). On the action of adrenaline. *Journal of Physiology* **31**, xx–xxi.

Ferrier D. (1875). Experiments in the brain of monkeys. *Proceedings of the Royal Society of London*, Ser B **23**, 409–430.

Ferrier D. (1876). *The Functions of the Brain*. London: Smith, Elder.

Ferrier D. (1878). *The Localization of Cerebral Disease*. London: Smith, Elder.

Ferrier D. (1890). *The croonian lectures on cerebral localisation*. London: Smith, Elder and Co.

Fishman RS. (1995). Brain wars: passion and conflict in the localization of vision in the brain. *Documenta Ophthalmologica* **89**(1–2) 173–84.

Fludd R. (1617–1621). *Utriusque cosmi majoris scilicet et minoris metaphysica, physica atque technica historia in duo volumina secundum cosmi differentiam divisa. Tomus primus de macrososmi historia in duo tractatus divisa*. Frankfurt: Oppenhemii, Aere Johan-Theodori de Bry, typis Hieronymi Galleri.

Ford BJ. (1992). Brownian movement in clarkia pollen: A reprise of the first observation. *The Microscope* **40**, 235–241.

Fowler OS, Fowler LN. (1875). *The Self-Instructor In Phrenology And Physiology; With Over One Hundred New Illustrations, Including A Chart For The Use Of Practical Phrenologists*. New York: Fowler & Wells/L.N. Fowler & Co.

Frank K, Tauc L. (1963). Voltage clamp studies on molluscan neuron membrane properties. In: Hoffman J. (ed). *The Cellular Function of Membrane Transport*. Englewood Cliffs, New Jersey: Prentice Hall.

Fritsch GT, Hitzig E. (1870). Über die electrische Erregbarkeit des Grosshirns. *Arch Anat Physiol Wiss Med* **37**, 300–322.

Frommann C. (1878). *Untersuchungen über die Gewebsveränderungen bei der Multiplen Sklerose des Gehirns und Rückenmarks*. Jena: Verlag von Gustav Fischer.

Frourens P. (1846). *Phrenology examined* (translated from the 2nd edition of 1845 by Charles de Lugena Meigs) Philadelphia: Hogan & Thompson.

Galambos R. (1961). A glia-neural theory of brain function. Proceedings of The National Academy of Sciences of the United States of America **47**, 129–36.

Galen C. (1821–1833). *Galeni Opera Omnia*. Leipzig: C. Nobloch.

Gall FJ. (1835). *On the Functions of the Brain and Each of Its Parts: With Observations on the Possibility of Determining the Instincts, Propensities and Talents, or the Moral and Intellectual Dispositions of Men and Animals, by the Configuration of the Head*, trans, Winslow Lewis, Jr. Boston: Marsh, Capen & Lyon.

Gall FJ, Spurzheim JG. (1810 –1819). *Anatomie et physiologie du système nerveux en général et du cerveau en particulier avec des observations sur la possibilité de reconnaître plusieurs dispositions intellectuelles et morales de l'homme et des animaux par la configuration de leurs têtes, 4 vols., with an atlas of 100 engraved plates*. Paris: Schoell.

Galvani L. (1791). De viribus electricitatis in motu musculari commentarius. *Bon Sci Art Inst Acad Comm* **7**, 363–418.

Galvani L. (1794). *Dell'uso e dell'attività dell'arco conduttore*: S. Tommaso d'Aquino.

Galvani L. (1841). *Opere edite ed inedite del Professore Luigi Galvani raccolte e pubblicate dall'Accademia delle Science dell'Istituto di Bologna*. Bologna: Dall'Olmo.

Garcia-Marin V, Garcia-Lopez P, Freire M. (2007). Cajal's contributions to glia research. *Trends In Neurosciences* **30**(9), 479–87.

Gerlach Jv. (1871). Von den Rückenmarke. In: Stricker S. (ed). *Handbuch der Lehre von den Geweben*, p 665–693. Leipzig: Engelmann.

Glees P. (1955). *Neuroglia morphology and function*. Oxford: Blackwell.

Golgi C. (1870). Sulla sostanza connettiva del cervello (nevroglia). *Rendiconti del R Instituto Lombardo di Scienze e Lettere* serie 2, v.3 275–277.

Golgi C. (1873). Suella struttura della sostanza grigia del cervello (comunicazione preventiva). *Gazzetta Medica Italiana, Lombardia* **33**, 244–246.

Golgi C. (1875). Sulla fina struttura dei bulbi olfactorii. *Rivista Sperimentale di Freniatria e Medicina Legale* **1**, 405–425.

Golgi C. (1885). *Sulla fina anatomia degli organi centrali del systema nervoso. Studi di Camillo Golgi Professore di Pathologia Generale e Istologia nell'Universita di Pavia (con 24 tavole)* Reggio Emila: Tip. S. Calderini e Figlio.

Golgi C. (1903). *Opera Omnia*. Milano: Hoepli.

Gorter E, Grendel F. (1925). On bimolecular layers of lipids on the chromocytes of the blood. *Journal of Experimental Medicine* **41**, 439–443.

Gross CG. (1995). Aristotle on the brain. *Neuroscientist* **1**, 245–250.

Hamill OP, Marty A, Neher E, Sakmann B, Sigworth FJ. (1981). Improved patch-clamp techniques for high-resolution current recording from cells and cell-free membrane patches. *Pflugers Archiv* **391**, 85–100.

Harris H. (1999). *The Birth of the Cell*. New Haven: Yale University Press.

Hatai S. (1902). On the origin of neurglia tissue from mesoblast. *Journal of Comparative Neurology* **12**, 291–296.

Held H. (1909). Über die Neuroglia marginalis der menschlichen Grosshirnrinde. *Monatschr f Psychol u Neurol* **26** Rdg.-Heft, 360–416.

Helmholtz H. (1850). Note sur la vitesse de propagation de l'agent nerveux dans les nerfs rachidiens. *C R Acad Sci (Paris)* **30**, 204–206.

Helmholtz H. (1852). Messungen über fortpflanzungsgeschwindigkeit der reizung in den nerven– zweite reihe. *Arch Anat Physiol Wiss Med*, 199–216.

Henle J, Merkel F. (1869). Uber die sogenannte Bindesubstanz der Centralorgane des Nerven-systems. *Z Med* **34**, 49–82.

Hild W, Chang JJ, Tasaki I. (1958). Electrical responses of astrocytic glia from the mammalian central nervous system cultivated *in vitro*. *Experientia* **14**, 220–1.

Hippocrates. (1950). On the sacred disease. In: Chadwick J, Mann WNtrans. (eds). *The medical works of Hippocrates*, p 179–189. Oxford: Blackwell.

His W. (1889a). Die Formentwickelung des menschlichen Vorderhirns vom Ende des ersten bis zum Beginn des dritten Moknats. *Abh kgl sachs Ges Wissensch math phys Kl* **15**, 673–736.

His W. (1889b). Die Neuroblasten und deren Entstehung im embryonalen mark. *Abh kgl sachs Ges Wissensch math phys Kl* **15**, 311–372.

Hodgkin AL, Huxley AF. (1939). Action potentials recorded from inside a nerve fibre. *Nature* **144**, 710–711.

Hodgkin AL, Huxley AF. (1952). A quantitative description of membrane current and its application to conduction and excitation in nerve. *Journal of Physiology* **117**, 500–44.

Hodgkin AL, Huxley AF, Katz B. (1952). Measurement of current-voltage relations in the membrane of the giant axon of Loligo. *Journal of Physiology* **116**, 424–48.

Hooke R. (1665). *Micrographia: or, Some physiological descriptions of minute bodies made by magnifying glasses*. London: J. Martyn and J. Allestry.

Jacobson M. (2005). *Beginnings of the Nervous System*. In: Rao MS, Jacobson M. (eds). *Developmental Neurobiology*, pp. 365–413. New York: Kluwer Academic/Plenum Publishers.

Jastrowitz M. (1870). Encephalitis und Myelitis des ersten Kindersalters. *Arch f Psychiat* **2**, 389–414.

Kettenmann H, Verkhratsky A. (2008). Neuroglia: the 150 years after. *Trends In Neurosciences* **31**, 653–9.

Kettenmann H, Backus KH, Schachner M. (1984). Aspartate, glutamate and gamma-amino-butyric acid depolarize cultured astrocytes. *Neuroscience Letters* **52**, 25–9.

Kölliker A. (1852). Zur Anatomie und Physiologie der Retina. *Verh Physikal-Med Ges Würzburg* **3**, 316–336.

Kölliker A. (1893). *Handbuch der Gewebelchre des menschen*. Leipzig: Wilhelm Engelmann.

Kostyuk PG, Krishtal OA, Pidoplichko VI. (1981). Intracellular perfusion. *Journal of Neuroscience Methods* **4**, 201–10.

Kryshtal OA, Pidoplichko VI. (1975). Intracellular perfusion of the giant neurons of snails (in Russian). *Neirofiziologiia* **7**, 327–9.

Kryshtal OA, Pidoplichko VI. (1977). Analysis of current fluctuations shunted from small portions of the membrane of a nerve cell soma (in Russian). *Neirofiziologiia* **9**, 644–6.

Kuffler SW, Nicholls JG, Orkand RK. (1966). Physiological properties of glial cells in the central nervous system of amphibia. *Journal of Neurophysiology* **29**, 768–87.

Kühne W. (1862). *Über dieperipherischen Endorgane der motorischen Nerven*. Leipzig: Engelmann.

Langley JN. (1905). On the reactions of cells and nerve-endings to certain poisons, chiefly as regards the reaction of striated muscle to nicotine and curari. *Journal of Physiology* **33**, 374–413.

Langley JN. (1906). On nerve endings and on special excitable substances in cells. *Proceedings of The Royal Society Of London* **78**, 170–194.

Lee KS, Akaike N, Brown AM. (1980). The suction pipette method for internal perfusion and voltage clamp of small excitable cells. *Journal of Neuroscience Methods* **2**, 51–78.

Leeuwenhoek Av. (1673–1696). *Alle de Briefen van Antoni van Leeuwenhoek/The Collected Letters of Antoni van Leeuwenhoek 1673–1696* (eleven volumes), edited, illustrated, and annotated by committees of Dutch scientists (Swets and Zeitlinger, Amsterdam, published intermittently between 1939 and 1983).

Leeuwenhoek Av. (1798). *The select works of Antony Van Leeuwenhoek, containing his microscopical discoveries in many of the works of nature*. Translated from the Dutch and Latin editions published by the author by Samuel Hoole. London: G. Sidney.

Lenhossék Mv. (1895). Der feinere Bau des Nervensystems im Lichte neuester Forschung, 2nd Edition. Berlin: Fischer's Medicinische Buchhandlung H. Kornfield.

Ling GN, Gerard RW. (1949). The normal membrane potential of frog sartorius fibres. *Journal of Cellular and Comparative Physiology* **34**, 383–396.

Loewi O. (1921). Über humorale Übertragbarkeit der Herznervenwirkung. *Pflugers Archiv* **189**, 239–242.

Longrigg J. (1993). *Greek Rational Medicine: Philosophy and Medicine from Alcmaeon to the Alexandrians*. New York: Routledge.

Lopez-Munoz F, Boya J, Alamo C. (2006). Neuron theory, the cornerstone of neuroscience, on the centenary of the Nobel Prize award to Santiago Ramon y Cajal. *Brain Research Bulletin* **70**, 391–405.

Lugaro E. (1907). Sulle funzioni della nevroglia. *Riv Pat Nerv Ment* **12**, 225–233.

Macalister A. (1911). Phrenology. *Encyclopaedia Britannica*, 11th Ed. Cambridge, Edinburgh: Camridge University Press. Pp. 534–541.

Malpighi M. (1687). *Opera Omnia*. London: Ed. Royal SocietyTomis Duobus.

Manzoni T. (1998). The cerebral ventricles, the animal spirits and the dawn of brain localization of function. *Archives Italiennes de Biologie* **136**, 103–52.

Marinesco MG. (1896). Lesions des centres nerveux produites par la toxine du *Bacillus Botulinus C R Soc Biol (Paris)* **48**, 989–991.

Marmont G. (1949). Studies on the axon membrane. I. A new method. *Journal of Cellular and Comparative Physiology* **34**, 351–382.

Matteucci C. (1842). Deuxième mémoire sur le courant électrique propre de la grénouille et sur celui des animaux à sang chaud. *Ann Chim Phys* **6**, 301–339.

Mazzarello P. (2010). *Golgi*. Oxford: Oxford University Press.

McCarthy KD, de Vellis J. (1980). Preparation of separate astroglial and oligodendroglial cell cultures from rat cerebral tissue. *Journal of Cell Biology* **85**, 890–902.

Merzbacher L. (1909). *Untersuchungen über die Morphologie und Biologie der Abräumzellen im Zentralnervensystem*. Fischer Verlag.

Metz AuSH. (1924). Die Hortega'schen Zellen, das sogenannte "dritte Element" und uber ihre funktionelle Bedeutung. *Z Neur* **100**, 428–449.

Mueller P, Rudin DO. (1963). Induced excitability in reconstituted cell membrane structure. *Journal of Theoretical Biology* **4**, 268–80.

Müller H. (1851). Zur Histologie der Netzhaut. *Z Wissenschaft Zool* **3**, 234–237.

Müller J. (1838–1842). *Elements of Physiology*, trans. W. Baly. London: Taylor and Walton.

Nageotte J. (1910). Phenomenes de secretion dans le protoplasma des cellules nevrogliques de la substance grise. *C R Soc Biol (Paris)* **68**, 1068–1069.

Nansen F. (1886). *The structure and combination of the histological elements of the sentral nervous system*. Bergen: Bergens Museum Aarbs.

Nedergaard M. (1994). Direct signaling from astrocytes to neurons in cultures of mammalian brain cells. *Science* **263**, 1768–71.

Neher E, Lux HD. (1969). Voltage clamp on Helix pomatia neuronal membrane; current measurement over a limited area of the soma surface. *Pflugers Archiv* **311**, 272–7.

Neher E, Sakmann B. (1976). Single-channel currents recorded from membrane of denervated frog muscle fibres. *Nature* **260**, 799–802.

Newton I. (1713). *Principia Mathematica* (2nd edition). English translation by Andrew Motte, Sir Isaac Newton's Mathematical Principles of Natural Philosophy and his System of the World (1729, reprinted 1934 by the University of California Press).

Nilius B. (2003). *Pflugers Archiv*iv and the advent of modern electrophysiology. From the first action potential to patch clamp. *Pflugers Archiv* **447**, 267–71.

Nissl F. (1899). Ueber einige Beziehungen zwischen Nervenzellerkrankungen und gliiSsen Erscheinungen bei verschiedenen Psychosen. *Arch Psychiat* **32**, 1–21.

Nobili L. (1828). Comparaison entre les deux galvanometres les plus sensibles, la grenouille et le moltiplicateur a deux aiguilles, suivie de quelques resultats noveaux. *Ann Chim Phys* **38**, 225–245.

Overton CE. (1899). Über die Allgemeinen Osmotischen Eigenschaften der Zelle, ihre vermutlichen Ursachen und ihre Bedeutung für die Physiologie. *Vierteljahrsschrift der Naturforschenden Gesellschaft in Zürich* **44**, 88–135.

Overton CE. (1902). Betrage zur allgemaine Muskel- und Nervenphysiologie. II Uber die Unentbehrlichkeit von Natrium- (oder Litium-) Ionen fur den Contractionsact des Muskels. *Pflugers Archiv* **92**, 346–380.

Parpura V, Basarsky TA, Liu F, Jeftinija K, Jeftinija S, Haydon PG. (1994). Glutamate-mediated astrocyte-neuron signalling. *Nature* **369**, 744–7.

Penfield W. (1924). Oligodendroglia and its relation to classical neuroglia. *Brain* **47**, 430–452.

Penfield W, Bouldrey E. (1937). Somatic motor and sensory representation in the cerebral cortex of man as studied by electrical stimulation. *Brain* **60**, 389–443.

Penfield WRT. (1986). *The cerebral cortex of man: A clinical study of localization of function*. New York: Hafner Pub. Co.

Pevsner J. (2002). Leonardo da Vinci's contributions to neuroscience. *Trends In Neurosciences* **25**(4), 217–20.

Piccolino M. (1997). Luigi Galvani and animal electricity: two centuries after the foundation of electrophysiology. *Trends In Neurosciences* **20**, 443–8.

Piccolino M. (1998). Animal electricity and the birth of electrophysiology: the legacy of Luigi Galvani. *Brain Research Bulletin* **46**, 381–407.

Piccolino M. (2003). A "Lost time" betwen science and literature: the "Temps Perdu" from Hermann von Helmholtz to Marcel Proust. *Audiological Medicine* **1**, 1–10.

Pratt FH, Eisenberger JP. (1919). The quantal phenomena in muscle: Methods, with further evidence of teh all-or-none principle for the skeletal fiber. *Amer Journal of Physiology* **49**, 1–54.

Prochaska G. (1784). *Functions of the Nervous System* (English translation by T. Laycock, 1851) Sydenham's Society series.

Purkinje JE. (1837). *Neueste Beobachtungen uber die Struktur des Gehirns.* Opera Omnia.

Ramon P. (1891). El encefalo de los reptiles. *Trab Lab Histol Fac Zarag* **24**, 1–31.

Ramón y Cajal S. (1888). Estructura de los centros nerviosos de las aves. *Rev Trim Histol Norm Patol* **1**, 1–10.

Ramón y Cajal S. (1895). *Algunas conjeturas sobre el mechanismoanatomico de la ideacion, asociacion y atencion*: Imprenta y Libreria de Nicolas Moya.

Ramón y Cajal S. (1909–1911). *Histologie du Système Nerveux de l'Homme et des Vertébrés* (reviewed and updated by the author, translated from Spanish by L. Azoulay), Maloine, Paris, France; English translation: Ramon-y-Cajal, S. (1995): *Histology of the Nervous system System of Man and Vertebrates,* translated by N. Swanson & L. Swanson, OUP, New York.

Ramón y Cajal S. (1913a). Contribucion al conocimiento de la neuroglia del cerebro humano. *Trab Laboratory Investigation Biol Univ Madrid* **11**, 255–315.

Ramón y Cajal S. (1913b). Un nuevo proceder para la impregnación de la neuroglía. *Bol Soc Esp Biol* **II**, 104–108.

Ramón y Cajal S. (1916). El proceder del oro-sublimado para la coloracion de la neuroglia. *Trab Laboratory Investigation Biol Univ Madrid* **14**, 155–162.

Ramon y Cajal S. (1925). Contribution a la connaissance de la nevroglia cerebrale et cerebeleuse dans la paralyse generale progressive. *Trab Laboratory Investigation Biol Univ Madrid* **23**, 157–216.

Ramón y Cajal S. (1933). *¿Neuronismo o reticularismo? Las pruebas objetivas de unidad anat'omica de las c'elulas nerviosas* Arch Neurobiol **13**, 1–144.

Raspail FV. (1825). Developpement de la fecule dans les organes de la fructification des cereales. *Annales des Sciences Naturelles* **6**, 224.

Reisch G. (1503). *Margarita philosophica.* Freiburg: Johann Schott.

Remak R. (1838). *Observationes anatomicae et microscopicae de systematis nervosi structura.* Dissertation. University of Berlin.

Retzius G. (1894). *Biologishe Untersuchungen. Neue Folge, Vol VI. Mit 32 Tafeln.* Jena – Stockholm: Von Gustav Fischer.

Robertson W. (1899). On a new method of obtaining a black reaction in certain tissue-elements of the central nervous system (platinum method). *Scottish Med Surg* **J 4**, 23.

Robertson W. (1900a). A microscopic demonstration of the normal and pathological histology of mesoglia cells. *J Ment Sci* **46**, 733–752.

Robertson WF. (1900b). *A Textbook of Pathology in relation to mental diseases.* Edinburgh: William F. Clay.

Schleich CL. (1894). *Schmerzlose Operationen: Örtliche Betäubung mit indiffrenten Flüssigkeiten. Psychophysik des natürlichen und künstlichen Schlafes.* Berlin: Julius Springer.

Schleiden MJ. (1838). Beiträge zur Phytogenesis. *Archiv für Anatomie, Physiologie und wissenschaftliche Medicin*, 137–176.

Schulze M. (1859). *Observationes de retinae structura penitiori*. Published lecture at the University of Bonn.

Schwann T. (1839). *Mikroskopische Untersuchungen über die Übereinstimmung in der Struktur und dem Wachstum der Tiere und Pflanzen*. Berlin: Sanderschen Buchhandlung.

Schwann T, Schleiden MJ. (1847). *Microscopical researches into the accordance in the structure and growth of animals and plants*. London: Sydenham Society.

Shepherd GM. (1991). *Foundations of the Neuron Doctrine*. New York: Oxford University Press.

Spurzheim JG. (1826). *The Anatomy of the Brain, with a General View of the Nervous System. Translated at the request, and under the immediate superintendence of the author from the unpublished French M.S. by R[obert] Willis*. London: MRCS.

Stallcup WB. (1981). The NG2 antigen, a putative lineage marker: immunofluorescent localization in primary cultures of rat brain. *Developmental Biology* **83**, 154–65.

Stillings D. (1975). Did Jan Swammerdam beat Galvani by 134 years? *Medical Instrumentation* **9**(5), 226.

Strickholm A. (1961). Impedance of a small electrically isolated area of the muscle cell surface. *Journal of General Physiology* **44**, 1073–1088.

Strickholm A. (1962). Excitation currents and impedence of a small electrically isolated area of the muscle cell surface. *Journal of Cellular and Comparative Physiology* **60**, 149–67.

Swammerdam J. (1758). *The book of nature (Biblia naturae)* London: C.G. Seyfert. pp. 236.

Swanson LW. (2007). Quest for the basic plan of nervous system circuitry. *Brain Research Reviews* **55**, 356–72.

Tan SY, Brown J. (2006). Rudolph Virchow (1821–1902): "pope of pathology". *Singapore Medical Journal* **47**, 567–8.

Todd RB. (1845). *The Descriptive and Physiological Anatomy of the Brain, Spinal Cord, Ganglions and their Coverings*. London: Sherwood, Gilbert and Piper.

Valentin GG. (1836). Über den Verlauf und die letzten Enden der Nerven. *Nova Acta Phys-Med Acad Leopoldina (Bresluu)* **18**, 51–240.

Verkhratsky A, Parpura V, Rodriguez JJ. (2011). Where the thoughts dwell: the physiology of neuronal-glial "diffuse neural net". *Brain Research Reviews* **66**, 133–51.

Vesalius A. (1543). *Andreae Vesalii Bruxellensis de Humani corporis fabrica, Libri VII*.

Virchow R. (1856). *Gesammelte Abhandlungen zyr wissenschaftlischen Medizin*. Frankfurt a.M.: Verlag von Meidinger Sohn & Comp.

Virchow R. (1858). *Die Cellularpathologie in ihrer Begründung auf physiologische and pathologische Gewebelehre. Zwanzig Vorlesungen gehalten während der Monate Februar, März und April 1858 im pathologischen Institut zu Berlin*. Berlin: August Hirschwald. pp. 440.

Volta A. (1918). *Le opere di Alessandro Volta* (edizione nazionale, 2 vols). Milano: Hoepli.

Von Euler US. (1946). A specific sympathomimetic ergone in adrenergic nerve fibres (sympathin) and its relations to adrenaline and nor-adrenaline. *Acta Physiologica Scandinavica* **12**, 73–97.

Von Staden H. (1989). *Herophilus: the art of medicine in early Alexandria*. Cambridge: Cambridge University Press.

von Waldeyer HWG. (1891). Über einige neuere Forschungen im Gebiete der Anatomie des Centralnervensystems. *Deutsche Medizinische Wochenschrift* **44**, 1–44.

Weigert C. (1895). *Kenntnis der normalen menschlichen Neuroglia*. Frankfurt a.M.: Moritz Diesterweg.

Wells SB. (1894). *How to Read Character: New Illustrated Handbook of Physiology, Phrenology and Physiognomy, For Students and Examiners: With a Descriptive Chart*. New York: Fowler & Wells Co., Publishers.

Willis T. (1672). *De anima brutorum quae hominis vitalis ac sentitiva est: exercitationes duae.* London: Typis E.F. impensis Ric. Davis, Oxon.

Wills A. (1999). Herophilus, Erasistratus, and the birth of neuroscience. *Lancet* **354**(9191), 1719–20.

Woolam D. (1952). Cast of the ventricles of the brain. *Brain* **75**, 259–267.

Wright NA, Poulsom R. (2012). Omnis cellula e cellula revisited: cell biology as the foundation of pathology. *Journal of Pathology* **226**, 145–7.

Young JZ. (1936). Structure of nerve fibres and synapses in some invertebrates. *Cold Spring Harbour Symp Quant Biol* **4**, 1–6.

# 2
# General Overview of Signalling in the Nervous System

## 2.1   Intercellular signalling: wiring and volume modes of transmission

The fundamental question in understanding brain function is: 'How do cells in the nervous system communicate?' In principle, all communications in the living world are mediated by molecules that diffuse between cells or between cellular compartments. These diffusable molecules interact with proteins/enzymes, forcing these latter to change configuration and thus modulate their function. Meaningful communication, however, requires regulation of the movement of diffusable molecules, allowing them to conduct relevant information.

At the very dawn of experimental neuroscience, two fundamentally different concepts for intercellular communication were developed. The 'reticular' theory of von Gerlach and Camillo Golgi postulated the internal continuity of the brain cellular network, which works as a single global entity, while the 'neuronal-synaptical'

*Glial Physiology and Pathophysiology*, First Edition. Alexei Verkhratsky and Arthur Butt.
© 2013 by John Wiley & Sons, Ltd. Published 2013 by John Wiley & Sons, Ltd.

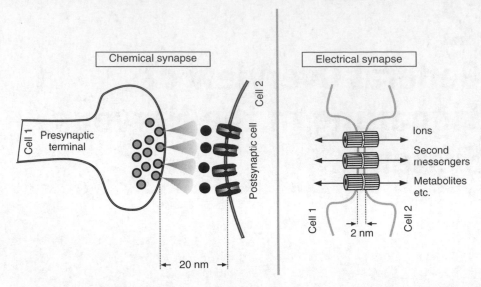

**Figure 2.1** Chemical and electrical synapses. Signals between neural cells are transmitted through specialised contacts known as synapses.

In the case of chemical synapses, cells are electrically and physically isolated. The chemical synapse consists of pre-synaptic terminal, synaptic cleft ($\approx$20 nm in width) and post-synaptic membrane. The pre-synaptic terminal contains vesicles filled with neurotransmitter which, upon elevation of intracellular free $Ca^{2+}$ concentration within the terminal, undergo exocytosis and expel the neurotransmitter into the cleft. Neurotransmitter diffuses through the cleft and interacts with ionotropic and/or metabotropic receptors located on the post-synaptic membrane, which in turn results in activation of the post-synaptic cell.

In the case of electric synapses, adjacent cells are physically and electrically connected through trans-cellular gap junction channels, each formed by two connexons (see Chapter 4). The trans-cellular channels permit passage of ions, hence providing for the propagation of electrical signalling, as well as larger molecules, hence providing for metabolic coupling.

doctrine of Santiago Ramón y Cajal and Charles Scott Sherrington implied that every neurone is a fully separate entity and cell-to-cell contacts are accomplished through a specialised structure (the synapse) which appears as the physical barrier (synaptic cleft) between communicating neurones (Figure 2.1A).

The latter theory postulated the focality of the intercellular signalling events, whereas Golgi thought about diffused transmission through the neural reticulum, which may affect larger areas of the CNS. The synaptic theory was victorious, yet the nature of the signal traversing the synaptic cleft was the subject of the second 'neuroscience' war, between followers of John Carew Eccles, who believed in purely electrical synapses (the electrical synapse is, in fact, a kind of chemical transmission, because it utilises diffusion of ions though intercellular channels – see Figure 2.1B), and supporters of Otto Loewi, Henry Dale and Bernhard Katz, who championed chemical transmission. This clash of ideas lasted for about 20 years before Eccles yielded and accepted the chemical theory fully.

For a while, everything calmed down and the neuronal chemical synapse theory looked unassailable. The cornerstone of this theory implied focal information transfer through synapses, and the brain can be relatively simply modelled as a precisely wired system of logical elements. As usual, however, nature appeared more complicated than our theories as, indeed, several different modes of cell-to-cell communication are operational within the CNS. Interestingly, the defeated reticular and electrical signalling theories of Golgi and Eccles more clearly describe glial signalling mechanisms, which, as slow waves of activity, lie in the background of the rapid neuronal synaptic signalling.

Direct physical connections between cells in the brain are of a ubiquitous nature. Gap junctions that form electrical synapses (Figure 2.1B) are, in essence, big intercellular channels that connect most of the neuroglial cells and some neurones, and possibly even neurones and glial cells. These gap junctions function both as electrical synapses (which allow electrotonic propagation of electrical signals due to diffusion of molecules) and as tunnels allowing intercellular exchange of important molecules, such as second messengers and metabolites. Moreover, neurotransmitters released at synaptic terminals as well as extra-synaptically, and neuro-hormones secreted by a multitude of neural cells, act not only locally but also distantly, by diffusing through the extracellular space.

These discoveries have led to the emergence of a more inclusive view of cell-to-cell signalling in the nervous system, which combines highly localised signalling mechanisms (through chemical and electrical synapses), generally termed as a 'wiring transmission', with more diffuse and global signalling, which occurs through diffusion in the extracellular space, as well as in the intracellular space within syncytial cellular networks. The latter way of signalling received the name of 'Volume Transmission', which be either extracellular or intracellular.

There are fundamental functional differences between wiring and volume transmission. Wiring transmission is rapid (hundreds of microseconds to several seconds), is extremely local, always exhibits a one-to-one ratio (i.e. signals occur only between two cells), and its effects are usually phasic (Figure 2.2).

In contrast, volume transmission is slow (seconds to many minutes/hours), is global, exhibits a one-to-many ratio (i.e. substance released by one cell may affect a host of receivers) and its effects are tonic. Extracellular volume transmission in the CNS is rather well characterised, for example in open synapses, in signalling mediated by gaseous neurotransmitters such as nitric oxide (NO), in the actions of neuropeptides, which are released extra-synaptically, in para-axonal transmission etc. (Figure 2.3).

The concept of intracellular volume transmission is relatively new, and so far it is believed to be confined mostly to the astroglial syncytium. The substrate of intracellular volume transmission is represented by gap junctions. Gap junctions also form electrical synapses, which are a classical example of wiring transmission (very focal and extremely fast). However, the same channels are instrumental for long-distance diffusion of molecules through glial networks, and as such they are

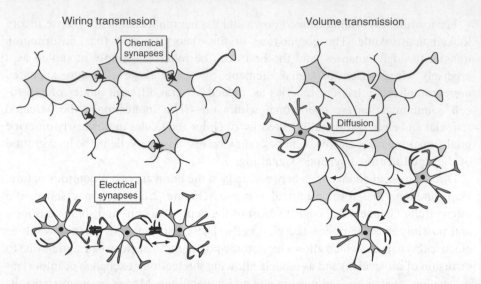

**Figure 2.2**   General principles of 'Wiring' and 'Volume' transmission.
Wiring transmission is represented by chemical synapses, the most typical of the CNS; synapses are tightly ensheathed by astroglial membranes, which prevents spillover of neurotransmitter from the synaptic cleft, and ensures focal signal transfer (arrows). Wiring transmission is also accomplished by electrical synapses, which allow rapid and local transfer of electrical signals. Volume transmission is generally produced by the diffusion of neurotransmitter from a focal point to several cells.

involved in signal propagation on a one-to-many (cells) ratio. The same mechanism may be instrumental in neuronal networks, particularly in the developing CNS, as neuroblasts and immature neurones exhibit high levels of gap junctional coupling.

These three principal pathways of signal transmission in the brain, working in concert, underlie CNS information processing by integrating all neural cells – neurones and glia – into highly effective information processing units.

# 2.2   Cellular signalling: receptors

Cellular signalling involves specific molecular cascades that sense, transmit and decode external stimuli. In the case of chemical neurotransmission, intracellular signalling invariably involves plasmalemmal *receptors*, which sense the external stimulus, and effector systems, which can be located either within the plasmalemma (ion channels) or in the cell interior. Often, the plasmalemmal receptors and the effector systems are linked through one or more second messengers.

**Ionotropic receptors** are essentially ligand-gated ion channels. Binding of a neurotransmitter to its receptor causes opening of the ion channel pore and generation of an ion flux, governed by the appropriate electrochemical driving force, determined by the transmembrane concentration gradient for a given ion and

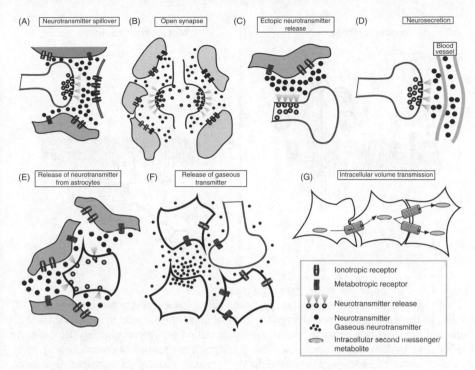

**Figure 2.3**   Examples of volume transmission in the nervous system.

A.   Neurotransmitter spillover: in synapses that are not perfectly covered by astroglial membranes, neurotransmitter may leak ('spillover') from the synapse and diffuse through the extracellular fluid to activate distant neuronal or glial cells.

B.   Open synapses: neurotransmitters or neurohormones may be released from open synapses, which do not have defined post-synaptic specialisations (e.g. catecholamine release from varicosities).

C.   Ectopic neurotransmitter release: neurotransmitters may be released from sites other than at the synapse (e.g. axons).

D.   Neurosecretion: neurohormones can be released directly into the extracellular fluid and enter the circulation.

E.   Release of neurotransmitters from astrocytes: neurotransmitters can be released from astroglia via vesicular or non-vesicular routes to diffuse through the extracellular fluid and act on neighbouring cells (glia, neurones, vasculature).

F.   Release of gaseous transmitters: e.g. nitric oxide, which act solely through volume transmission.

G.   Intracellular volume transmission: second messengers or metabolites can spread through gap junctions providing for intracellular volume transmission.

Adapted and redrawn from Sykova E. (2004). Extrasynaptic volume transmission and diffusion parameters of the extracellular space. *Neuroscience* **129**, 861–876; Zoli M, Jansson A, Sykova E, Agnati LF, Fuxe K. (1999). Volume transmission in the CNS and its relevance for neuropsychopharmacology. *Trends In Pharmacological Sciences* **20**, 142–150.

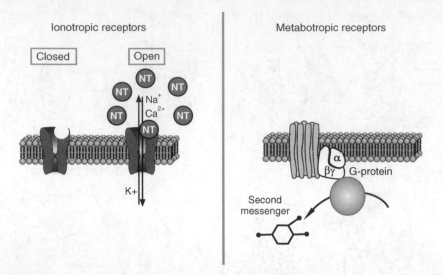

**Figure 2.4**   Ionotropic and metabotropic receptors.

Ionotropic receptors are represented by ligand-gated ion channels. Neurotransmitter (NT) binding to the receptor site directly opens the channel pore, which results in ion fluxes; these, in turn, shift the membrane potential, producing depolarization or hyperpolarisation, depending on the ion and transmembrane electrochemical gradients. Metabotropic receptors belong to an extended family of seven-transmembrane-domain proteins coupled to numerous G-proteins. Activation of metabotropic receptors results in indirect opening of ion channels or in activation/inhibition of enzymes responsible for synthesis of different intracellular second messengers.

the degree of membrane polarisation (Figures 2.4, 2.5). Activation of ionotropic receptors results in:

1.   a change in the membrane potential – depolarisation or hyperpolarisation; and

2.   changes in intracellular (cytosolic) ion concentrations.

Ionotropic receptors are represented by three major classes of channels which are topologically different, that is they differ in the number of subunits forming the functional ligand-gated channel and in the number of transmembrane domains forming each of the subunits (Figure 2.6).

The most diverse class of ionotropic receptors is represented by the pentameric receptors, which include receptors for acetylcholine (ACh), GABA, glycine and serotonin in vertebrates and many more receptors in invertebrates. The subunits of pentameric receptors have four fully developed transmembrane domains. The pentameric receptors form both cationic and anionic channels, which respectively provide for cell excitation (depolarisation) and inhibition (hyperpolarisation). This rule is not ubiquitous and, in some cells (e.g. in neuroglia or in developing neurones), the anionic channels produce depolarisation, which is determined by $Cl^-$ distribution across the membrane. Evolution of the pentameric receptors began in bacteria

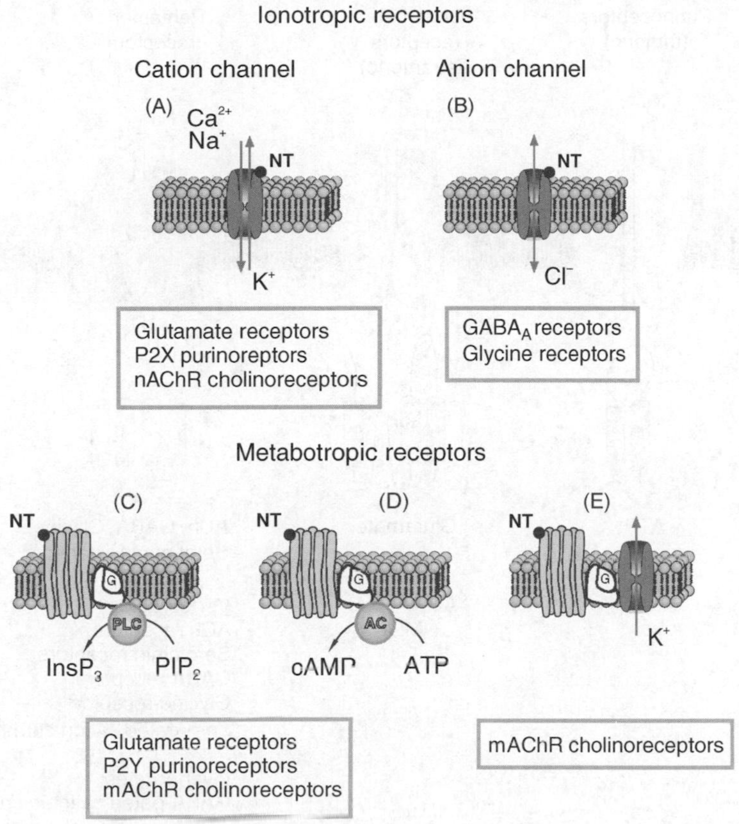

Ionotropic receptors

Cation channel                           Anion channel

(A)  $Ca^{2+}$                          (B)
     $Na^+$
              NT                                      NT

              $K^+$                                   $Cl^-$

| Glutamate receptors | GABA$_A$ receptors |
| P2X purinoreptors | Glycine receptors |
| nAChR cholinoreceptors | |

Metabotropic receptors

(C)                    (D)                    (E)
NT                     NT                     NT

PLC                    AC                                    $K^+$

InsP$_3$   PIP$_2$     cAMP   ATP

| Glutamate receptors | mAChR cholinoreceptors |
| P2Y purinoreceptors | |
| mAChR cholinoreceptors | |

**Figure 2.5**  Specific examples of ionotropic and metabotropic receptors.

**Ionotropic receptors**: Ionotropic receptors in the nervous system are represented by ligand-gated *cation channels* and *anion channels*. Ligand-gated cation channels are permeable to $Na^+$, $K^+$ and, to various extents, $Ca^{2+}$, e.g. ionotropic glutamate receptors, ionotropic P2X purinoreceptors and nicotinic cholinoreceptors (nAChRs). Activation of these receptors depolarizes and hence excites cells. Ligand-gated anion channels are permeable to $Cl^-$, e.g. GABA$_A$ and glycine receptors. Activation of these receptors in neurones causes $Cl^-$ influx, hence hyperpolarising and inhibiting the cells; but in glia (and immature neurones), their activation results in $Cl^-$ efflux, because intracellular $Cl^-$ concentration is high, and hence cell depolarisation.

**Metabotropic receptors**: In the CNS, these are coupled to *phospholipase C* (PLC), *adenylate cyclase* (AC), and *ion channels*. Metabotropic receptors coupled to PLC produce the second messengers *InsP$_3$* (inositol-1,4,5-trisphosphate) and *DAG* (diacylglycerol) from *PIP$_2$* (phosphoinositide-diphosphate), e.g. group I metabotropic glutamate receptors and most P2Y metabotropic purinoreceptors. Metabotropic receptors coupled to AC produce *cAMP* (cyclic adenosine-monophosphate), e.g. group II and III metabotropic glutamate receptors, and some muscarinic cholinoreceptors (mAChRs). Metabotropic receptors coupled to potassium channels are represented by muscarinic cholinoreceptors.

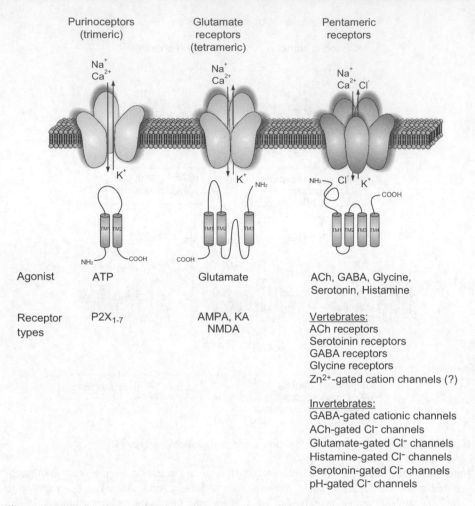

**Figure 2.6**  Three classes of ionotropic receptors.

Purinoceptors (trimeric P2X receptors; every subunit is assembled from two transmembrane domains), glutamate receptors (tetrameric AMPA, kainate [KA] and NMDA receptors; each subunit is assembled of three transmembrane domains), and pentameric receptor channels for acetylcholine (ACh), GABA, glycine and serotonin (each subunit is composed of four transmembrane domains). Vertebrate P2X and ionotropic glutamate receptors are non-selective cation channels, whereas pentameric receptors are either non-selective cation channels (nicotinic ACh (nACh), serotonin (5-HT$_3$)) or chloride channels (GABA$_A$, glycine). Invertebrate tissues express a range of pentameric channels with unusual properties.

(where pentameric channels are activated by protons) and it is characterised by sensitivity to many ligands. In invertebrates, the pentameric ionotropic receptors are remarkably diverse and include glutamate, acetylcholine, histamine, serotonin and pH gated Cl$^-$ channels and GABA-gated cation channels.

Two other classes of ligand-gated channels are represented by ionotropic receptors to glutamate and to ATP. Glutamate-gated channels are tetrameric, and each subunit has one rudimentary and three fully developed transmembrane domains, whereas P2X purinoceptors are trimers and every subunit is assembled from two trans-membrane domains. Incidentally, these two types of receptors also have ancient phylogenetic roots, as, indeed, ancestral forms of glutamate receptors appear in bacteria and P2X receptors are functional in the earliest eukaryotes. Interestingly, ionotropic purinoceptors and glutamate receptors exist in plants, indicating their emergence prior to the divergence of the plant and animal kingdoms. Most impor-tantly, however, both P2X and glutamate receptors retain strict adherence to their natural agonists (ATP and glutamate, respectively) throughout the phylogenetic tree.

**Metabotropic receptors** are coupled to intracellular enzymatic cascades and their activation triggers the synthesis of various intracellular second messengers, which in turn regulate a range of intracellular processes (Figures 2.4, 2.5). The most abundant type of metabotropic receptors are seven-transmembrane-domain-spanning receptors. These receptors are coupled to several families of G-proteins, which control the activity of phospholipase C (PLC) and adenylate cyclase (AC) or guanylate cyclase (GC). These enzymes, in turn, control synthesis of the intracellular second messengers inositol-trisphosphate ($InsP_3$) and diacylglycerol (DAG), cyclic adenosine 3',5'-monophosphate (cAMP) or cyclic guanosine 3'5'-monophosphate (cGMP). The G-proteins may also be linked to plasmalemmal channels, and often activation of metabotropic receptors triggers opening of the latter.

## 2.3    Intracellular signalling: second messengers

**Second messengers** are small (and therefore easily diffusible) molecules that act as information transducers between the plasmalemma and cell interior (Figure 2.7). The most ubiquitous and universal second messenger is the calcium ion ($Ca^{2+}$), which controls a multitude of intracellular reactions from exocytosis to gene expression. Other important second messengers include $InsP_3$, cAMP and cGMP, cyclic ADP ribose and NAADP. Second messengers interact with intra-cellular receptors, usually represented by proteins/enzymes, and either up- or down-regulate their activity, therefore producing cellular physiological responses.

## 2.4    Calcium signalling

Calcium ions are the most versatile and universal intracellular messengers. They are involved in the regulation of almost all known cellular functions and reactions. The exceptions are few, the most notable probably being the propagation of nerve action potentials, which depends on $Na^+$ and $K^+$ channels that are not acutely $Ca^{2+}$-regulated. The most important properties of $Ca^{2+}$ signalling are the promiscuity with respect to its effector systems and its auto-regulation. Indeed, $Ca^{2+}$ regulates a truly remarkable variety of intracellular processes, within extremely different temporal domains, from microseconds (e.g. exocytosis) to months or even years (e.g. memory processes).

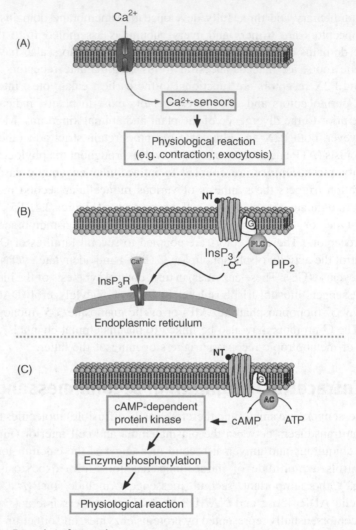

**Figure 2.7**   Examples of second messenger systems.

**Calcium signalling system:** $Ca^{2+}$ enters the cytoplasm, either through plasmalemmal $Ca^{2+}$ channels or through intracellular $Ca^{2+}$ channels located in the membrane of endoplasmic reticulum. Once in the cytoplasm, $Ca^{2+}$ binds to numerous $Ca^{2+}$-sensitive enzymes (or $Ca^{2+}$ sensors) to affect their activity and trigger physiological responses.

**InsP$_3$ signalling system:** $InsP_3$, produced following activation of metabotropic receptors/PLC, binds to $InsP_3$ receptors (which are intracellular $Ca^{2+}$ release channels) on the endoplasmic reticulum. Activation of these receptors triggers $Ca^{2+}$ release from intracellular stores and turns on the calcium signalling system.

**cAMP signalling system:** cAMP, produced following activation of metabotropic receptors/AC, binds to and activates a variety of cAMP-dependent protein kinases. These enzymes, in turn, phosphorylate effector proteins (e.g. plasmalemmal $Ca^{2+}$ channels), thus affecting their function and regulating physiological cellular responses.

Physiological effects of $Ca^{2+}$ are produced by intracellular *$Ca^{2+}$ sensors*, represented by enzymes which, upon $Ca^{2+}$ binding, change their activity. These enzymes have different affinities and, therefore, sensitivities to $Ca^{2+}$ (e.g. $Ca^{2+}$ sensors in the cytosol are regulated by $Ca^{2+}$ in concentrations of hundreds of nM, whereas $Ca^{2+}$-dependent enzymes in the endoplasmic reticulum are sensitive to $Ca^{2+}$ concentrations in the range of 100–1000 μM). Furthermore, intracellular $Ca^{2+}$ sensors are localised in different parts of the cell, and therefore local $Ca^{2+}$ gradients may specifically regulate particular sets of $Ca^{2+}$-dependent processes. These peculiarities of intracellular $Ca^{2+}$ effector systems allow for amplitude and spacial encoding of $Ca^{2+}$ signals, and solve the problem of specificity of such an intrinsically promiscuous system.

The actual molecular systems responsible for controlling intracellular $Ca^{2+}$ homeostasis and producing $Ca^{2+}$ signalling events are limited to several protein families represented by *$Ca^{2+}$ channels* and *$Ca^{2+}$ transporters* (Figure 2.8). These systems are very much conserved and ubiquitously expressed within the cellular kingdom. Most importantly, all of these systems are regulated by $Ca^{2+}$ itself, thus making a very robust, albeit versatile and adaptable, piece of molecular machinery.

## 2.4.1 Cellular $Ca^{2+}$ regulation

Free intracellular $Ca^{2+}$ represents only a small ($\approx$0.001 per cent) fraction of total cellular calcium. Within the cells, free $Ca^{2+}$ is very unevenly distributed between intracellular compartments. Cytosolic free $Ca^{2+}$ concentration ($[Ca^{2+}]_i$) is very low, being in the range of 50–100 nM. Calcium concentration within the ER is much higher, varying between 0.2 and 1.0 mM, and therefore similar to extracellular $Ca^{2+}$ concentration, which lies around 1.5–2.0 mM. As a result of these concentration differences, an extremely large electrochemical driving force keeps the cytosol under continuous '$Ca^{2+}$ pressure', as $Ca^{2+}$ tries to diffuse from the high concentration regions to the compartments with low free $Ca^{2+}$.

These distinct compartments, however, are separated by biological membranes (the plasma membrane and endomembrane separate the cytosol from the extracellular and ER compartments, respectively). Movement of $Ca^{2+}$ between the compartments therefore requires specific systems, represented by several superfamilies of transmembrane $Ca^{2+}$-permeable channels, ATP-driven $Ca^{2+}$ pumps and electrochemically-driven $Ca^{2+}$ exchangers. The $Ca^{2+}$ fluxes resulting from the activity of these systems may either deliver or remove $Ca^{2+}$ from the cytoplasm (Figure 2.8).

Major routes for plasmalemmal $Ca^{2+}$ entry are provided by *voltage-operated, ligand-gated and nonspecific channels* (Figure 2.8), which have distinct activation mechanisms and differ in their $Ca^{2+}$ permeability. Plasmalemmal voltage-operated $Ca^{2+}$ channels are the most selective for $Ca^{2+}$, whereas other channels allow the passage of $Ca^{2+}$ and other cations. For example, AMPA type glutamate

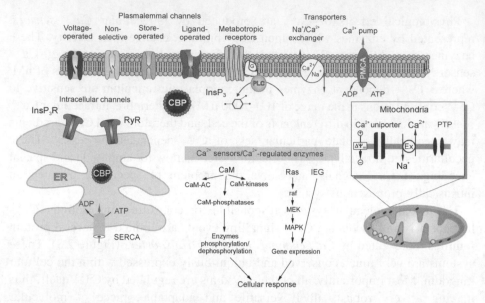

**Figure 2.8**  Molecular cascades of cellular calcium homeostasis.

Calcium homeostasis and the calcium signalling system are regulated by the concerted interaction of $Ca^{2+}$ channels (which include plasmalemmal and intracellular $Ca^{2+}$ channels), $Ca^{2+}$ transporters ($Ca^{2+}$ pumps and $Na^+/Ca^{2+}$ exchanger, NCX) and cellular $Ca^{2+}$ buffers. $Ca^{2+}$ channels provide pathways for $Ca^{2+}$ entry into the cytosol, whereas $Ca^{2+}$ transporters accomplish $Ca^{2+}$ translocation against concentration gradients either back to extracellular space or into the lumen of the ER. Mitochondria also act as dynamic $Ca^{2+}$ buffers; mitochondrial $Ca^{2+}$ accumulation occurs through the $Ca^{2+}$ uniporter (highly selective $Ca^{2+}$ channel) down the electro-chemical gradient (intra-mitochondrial potential is $\approx-200$ mV relative to the cytosol), whereas $Ca^{2+}$ can be released from mitochondria via NCX or (especially in pathological conditions) via permeability transition pores (PTP). See the text for further details.

**Abbreviations**: NCX – $Na^+/Ca^{2+}$ exchanger; PMCA – Plasmalemmal Calcium ATP-ase; CBP – $Ca^{2+}$ binding proteins; $InsP_3R$ – Inositol-1,4,5-trisphosphate Receptor/Inositol-1,4,5-trisphosphate-gated $Ca^{2+}$ channel; RyR – Ryanodine Receptors/$Ca^{2+}$-gated $Ca^{2+}$ channel; SERCA – Sarco(Endo) plasmic Reticulum Calcium ATP-ase. Intra-ER $Ca^{2+}$ binding proteins also act as $Ca^{2+}$ dependent chaperones, which are enzymes controlling protein folding into the tertiary structure. Intracellular $Ca^{2+}$ sensors are: CaM – calmodulin; CaM kinase – calcium-calmodulin-dependent protein kinase; CaM AC – calcium-calmodulin-dependent-adenylate cyclase; CaM-phosphatase – calcium-calmodulin-dependent-protein phosphatase; Ras – p21ras guanine nucleotide binding proteins; Raf – raf protein kinase; MEK – mitogen-activated/extracellular regulated kinase; MAPK – mitogen-activated protein kinase; IEG – immediate early genes. (Full colour version in plate section.)

receptors are principally ligand-gated $Na^+$ channels, but also have permeability to $Ca^{2+}$ and $K^+$.

Due to a very steep concentration gradient for $Ca^{2+}$ between the extracellular space and the cytosol, opening even a small number of plasmalemmal $Ca^{2+}$ channels results in a relatively large $Ca^{2+}$ influx, which may rapidly change cytosolic free $Ca^{2+}$. The second important source of cytosolic $Ca^{2+}$ is associated with release from the ER, which serves as an intracellular $Ca^{2+}$ store and represents the main source of cytoplasmic $Ca^{2+}$ signals in non-excitable cells. From the ER, $Ca^{2+}$ is delivered to the cytosol via two classes of ligand-gated $Ca^{2+}$ channels residing in the endomembrane, namely *ryanodine receptors (RyRs)* and *InsP₃ receptors (InsP₃Rs)*.

**RyRs** are activated by cytosolic $Ca^{2+}$, and therefore act as an amplifiers of $Ca^{2+}$ signals; these $Ca^{2+}$ channels are generally known as RyR because they are selectively activated (at low concentrations, $< 10\,\mu M$) or inhibited (at 50–100 μM) by the plant alkaloid ryanodine. The activation of RyR is also regulated by the naturally occurring intracellular second messenger cyclic ADP-ribose.

There are three types of RyRs: the RyR1 (or 'skeletal muscle' type); the RyR2 (or 'cardiac muscle' type); and the RyR3 (or 'brain' type). Note that these names are misleading, as they are not only expressed in these tissues; moreover, RyR3 expression in the CNS is actually relatively minor. RyR1 can establish direct contacts with plasmalemmal voltage-operated $Ca^{2+}$ channels, and the opening of the latter upon depolarisation will also open RyR1 and trigger *depolarisation-induced $Ca^{2+}$ release* (which does not require $Ca^{2+}$ entry and $Ca^{2+}$ interactions with the ER channel). RyR2 and RyR3 can be activated only by an increase in cytosolic $[Ca^{2+}]_i$, thus producing *calcium-induced $Ca^{2+}$ release*.

**InsP₃Rs** are activated by the intracellular second messenger InsP₃, which triggers *InsP₃-induced $Ca^{2+}$ release*. Importantly, InsP₃Rs are also regulated by cytosolic free $Ca^{2+}$, so that elevation of the latter increases the sensitivity of the receptors to InsP₃; high ($>1\,\mu M$) $[Ca^{2+}]_i$ inhibits type 1 InsP₃R, but not types 2 and 3.

Elementary $Ca^{2+}$ release events associated with opening of single RyR or InsP₃R are respectively known as $Ca^{2+}$ *sparks* or *puffs*; summation of the local events produces a global cytosolic increase in $[Ca^{2+}]_i$. Release of $Ca^{2+}$ from several ER channels is able to activate neighbouring RyRs and InsP₃Rs, thereby creating a propagating wave of ER excitation. By this means, $Ca^{2+}$ signals are able to travel intracellularly for long distances within polarised cells.

Importantly, the ER and plasmalemma are functionally linked through a specific class of plasmalemmal channels known as '*store-operated $Ca^{2+}$ channels*' (SOCCs; this pathway is also known as a 'capacitative' $Ca^{2+}$ entry). The latter provide for additional $Ca^{2+}$ influx in conditions when the ER is depleted from $Ca^{2+}$. This additional influx helps to replenish the ER $Ca^{2+}$ stores and produces plateau phase of $Ca^{2+}$ signals.

Upon entering the cytoplasm, $Ca^{2+}$ is immediately bound by *$Ca^{2+}$-binding proteins* (e.g. calbindin 28K), which determine the $Ca^{2+}$-buffering capacity of the cytoplasm. $Ca^{2+}$ that escapes binding, and therefore stays free, generates an intracellular $Ca^{2+}$ signalling event. The cytoplasmic buffering capacity of different cells varies substantially. For example, in cerebellar Purkinje neurones, only one out of $4,000\ Ca^{2+}$ ions remains free, whereas in hippocampal neurones, this ratio equals 1: 70–150.

Excess $Ca^{2+}$ entering the cytoplasm during stimulation is removed by several plasmalemmal and intracellular transporters, which expel $Ca^{2+}$ from the cytosol against a concentration gradient and prevent the system from overloading. Plasmalemmal $Ca^{2+}$ extrusion is achieved by $Ca^{2+}$ pumps (*PMCA, plasmalemmal $Ca^{2+}ATP$-ase*), which use the energy of ATP hydrolysis to transport $Ca^{2+}$, and by *sodium-calcium exchange (NCX)*, which uses the electrochemical gradient of $Na^+$ ions as the driving force for $Ca^{2+}$ efflux (extrusion of every $Ca^{2+}$ ion requires entry of 3–4 $Na^+$ ions into the cell, and is dependent on the $Na^+$ concentration gradient maintained by the activity of $Na^+$-$K^+$ pumps).

A sizeable amount of $Ca^{2+}$ is also removed from the cytosol by active uptake into the lumen of the ER via the *SERCA pumps (Sarco(Endo)plasmic Reticulum $Ca^{2+}ATP$-ases*) residing in the endomembrane. The activity of SERCA pumps is strongly regulated by the free $Ca^{2+}$ concentration within the ER, and depletion of the ER from $Ca^{2+}$ ions significantly increases the rate of $Ca^{2+}$ uptake by the SERCA pumps.

All of these extrusion systems are assisted by the mitochondria, which are endowed with a very selective $Ca^{2+}$ channel known as the '$Ca^{2+}uniporter$'. As the mitochondrial inner membrane is very electronegative compared to the cytosol (up to –200 mV), elevations of cytosolic $Ca^{2+}$ above $\approx 0.5$ μM drive $Ca^{2+}$ ions along the electrochemical gradient into the mitochondria. On entering mitochondria, $Ca^{2+}$ activates ATP synthesis and provides a mechanism for coupling cell stimulation with energy production.

Finally, it should be noted that excessive stimulation of $Ca^{2+}$ influx into the cytosol has a detrimental effect, being the main mechanism of so-called '$Ca^{2+}excitotoxicity$'. The latter occurs during long-lasting excessive stimulation of $Ca^{2+}$ entry (e.g. by pathological release of glutamate during brain ischaemia) or by failure of $Ca^{2+}$ extrusion systems, usually through lack of energy. Long-lasting increases in $[Ca^{2+}]_i$ in turn stimulate various enzymatic pathways that initiate apoptotic or necrotic cell death.

## 2.5   Concluding remarks

Despite the complexity of the human brain, it is remarkable that the complexity, versatility and adaptability of intercellular signalling in neural networks is defined by combining a relatively small number of few basic molecular cascades responsible for regulating the transport of several signalling molecules (ions, neurotransmitters, neurohormones and second messengers).

# 3
# Neuroglia: Definition, Classification, Evolution, Numbers, Development

*Glial Physiology and Pathophysiology*, First Edition. Alexei Verkhratsky and Arthur Butt.
© 2013 by John Wiley & Sons, Ltd. Published 2013 by John Wiley & Sons, Ltd.

## 3.1    Definition of neuroglia as homeostatic cells of the nervous system

*'THE NEUROGLIA is the delicate connective tissue which supports and binds together the nervous elements of the central nervous system. One part of it, which lines the central canal of the cord and ventricles of the brain, is formed from columnar cells, and is called ependyma, while the rest consists of small cells with numerous processes which sometimes branch and sometimes do not.'*

Encyclopaedia Britannica, 1910, 11th Ed., v. 19, p. 401

*'As the Greek name implies, glia are commonly known as the glue of the nervous system; however, this is not fully accurate. Neuroscience currently identifies four main functions of glial cells: to surround neurons and hold them in place, to supply nutrients and oxygen to neurons, to insulate one neuron from another, and to destroy pathogens and remove dead neurons. For over a century, it was believed that they did not play any role in neurotransmission. That idea is now discredited; they do modulate neurotransmission, although the mechanisms are not yet well understood.'*

Wikepedia, June 15th 2012 (http://en.wikipedia.org/wiki/Neuroglia)

To the continual surprise and confusion of everybody working in neuroglial research, the proper definition of 'neuroglia' has not hitherto been agreed upon. Many existing definitions highlight the supportive role of these cells, and some rests on their process branching and delicate morphology, but the most common definition assigned to neuroglia is "cells residing in the brain that are not electrically excitable neurones or vascular cells".

For example, Ted Bullock and Adrian Horridge defined neuroglia as *'Any non-nervous cell of the brain, cords . . . ganglia . . . and . . . peripheral nerves, except for cells comprising blood vessels, trachea, muscle fibers, glands, and epithelia . . .'* (Bullock & Horridge, 1965). As a result, 'neuroglia' has become a generalised term that covers cells with different origins (ectodermal for macroglia and mesodermal for microglia), morphology, physiological properties and functional specialisation. Indeed, in the CNS, neuroglia include the cells of the choroid plexus, the oligodendrocytes, the ependymal cells, the radial glia of the retina, the immunocompetent microglia/innate macrophages and the hugely diverse astrocytes; whereas, in the PNS, they include the diverse kinds of Schwann cells, satellite glia, olfactory ensheathing cells and the highly numerous enteric glia. All belong to the family neuroglia.

There is, however, one unifying fundamental property common for all these cell types and this is their ultimate function – homeostasis of the nervous system. Indeed, as we shall see below, the evolution of the nervous system led to a specialisation of neurones, which become perfect elements for signalling and information processing. This came at the price of losing essential housekeeping functions, as neurones are generally incapable of regulating their own immediate environment and are vulnerable to many kinds of environmental insults. These main housekeeping functions went to the neuroglia, which have themselves specialised into many types of cells to perform specific aspects of nervous system homeostasis.

This homeostatic function of neuroglia is executed at many levels, and includes:

- whole body and organ homeostasis (e.g. astrocytes control the emergence and maintenance of the CNS, peripheral glia are essential for communication between the CNS and the body, and enteric glia are essential for every aspect of gastrointestinal function);

- cellular homeostasis (e.g. astroglia and NG2-glia are both stem elements);

- morphological homeostasis (glia define the migratory pathways for neural cells during development, shape the nervous system cyto-architecture and control synaptogenesis/synaptic pruning, whereas myelinating glia maintain the structural integrity of nerves);

- molecular homeostasis (which is represented by neuroglial regulation of ion, neurotransmitter and neurohormone concentrations in the extracellular spaces around neurones);

- metabolic homeostasis (e.g. neuroglial cells store energy substrates in a form of glycogen and supply neurones with lactate);

- long-range signalling homeostasis (by myelination provided by oligodendroglia and Schwann cells);

- defensive homeostasis (represented by astrogliosis and activation of microglia in the CNS, Wallerian degeneration in CNS and PNS, and immune reactions of enteric glia; all these reactions provide fundamental defence for neural tissue).

Moreover, some neuroglial cells act as chemosensitive elements of the brain that perceive systemic fluctuations in $CO_2$, pH and $Na^+$ and thus regulate behavioural and systemic homeostatic physiological responses.

Therefore, the neuroglia can be broadly defined as *homeostatic cells of the nervous system*, represented by highly heterogeneous cellular populations of different origin, structure and function.

## 3.2 Classification

Generally (Figure 3.1), the neuroglia in the mammalian nervous system are sub-classified into peripheral nervous system (PNS) glia and central nervous system (CNS) glia. The PNS glial cells (see Chapter 8) include:

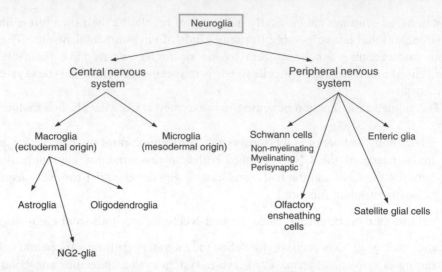

**Figure 3.1**    Classification of neuroglia.

1. *myelinating Schwann cells* that myelinate peripheral axons;

2. *non-myelinating Schwann cells* that surround multiple non-myelinating axons; and

3. *perisynaptic Schwann cells*, which enwrap peripheral synapses (for example neuro-muscular junctions).

The PNS glial cells which surround neurones in peripheral ganglia are known as *satellite glial cells*, and those in the olfactory system are known as *olfactory ensheathing cells*. Finally, the PNS includes *enteric glia*, which reside in the enteric nervous system.

CNS glia are generally subdivided into *astrocytes, oligodendrocytes, NG2-glia and microglia*. Astrocytes, which are the main homeostatic cells of the grey matter are, in turn, subdivided into many different types, which will be discussed in detail in Chapter 4. Oligodendrocytes are the myelinating cells in the CNS (see Chapter 5), and NG2-glia act as oligodendroglial precursors (Chapter 6). Finally, microglia represent the innate brain immunity and defence (Chapter 7).

## 3.3    Evolution of neuroglia

The 'Tree of Life' (visit the *Tree of Life* project at http://tolweb.org/tree/phylogeny. html) is in constant change, as the taxonomy is being continuously revised (the literature on this topic is immense and the reader is advised to look for details in several papers published during last decade, e.g. Cavalier-Smith, 1998; Cavalier-Smith, 2009; Ding *et al.*, 2008; Dunn *et al.*, 2008; Keeling *et al.*, 2005; Parfrey *et al.*, 2006; Yoon *et al.*, 2008). Whatever taxonomic chart we may use (either dividing all

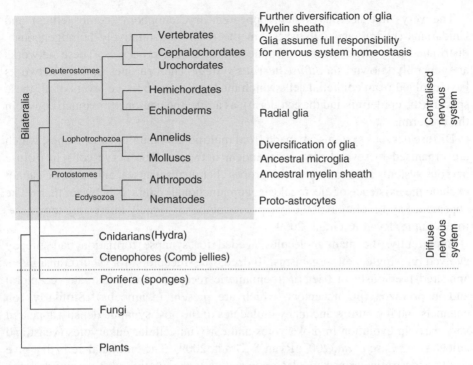

**Figure 3.2** Evolution of nervous systems and of neuroglia.

living forms into Domains of Bacteria, Archea and Eucarua, or that using Empires of Prokaryota and Eukaryota), the nervous system of which neuroglia are a part are a sole property of the Kingdom of Animalia. The cladogram of the latter is relatively well defined (Figure 3.2) and broadly comprises radially symmetrical Cnidaria and Ctenophora (which previously were regarded as members of a common family of Coelentarata, but are now considered as separate phyla) and Bilateralia that encompass the vast majority of phyla. The bilateralia are represented by Protostomia (further subdivided into Ecdysozoa and Lophotrochozoa; some taxonomists also recognise the Platyzoa as separate superphyla) and Deuterostomia, which include Echinodermata, Hemichordata and Chordata (to which vertebrates belong).

The early evolution of the nervous system can only be speculated upon, because fossils do not provide much material for analysis, and it is likely that many early life forms have not survived to our time. Nonetheless, certain generalisations can be drawn, and overall we are in possession of a rather logical system of views on the milestones of nervous system phylogeny. In this matter, of course, we shall restrict our narrative only to the very general outline of the evolutionary routes of the nervous system; for a more detailed account, readers are referred to numerous comprehensive reviews (e.g. Arendt *et al.*, 2008; Ghysen, 2003; Holland, 2003; Stollewerk & Simpson, 2005).

The very first nervous system appeared in Ctenophora (comb jellies) and Cnidarians (hydras and jellyfishes), in the form of a relatively homogeneously distributed network of neurones connected with their processes. These networks are generally known as a *diffuse nervous system*. The neurones in these networks have evolved from epithelial cells which made up the two tissue layers of all these species (the epidermis and the ectoderm); as a rule, the neurones are much denser in the epidermis.

Diffuse nervous systems are made from multipolar and unipolar neurones, which are organised in several semi-independent networks. The ncrve cells in diffuse nervous systems are connected with proper chemical synapses, although we cannot exclude the existence of electrical (i.e. gap junctional) contacts between them. The appearance and evolution of the synapse is another extremely interesting topic (see, for example, Ryan & Grant, 2009).

Importantly, the main molecules needed for synapse formation had already evolved in single cell organisms. Indeed, the receptors for neurotransmitters appeared previously in bacteria (pentameric receptors and glutamate receptors) and in protozoa (purinoceptors, which are present in amoeba). Similarly, ion channels and ion pumps and many molecules of the post-synaptic density appeared very early in evolution in prokaryotes and early unicellular eukaryotes (yeast and amoeba; see Case *et al.*, 2007; Ryan & Grant, 2009). The epithelial cells that give rise to ancestral neurones are also endowed with exocytotic machinery underlying vesicular release of proto-neurotransmitters.

The next step in evolution of the nervous system is associated with the appearance of neuronal masses known as ganglia. This signalled the appearance of the *centralised nervous system*. In some Cnidarian polyps, the nerve networks already showed some concentration around the oral opening, and this was likely the beginning of the centralisation process. How this process of centralisation proceeded remains generally unknown, but several hypotheses are currently in existence.

Notably, centralisation coincided with the appearance of bilateral symmetry and emergence of Bilateralia. Initially, for example in Nematoda, the centralised nervous system was made of several ganglia localised around the oral orifice. The centralisation continued in phylogeny, and in more advanced protostomes (for example in insects and crustacea), the central nervous system is present in the form of a polyganglionic brain. Further developments led to the appearance of a layered nervous system, which evolved in Echinoderma and Hemichordata and become fully organised in Chordata.

The evolutionary origins of glial cells are obscure. There are some indications that glia have appeared in phylogeny on several occasions, and parallel evolution is likely. There is no evidence for the existence of glial cells in diffuse nervous systems and no cells associated with neurones or their processes have been detected in the comb jellies. Similarly, no glial cells were found in Cnidaria polyps, with the exception of scyphomedusae, in which some glia-like cells were apparently reported – although neither their function nor, indeed, their glial identity, has been analysed in detail (Hartline, 2011).

Most probably, the neuroglia appeared with the emergence of a centralised nervous system, when neurones acquired specialisation and subsequently began to amass into sensory organs and ganglia. The very first glial cells are associated with sensory organs and have the same epithelial origin as neurones. These glia-like cells are described in Acoelomorpha, the primitive flat-worms, which are generally considered to be the earliest (or one of the first) Bilateralia. More advanced and much more characterised are glial cells in nematodes (in particular in *Caenorhabditis elegans*), whose properties we shall discuss below.

In Platyzoa, which are also considered to be primitive Bilateralia, appearance of glial cells is mosaic: glial cells are absent in Rotifera (wheel animals) and in many platyhelminthes (for example in tubellarian flatworms, Catenulida or Macrostomida). At the same time, glial (or accessory) cells have been found in polyclad flat-worms and in some (but not in all) triclad planaria. Neuroglia are generally present throughout Ecdysozoa and Lophotrochozoa, being well developed in molluscs, in Annelids, and even more so in Arthropods (insects and crustaceans).

In Deuterostomes, at the very base of Chordata, a new type of neuroglia emerge, the radial glial cells, which is most likely directly associated with the appearance of a layered nervous system. In many early Chordata, the radial glial cells dominate and are present throughout life, while parenchymal glia (i.e. astrocytes) are either completely absent, or remain in the minority. An increase in brain thickness triggered further development of parenchymal glia, which became increasingly heterogeneous and assumed a full homeostatic responsibility in the CNS of mammals, while the radial glia instead became mostly confined to the prenatal period and largely disappeared from the adult brain parenchyma.

All in all, the full story of glial evolution is complex and not fully understood; there are several comprehensive reviews (Hartline, 2011; Heiman & Shaham, 2007; Oikonomou & Shaham, 2011; Radojcic & Pentreath, 1979; Reichenbach & Pannicke, 2008), to which readers are referred for further details. Below, we shall provide an account of the evolution of the main types of neuroglia.

## 3.3.1   Evolution of astrocytes

(i)  **Nematoda: neuroglia in *Caenorhabditis elegans***   The nervous system of *C. elegans* is very well characterised morphologically and functionally. It contains 302 neurones and some 56 supportive/glial cells, which can be considered as proto-astrocytes; 50 of these glia are of epithelial origin, and six specialised glial cells are of mesodermal origin. The nervous system of *C. elegans* has major signs of centralisation. The sensory neurones distributed in the periphery send their pro-cesses to the nerve ring located in the frontal part of the body. The nerve ring also contains cephalic and motor neurones, which send efferent signals through the ventral and dorsal nerve cords. The sensory neurones in *C. elegans* have remarkable specialisation and diverse modality, being sensitive to soluble and volatile chemicals (analogues of taste and olfaction), temperature, mechanical stimulation, osmotic pressure, oxygen and even pheromones.

Most of the glial cells of the worm, 46 out of 50, are associated with the endings of these sensory neurones. These dendritic endings, together with glia, form sensory organs known as *sensilla*. Incidentally, males have specific sensilla (23 in total, composed of endings from 46 neurones) concentrated in the tail and imperative for mating; their particular function is physical sensation of the vulva of a mating partner (Heiman & Shaham, 2007). The number of neurites in sensilla varies between 1 and 12, but each sensilla has a pair of glial cells known as the sheath and socket cells (Figure 3.3). Sensilla in the male tail, as a rule, contain only a single glial cell classified as the structural cell. The remaining four glial cells, known as

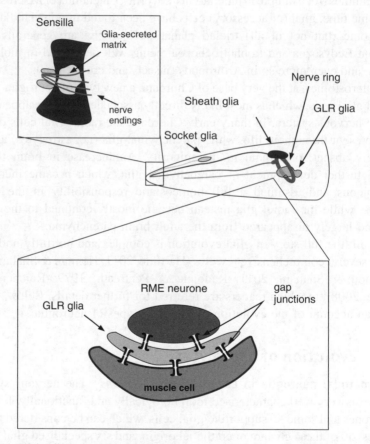

**Figure 3.3**  Glial cells in *Caenorhabditis elegans*.
The 'brain' of *C. elegans* is represented by a nerve ring. Most of the glial cells are part of sensory organs known as sensilla. Each sensilla has two glial cells: the sheath cell and socket cell. In the anterior part, there are four CEP (cephalic) glial cells that ensheath the nerve ring. The nerve ring also has six GLR glial cells which establish gap junctional contacts between motor neurones (RME) and muscle cells. (Full colour version in plate section.)

CEP sheath cells (because of their association with cephalic neurones), ensheath the nerve ring and send processes contacting synapses in the neuropil. Finally, the six mesodermally derived glia, known as GLR cells, are located around the nerve ring, where they make gap junctions with neurones and muscle cells.

The functional role of glial cells in *C. elegans* is not entirely clear, but they include: proper functioning of sensilla, possibly through increasing sensory efficacy; enwrapping and encapsulating synapses, possibly controlling ion homeostasis in perisynaptic regions; neuronal development and morphogenesis; and active neuronal-glial interactions. In addition, glial cells in *C. elegans* are also able to phagocytose dying cells during embryogenesis. At the same time, glial cells are not obligatory for *C. elegans* survival. Genetic or physical ablation of glia, although affecting sensory efficacy and neuronal morphogenesis, does not prevent the worm's nervous system from functioning and does not substantially affect animal survival (Bacaj *et al.*, 2008). Glial cells in *C. elegans* are not involved in neuronal metabolic support, either. Physiologically, glia of *C. elegans* show many neuronal features; for example, they generate $Ca^{2+}$ signals through activation of voltage-operated channels and do not have developed intracellular $Ca^{2+}$ stores (Stout & Parpura, 2011).

**(ii)  Annelida: astroglia in leech**  The medicinal leech *Hirudo medicinalis* was one of the very first animal models for studying neuroglia, as Stephen Kuffler and Richard Orkand used them for their pioneering electrophysiological experiments in the mid-1960s (Kuffler & Potter, 1964; Orkand *et al.*, 1966). The medicinal leech belongs to the Annelids and has a well defined centralised and segmented nervous system. The leech nervous system is composed of 34 ganglia. Six fused ganglia form the anterior brain, seven fused ganglia form the posterior brain and in between lies a chain of 21 ganglia, with each segment of the worm body being innervated with a single ganglion (Figure 3.4). In the frontal part of the nerve chain, four ganglia (two supra-oesophageal and two sub-oesophageal) are fused to form two neuronal masses that can be regarded as the animal's quasi-brain. These two frontal masses are linked together and form a peri-oesophageal ring. At the rear end of the leech body, another seven ganglia are fused into a caudal ganglion.

Leech neuroglia show a degree of specialisation, represented by several main types. Every single ganglion contains about 400 neurones (with the exception of the 5th and 6th ganglia innervating the reproductive system, which have ≈700 nerve cells) and ten glial cells. The glial cells comprise two giant glial cells, two connective glial cells which ensheath axons, and six packet cells which cover neuronal cell bodies. The giant glial cells, located in the ganglion central neuropil, are quite unique in their size and physiology. The somata of these glial cells have a diameter of ≈100 μm and their processes extend through the whole of the neuropil, being ≈300 μm in length.

The giant glial cells have an extensive complement of receptors, ion channels and transporters (Deitmer *et al.*, 1999; Lohr & Deitmer, 2006). The receptor palette includes ionotropic and metabotropic glutamate receptors, nicotinic acetylcholine

(A)

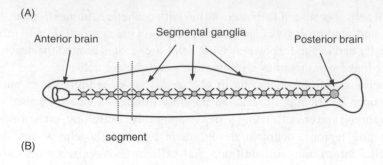

(B)

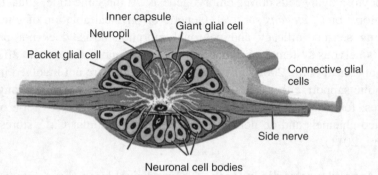

**Figure 3.4** Neuroglia in the medicinal leech, *Hirudo medicinalis*.

A.  General structure of the nervous system.

B.  Structure of the segmental ganglia, which contains three types of glial cells: the giant glial cell, packet glial cells and connective glial cells. (B - modified from Deitmer et al., 1999 with permission)

receptors, ionotropic and metabotropic serotonin receptors, metabotropic purino-ceptors linked to ER $Ca^{2+}$ release, and metabotropic receptors linked to myomo-dulin. The main type of ion channels are represented by potassium channels. In addition, giant glial cells express voltage-operated $Ca^{2+}$ channels and chloride channels. Multiple transporters are involved in regulation of extracellular gluta-mate, choline and pH.

The giant glial cells have complex $Ca^{2+}$ signalling, with a high degree of compartmentalisation; the $Ca^{2+}$ signals are mainly generated by membrane chan-nels and $Ca^{2+}$ permeable ionotropic receptors, whereas the contribution of intra-cellular $Ca^{2+}$ stores to $Ca^{2+}$ signalling is relatively small. Neuronal activity in the neuropil activates glial receptors and triggers local $Ca^{2+}$ fluxes which, in turn, produce highly localised $Ca^{2+}$ signals.

Most likely, the main physiological role of giant glial cells is the regulation of ions (mostly $K^+$ and $H^+$) and neurotransmitter homeostasis in the neuropil. In Annelids (similar to many other invertebrates, such as Arthropods and Molluscs), nerve cell somata are often invaginated by glial cells processes. This structure is known in histology as the '*trophospongium*' (Holmgren, 1901), and it is likely to be involved in trophic support of neurones.

The connective glial cells ensheath axons and are possibly involved in mechanical and metabolic support of the latter. The packet cells enwrap neuronal cell bodies and segregate neurones in architectural microdomains known as packets; in addition, packet cells are probably involved in regulation of the perineuronal microenvironment. Therefore, neuroglia in Annelids contribute to functional compartmentalisation of the neuronal groups, a function which is present in all subsequent evolutionarily more advanced life forms. All three types of glia in the leech are coupled through gap junctions (formed by innexins, two types of which are specifically expressed in glial cells) and form a panglial syncytium embracing the whole of the nervous system. This syncytium may provide for long-range molecular diffusion through the nerve cord.

**(iii)  Arthropods: astrocytes in *Drosophila* and other insects**  The Arthropods and, in particular, insects, developed highly diversified neuroglia. In *Drosophila*, the nervous system has been investigated in detail, and we have reasonably deep knowledge on neuroglial morphology and function. The *Drosophila* brain is constructed from three pairs of ganglia fused into one frontally located mass. It is divided into the paired visual protocerebrum (receiving visual information), paired deuterocerebrum (receiving sensory input from antennae) and tritocerebrum (which is believed to integrate information from other parts of CNS). Each part of the CNS has several relatively independent neuropil regions.

There are several classifications of *Drosophila* neuroglia, which divide these cells according to their anatomical location and morphology. Here, we adopt the classification presented by Edwards & Meinertzhagen (2010) (see also Hartenstein, 2011; Parker & Auld, 2006 for further details). The total number of neuroglial cells in *Drosophila* CNS (which comprise ≈90,000 cells) does not exceed ten per cent.

- The first type of CNS glia is the *surface glia*, which makes the haemolymph-brain barrier and is subdivided into *perineural glia* (relatively small cells lying on the ganglionic surface) and *subperineural* or *basal glia* (represented by large sheet-like cells connected with a septate junction that forms the actual barrier).

- The second type is the *cortex glia* that contact neuronal cell somata in the CNS; each glial cell establishes contacts with many neurones.

- The third type is *neuropil glia*, which are located in the neuropil and cover axons and synapses. The neuropil glia are further subdivided into *ensheathing* or *fibrous cells* that enwrap axons, and *astrocyte-like glia*, which form a peri-synaptic glial cover.

- Finally, there are *tract glial cells*, which cover axonal tracts connecting different neuropils.

There is further diversity of neuroglia in different regions of the *Drosophila* nervous system. For example, in the optic lamina (the optic neuropil), as many as six different glial cell types are distinguished (*fenestrated glia, pseudocartridge glia, distal and proximal satellite glia, epithelial glia* and *marginal glia*). Similarly, several classes of neuroglial cells have been described in the deep optic lobe. These include *giant optic chiasm glia, small outer optic chiasm glia, medulla satellite glia* and *medulla neuropil glia*. Several other small sub-populations of glia have been identified in the eye disk, optic stalk, and in the antennae. Finally, the peripheral nervous system of *Drosophila* contains *wrapping glia* that cover peripheral axons. A similar degree of complexity is also found in other insects, such as, for example, in the housefly *Musca domestica*, or in tobacco hornworn *Manduca sexta*.

When comparing Arthropods with Annelids, we see a rather significant development of glial diversity; these heterogeneous glia assume many new functions compared to lower phyla. An important new function of glia in Arthropods is the formation of the blood-brain barrier (or, to be precise, the haemolymph-brain barrier, because Arthropods do not have a closed circulatory system, nor do they have proper blood) that effectively separates the CNS from the rest of the body and segregates molecules allowed to enter the nervous system. In addition, glia separate the intra-brain tracheoles that supply CNS with air/oxygen.

As has already been mentioned, the haemolymph-brain barrier is sealed by septate junctions that play a role similar to tight junctions between endothelial cells of the blood-brain barrier in higher vertebrates. The haemolymph-brain barrier is formed solely by neuroglia and it is critical in controlling transport of ions (especially $K^+$, whose concentration rises high during feeding) and various nutrients. There are some indications that nutrients can cross the glial barrier by regulated endo/exocytosis. The glial cells also define the architecture of the insect CNS, by separating functionally distinct neuronal ensembles.

In insects, glial cells regulate ion balance in the intra-CNS fluids through the activity of $Na^+$ and $K^+$ ion pumps. In addition, glial cells redistribute ions from regions of high concentration through intercellular diffusion via gap junctions (formed by innexins) that connect glial cells into syncitia. Insect CNS glial cells are critical for homeostasis (clearance and recycling) of the principal neurotransmitter histamine in the retina, which is achieved through a shuttle operating between photoreceptors and surrounding glial cells.

In the CNS, glial cells also control glutamate homeostasis; *Drosophila* glia specifically express two types of excitatory amino acid transporters – dEAAT1and dEAAT2 – which belong to the extended family of EAAT transporters, also present in vertebrates. Furthermore, insect neuroglia also express glutamine synthetase and thus may be involved in glutamate-glutamine shuttling with neurones. Incidentally, glutamate is a main neurotransmitter controlling sexual behaviour, and especially courtship, in *Drosophila*, and specific glial disruption of the glutamate transporter alters courtship behaviour though disrupting proper apprehension of male-associated pheromones, resulting in homosexual courtship attempts. *Drosophila* glia also express an enzyme, dopa decarboxylase, which is needed for synthesis of 5-HT (serotonin) and may act as a supply of the latter. *Drosophila* glia are intimately involved in controlling circadian rhythms.

Trophic support of neurones is another fundamental function of insect glia. For example, in the honeybee retina, the glial cells (known as pigment cells) convert glucose/glycogen into alanin, which is then released and taken up by neurones and acts as an energy substrate. Neuroglial cells in insects are involved in various aspects of CNS development, for example by presenting localisation clues for migrating neurones. The neuroglia in insects are obligatory for neuronal survival, and neurones degenerate in several *Drosophila* mutants with altered glial functions. Finally, glial cells in insects are involved in brain defence and are already endowed with astrogliosis capabilities; in addition, insect neuroglia are capable of phagocytosis.

### (iv) Neuroglia in early Deuterostomia (Hemichordata and Echinodermata)
The Hemichordata (Acorn worms) and Echinodermata (e.g. sea urchin, starfishes, sea cucumber) are currently considered to be sister phyla of Chordata; it is still unclear whether they represent a parallel evolutionary trait or are related to Chordata. The nervous system of Echinoderms consists of a circumoral nerve ring and radial nerve cords (five in most of the species).

When comparing neuroglia of Echinoderms to the Arthropods or Molluscs, the most surprising feature is an almost complete disappearance of different glial forms and an emergence of a new type of glia. These new glia are characterised by an elongated shape, long processes that span the whole thickness of the neural parenchyma, perpendicular orientation to the surface of the neuroepithelium and high level of expression of intermediate filaments in the cytoplasm. All in all, these cells are very similar to radial glia of higher vertebrates (Mashanov *et al.*, 2009).

The function of these radial glial cells is not really known, although they are actively involved in regeneration of the nervous system, being the precursors of newborn neurones and assisting migration of these neurones through the CNS tissue. These features very much resemble the main functions of radial glia in the vertebrate brain, and we may expound that the Deuterostomia developed a new organisation of the nervous system, relying on radial glia, that determines the layered organisation of the CNS. In addition, in some Echinoderms (e.g. sea cucumber), a few glia-like cells located in CNS parenchyma have been discovered, although neither their function, nor indeed their glial identity, are yet known. We know next to nothing about neuroglia in Hemichordata. The ganglia of *Cephalodiscus gracilis*, for example, were reported to contain no glia at all (Rehkamper *et al.*, 1987).

### (v) Neuroglia in low vertebrates
In the early vertebrates, the same tendency of prevalence of radial glia in some species can be observed. In elasmobranchii (chondrichthian fish such as sharks and rays), for example, two types of brains are distinguished – the 'laminar' type I and 'elaborated' type II. The type I brains are

relatively thin with large ventricles; in this type of the brain neurones are mostly confined to the periventricular zone. The 'elaborated' brains are larger and thicker and neurones migrate away from the periventricular zone and form nuclei. Neuroglia in the 'laminar' brains are represented mainly by radial glia (also known as ependymoglia or tanycytes), whereas the parenchyma of 'elaborated' brains contains numerous astrocytes/astrocyte-like cells (Ari & Kalman, 2008).

The increase in parenchymal astrocytes in elaborated brains can be explained by an increase in surface-volume ratio of radial glial cells, with an increase in the thickness of the brain. This constrains homeostatic capabilities of the radial glia and, hence, prompts increase in the number/complexity of parenchymal astrocytes (Reichenbach et al., 1987). Alternatively, the emergence of parenchymal astrocytes is explained in terms of increased complexity of vascularisation, requiring perivascular glial support that cannot be provided by radial glia (Wicht et al., 1994). It is worth noting that astrocytes/neuroglia in sharks form the blood-brain barrier, and some of the capillaries are completely surrounded by astroglial process, being thus endocellular vessels (Abbott, 2005; Long et al., 1968).

A similar preponderance of radial glia is observed in bony fish and in particular in teleosts (e.g. zebrafish). In zebrafish, radial glial cells extend through the entire width of the brain, from the ependymal coating of the ventricles to the pial surface of the brain. These radial glial cells express GFAP, have glutamine synthetase (indicating their possible role in glutamate homeostasis and metabolism) and express aquaporin-4 (indicating their role in water homeostasis – see Grupp et al., 2010). The absence of parenchymal glia (astrocytes) is particularly important for the reactions of fish brains to injury. Insults to the teleost fish brain do not trigger astrogliosis; stab wounds, for example, are closed rapidly (in several days) without formation of the scar. Instead of an astrogliotic response, the zebra fish increase neurogenesis, which most likely provides new cells to fill the wound (Baumgart et al., 2010). Importantly, in teleosts, the blood-brain barrier is shifted to ependymal cells. This arrangement remains in all higher vertebrates, although tight junction proteins are found in glia in the optic nerve of some species.

**(vi)    Glial advance in higher vertebrates**    Neuroglia attained maximal development in mammals. Moreover, an increased complexity of the brain, together with an increased intellectual power, was accompanied by remarkable increases in the numbers and complexity of glia (Oberheim et al., 2006; Reichenbach, 1989). This coincided with similarly remarkable increases in glial diversity and in glial functions. The evolutionary increase in astroglial complexity is particularly obvious in the brains of primates, and especially in the brain of humans (Oberheim et al., 2009).

Human astrocytes are much larger and far more complex than those in the rodent brain (Figure 3.5). In the human brain, the average diameter of belonging to a human protoplasmic astrocyte is ≈2.5 times larger than that formed by an equivalent rat astrocyte (142 μm vs. 56 μm). The volume of the human

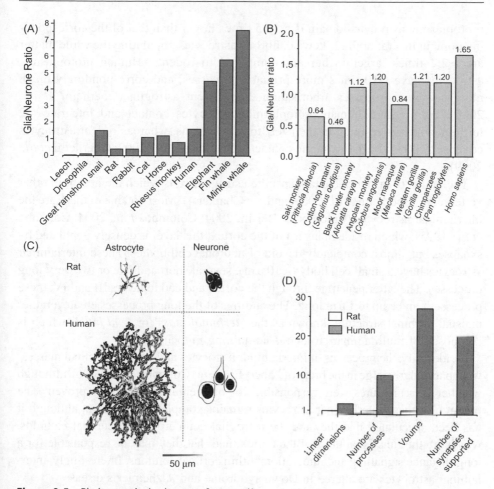

**Figure 3.5**  Phylogenetical advance of neuroglia.

A.  Glia-to-neurone ratio in the nervous system of invertebrates and in the cortex of vertebrates. Glia-to-neurone ratio is generally increased in phylogeny; this ratio more or less linearly follows an increase in the size of the brain.

B.  The glia/neurone ratio in the cortex of higher primates; this ratio is highest in humans (Data taken from Sherwood *et al.*, 2006).

C.  Graphic representation of neurones and astroglia in mouse and in human cortex. Evolution has resulted in remarkable changes in astrocytic dimensions and complexity.

D.  Relative increase in glial dimensions and complexity during evolution. Linear dimensions of human astrocytes, when compared with mice, are ≈2.75 times larger, and their volume is 27 times larger; human astrocytes have ≈10 times more processes and every astrocyte in human cortex enwraps ≈20 times more synapses.

C, D adapted, with permission, from Oberheim *et al.*, 2006.

protoplasmic astrocyte domain is ≈16.5 times larger than that of the correspond-ing domain in a rat brain. Likewise, fibrous astrocytes populating the white matter are ≈2.2 times larger in humans compared to rodents. Human protoplasmic astrocytes have ≈10 times more primary processes, and correspondingly much more complex processes arborisation than rodent astroglia (Oberheim *et al.*, 2006). As a result, human protoplasmic astrocytes contact and integrate ≈2 million synapses residing in their territorial domains, whereas rodent astrocytes cover ≈20,000–120,000 synaptic contacts (Bushong *et al.*, 2002; Oberheim *et al.*, 2009).

The brains of primates contain specific astroglial cells which are absent in other vertebrates (Oberheim *et al.*, 2009; and see Chapter 4). Most notable of these are the interlaminar astrocytes (Colombo & Reisin, 2004; Colombo *et al.*, 2004; Colombo *et al.*, 1995), which reside in layer I of the cortex; this layer is densely populated by synapses but almost completely devoid of neuronal cell bodies. These interlaminar astrocytes have a small cell body (≈10 μm), several short and one or two very long processes. The latter penetrate through the cortex and end in layers III and IV; these processes can be up to 1 μm long. The endings of the long processes create a rather unusual terminal structure, known as the '*terminal mass*' or '*end bulb*', which is composed of multilaminar structures containing mitochondria.

Incidentally, the processes of interlaminar astrocytes and size of 'terminal masses' were particularly large in the brain of Albert Einstein (Colombo *et al.*, 2006), although whether these features were responsible for his genius is not really proven. The function of these interlaminar astrocytes remains completely unknown, although it has been speculated that they are the astroglial counterpart of neuronal columns, which are the functional units of the cortex, and that they may be responsible for a long-distance signalling and integration within cortical columns. Interestingly, inter-laminar astrocytes are altered in Down syndrome and Alzheimer's disease.

Human brains also contain polarized astrocytes, which are uni- or bipolar cells that dwell in layers V and VI of the cortex, quite near to the white matter; they have one or two very long (up to 1 μm) processes that terminate in the neuropil. The processes of these cells are thin (2–3 μm in diameter) and straight, and they also have numerous varicosities. Once more, the function of polarized astrocytes remains enigmatic, although they might be involved in para-neuronal long-distance signalling.

The evolution of neurones produced fewer changes in their appearance – that is, the density of synaptic contacts in rodents and primates is very similar (in the rodent brain, the mean density of synaptic contacts is ≈1397 millions/$\mu m^3$, which is not much different from humans, where synaptic density in the cortex is ≈1100 millions/$\mu m^3$). Similarly, the number of synapses per neurone does not differ significantly between primates and rodents. The shape and dimensions of neurones also have not changed dramatically over the phylogenetic ladder. Human neurones are certainly larger, yet their linear dimensions are only about 1.5 times greater than in rodents. Thus, at least morphologically, evolution resulted in far greater changes in glia than in neurones, which most likely has important, although yet undetermined, significance.

## 3.3.2   Evolution of myelination

The problem of nerve impulse propagation was always a challenge to evolutionary development of multicellular organisms. Increase in animal size obviously requires faster nerve conductance, which in the simplest way, could be achieved through an increase in axon diameter (Hartline & Colman, 2007). Indeed, increase in axon diameter reduces resistance of the axon proportionally to the square of diameter, and the conductance velocity is directly proportional to the square root of the axon diameter (Hodgkin, 1954). This strategy was employed by many invertebrates, including Annelids, certain crustacea and Molluscs. In *Loligo* squid, for example, large axons (0.5 mm in diameter) propagate action potentials with a velocity of up to 30 m/s.

Increase in axon diameter, however, implies at least two fundamental limitations which are incompatible with complex nervous systems. First, the conduction through large axons is energetically costly, because substantial $Na^+/K^+$ pumping is needed to maintain the ion gradients. Second, large axons apply severe space constrains; for example, if the human optic nerve were composed from large axons similar to those of the squid, the diameter of the nerve would have to exceed 0.75 m (see Chapter 5).

An alternative strategy was the development of the myelin sheath, in which axons are coated with multiple layers of lipid membranes. These membranes are interrupted by gaps known as nodes of Ranvier (see Chapters 5 and 7 for details), in which the axolemma is rich in voltage-operated ion channels that generate the action potential. These lipid rich membranes insulate parts of the axons between the nodes, thus increasing axonal transverse resistance and reducing transverse capacitance. This allows saltatory propagation of action potentials, which substantially increases the conduction velocity in relatively small diameter axons (with maximal conduction velocity in vertebrates reaching 100–120 m/s). It has been generally accepted that myelination first occurred in vertebrates, which represented a fundamental evolutionary step that allowed development of compact nervous systems with many commissural axons, connecting neurones from different parts of the CNS and allowing rapid propagation through intra-CNS tracts and peripheral nerves (Zalc, 2006).

Myelin proper is, indeed, found only in relatively developed vertebrates. Compacted myelin sheaths are absent in lower vertebrates, such as hagfish and lampreys, and began to develop in sharks and bony fish. It has been suggested that myelination emerged for the first time in placoderms (extinct early jawed armoured fish that lived in the early Silurian period, $\approx$420 million years ago), which are phylogenetically placed at the base of Chondrichtian and bony fishes. This suggestion is based on the fossil record which compared the foramina for occulomotor nerves in jawless primitive Osteostraci fishes (that are believed to lack myelination) and Placoderms. The diameter of nerve foramina between these two fishes is the same (about 0.1 μm), whereas the length of nerve in Placoderms was 10 times larger, which logically incurred the need for myelin to preserve the same duration of action potential-mediated signal transduction (Zalc et al., 2008).

Further reasoning suggests the connection between appearance of the jaw in early Gnatostomata (the jawed vertebrates, which embrace all higher vertebrates living today, including mammals) and myelination. By acquiring myelinated nerves, these fishes arguably acquired better ability to hunt their prey, while keeping the axonal diameter the same or even smaller compared to their jawless predecessors (Zalc et al., 2008). This is all speculation, but what we know is that Agnathans do not have myelin, whereas even the most primitive Elasmobranchii and Holocephalans (i.e. sharks, ratfishes and chimera fish) have well developed myelin sheaths with nodes of Ranvier, this general structure persisting in all higher vertebrates.

The ensheathing of axons (which does not really involve compacted myelin) had, however, appeared much earlier in evolution (see reviews of Bullock, 2004; Hartline & Colman, 2007; Roots, 2008). Several invertebrate species (most notably some Annelids and Crustaceans) have well defined periaxonal coverage, and these covered axons conduct action potentials with high velocity. For example, in the earthworm *Lumbricus terrestrils*, the central axons of 50–100 μm in diameter are ensheathed with more than 60–200 layers of cell membranes produced by many cells, nuclei of which are scattered along the axon. These are glial cells which send processes to wrap the axon. The whole structure does not have clearly identifiable nodes, yet the conductance velocity of 20–45 m/s is greater than that in the much thicker giant axons of the *Loligo* squid. Similar axonal coverage has been found in another group of marine Annelids, Phoronids, in which axons are wrapped with many (9–20) layers of membranes. In the aquatic sludge worm, *Branchiura sowerbyi*, the axon is enwrapped by about 50 membrane layers.

The most striking example of invertebrate axonal ensheathment is found in Crustaceans – in particular, in prawns, shrimps and crabs. In the prawns of the genus *Penaeus* (e.g. Japanese tiger shrimp or Chinese white shrimp), the axonal-glial structure is quite peculiar. First, the diameter of the axon is much smaller compared to the overall fibre diameter. The axon is surrounded by glial membranes and by a large, so-called, submyelinic space, lying between the axonal membrane and the first layer of glial membranes (Figure 3.6). During excitation, the ion currents are trapped in this space as if the normal axon is surrounded by a giant axon (the submyelinic space acts, in essence, as a low-resistance pathway), which gives an unprecedented functional result as the prawn's fibres (120 μm in diameter) conduct action potentials with the speed of up to 210 m/s (Kusano, 1966; Xu & Terakawa, 1993, 1999). The submyelinic spaces are tightly sealed at nodes, known as '*fenestration nodes*', thus allowing for saltatory conduction. The nodal diameter and internodal distance are proportional to the axon diameter, and in prawns vary between 5–50 μm and 3–12 μm, respectively. The thickness of the glial membranous sheath is ≈10 μm, and it is comprised of 10–60 layers, with 8–9 nm distance between them. Similar to vertebrates, voltage-operated sodium channels in prawns are concentrated at the nodes, where their density can reach in the order of thousands of channels/μm$^2$.

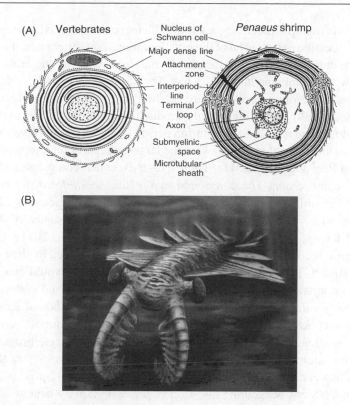

**Figure 3.6** Myelin-like sheath in shrimps.

A. Structure of the myelin sheath in vertebrates and myelin-like sheath in *Penaeus* shrimp. The myelin sheath of vertebrates is tightly wrapped around the axon and forms a continuous spiral of membrane, with the nucleus of the Schwann cell on the outer edge of the sheath. The myelin-like sheath of the shrimp is separated from the axon by the submyelinic space, which acts as an outer axon; the nuclei of the Schwann cells are located within the sheath.

B. The predecessor of modern shrimps was the metre-long swimming invertebrate *Anomalocaris*, the top predator in the Cambrian ocean more than 500 million years ago. These giant shrimps had exceptionally complex external eyes, composed of many tens of thousands of lenses. Arguably, these predators require fast propagating and compact axons, which could indicate that they were the first to develop myelin-like sheath.

(A) Reproduced, with permission, from Xu, K. and Terakawa, S. Fenestration nodes and the wide submyelinic space form the basis for the unusually fast impulse conduction of shrimp myelinated axons. J Exp Biol, 202 (Pt 15), 1979–1989 (1999) © the Company of Biologists. The Journal of Experimental Biology: jeb.biologists.org, (B) Reproduced with permission from Nature (cover picture for v. 480). (Full colour version in plate section.)

There is a fundamental difference between vertebrates and prawn axonal coverage. In vertebrates, the single Schwann cell or process of oligodendrocyte spirals around the axon, forming multiple membranous lamellae; in prawns, a single myelinating glial cell sends multiple processes, each of which encircles the axon once. Another difference is location of the nuclei of the myelinating cell. In vertebrates, this is always located at the outer edge of myelin sheath, whereas in prawns, the nuclei are randomly located between membrane laminae (Xu & Terakawa, 1999).

What was the evolutionary pressure leading to the appearance in prawns of axonal systems with exceedingly high conduction velocities? This may have an ancient phylogenetic root. In the Cambrian period (500–540 millions years ago), the giant prawns, the *Anomalocaridids*, were the largest and most ferocious predators of the sea (Van Roy & Briggs, 2011). Their length exceeded one metre and they had particularly acute vision. The compound eye of the *Anomalocaridid* was exceptionally big (according to fossil measurements, the visual surface was 22 mm long and 12 mm wide) and it was composed of tens of thousands of hexagonal ommatidial lenses, ≈70–110 μm in diameter (Paterson *et al.*, 2011). Obviously, the rapid nervous conductance and the reduction in size provided by the appearance of a glial sheath, in conjunction with submyelinic space, would have been of paramount importance for the evolution of such a complex visual system, with the need to rapidly collect information from these tens of thousands of lenses and to support the successful predatory behaviour of such a large animal.

Notably, mammals also retain a population of oligodendrocyte progenitor cells (OPCs) in the adult, that are capable of regenerating oligodendrocytes throughout life (see Chapters 5 and 6). The abundance of these NG2-glia in the adult mammalian CNS has begged the question of the evolutionary benefit of retaining such a substantive surplus of cells. The brain of adult non-mammalian vertebrates exhibits a high proliferative and neurogenic activity, which is the function of radial glia in the telencephalic ventricular zones. In adult mammals, parenchymal NG2-glia are the main proliferating cells. Although there is evidence for NG2-glia or adult OPCs in fish and frogs, they do not appear to respond to insults by increased proliferation. It is possible that the remyelinating capacity of NG2-glia (adult OPCs) is a mammalian evolutionary development and reflects the greater complexity and cellular specialization in the mammalian brain.

In conclusion, myelination emerged early in evolution. Most likely, it developed from the neuroglia that contacted axons with purely structural and metabolic purposes. Once it had occurred, myelination gave obvious evolutionary advantages, the most important being an increase in compactness of the nervous system and reduction in energy expenditure for restoring ion balances. Parallel evolution is evident, and different phyla developed their own arrangements. The most peculiar of these are the prawn nerve fibres which, at the same time, are characterised by the fastest conduction velocities.

### 3.3.3 Evolution of microglia

The evolutionary origins of microglia remain largely unexplored. However, it is conceivable to assume that they appear in response to formation of the ancient nervous system barriers following the emergence of compact neuronal masses. The appearance of these body/nervous system barriers obviously restricted immune/defence cells from entering the neural masses, thus leaving nervous tissue unprotected against possible insults. The evolutionary response was achieved by migration of immune cells into neuronal ganglia, where they changed their phenotype and become innate immune/defence cells of the nervous tissue. The evidence for phylogenetically early microglial cells is available for Annelids (leech), Molluscs (bivalva and snails) and some Arthropods (insects) (see Kettenmann *et al.*, 2011 for detailed review).

The leech nervous system has a surprisingly high density of microglial cells. In other cases, microglia are small with a spindle-like shape. Following injury, leech microglia migrate to the site of lesion, change their morphology and acquire phagocytic properties. Activated microglia in the leech can be stained by weak silver carbonate, a classical probe for vertebrate microglia. The leech microglial cells are also implicated in production of antimicrobial peptides in response to infectious attack (Schikorski *et al.*, 2008).

Microglial cells are present in the ganglia of Molluscs. For example, microglia in the mussel *Mytilus edulis*, a marine bivalve, can migrate in response to various signals, including NO, opioid peptides, cannabinoids and cytokines. Similarly, migrating microglia have been found in the snail *Planorbarius corneus* and in the insect *Leucophaea maderae*. In another snail, *Planorbis corneus*, the microglial cells (morphologically distinguished by phagocytic inclusions) are concentrated in the ganglia neuropil and subcapsular cortex, and the number of these phagocytic cells increases substantially after mechanical lesion (Pentreath *et al.*, 1985).

## 3.4   Numbers: how many glial cells are in the brain?

How many glial cells are there in the nervous system and, in particular, how many glial cells are in the human brain? Numerous papers and monographs (including the first edition of our book *Glial Neurobiology*) stated that, in the human brain, glial cells outnumber neurones by a factor of ten. However, this statement seems to be incorrect. In principle, we still do not know the exact number of neural cells in the human brain, but the experimental data obtained from stereological and nuclear counts indicate that, overall, the numbers of neurones and non-neuronal cells in the human brain is roughly equal.

In general, there is an assumption that the evolution of the nervous system resulted in an increase in the number of glia. Indeed in *C. elegans*, ≈50 neuroglia coexist with ≈300 neurones; in the leech, each ganglia contains ≈400 neurones and only 10–12 neuroglial cells; in *Drosophila*, only about 9000 neuroglia populate the CNS, containing ten times more neurones. There are exceptions, however; for example, the buccal ganglia of the great ramshorn snail *Planorbis corneus* contains 298 neurones and 391 glial cells, giving the glia to neurone ratio ≈1.5 (Pentreath *et al.*, 1985), with glial cells occupying about 43 per cent of the ganglia volume and neurones about 33 per cent.

In vertebrates, it is generally agreed that glia to neurone ratios in the cortex increase with an increase of the size of the brain. According to different estimates, the glia to neurone ratio in the cortex is about 0.3–0.4 in rodents, ≈1.1 in the cat; ≈1.2 in the horse, 0.5–1.0 in the Rhesus monkey, somewhere between 1.5–1.7 in humans, and as high as 4–6 in elephants and in the fin whale *Balaenoptera physalus* (Figure 3.5; for details see Christensen *et al.*, 2007; Dombrowski *et al.*, 2001; Friede, 1954; Hawkins & Olszewski, 1957; Lidow & Song, 2001; Oberheim *et al.*, 2006; Reichenbach, 1989; Tower, 1954).

Rather surprising counts have been obtained for cortices of Göttingen miniature pigs, which (in adulthood) contain 324 million neurones and 714 million neuroglia, with a glia to neurone ratio of 2.2 (Jelsing *et al.*, 2006). The largest number of glia have been found in the neocortex of the common Minke whale (*Balaenoptera acutorostrata*), which contains ~ 12.8 billion neurones and 98 billion glia, giving therefore a glia to neurone ratio of ~ 7.6 (Eriksen & Pakkenberg, 2007).

The total cellular count of the cells in the human brain, however, remains quite enigmatic, because of many methodological difficulties. Stereological counts of neurones in the human cortex, for example, have yielded rather different results, with overall numbers of neurones varying between 7–10 and 28–39 billion (Lent *et al.*, 2012; Pakkenberg, 1966). The number of cells in the cerebellum has been estimated to be the largest in the brain, with counts ranging between 70–109 billion (Andersen *et al.*, 1992; Lange, 1975).

A direct approach to this problem was taken in recent years by Brazilian neuroanatomists, who used the so-called 'isotropic fractionation' for counting the total number of neuronal and non-neuronal cells in mammalian brains (Azevedo *et al.*, 2009; Herculano-Houzel & Lent, 2005). In this technique, the brains are homogenized and the total number of nuclei is counted; subsequently, the neuronal nuclei are stained with antibodies against neurone-specific neuronal Nuclei protein (NeuN) and counted. The remaining non-stained nuclei apparently reflect the total number of non-neuronal cells (which naturally include glia as well as other non-neuronal cells, such as vascular cells).

Using this technique, the total number of cells in the rat brain was estimated at 330 million, of which 200 million are neurones, thus giving a non-neuronal (glial) cells to neurone ratio of ≈0.65. When the same technique was applied to the human brain, the total number of neurones and non-neuronal cells appeared to be almost equal: there were on average 86 billion neurones and about 84 billion non-neuronal cells in the brains of adult (50–70 years old) human males (Figure 3.7; Azevedo *et al.*, 2009).

Of course, the total numbers do not reflect the diversity of the nervous system, different regions of which have a very different cytoarchitecture. The nuclear counts confirmed this diversity by showing very different numbers for the glia to neurone ratio for different parts of the brain. The lowest ratio (≈0.22) was found for the

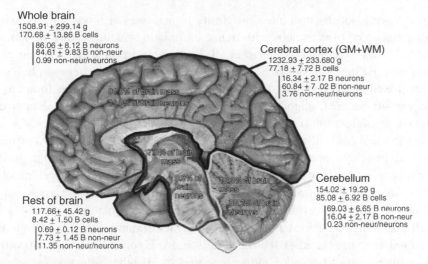

**Figure 3.7**   Cell numbers (neurones vs. non-neuronal cells) in different regions of the human brain. Values represent mean ± standard deviation. Cell numbers were determined by isotopic fractionation, which determines total number of nuclei, and counts of NeuN positive nuclei give the number of neurones.
Reproduced, with permission, from Azevedo, F. A. C. et al. (2009) Equal numbers of neuronal and nonneuronal cells make the human brain an isometrically scaled-up primate brain. Journal of Comparative Neurology pp.532-541 © John Wiley & Sons Ltd.

cerebellum, with 70 billion neuronal nuclei and only 16 billion non-neuronal ones. In the cerebral cortex (i.e. in both grey and white matters), the ratio was ≈3.76, with 60 billion non-neuronal cells and 16 billion neurones, whereas in basal ganglia the non-neuronal cells to neurones ratio was ≈11.3 with 0.69 billion neurones and 7.73 billion non-neuronal cells (Azevedo *et al.*, 2009; Lent *et al.*, 2012).

This 'isotropic fractionation' technique can not be considered flawless, of course. We do not know how many nuclei are lost in the process, how accurate is the staining, or how good is the spatial resolution. The numbers also have to be treated with caution; they were obtained from analysing only four different brains, from relatively old humans. Finally, this technique does not discriminate between subtypes of non-neuronal cells, and neither does it provide information about numbers of astrocytes, oligodendrocytes, NG2-glia and microglia.

Stereological counts from 31 human post-mortem tissues provided the following numbers of neurones and glia for neocortex (Pelvig *et al.*, 2008). The total number of neurones was 21.4 billion in females and 26.3 billion in males; the total number of glial cells was 27.9 billion in females and 38.9 billion in males. This gives an overall glia to neurone ratio of ≈1.3. In this work, the authors also tried to calculate the relative numbers of glial cell types, and they found that astrocytes accounted for ≈20 per cent, oligodendrocytes for 75 per cent and microglia for 5 per cent of the total glial cell population. The identifying criteria, however, were rather doubtful, since no specific staining was employed. For example, oligodendrocytes were defined as cells localised in close proximity to neurones or blood vessels, with a small rounded or oval nucleus with dense chromatin structure and a perinuclear halo; NG2-glia were not considered at all. In the absence of specific staining, the counts for glial subtypes should be taken with caution. In the earlier morphological studies, based on 2D counting, the distribution of glial cell types was found to be: astrocytes 40 per cent, oligodendrocytes 50 per cent and microglia 5–10 per cent (Blinkow & Glezer, 1968).

Detailed analysis of the glia to neurone ratio was performed on several primates from very primitive monkeys, such as tamarins and Saki monkey, through gorillas and chimpanzees, to humans (Sherwood *et al.*, 2006). In this study, the cell numbers were counted in special areas of cortex associated with complex tasks such as memory (area 9L in prefrontal cortex), speech-related Broka area (area 44) and anterior paracingulate cortex associated with theory of mind (area 32), as well as in primary motor cortex (area 4). It turned out (see also Figure 3.6) that human cortices have a higher glia to neurone ratio compared to all other primates, which was paralleled by a very substantial increase in human brain size (the heaviest primate brain, i.e. gorilla, weighs on average 509 gm, whereas the average human brain weighs $\approx$1,373 g).

An increase in glia to neurone ratio in mammalian evolution most likely reflects an increase in neuronal energy expenditure and, hence, a need for more support provided by glia. Indeed, it has been calculated that human neurones need about 3.3 times more energy to fire a single spike and 2.6 times more energy to maintain the resting membrane potential, when compared to rodents (Lennie, 2003). Another pressure is certainly provided by an increased activity of synaptic transmission and, hence, higher demand for homeostatic clearance/maintenance of balance of neurotransmitters and ions.

## 3.5   Embryogenesis and development of neuroglia in mammals

### 3.5.1   Macroglial cells

All neural cells (i.e. neurones and macroglia) derive from the neuroepithelium, which forms the neural tube. These cells are pluripotent, in a sense that their progeny may differentiate into neurones or macroglial cells with equal probability, and therefore these *neuroepithelial cells* may be defined as true '*neural progenitors*'. These neural progenitors give rise to neuronal or glial precursors cells ('neuroblasts' and 'glioblasts', respectively), which in turn differentiate into neurones or macroglial cells. For many years, it was believed that the neuroblasts and glioblasts appear very early in development, and that they form two distinct and non-interchangeable pools, committed, respectively, to producing strictly neuronal or glial lineages. It was also taken more or less for granted that the pool of precursor cells is fully depleted around birth, and that neurogenesis is totally absent in the mature brain.

In recent decades, however, this paradigm has been challenged as it appears that neuronal and glial lineages are much more closely related than was previously thought, and that the mature brain still has numerous stem cells which may provide for neuronal replacement. Moreover, it turns out that neural stem cells have many properties of astroglia. All these matters will be discussed in more detail in Chapter 4.

The modern scheme of neural cell development is as follows. At the origin of all neural cell lineages lie neural progenitors in the form of neuroepithelial cells. Morphologically, neural progenitors appear as elongated cells extending between the two surfaces (ventricular and pial) of the neuronal tube. Very early in development, the neural progenitors give rise to *radial glial cells*, which are the first cells that can be distinguished from neuroepithelial cells. The somata of radial glial cells are located in the ventricular zone and their processes extend to the pia. These radial glial cells are the central element in subsequent neurogenesis, because they act as the main neural progenitors during development, giving rise to neurones, astrocytes and some oligodendrocytes. The majority of oligodendrocytes, however, originate from glial precursors that are generated in specific sites in the brain and spinal cord (see below).

Astrocytes are generated both from radial glia and, later, in development from specific glial precursors that also give rise to oligodendrocytes; the proportion of the final population of astrocytes derived from radial glia and glial precursors depends on the region of the CNS. Radial glia not only produce neurones, they also form a scaffold along which newborn neurones migrate from the ventricular zone to their final destinations (see Chapter 4). Moreover, descendants of radial glia persist in specific neurogenic regions of the adult brain and retain the function of stem cells.

Oligodendrocytes develop from committed glial precursors through several intermediate stages (Goldman, 2007), which have been thoroughly characterized in culture systems, by using several specific antibodies (see Chapter 5). The developmental origins of astrocytes is less clear than that of neurones and oligodendrocytes. Some astrocytes appear to arise from astrocyte progenitors that migrate to their different sites in the brain, while others are derived from radial glia. In the perinatal cortex astrocytes retain proliferative capabilities and most new astroglial cells arise from symmetric division of differentiated astrocytes (Ge *et al.*, 2012). Some astrocytes derive embryonically from glial precursors with the phenotype of oligodendrocyte progenitor cells (OPCs), which fate-mapping studies show generate protopalsmic astrocytes as well as oligodendrocytes in the forebrain. In the forebrain, glial precursors from the subventricular zone migrate into both white matter and cortex, to become astrocytes, oligodendrocytes and NG2-glia (as well as some interneurones).

In the cerebellum, some Bergmann glia and other astrocytes arise from radial glia (and some share a common lineage with Purkinje neurones) and, later in development, glial progenitors migrate from an area dorsal to the IV$^{th}$ ventricle to give rise to all types of cerebellar astrocytes, myelinating oligodendrocytes and NG2-glia (as well as interneurones). In the embryonic retina, common precursors give rise to both neurones and Müller glia. Glial precursors that migrate into the retina via the optic nerve give rise to astrocytes, but oligodendrocytes and NG2-glia are absent from the retina of most mammals. Astrocytes and oligodendrocytes in the spinal cord appear to arise from different precursors in separate areas of the ventricular zone. The ventral neuroepithelium of the embryonic cord is divided into a number of domains, which contain precursors that first generate neurones (motor neurones and inter-neurones) and then oligodendrocytes. Astrocytes most likely arise from radial glia.

### 3.5.2   Astroglial cells are brain stem cells

Neurogenesis in the mammalian brain occurs throughout the life span in specific neurogenic regions. New neurones that continuously appear in the adult brain are added to neural circuits, and these may even be responsible for the considerable plasticity of the latter. The appearance of new neurones does not happen in all brain regions of mammals; it is mainly restricted to hippocampus and olfactory bulb (although, in many non-mammalian vertebrates, neurogenesis occurs in almost every brain region).

In both hippocampus (in its subgranular zone) and in the subventricular zone (the latter produces neurones for the olfactory bulb), the stem cells have been identified as astrocytes. It remains unclear whether astroglial cells in other brain regions may also retain these stem cell capabilities (See Chapter 4 for more detailed discussion).

### 3.5.3   Peripheral glia and Schwann cell lineage

Peripheral glia arise from neural crest cells (see Chapter 8). The Schwann cell lineage starts from *Schwann cell precursors*, which are the progeny of neural crest cells. Neural crest cells also give rise to peripheral sensory and autonomic neurones and their associated satellite glia, as well as the neurones and glia of the enteric nervous system. By around the time of birth, Schwann cell precursors have developed into *immature Schwann cells*, and the latter differentiate into myelinating or non-myeli-nating Schwann cells. An important juncture in the progression of the Schwann cell lineage occurs when some of the immature cells establish contacts with large-diameter axons and commence the process of myelination (see Chapter 8). Immature Schwann cells that happen to associate with small diameter axons remain non-myelinated. An important difference between non-myelinating and myelinating Schwann cells is that the former maintain contacts with several thin axons, whereas myelinating Schwann cells always envelop a single axon of large diameter.

Schwann cell precursors and immature Schwann cells are capable of frequent division, and proliferation stops only when cells arrive at their terminal differentiation stage. However, mature Schwann cells (both myelinating and non-myelinating) can swiftly de-differentiate and return into the proliferating stage, similar to immature cells. This de-differentiation process underlies the Wallerian degeneration that follows injury of peripheral nerves (see Chapter 9). After completion of nerve regeneration, Schwann cells once more re-differentiate.

### 3.5.4   Microglial cell lineage

Microglial cells derive from the myelomonocytic lineage, which in turn develops from hemangioblastic mesoderm (see Chapter 7). The progenitors of microglial cells, the primitive myeloid progenitors originating from the extraembryonic yolk sac enter the neural tube at early embryonic stages (e.g. at embryonic day 8 in rodents). These *foetal macrophages* are tiny rounded cells which, in the course of development, transform into embryonic microglia that have a small cell body and several short processes. The second wave of myeloid cell migration into the brain occurs in the early postnatal period, mainly in the corpus callosum where the dense groups of *amoeboid microglial cells* are defined as *fountains of microglia*. The amoeboid microglial cells proliferate very rapidly and migrate into the cortex, where they settle and turn into *ramified resting microglia*.

Microglia play an essential phagocytic role during development, removing the debris that arises from the large degree of neural apoptosis during development. Microglia can be 'killers' as well as 'cleaners' in the developing CNS. For example, in the embryonic retina, immature neurones express low affinity p75 receptors for nerve growth factor (NGF), which are down-regulated as neurones mature, but excess neurones do not lose their receptors and die by apoptosis in response to NGF released by microglia. Microglia are also responsible for immune tolerance to CNS antigens, by migrating into the embryonic CNS and providing a memory of 'self' before the blood-brain barrier is formed, after which the CNS becomes immune privileged and largely isolated from the systemic immune system. Amoeboid microglia in the developing CNS express many antigenic markers in common with systemic macrophages, but these are down-regulated as they differentiate into resting microglia. Any insult to the CNS results in the activation of microglia, which regain an amoeboid morphology, macrophage antigens and a phagocytic function.

Microglial cells retain their mitotic capabilities and they continue to divide (albeit at a very slow rate) in the adult.

Following insults to the adult CNS, macrophages may again enter the brain and are often indistinguishable from resident activated microglia. In these cases, most studies do not distinguish between microglia and macrophages (generally identified antigenically), and the terms are used interchangeably.

## 3.6   Concluding remarks

Glial cells appeared and evolved several times in phylogeny. The very first neuroglia were associated with sensory organs, where they assisted neuronal function. Increase in the complexity of the nervous system and its centralisation and cephalisation increased the demand for homeostatic support that was provided by more complex neuroglia. In invertebrates, glial cells diversified and assumed many homeostatic functions related to control of ion and neurotransmitter homeostasis, metabolic support, and regulation of neuronal development.

Glial cells also formed the ancestral blood-brain barrier, thereby isolating the nervous system from the rest of the body. This isolation stipulated the further development of glial cell defensive functions, which led to an appearance of the astrogliotic response and emergence of phagocytotic microglia. In parallel, increases in animal size and complexity of interneuronal connections stimulated the development of the myelin sheath, which first appeared in invertebrates in several primitive forms, then was further developed in vertebrates. The evolution of myelination formed the basis for increased complexity of the nervous system that relies on interneuronal connections.

In early ancestors of vertebrates, and in early Chordata, a new type of glia – the radial glia – appeared; this was connected with the appearance of a multilayered brain. In the early forms, the radial glia dominated. An increase in brain thickness triggered another wave of evolution of astroglia that developed into the main homeostatic cell of the brain. Increased brain size coincided with an increase in the total glia to neurone ratio to provide increased support to mammalian neurones. Finally, in the brains of primates, and especially in the brains of humans, the astrocytes become exceedingly complex, and new types of astroglial cells, involved in interlayer communication/integration, have evolved.

# References

Abbott NJ. (2005). Dynamics of CNS barriers: evolution, differentiation, and modulation. *Cellular and Molecular Neurobiology* **25**(1), 5–23.

Andersen BB, Korbo L, Pakkenberg B. (1992). A quantitative study of the human cerebellum with unbiased stereological techniques. *Journal of Comparative Neurology* **326**(4), 549–60.

Arendt D, Denes AS, Jekely G, Tessmar-Raible K. (2008). The evolution of nervous system centralization. *Philosophical Transactions of The Royal Society Of London. Series B: Biological Sciences* **363**(1496), 1523–8.

Ari C, Kalman M. (2008). Evolutionary changes of astroglia in Elasmobranchii comparing to amniotes: a study based on three immunohistochemical markers (GFAP, S-100, and glutamine synthetase). *Brain, Behavior and Evolution* **71**(4), 305–24.

Azevedo FA, Carvalho LR, Grinberg LT, Farfel JM, Ferretti RE, Leite RE, Jacob Filho W, Lent R, Herculano-Houzel S. (2009). Equal numbers of neuronal and nonneuronal cells make the human brain an isometrically scaled-up primate brain. *Journal of Comparative Neurology* **513**(5), 532–41.

Bacaj T, Tevlin M, Lu Y, Shaham S. (2008). Glia are essential for sensory organ function in C. elegans.*Science* **322**(5902), 744–7.

Baumgart EV, Barbosa JS, Bally-Cuif L, Gotz M, Ninkovic J. (2010). Stab wound injury of the zebrafish telencephalon: a model for comparative analysis of reactive gliosis. *Glia* **60**(3), 343–57.

Blinkow S, Glezer I. (1968). *The neuroglia.* In: *Blinkow SM, Gleser II, editors. The Human Brain in Figures and Tables; A quantitative handbook.* New York: Plenum Press. p 237–253.

Bullock TH. (2004). The natural history of neuroglia: an agenda for comparative studies. *Neuron Glia Biology* **1**(2), 97–100.

Bullock TH, Horridge GA. (1965). *Structure and function in the nervous systems of invertebrates*. San Francisco, London: W. H. Freeman.

Bushong EA, Martone ME, Jones YZ, Ellisman MH. (2002). Protoplasmic astrocytes in CA1 stratum radiatum occupy separate anatomical domains. *Journal of Neuroscience* **22**(1), 183–92.

Case RM, Eisner D, Gurney A, Jones O, Muallem S, Verkhratsky A. (2007). Evolution of calcium homeostasis: from birth of the first cell to an omnipresent signalling system. *Cell Calcium* **42**(4-5) 345–50.

Cavalier-Smith T. (1998). A revised six-kingdom system of life. *Biological Reviews of The Cambridge Philosophical Society* **73**(3), 203–66.

Cavalier-Smith T. (2009). Megaphylogeny, cell body plans, adaptive zones: causes and timing of eukaryote basal radiations. *Journal of Eukaryotic Microbiology* **56**(1), 26–33.

Christensen JR, Larsen KB, Lisanby SH, Scalia J, Arango V, Dwork AJ, Pakkenberg B. (2007). Neocortical and hippocampal neuron and glial cell numbers in the rhesus monkey. *Anatomical Record (Hoboken, NJ)* **290**(3), 330–40.

Colombo JA, Reisin HD. (2004). Interlaminar astroglia of the cerebral cortex: a marker of the primate brain. *Brain Research* **1006**(1), 126–31.

Colombo JA, Yanez A, Puissant V, Lipina S. (1995). Long, interlaminar astroglial cell processes in the cortex of adult monkeys. *Journal of Neuroscience Researchearch* **40**(4), 551–6.

Colombo JA, Sherwood CC, Hof PR. (2004). Interlaminar astroglial processes in the cerebral cortex of great apes. *Anatomy and Embryology* **208**(3), 215–8.

Colombo JA, Reisin HD, Miguel-Hidalgo JJ, Rajkowska G. (2006). Cerebral cortex astroglia and the brain of a genius: a propos of A. Einstein's. *Brain Research Reviews* **52**(2), 257–63.

Deitmer JW, Rose CR, Munsch T, Schmidt J, Nett W, Schneider HP, Lohr C. (1999). Leech giant glial cell: functional role in a simple nervous system. *Glia* **28**(3), 175–82.

Ding G, Yu Z, Zhao J, Wang Z, Li Y, Xing X, Wang C, Liu L. (2008). Tree of life based on genome context networks. *PLoS One* **3**(10), e3357.

Dombrowski SM, Hilgetag CC, Barbas H. (2001). Quantitative architecture distinguishes prefrontal cortical systems in the rhesus monkey. *Cerebral Cortex* **11**(10), 975–88.

Dunn CW, Hejnol A, Matus DQ, Pang K, Browne WE, Smith SA, Seaver E, Rouse GW, Obst M, Edgecombe G.D. et al. (2008). Broad phylogenomic sampling improves resolution of the animal tree of life. *Nature* **452**(7188), 745–9.

Edwards TN, Meinertzhagen IA. (2010). The functional organisation of glia in the adult brain of Drosophila and other insects. *Progress In Neurobiology* **90**(4), 471–97.

Eriksen N, Pakkenberg B. (2007). Total neocortical cell number in the mysticete brain. *Anatomical Record (Hoboken, NJ)* **290**(1), 83–95.

Friede R. (1954). Der quantitative Anteil der Glia an der Cortexentwicklung. *Acta Anatomica* **20** (3), 290–6.

Ge WP, Miyawaki A, Gage FH, Jan YN, Jan LY (2012). Local generation of glia is a major astrocyte source in postnatal cortex. *Nature* **484**, 376–80.

Ghysen A. (2003). The origin and evolution of the nervous system. *International Journal of Developmental Biology* **47**(7-8) 555–62.

Goldman JE. (2007). *Astrocyte lineage*. In: Lazzarini RA. (ed). *Myelin Biology and Disorders*, pp. 311–328. New York: Elsevier Academic Press.

Grupp L, Wolburg H, Mack AF. (2010). Astroglial structures in the zebrafish brain. *Journal of Comparative Neurology* **518**(21), 4277–87.

Hartenstein V. (2011). Morphological diversity and development of glia in Drosophila. *Glia* **59**(9), 1237–52.

Hartline DK. (2011). The evolutionary origins of glia. *Glia* **59**(9), 1215–36.

Hartline DK, Colman DR. (2007). Rapid conduction and the evolution of giant axons and myelinated fibers. *Current Biology* **17**(1), R29–35.

Hawkins A, Olszewski J. (1957). Glia/nerve cell index for cortex of the whale. *Science* **126**(3263), 76–7.

Heiman MG, Shaham S. (2007). Ancestral roles of glia suggested by the nervous system of Caenorhabditis elegans. *Neuron Glia Biology* **3**(1), 55–61.

Herculano-Houzel S, Lent R. (2005). Isotropic fractionator: a simple, rapid method for the quantification of total cell and neuron numbers in the brain. *Journal of Neuroscience* **25**(10), 2518–21.

Hodgkin AL. (1954). A note on conduction velocity. *Journal of Physiology* **125**(1), 221–4.

Holland ND. (2003). Early central nervous system evolution: an era of skin brains? *Nature Reviews Neuroscience* **4**(8), 617–27.

Holmgren E. (1901). Beiträge zur Morphologie der Zelle: I. Nervenzellen. *Anat Hefte* **18**, 267–326.

Jelsing J, Nielsen R, Olsen AK, Grand N, Hemmingsen R, Pakkenberg B. (2006). The postnatal development of neocortical neurons and glial cells in the Gottingen minipig and the domestic pig brain. *Journal of Experimental Biology* **209**(Pt 8) 1454–62.

Keeling PJ, Burger G, Durnford DG, Lang BF, Lee RW, Pearlman RE, Roger AJ, Gray MW. (2005). The tree of eukaryotes. *Trends In Ecology & Evolution* **20**(12), 670–6.

Kettenmann H, Hanisch UK, Noda M, Verkhratsky A. (2011). Physiology of microglia. *Physiological Reviews* **91**(2), 461–553.

Kuffler SW, Potter DD. (1964). Glia in the Leech Central Nervous System: Physiological Properties and Neuron-Glia Relationship. *Journal of Neurophysiology* **27**, 290–320.

Kusano K. (1966). Electrical activity and structural correlates of giant nerve fibers in Kuruma shrimp (*Penaeus japonicus*). *Journal of Cellular Physiology* **68**, 361–383.

Lange W. (1975). Cell number and cell density in the cerebellar cortex of man and some other mammals. *Cell and Tissue Research* **157**(1), 115–24.

Lennie P. (2003). The cost of cortical computation. *Current Biology* **13**(6), 493–7.

Lent R, Azevedo FA, Andrade-Moraes CH, Pinto AV. (2012). How many neurons do you have? Some dogmas of quantitative neuroscience under revision. *European Journal of Neuroscience* **35**(1), 1–9.

Lidow MS, Song ZM. (2001). Primates exposed to cocaine in utero display reduced density and number of cerebral cortical neurons. *Journal of Comparative Neurology* **435**(3), 263–75.

Lohr C, Deitmer JW. (2006). Calcium signaling in invertebrate glial cells. *Glia* **54**(7), 642–9.

Long DM, Bodenheimer TS, Hartmann JF, Klatzo I. (1968). Ultrastructural features of the shark brain. *American Journal of Anatomy* **122**(2), 209–36.

Mashanov VS, Zueva OR, Heinzeller T, Aschauer B, Naumann WW, Grondona JM, Cifuentes M, Garcia-Arraras JE. (2009). The central nervous system of sea cucumbers (Echinodermata: Holothuroidea) shows positive immunostaining for a chordate glial secretion. *Frontiers in Zoology* **6**, 11.

Oberheim NA, Wang X, Goldman S, Nedergaard M. (2006). Astrocytic complexity distinguishes the human brain. *Trends In Neurosciences* **29**(10), 547–53.

Oberheim NA, Takano T, Han X, He W, Lin JH, Wang F, Xu Q, Wyatt JD, Pilcher W, Ojemann JG and others. (2009). Uniquely hominid features of adult human astrocytes. *Journal of Neuroscience* **29**(10), 3276–87.

Oikonomou G, Shaham S. (2011). The glia of Caenorhabditis elegans. *Glia* **59**(9), 1253–63.

Orkand RK, Nicholls JG, Kuffler SW. (1966). Effect of nerve impulses on the membrane potential of glial cells in the central nervous system of amphibia. *Journal of Neurophysiology* **29**(4), 788–806.

Pakkenberg H. (1966). The number of nerve cells in the cerebral cortex of man. *Journal of Comparative Neurology* **128**(1), 17–20.

Parfrey LW, Barbero E, Lasser E, Dunthorn M, Bhattacharya D, Patterson DJ, Katz LA. (2006). Evaluating support for the current classification of eukaryotic diversity. *PLoS Genetics* **2**(12), e220.

Parker RJ, Auld VJ. (2006). Roles of glia in the Drosophila nervous system. *Seminars in Cell and Developmental Biology* **17**(1), 66–77.

Paterson JR, Garcia-Bellido DC, Lee MS, Brock GA, Jago JB, Edgecombe GD. (2011). Acute vision in the giant Cambrian predator Anomalocaris and the origin of compound eyes. *Nature* **480**(7376), 237–40.

Pelvig DP, Pakkenberg H, Stark AK, Pakkenberg B. (2008). Neocortical glial cell numbers in human brains. *Neurobiology of Aging* **29**(11), 1754–62.

Pentreath VW, Radojcic T, Seal LH, Winstanley EK. (1985). The glial cells and glia-neuron relations in the buccal ganglia of Planorbis corneus (L.): cytological, qualitative and quantitative changes during growth and ageing. *Philosophical Transactions of The Royal Society Of London. Series B: Biological Sciences* **307**(1133), 399–455.

Radojcic T, Pentreath VW. (1979). Invertebrate glia. *Progress In Neurobiology* **12**(2), 115–79.

Rehkamper G, Welsch U, Dilly PN. (1987). Fine structure of the ganglion of Cephalodiscus gracilis (Pterobranchia, Hemichordata). *Journal of Comparative Neurology* **259**(2), 308–15.

Reichenbach A. (1989). Glia, neuron index: review and hypothesis to account for different values in various mammals. *Glia* **2**(2), 71–7.

Reichenbach A, Pannicke T. (2008). Neuroscience. A new glance at glia. *Science* **322**(5902), 693–4.

Reichenbach A, Neumann M, Bruckner G. (1987). Cell length to diameter relation of rat fetal radial glia – does impaired K+ transport capacity of long thin cells cause their perinatal transformation into multipolar astrocytes? *Neuroscience Letters* **73**(1), 95–100.

Roots BI. (2008). The phylogeny of invertebrates and the evolution of myelin. *Neuron Glia Biology* **4**(2), 101–9.

Ryan TJ, Grant SG. (2009). The origin and evolution of synapses. *Nature Reviews Neuroscience* **10**(10), 701–12.

Schikorski D, Cuvillier-Hot V, Leippe M, Boidin-Wichlacz C, Slomianny C, Macagno E, Salzet M, Tasiemski A. (2008). Microbial challenge promotes the regenerative process of the injured central nervous system of the medicinal leech by inducing the synthesis of antimicrobial peptides in neurons and microglia. *Journal of Immunology* **181**(2), 1083–95.

Sherwood CC, Stimpson CD, Raghanti MA, Wildman DE, Uddin M, Grossman LI, Goodman M, Redmond JC, Bonar CJ, Erwin JM and others. (2006). Evolution of increased glia-neuron ratios in the human frontal cortex. *Proceedings of The National Academy Of Sciences Of The United States Of America* **103**(37), 13606–11.

Stollewerk A, Simpson P. (2005). Evolution of early development of the nervous system: a comparison between arthropods. *Bioessays* **27**(9), 874–83.

Stout RF, Jr., Parpura V. (2011). Voltage-gated calcium channel types in cultured *C. elegans* CEPsh glial cells. *Cell Calcium* **50**(1), 98–108.

Tower DB. (1954). Structural and functional organization of mammalian cerebral cortex; the correlation of neurone density with brain size; cortical neurone density in the fin whale (Balaenoptera physalus L.) with a note on the cortical neurone density in the Indian elephant. *Journal of Comparative Neurology* **101**(1), 19–51.

Van Roy P, Briggs DE. (2011). A giant Ordovician anomalocaridid. *Nature* **473**(7348), 510–3.

Wicht H, Derouiche A, Korf HW. (1994). An immunocytochemical investigation of glial morphology in the Pacific hagfish: radial and astrocyte-like glia have the same phylogenetic age. *Journal of Neurocytology* **23**(9), 565–76.

Xu K, Terakawa S. (1993). Saltatory conduction and a novel type of excitable fenestra in shrimp myelinated nerve fibers. *Japanese Journal of Physiology* **43**(Suppl 1), S285–93.

Xu K, Terakawa S. (1999). Fenestration nodes and the wide submyelinic space form the basis for the unusually fast impulse conduction of shrimp myelinated axons. *Journal of Experimental Biology* **202**(Pt 15) 1979–89.

Yoon HS, Grant J, Tekle YI, Wu M, Chaon BC, Cole JC, Logsdon JM, Jr., Patterson DJ, Bhattacharya D, Katz LA. (2008). Broadly sampled multigene trees of eukaryotes. *BMC Evolutionary Biology* **8**, 14.

Zalc B. (2006). *The acquisition of myelin: a success story*. In: Chadwick DJ, Goode J. (eds.). *Purinergic Signalling in Neuron-Glia Interactions*, pp. 15–25. *Chichester*: Wiley.

Zalc B, Goujet D, Colman D. (2008). The origin of the myelination program in vertebrates. *Current Biology* **18**(12), R511–2.

# 4
# Astroglia

*Glial Physiology and Pathophysiology*, First Edition. Alexei Verkhratsky and Arthur Butt.
© 2013 by John Wiley & Sons, Ltd. Published 2013 by John Wiley & Sons, Ltd.

# 4.1   Definition and heterogeneity

As has already been mentioned in Chapter 1, the term 'astrocyte' means 'star-like cell'. Astrocytes arguably are the most diverse glial cells in the CNS. The classic, most generally acknowledged definition of astrocyte is based on the morphology and on the expression of specific astroglial markers. Indeed, it is commonly believed that an archetypal feature of astrocytes is their expression of intermediate filaments, which form the cytoskeleton. The main types of astroglial intermediate filament proteins are *Glial Fibrillary Acidic Protein* (GFAP) and *vimentin*; expression of GFAP is commonly used as a specific marker for identification of astrocytes. The astrocyte is therefore generally defined as a cell with star-like appearance expressing GFAP.

In reality, most of the astrocytes do not have a star-like morphology and many astrocytes do not express GFAP (Kimelberg, 2004); indeed, the normal levels of GFAP expression vary quite considerably between brain regions. For example, GFAP is expressed by virtually every Bergmann glial cell in the cerebellum and by fibrous astrocytes in white matter, whereas only about 15–20 per cent of protoplasmic astrocytes express GFAP in the cortex of mature animals.

In general, the name 'astroglia' is an umbrella term that covers many types of glial cells (Figures 4.1–4.4 ). Some astrocytes do, indeed, have a star-like appearance, with several primary (also called stem) processes originating from the soma, although most of them have more complex morphology. Possibly the largest groups

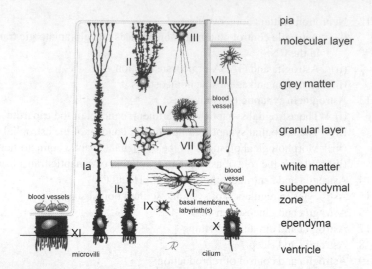

**Figure 4.1**   Morphological diversity and subtypes of astrocytes.
Ia - pial tanycyte
Ib - vascular tanycyte
II - radial astrocyte (Bergmann glial cell)
III - marginal astrocyte
IV - protoplasmic astrocyte
V - velate astrocyte
VI - fibrous astrocyte
VII - perivascular astrocyte
VIII - interlaminar astrocyte
IX - immature astrocyte
X - ependymocyte
XI - choroid plexus cell

From Rechenbach & Wolburg, 2005.

of astrocytes are represented by the *protoplasmic astrocytes* and *fibrous astrocytes* of the grey and white matter, respectively.

The second big group of astroglial cells is the *radial glia*. These are bipolar cells with an ovoid cell body and elongated processes. Radial glia usually produce two main processes, one of them forming endfeet on the ventricular wall and the other at the pial surface. They are a common feature of the developing brain, as they are the first cells to develop from neural progenitors. From very early embryonic stages, radial glia also form a scaffold which assists neuronal migration (see following sections for details). After maturation, radial glia disappear from many brain regions and transform into stellate astrocytes, although radial glia-like cells remain in the retina (*Müller glia*) and the cerebellum (*Bergmann glia*).

In addition to the two major groups of astroglial cells, there are smaller populations of specialised astroglia localised to specific regions of the CNS, namely the *velate astrocytes* of the cerebellum, the *interlaminar and polarised astrocytes* of the primate cortex, *tanycytes* (found in the periventricular organs, the hypophysis

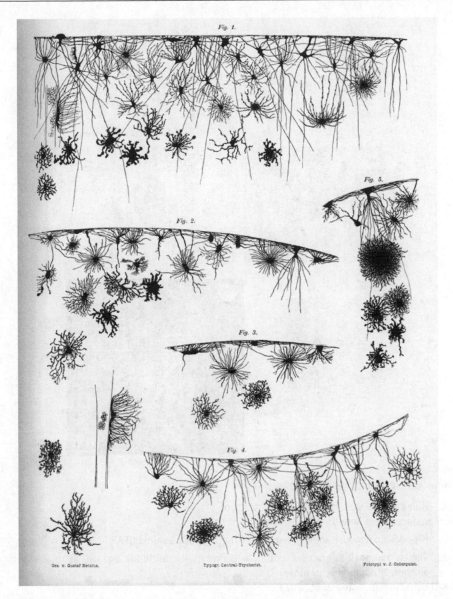

**Figure 4.2** Morphological diversity of human glial cells. Neuroglial cells from the human cortex.
(Fig. 1) Vertical slice of one of the gyrus of the frontal lobe obtained from 42-year-old women.
(Figs 2–5) Vertical slices of the parietal region obtained from a 70-year-old man.

In all parts, the upper surface of the cortex is oriented towards the top of the image. Superficial glial cells send their processes towards the surface of the slice, where they spread; glial cells located in the deeper layers are represented by many different types. All images are obtained from Golgi-stained preparations.

Reproduced from Retzius, 1894.

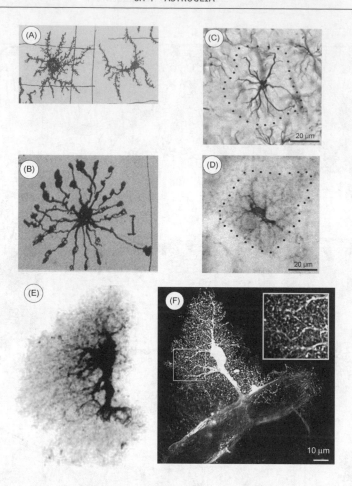

**Figure 4.3**   Visualisation of astrocytes.

A,B.   Human astrocytes stained by Golgi method
(A: reproduced from Retzius, 1894; B: drawing of Cajal).

   C.   Hippocampal mouse astrocyte stained with antibody against GFAP.

   D.   Similar mouse hippocampal astrocyte stained with antibody against astroglia-specific
        enzyme, glutamine synthetase
(C & D both from Olabarria *et al.*, 2011).

   E.   A single astrocyte labelled with enhanced green fluorescent protein (eGFP). The fine
        intricate processes of protoplasmic astrocytes are visualised by eGFP fluorescence. Insert
        shows the eGFP labelled astrocytic processes in higher magnification. The astrocytes were
        transfected *in situ* by an intracortical injection of adenoviral eGFP. The brains were
        processed for histology 2–4 days later
(reproduced, with permission, from Wilhelmsson *et al.*, 2006).

   F.   Image of hippocampal astrocyte injected with fluorescent dye Alexa Fluor 568; dye filling
        reveals a cloud of fine spongiform processes

Reproduced with permission from Nedergaard, M., Rodriguez, J. J. and Verkhratsky, A. (2010)
Glial calcium and diseases of the nervous system in Cell Calcium 47:2, pp. 140–150 © Elsevier.
(Full colour version in plate section.)

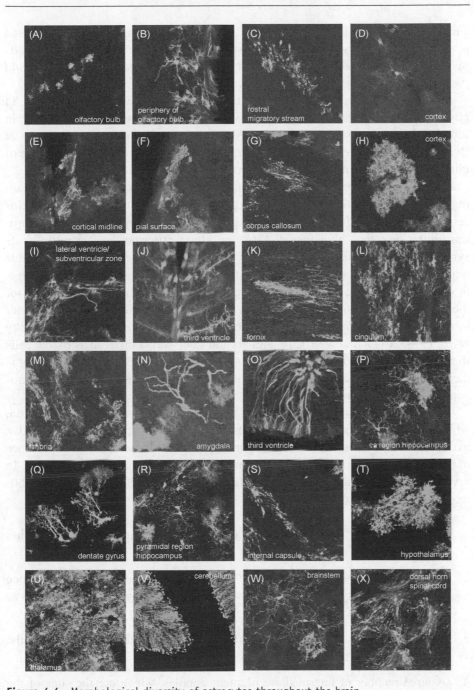

**Figure 4.4** Morphological diversity of astrocytes throughout the brain.

Collection of images (reconstructions from confocal images stacks) taken from different regions of the brain and the spinal cord of the adult transgenic mouse expressing enhanced green fluorescence protein under control of glia-specific promoter.

Reproduced with permission from authors (Emsley and Macklis, 2006; open access paper). (Full colour version in plate section.)

and the raphe part of the spinal cord), *pituicytes* in the neuro-hypophysis, and *perivascular* and *marginal* astrocytes. Astroglia also include several types of cells that line the ventricles or the subretinal space, namely *ependymocytes*, *choroid plexus cells* and *retinal pigment epithelial cells*.

All these diverse cell types differ in their morphology and gene expression, in physiological properties, sensitivity to various neurotransmitters and finally in functional features (see, for example, Matyash & Kettenmann, 2010; Wang & Bordey, 2008; Zhang & Barres, 2010 for recent reviews and references; the issue of glial heterogeneity will be referred to frequently throughout this book).

Studies over recent decades have found that astrocytes from different brain regions differ substantially in expression of genes for the most fundamental proteins responsible for glial function, including genes encoding ion channels and neuro-transmitter receptors, glutamate, GABA and glycine transporters, for nitric oxide synthase and for enzymes catabolising dopamine and serotonin (monoamine oxidase) and GABA (GABA transaminase). Physiological experiments *in vitro*, *in situ* and *in vivo* have revealed similar regional differences throughout the brain for the functional expression of ion channels and neurotransmitter receptors, the latter most likely being regulated by the local neurotransmitter environment (Verkhratsky *et al.*, 1998, 2011). Likewise, $Ca^{2+}$ signals and $Ca^{2+}$ waves differ in astroglial cells in different brain regions (Nimmerjahn *et al.*, 2009). Similarly region dependent is the ability of astrocytes to uptake glutamate and GABA, to secrete various neuro-peptides, to affect neuronal growth, etc.

Identification of astrocytes, therefore, requires a rather complex set of criteria, which is difficult not only because of the huge astroglial heterogeneity, but also due to developmental changes in astroglial phenotype and because of the wide presence of NG2-glia, which in some past studies were considered a subtype of astrocyte. In several systematic studies, Harald Kimelberg (Kimelberg, 2009, 2010) has elabo-rated eight criteria for identifying astrocytes, as follows:

1. Absence of electrical excitability (i.e. astrocytes cannot generate action potential).

2. A very negative membrane potential ($-80$ to $-90$ mV) because of a prevalence of $K^+$ permeability of the plasmalemma; the membrane of astrocyte behaves as an almost ideal $K^+$ electrode.

3. Functional expression of transporters for GABA and glutamate that permits the astroglial role in neurotransmitter homeostasis.

4. A large number of intermediate filament bundles, which are the sites of the astrocyte specific protein GFAP.

5. Glycogen granules.

6. Processes from each cell contacting and surrounding blood vessels.

7.   Elaborated perisynaptic processes.

8.   Linkage to other astrocytes by gap junctions formed by connexin 43 and/or 30.

Despite the fact that many astroglial cells indeed conform to these criteria, there are equally numerous exceptions. For example, there are many GFAP-positive cells which do not form gap junctions with neighbouring astrocytes and, *vice versa,* there are cells with a typical astroglial electrophysiological signature and extensive gap junction coupling, but with no immunoreactivity to GFAP (Wang & Bordey, 2008). Furthermore, according to these above criteria there is a substantial trimming of cell types covered by the definition of astroglia to two major cell types (Kimelberg, 2010), star-shape astroglia (protoplasmic and fibrous astrocytes) and elongated astroglia (retinal Müller glia and cerebellar Bergmann glia).

This classification, although being straightforward and conceptually simple, omits too many classes of cells that share functional properties considered fundamental and defining for astrocytes. This fundamental property of astrocytes is the maintenance of CNS homeostasis. In this respect, we propose that the family of astrocytes can be functionally defined as '*the true homeostatic cells of the CNS that provide for molecular, cellular and organ homeostasis*'.

## 4.2   Morphology of the main types of astroglia

(i) *Protoplasmic astrocytes* are present in grey matter of the brain and in the spinal cord. In rodents, they are endowed with several (5–10) primary processes (on average ≈50 μm long), which in turn extend extremely elaborate branches to form complex process arborisations. Protoplasmic astrocyte density in the cortex varies between 10,000 and 30,000 per mm$^3$.

The classical staining techniques, such as Golgi impregnation or gold chloride-sublimate staining method of Cajal, as well as immunohistochemical staining with GFAP antibodies (see Figures 4.3–4.4) have provided oversimplified images of protoplasmic astrocytes. These techniques mostly revealed the main astroglial processes, which contributed to our image of astroglia as star-like cells. The introduction of staining techniques that utilised either filling astrocytes with fluorescent dyes, staining with rhodamin 101 (which preferably accumulates in the astrocyte cytosol), or using targeted expression of cytoplasmic fluorescent proteins (see below for further details), have revolutionised morphological studies of astroglia. Indeed, protoplasmic astrocytes have an incredibly complex process arborisation that cannot be seen by GFAP immunolabelling (Figure 4.3 E,F; Figure 4.4). The bulk of this arborisation is made of short, 'feather-like', ultra-fine and extensively ramified processes, 2–10 μm long, extending from principal processes to endow protoplasmic astrocytes with a spongiform appearance (Figure 4.3). These fine processes also exhibit rapid structural plasticity, especially at the sites contacting to synapses, where astrocytes extend lamellipodia-like membrane protrusions along neuronal surfaces, or filiopodia-like extensions, which protrude and retract within tens of seconds (Hirrlinger *et al.*, 2004).

The arborisation of protoplasmic astrocytes delineates discrete territorial domains, and there is little overlap (<10 per cent) between neighbouring cells. On average protoplasmic astrocyte in rodent hippocampus of rats occupies the volume of ≈43,000–66,000 $\mu m^3$ (Bushong *et al.*, 2002; Wilhelmsson *et al.*, 2006). The process surface area of protoplasmic astrocytes may reach up to 80,000 $\mu m^2$ and cover most of neuronal membranes within their domain. Some processes of protoplasmic astrocytes contact blood vessels, forming so-called *perivascular endfeet*, and some protoplasmic astrocytes also send processes to the pial surface, where they form *subpial endfeet*, which contribute to *glia limitans*.

The density of protoplasmic astrocytes is different in various brain regions. A single protoplasmic astrocyte in rodent cortex contacts 4–8 neurones, surrounds ≈300–600 neuronal dendrites and provides cover for up to 20,000–120,000 synapses residing within its domain (Bushong *et al.*, 2002; Halassa *et al.*, 2007b). As has been already discussed in Chapter 3, human protoplasmic astrocytes are 2–3 times larger and exceedingly more complex; the processes of a single human protoplasmic astrocyte cover approximately 2 million synapses.

The morphology of protoplasmic astrocytes across the brain is highly heterogeneous (Figure 4.4). Even within the same CA1 hippocampal area, protoplasmic astrocytes have different shapes, with sub-populations of fusiform cells, spherical or markedly elongated astrocytes (Bushong *et al.*, 2002). Protoplasmic astrocytes in the entorhinal cortex are elongated cells with several main processes, whereas astrocytes in other brain regions have distinctly different morphology (Figure 4.5). These differences are clearly revealed by both immunocytochemistry with GFAP (which visualises cytoskeleton) and with genetically targeted green fluorescent protein (that is distributed within the cytosol and therefore also shows fine processes)

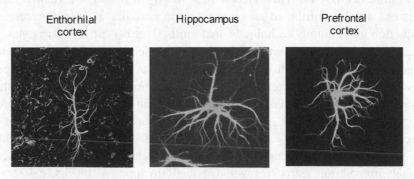

| Enthorhilal cortex | Hippocampus | Prefrontal cortex |

**Figure 4.5**  GFAP immunostaining of protoplasmic astrocytes in enthorhinal cortex, hippocampus and prefrontal cortex, showing their distinct morphology. (Rodriguez and Verkhratsky, own observations; Full colour version in plate section.)

(ii) *Fibrous astrocytes* are present in white matter tracts in the brain and in the spinal cord, in the optic nerve and in the nerve fibre layer of the retina. Their processes are long (up to 300 μm), though much less elaborate compared to protoplasmic astroglia. The somata of fibrous astrocytes are organised in rows between the axonal bundles. The processes of fibrous astrocytes establish several perivascular or subpial endfeet and send numerous extensions (*perinodal processes*) that contact axons at nodes of Ranvier, the sites of action potential propagation in myelinated axons.

The density of fibrous astrocytes in the white matter is ≈200 cells per mm$^3$. In contrast to protoplasmic astrocytes, the fibrous astrocytes do not form separate territorial domains and show a high degree of overlap. They also show diverse morphology; for example, in the rodent optic nerve, fibrous astrocytes arc subdivided into transverse, random, and longitudinal, depending on the orientation of processes with respect to the long axis of the nerve (Butt *et al.*, 1994).

(iii) In the posterior prefrontal cortex and amygdaloid cortex, a specific subpopulation of astrocytes associated with the cortical surface has been defined as *surface-associated astrocytes*. The somata of these cells lie at the cortical surface and send two types of processes - the descending processes to the layer I, and superficial processes that extend to surround pial vessels (Feig & Haberly, 2011).

(iv) *Velate astrocytes* are a subtype of protoplasmic astrocyte, which occur in brain regions densely packed with relatively small neurones (Chan-Palay & Palay, 1972). These cells are much smaller compared to astrocytes in the cortex and hippocampus, although they have very high surface to volume ratio In the cerebellum, velate astrocytes form membranous sheaths that enwrap several granule neurones (hence their name: 'velate' means being enwrapped with vellum). A similar type of velate astrocyte is also present in the olfactory bulb.

(v) *Interlaminar astrocytes* are found specifically in the cerebral cortex of higher primates (Colombo & Reisin, 2004; Oberheim *et al.*, 2009, 2012). Their characteristic peculiarity is that they extend one or two very long (up to 1 mm) unbranched processes from the soma located within the supragranular layer to cortical layers III to V (Figure 4.6). The interlaminar astrocytes also extend several shorter processes. The long 'interlaminar' processes terminate with specific bouton-like structures, also known as terminal masses, which usually contain single mitochondria. As a matter of anecdotal evidence, it has been shown that Albert Einstein's brain had unusually large terminal masses (up to 15 μm in diameter), which, however are likely to indicate some neurodegenerative changes (Colombo *et al.*, 2006).

The processes of interlaminar astrocytes run parallel to each other, forming the 'palisade'. Interlaminar astrocytes exist exclusively in higher primates, being mostly present in old world monkeys, apes and humans. The phylogenetic origin of this type of astrocyte is obscure, although there are some indications that they could have appeared about 30 million years ago in prosimians (at least they have been found in brown lemur, *Eulemur fulvus* (Colombo *et al.*, 2000). The interlaminar astrocytes appear postnatally and are thought to originate from some

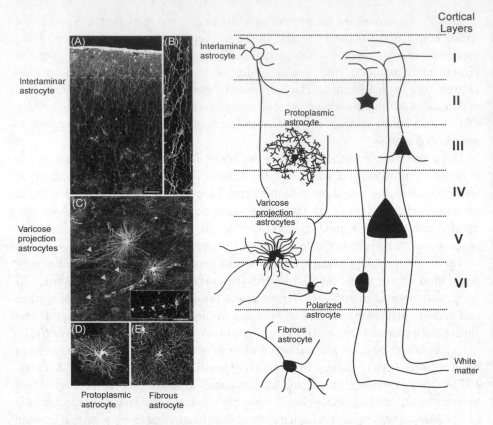

**Figure 4.6**  Morphological heterogeneity and subtypes of astrocytes in primate cortex.

A.  Pial surface and layers 1–2 of human cortex. GFAP staining in white; DAPI, in blue. Scale bar, 100 μm. Yellow line indicates border between layer 1 and 2.

B.  Interlaminar astrocyte processes. Scale bar, 10 μm.

C.  Varicose projection astrocytes reside in layers 5–6 and extend long processes characterised by evenly spaced varicosities. Inset: Varicose projection astrocyte from chimpanzee cortex. Yellow arrowheads indicate varicose projections. Scale bar, 50 μm.

D.  Typical human protoplasmic astrocyte. Scale bar, 20 μm.

E.  Human fibrous astrocytes in white matter. Scale bar, 10 μm.
    Modified with permission from Oberheim *et al.*, 2012.
    Left panel schematically shows different astrocytes and their relations to cortical layers. (Full colour version in plate section.)

astroglial precursors and not from radial glia (Colombo & Reisin, 2004). The specific function of these cells is unknown, although they may be involved in delineating cortical columnar modules spanning across layers.

(vi) *Polarised astrocytes* are another class of cells possibly confined to the brains of primates, which are positioned in the deep cortical layers very near to the white matter. These cells have one or two long (up to 1 mm in length) processes that penetrate into superficial cortical layers (Figure 4.6 and (Oberheim *et al.*, 2012, 2006).

(vii) *Varicose projection astrocytes* appear to exist only in the brains of humans. These cells are characterised by several (up to 5) long (up to 1 mm) unbranched processes that extend in all directions through the deep cortical layers. These processes are endowed with evenly spaced varicosities. Once more, the role of these type of cells remains unknown (Figure 4.6 and Oberheim *et al.*, 2009).

In addition to these 'classical' astrocytes, more types of astroglia, represented by radial-like glia and glia in specific organs, are distinguished in the brains of mammals.

(viii) The retina contains specialised radial glia called *Müller cells*, which make extensive contacts with retinal neurones. The majority of Müller glial cells have a characteristic morphology (Figure 4.7), extending longitudinal processes along the line of rods and cones. In certain areas of the retina (e.g. near the optic nerve entry site), Müller cells are very similar to protoplasmic astrocytes. In human retina, Müller glial cells occupy up to 20 per cent of the overall volume, and the density of these cells approaches 25,000 per mm$^2$ of retinal surface area. Each Müller cell forms contacts with a clearly defined group of neurones organised in a columnar fashion; a single Müller cell supports $\approx$16 neurones in human retina and up to 30 in rodents.

(ix) The cerebellum contains specialised radial glia called *Bergmann glia* (historically also known as Golgi epithelial cells). They have relatively small cell bodies ($\approx$15 μm in diameter) and 3–6 processes that extend from the Purkinje cell layer to the pia (Figure 4.7). Usually, several ($\approx$8 in rodents) Bergmann glial cells surround a single Purkinje neurone and Bergmann glial processes form a 'tunnel' around the dendritic arborisation of Purkinje neurones. The processes of Bergmann glial cells are extremely elaborated, and they form very close contacts with synapses formed by parallel fibres on Purkinje neurone dendrites; each Bergmann glial cell provides coverage for up to 8,000 of such synapses.

(x) *Radial-like glia of the supra-optic nucleus* have been described in rodents. The cell bodies of these glia are located at the ventral borders of the nuclei in the ventral glia lamina. These cells send several thick processes in a dorsoventral direction, often spanning the entire nucleus (Bonfanti *et al.*, 1993).

(xi) *Tanycytes* (name derives from Greek 'tanus', meaning elongated) are bipolar specialised astrocytes found in the periventricular organs, in the hypothalamus, in the hypophysis and in the raphe part of the spinal cord (see Rodriguez *et al.*, 2005 for a detailed review). Tanycytes differentiate from radial glia in the perinatal period. In the periventricular organs, tanycytes form a brain-blood barrier by establishing tight junctions with capillaries (the blood-brain barrier is normally formed by tight junctions between the endothelial cells, but capillaries in the periventricular organs are 'leaky' and the tanycytes form a permeability barrier between neural parenchyma and the CSF). In the hypothalamus, four sub-types of tanycytes are distinguished, with different functional and barrier properties. Tanycytes' processes contact the ventricular wall and portal capillaries, thus providing a link between cerebrospinal fluid and neurosecretion.

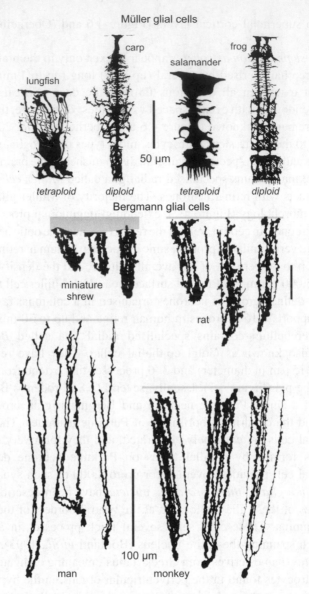

**Figure 4.7**  Radial glial cells. These *camera lucida* drawings were kindly provided by Professor Andreas Reichenbach, Leipzig University.

(xii) Another type of astroglia in neuro-endocrine organs are known as *pituicytes*, which are localised to the neuro-hypophysis (Hatton, 1988). The processes of these cells surround neuro-secretory axons and axonal endings under resting conditions, and they retreat from neural processes when increased hormone output is required. These cells are believed to modulate the hormonal output from the neuro-hypophysis (Rosso & Mienville, 2009).

(xiii) *Perivascular and marginal astrocytes* are localised very close to the *pia mater*, where they form numerous endfeet with blood vessels. As a rule, they do not form contacts with neurones, and their main function is in forming the pial and perivascular *glia limitans barrier*, which assists in isolating the brain parenchyma from the vascular and subarachnoid compartments.

(xiv) *Ependymocytes, choroid plexus cells* and *retinal pigment epithelial cells* line the ventricles and the subretinal space. These are secretory epithelial cells, which have been covered under the umbrella term 'glia' because they are not neurones. The choroid plexus cells produce the cerebro-spinal fluid, CSF, which fills the brain ventricles, spinal canal and the subarachnoid space. The ependymocytes and retinal pigment cells are endowed with numerous very small movable processes (microvilli and kinocilia) which, by regular beating, produce a stream of CSF and vitreous humour, respectively.

# 4.3   How to identify astrocytes in the nervous tissue

The great phenotypical differences between the different classes of astroglia makes the definitive identification of astrocytes in the CNS far from trivial. The classical histological procedures and immunostaining with antibodies against GFAP do not label all astrocytes and often reveal only their major processes (Figure 4.3A,B). *In situ* the levels of GFAP expression vary quite considerably between astrocytes in different brain regions. For example, GFAP is expressed by virtually every Bergmann glial cell in the cerebellum and in about 80 per cent of protoplasmic astrocytes in the juvenile hippocampus, whereas only about 15–20 per cent of astrocytes in the cortex of mature animals express GFAP. In addition, GFAP antibodies stain only the main processes where the filaments are concentrated (Figure 4.3C).

Astrocytes can be also visualised with other markers. One of these markers is the calcium binding protein S100β, but this protein is expressed only in a subpopulation of mainly perivascular astroglial cells and also labels NG2-glia. Immunostaining using antibodies against glutamate synthetase provides nice images, since the enzyme is cytosolic and, therefore, many fine processes of astrocytes can be faithfully visualised (Figure 4.3D). However, glutamate synthetase is also expressed in some oligodendrocytes. Other astroglial markers include the glutamate trans-porter GLT-1 (EAAT2), the inward rectifier channel $K_{ir}4.1$ subtype and aquaporin AQP4, but these molecules are usually concentrated in specific parts of astroglial membranes (e.g. in endfeet), which often results in a punctate staining.

Alternatively, astrocytes can be visualised by fluorescent dyes. The simplest way of astroglia-specific delivery of the dye is intracellular injection or perfusion via patch-clamp pipette, which is used for membrane-impermeable probes such as Lucifer yellow, Alexa dyes or biocytin (Figure 4.3E). Astrocytes *in situ* and *in vivo* can also be loaded with membrane-permeable fluorescent dyes. A rather reliable vital staining can be achieved with a cationic dye sulforhodamine 101 and its analogues Rhodamine B or Rhodamine G (Nimmerjahn *et al.*, 2004). Sulforhodamine is selectively taken up by astroglia and stains the cytoplasm, giving bright and detailed images. Moreover, the staining can be achieved even by intravenous injections of sulforhodamine (20 mg/kg). The astrocytes become fluorescent about 40 minutes after injection and the staining persists for up to five hours (Appaix *et al.*, 2012). Incidentally, astrocytes are also preferentially stained by classical $Ca^{2+}$-sensitive probes, such as fura-2 and fluo-3/4; when incubating slices with these dyes, astrocytes are stained before neurones, which can be used for selective labelling (Kirischuk & Verkhratsky, 1996).

Perhaps the best method for labelling astrocytes is the use of transgenic mice, in which various fluorescent soluble proteins are expressed under the control of astroglia-specific promoter (GFAP, GLT-1 or S100β). The fluorescent proteins include green fluorescent protein or its enhanced analogue, GFP and eGFP, as well as other members of the GFP family with different emission characteristics, such as cyan, or yellow fluorescent proteins, CFP and YFP, reef coral fluorescent proteins etc. (see, for example, Hirrlinger *et al.*, 2005). The most popular are the mouse models that express fluorescent proteins under control of the human GFAP promoter (Nolte *et al.*, 2001).

The problem with this approach is related to the difference in expression of GFAP around the brain, which determines the differences in expression of fluorescent reporter. Nonetheless, the fluorescent proteins are cytoplasmic and they visualise the full extent of astroglial processes arborisations (Figures 4.3F, 4.4.) - and, of course, the transgenic mice can be used for *in vivo* studies, including longitudinal observations.

## 4.4    Astroglial syncytial networks

A characteristic physiological feature of astrocytes is that they are physically connected to form a functional cellular syncytium, or reticular component of the CNS. This represents a fundamental difference between neuronal and glial networking. For the vast majority of neurones, networking is provided by synaptic contacts, which preclude physical continuity of the neuronal network while providing for functional inter-neuronal signal propagation. In contrast, glial networks are supported by direct intercellular contacts, generally known as *gap junctions*.

### 4.4.1    Gap junctions, connexons and connexins

Gap junctions are specific structures connecting cells of many types, being arguably the most common form of cell to cell communication. Gap junctions are ubiquitous, connecting epithelial cells of the gastrointestinal tract and kidney, providing metabolic coupling in the liver, electrical coupling in the heart, intercellular signalling in endocrine tissues, and also defining cochlear physiology and, hence, hearing (see, for example (Bosco *et al.*, 2011; Brisset *et al.*, 2009; Hanner *et al.*, 2010; Nickel & Forge, 2008).

At the ultrastructural level (seen by electron microscopy, EM, and freeze fracture EM), gap junctions appear as specialised areas where two apposing membranes of adjacent cells come very close together, so that the intercellular cleft is reduced to a width of about 2–3 nm. Within these areas, each gap junction is made up of many hundreds of intercellular channels, referred to as gap junction channels (Figure 4.8); these clusters of channels are known as *gap junction plaques*. These channels span through the membranes of adjacent cells and form an aqueous channel with a pore diameter between 6.5 and 15 Å that is permeable to hydrophilic molecules with molecular weight < 1 kDa. This is a very important feature, as it provides a conduit

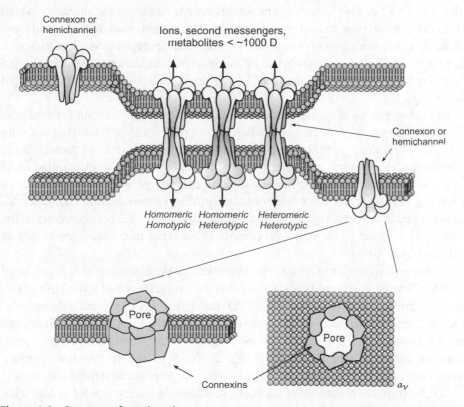

**Figure 4.8**   Structure of gap junctions.
  Gap junctional plaques are composed from several hundreds of intercellular gap junctional channels between two closely apposed cellular membranes, with the gap between cells ≈2–3 nm wide. The intercellular channels are formed by two apposed hemichannels or connexons. Each connexon, in turn, is composed from six subunits known as connexins (see the text for further explanation). The gap junction channels permit intercellular movement of solutes with a molecular weight up to 1000 Da, such as ions, second messengers and metabolites.

for intercellular diffusion of ions for effective electrical coupling, as well as many cytoplasmic second messengers (e.g. InsP$_3$), nucleotides (ATP, ADP), gluthatione, prostgalandins, metabolites and even vitamins.

Gap junction channels are composed from two precisely aligned hexameric hemichannels or *connexons*, one of each from the two adjacent coupled cells (Figure 4.8; for references and details, see Dermietzel *et al.*, 1990; Peters, 2006; Saez *et al.*, 2003). Each connexon, in turn, is composed of six symmetrical subunits, named *connexins*. Hence, a functional gap junction channel contains two connexons made up of 12 connexins. The connexins belong to an extended family and are present only in vertebrates; in the invertebrates, the homologous channels are made out of similar proteins called innexins.

There are 21 connexin genes in the human genome, 20 in rodents and up to 37 in teleost fishes. Connexins differ in molecular weight (varying between 26–62 kDa), which is used in connexin nomenclature, generally depicted as Cx m.w., for example Cx32 or Cx45. Each connexin has four transmembrane domains, which form the channel pore and gating mechanism. The connexons may be formed from identical connexins (*homomeric*) or from several different connexins (*heteromeric*). Similarly, gap junction channels can be made from identical connexons (making a *homotypic* gap junctional channel) or different (when the channel is called *heterotypic*).

Not all connexins are compatible to form an intercellular channel; for example, Cx32 forms gap junction channels when paired with Cx26 or Cx30, but not with Cx43. To produce a functional gap junction, several tens to hundreds of connexons must form a cluster. These clusters may connect similar cells (e.g. astrocyte to astrocyte), making a *homocellular gap junction*, or different cells (e.g. astrocyte and oligodendrocyte), forming a *heterocellular gap junction*. In addition, in astrocytes, gap junctional channels are formed between parts of the same cell, connecting astroglial processes. These types of contacts are known as *reflexive gap junctions*.

An interesting feature of connexins is their extremely fast turnover, with a typical half-life limited to several hours. Connexins are synthesised and folded in the ER, and are trafficked to the membrane via the Golgi complex and microtubule-facilitated transport. After spending several hours in the membrane, gap junctions are internalised into specific double-membrane vacuoles known as annular junctions or connexosomes (Kjenseth *et al.*, 2010). Why the cell spends so much material and energy on constantly synthesising large proteins remains unclear.

The biophysical behaviour of intercellular channels is very similar to any other type of the membrane ion channel, in that they undergo rapid transition between 'open' and 'closed' states. Importantly, the permeability and opening of gap junctional channels are controlled by many intracellular factors. For example, large increases in cytoplasmic Ca$^{2+}$ ($>10\,\mu$M) and intracellular acidification effectively inhibit junctional conductance. Junctional permeability is also controlled by intracellular second messengers such as cAMP, or by intracellular kinases such as PKC. The pharmacology of gap junctions is poorly defined, although they can be effectively blocked by volatile anaesthetics (halothane) and several alcohols (octanol or heptanol).

Some of the connexons do not form the intercellular channels, but rather are present in the plasmalemma as hemichannels, which can also be activated by various stimuli and form a pathway for different molecules to enter or exit the cell (Spray *et al.*, 2006; Thompson & Macvicar, 2008). Hemichannels are particularly implicated in the release of various neurotransmitters from astroglia, which will be discussed in detail later. It is important to mention that another class of channel-forming proteins, the pannexins, is widely considered to form hemichannels. In fact pannexins, although being widespread in the mammalian CNS, do not form functional gap junctions and, therefore (semantically), cannot exist as hemichannels. Similarly, there are no data favouring pannexin-associated formation of large transmembrane pores. On the contrary, in-depth analysis of Pannexin-1 mediated currents found them to be anion-selective (Ma *et al.*, 2012), and therefore it can be argued that pannexins are transmembrane channels rather than hemichannels.

In the CNS of mammals, at least 11 different connexins are expressed including Cx26, Cx29, Cx30, Cx32, Cx36, Cx37, Cx40, Cx43, Cx45, Cx46 and Cx47 (see Dermietzel & Spray, 1998; Nagy & Rash, 2000; Theis *et al.*, 2005) for extended review). Astrocytes in the CNS have the highest density of gap junctions, and the main astroglial connexins are Cx43 and, to a lesser extent, Cx30, together possibly with Cx40 and Cx45 (Dermietzel & Spray, 1998). The Cx26 connexins are present in subpial and subependymal astrocytes and are more abundant in astrocytes at early developmental stages.

Astroglial gap junctions underlie a relatively high degree of functional coupling. On average, pairs of astrocytes in the grey matter are connected by ≈230 gap junctions, and injection of relatively small fluorescent molecules (e.g. Lucifer yellow, m.w. ≈450–500 Da, or Alexa dyes with m.w. ≈450 Da) into a single astrocyte in some brain regions results in staining of about 50–100 neighbouring astroglial cells. This spread, however, is limited by the confines of individual astroglial networks.

The gap junctional connectivity of astroglia is instrumental for many of their functions, including generation of $Ca^{2+}$, $Na^+$ and metabolic waves, water transport, $K^+$ buffering, control of vasculature etc. (see below for detailed discussion). Finally, the gap junctional connectivity of astroglia may represent an 'analogue' inter-cellular signalling system (alternative to 'binary' interneuronal communication) which, by utilising intercellular diffusion of multiple molecules, can provide a second level of information processing in the CNS.

## 4.4.2   Astroglial networks

Initial discoveries of the high degree of gap junctional connections between astro-cytes, as well as identification of heterocellular glial gap junctions interconnecting astrocytes, oligodendrocytes and ependymal cells, led to the concept of a *panglial syncytium*. This envisaged an extended reticulum embracing all macroglial cells, with astrocytes acting as a sort of relay station or 'universal intermediaries' (Mugnaini, 1986). Early experiments seemingly corroborated this idea by demonstrating a high degree of coupling in purified astroglial cultures and heterocellular coupling in astro-oligodendroglial co-cultures. Heterocellular coupling was also observed in retinal preparations, and coupling between astrocytes and oligodendrocytes has been confirmed in the corpus callosum.

Generally, however, experiments *in situ* and *in vivo* have failed to identify far reaching heterocellular glial connectivity. In the majority of cases, dyes injected into a single astrocyte (in cortex, hippocampus, striatum, and inferior colliculus) were spread between groups of tens or even hundreds of cells, all of which were astroglial. This, of course, does not completely exclude heterocellular contacts and, indeed, dye coupling between astrocytes and other cell types, including oligodendrocytes and neurones, can be visualised. However, these contacts are much rarer than thought previously and often are restricted to early developmental stages. Furthermore, extended coupling experiments utilising various fluorescent dyes and high resolution microscopy in acute slices and in live brain tissues have demonstrated an anatomical segregation of glial networks. As a result, the concept of one panglial syncytium has been modified into a concept of multiple *astroglial syncytial networks* that are segregated within defined anatomical structures (Figure 4.9 and Giaume *et al.*, 2010; see Giaume & Liu, 2011 for overview).

Initially, segregated astroglial networks were identified in the somatosensory cortex in rodents, in which astrocytes localised within individual barrels demonstrated a high degree of coupling - whereas astrocytes positioned between barrels were weakly coupled, if at all (Figure 4.9). Furthermore, within barrels, the coupling was oriented towards the barrel centre. As a result, segregated astroglial syncytia are confined to a single barrel and have little connection to syncytia formed in neighbouring barrels. In the olfactory bulb, coupling was confined to astrocytes within single glomeruli, with little connectivity between astrocytes from different glomeruli. In addition, cell bodies of glomerular astrocytes are localised at the periphery, with their processes projecting into the glomerula centre. In the hippo-campus, the size of astroglial networks seems to be larger, yet there is still a degree of segregation between them.

This adds another dimension of complexity to networking in the CNS because, indeed, neuronal and astroglial networks show similar and overlapping anatomical and functional segregation. This allows building of multicellular domains that represent functionally segregated neural units. The size of astroglial networks and connectivity within them is controlled by numerous factors, including those released during neuronal activity, by local neurohormones, endocrine factors, and factors released from astrocytes. This, in turn, considerably increases the degree of plasticity of these structures and opens new possibilities for intercellular integration and information processing.

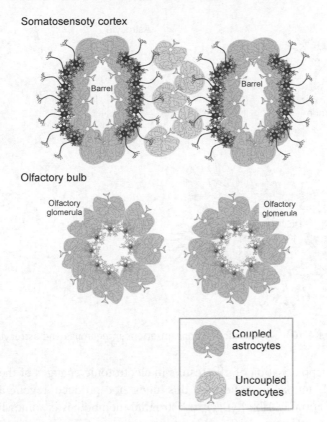

Somatosensoty cortex

Barrel

Barrel

Olfactory bulb

Olfactory
glomerula

Olfactory
glomerula

Coupled
astrocytes

Uncoupled
astrocytes

**Figure 4.9** Astroglial syncytial networks in different brain regions. The astroglial coupling is colour coded, i.e. astrocytes with the same colour are coupled into single network. See text for explanation. (Full colour version in plate section.)

# 4.5 Physiology of astroglia

## 4.5.1 Membrane potential and ion distribution

In general, mature astrocytes have a rather negative resting membrane potential ($\approx -80$ to $-90\,\text{mV}$) because of the predominance of potassium conductance, which maintains the membrane potential close to the potassium equilibrium potential ($E_K$). Astrocytes, however, are heterogeneous with respect to membrane potentials and potassium conductances, and the 'textbook' view of astrocytes as a homogeneous population of cells with a highly negative membrane potential close to the $E_K$ is an oversimplification. In hippocampal organotypic cultures, and in the optic nerve, the resting potential of astrocytes was shown to vary between $-85$ and $-25\,\text{mV}$ (Bolton et al., 2006; McKhann et al., 1997). The resting potential of astrocytes in the optic nerve is regulated by cAMP (which hyperpolarises cells by $\approx 15\,\text{mV}$) and by cAMP-dependent protein kinase, inhibition of which depolarised these astrocytes by $\approx 40\,\text{mV}$ (Bolton et al., 2006).

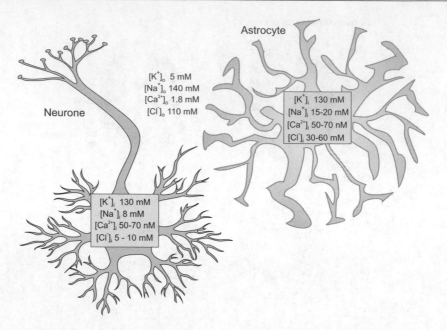

**Figure 4.10** Cytoplasmic ion concentrations in neurones and astrocytes.

Electrical depolarisation of glia results in electrotonic changes of the membrane potential and, unlike in neurones, this does not produce regenerative action potentials. The ion distribution across astroglial membranes is somewhat different from neurones (Figure 4.10). While intracellular $K^+$ concentration ($\approx$120–140 mM), and $Ca^{2+}$ (<0.0001 mM) is generally the same as in neurones, astrocytes contain substantially more $Na^+$ (cytoplasmic $Na^+$ concentration in astrocytes *in vitro* and *in situ* could be as high as 15–20 mM (Kirischuk *et al.*, 2012). Another difference is in $Cl^-$ distribution; the cytoplasmic $Cl^-$ concentration is unusually high in astrocytes and oligodendrocytes, being in the range of 30–60 mM (Deitmer & Rose, 2010; Kettenmann, 1990). This is due to the high activity of $Na^+/K^+/2Cl^-$ co-transporters that transport $2Cl^-$ into the cell in exchange for $1\,K^+$ and $1\,Na^+$. As a result, the reversal potential for $Cl^-$ is $\approx -40$ mV, and activation of $Cl^-$ permeable channels triggers $Cl^-$ efflux and depolarisation of astrocytes.

## 4.5.2   Ion channels

Glial cells express all major types of ion channels, including $K^+$, $Na^+$ and $Ca^{2+}$, non-selective channels and various types of anion channels (see Table 4.1). Biophysically, these channels are similar to those found in other types of cells, such as nerve or muscle cells.

**(i)   Potassium channels**   Resting membrane conductance of astroglial cells is dominated by passive $K^+$ currents. Astroglial cells express several types of *voltage-*

**Table 4.1** Ion channels in astroglia

| Ion channel | Molecular identity | Localisation | Main function |
|---|---|---|---|
| Potassium channels | | | |
| Voltage-independent $K^+$ channels | Two-pore domain $K^+$ channels: TREK1, TREK2 and TWIK1 | Hippocampus | Contribute to resting membrane potential |
| Inward rectifier potassium channels | $K_{ir}$ 4.1 (predominant) $K_{ir}$ 2.1, 2.2, 2.3 $K_{ir}$ 3.1 $K_{ir}$ 6.1, 6.2 | Ubiquitous | Maintenance of resting membrane potential; $K^+$ buffering |
| Outward rectifying $K^+$ channels | | | |
| Delayed rectifier potassium channels $K_D$ | $K_v 1.1$, $K_v 1.2$, $K_v 1.5$ and $K_v 1.6$ | Ubiquitous | Generally unknown; may be involved in regulation of proliferation |
| Rapidly inactivating A-type potassium currents ($K_A$) | $K_v 1.4$ | Hippocampus; astrocytes *in vitro* | Unknown |
| $Ca^{2+}$-dependent $K^+$ channels | $K_{Ca}3.1$ | Cortex | Unknown |
| Sodium channels | $Na_v 1.1$, $Na_v 1.2$ and $Na_v 1.3$ | Spinal cord cultured astrocytes; only $Na_v 1.2$ were detected in spinal cord astrocytes *in situ* | Regulation of differentiation, proliferation and migration(?) Can be up-regulated in pathological conditions |
| Calcium channels | L- ($Ca_v 1.2$), N- ($Ca_v 2.2$), P/Q- ($Ca_v 2.1$), R- ($Ca_v 2.3$) and T ($Ca_v 3.1$) | Astrocytes *in vitro*; functional expression *in situ* remains controversial. | Unknown |
| Transient receptor potential, TRP, channels | TRPC1, TRPC4, TRPC5 | Region distribution is unknown | Store-operated $Ca^{2+}$ entry |
| Chloride channels | CLC1, CLC2, CLC3 Volume-regulated anion channels of unknown identity | Ubiquitous | Chloride transport; regulation of cell volume |
| Aquaporins (water channels) | AQP4 (predominant) AQP9 | AQP4 - ubiquitous AQP9 - astrocytes in brain stem; ependymal cells; tanycytes in hypothalamus and in subfornical organ | Water transport |

*independent* $K^+$ *channels* (of TREK family), voltage-dependent $K^+$ channels represented by the *inward rectifier* $K^+$ *channels* ($K_{ir}$), *delayed rectifier potassium channels* ($K_D$), *rapidly inactivating A-type channels* ($K_A$) and also *calcium-activated* $K^+$ *channels* ($K_{Ca}$). Astrocytes' membranes always contain high densities of $K^+$ channels, although the molecular identity of these channels can vary substantially between cells from different brain regions (Matyash & Kettenmann, 2010).

The *voltage-independent* $K^+$ *channels* in astrocytes are represented by two-pore forming domains channels. The TREK1, TREK2 and TWIK1 channels were found in cultured astrocytes and in astrocytes in hippocampal slices (Seifert *et al.*, 2009; Zhou *et al.*, 2009). TWIK channels contribute significantly to the passive conductance in a subpopulation of hippocampal astrocytes. The TREK channels, in principle, can be activated by a wide variety of factors, which include mechanical stretch, protons (acidosis) and temperature; they are also sensitive to polyunsaturated fatty acids, and lysophospholipids. All of these factors therefore can (at least theoretically) affect membrane potential of astroglia, although the direct evidence is still lacking.

The *inward rectifier potassium channels,* $K_{ir}$ are abundantly expressed in astrocytes and are generally responsible for setting the resting membrane potential (Butt & Kalsi, 2006; Olsen & Sontheimer, 2008). They are called inwardly (or anomalously) rectifying because of their peculiar voltage-dependence. These channels tend to be closed when the membrane is depolarised and are activated when the membrane is hyperpolarised to the levels around, or more negative than, the $E_K$. In other words, these channels favour potassium diffusion in the inward direction over the outward one.

The voltage-dependence of $K_{ir}$ currents is determined by their sensitivity to intracellular $Mg^{2+}$ and/or polyamines, rather than by the existence of a true voltage sensor. Upon depolarisation, $Mg^{2+}$ and polyamine ions enter the permeation pathway and inhibit the channel (Lu, 2004). The $K_{ir}$ channels are regulated by extracellular $K^+$ concentration, and increases in the latter result in inward flow of $K^+$ ions, which is important for $K^+$ removal from the extracellular space which is considered one of the primary physiological function of astrocytes. Importantly for this process, an increase in extracellular $K^+$ concentration increases the inward $K^+$ currents proportionally to the square root of $[K^+]_o$ (Olsen & Sontheimer, 2008). All $K_{ir}$ channels are inhibited by $Ba^{2+}$ in micromolar concentrations, so $Ba^{2+}$ is generally used as a pharmacological probe for $K_{ir}$ channels.

There are at least 16 different $K_{ir}$ channel subunits, encoded by distinct genes (grouped into seven families, designated $K_{ir}1.xx$ to $K_{ir}7.xx$), and glia express representatives of most kinds (see Butt & Kalsi, 2006; Olsen & Sontheimer, 2008 for details and references). Generally, the $K_{ir}1.x$, $K_{ir}4.x$, $K_{ir}5.x$ and $K_{ir}7.x$ channels have a weak rectification and pass a substantial outward $K^+$ current upon depolarisation.

Protoplasmic and fibrous astrocytes, as well as radial-like Müller glia and Bergmann glia, are generally characterised by expression of the $K_{ir}4.1$ channel.

This channel is almost exclusively glial in the CNS, and a critical role for $K_{ir}4.1$ in setting the negative glial membrane potential has been demonstrated in $K_{ir}4.1$ knockout mice. The $K_{ir}4.1$ channel is quite sensitive to extracellular $Na^+$ concentration, and reduction of the latter by only 15 mM substantially increases current amplitude and reduces its time-dependent inactivation.

In addition to $K_{ir}4.1$, glia express diverse $K_{ir}$, including:

- $K_{ir}5.1$, which do not form functional homomeric channels but form heteromeric channels by co-assembly with other subunits of the same family, most notably $K_{ir}4.1$;

- members of the strongly rectifying and constitutively active $K_{ir}$ 2.0 family (e.g. $K_{ir}2.1$, 2.2 and 2.3), which may also co-assemble with $K_{ir}4.1$;

- $K_{ir}3.0$ channels (e.g. $K_{ir}3.1$), which are coupled to a range of G-protein linked neurotransmitter receptors ($K_{ir}3.0$ channels are generally formed by co-assembly of $K_{ir}3.1$ subunits with other members of the same family, such as the $K_{ir}3.1/K_{ir}3.4$ heteromers in atrial myocytes, which are responsible for the acetylcholine (ACh)-induced deceleration of heart beat); and

- ATP-dependent $K_{ir}$ ($K_{ir}6.1$ and 6.2), which are only active when intracellular concentrations of ATP fall to very low levels and therefore serve to maintain the high $K^+$ conductance and hyperpolarised resting membrane potential in glia during metabolic challenge.

Expression of $K_{ir}$ channels varies between different brain regions. In hippocampal astrocytes, for example, $K^+$ conductance is dominated by inwardly rectifying $K_{ir}4.1$ channels, with some contribution of TREK channels (Seifert *et al.*, 2009). In the spinal cord $K_{ir}4.1$, expression is the highest in astrocytes from ventral horn, and the lowest in the apex of the dorsal horn, which correlates with amplitudes of inwardly rectifying $K^+$ currents (Olsen *et al.*, 2007).

Expression of $K_{ir}$ channels is developmentally regulated. In general, up-regulation of $K_{ir}4.1$ channel expression in astrocytes may be regarded as a sign of their maturation. Functional expression of $K_{ir}4.1$ begins postnatally; in rodent hippocampus, for example, several-fold increases in $K_{ir}4.1$ channel protein, and inward $K^+$ currents, occur during the first 10–20 days of life (Seifert *et al.*, 2009; Sontheimer *et al.*, 1989). There are incidental observations that $K_{ir}4.1$ channels may provide a pathway for $Ca^{2+}$ entry after lowering extracellular $K^+$ concentration below 2 mM, although the underlying mechanism and significance remain unknown (Hartel *et al.*, 2007).

The outwardly rectifying (or voltage-dependent) potassium channels represent a diverse gene family made up of at least 15 subfamilies that cover $\approx 40$ $K_v$ channels. These channels are closed at resting potential and are activated in response to depolarisation, mediating outward currents (hence 'outwardly rectifying'). These channels are sensitive to the broad spectrum $K^+$ channel blockers tetraethylammonium

(TEA) and 4-amynopyridine (4-AP). The *delayed rectifier channels* are abundant in glia (see Olsen & Sontheimer, 2005 and references therein). Astrocytes express mainly channels of the $K_v1.x$ subfamily - e.g. $K_v1.1$, $K_v1.2$, $K_v1.5$ and $K_v1.6$ channels were identified in cultured astrocytes. $K_v$ channel expression correlates with differentiation status, whereby they are down-regulated during astrocyte maturation, and de-differentiation and astrogliois is associated with a reappearance of $K_v$ channels (and decrease in $K_{ir}$).

The *rapidly inactivating A-type potassium currents (KA)* are mostly responsible for fast hyperpolarisation and are abundant in excitable cells. In astrocytes, the $K_A$ currents have been recorded *in vitro* and in rat hippocampal slices, and the underlying channel seems to be of $K_v1.4$ variety (Olsen & Sontheimer, 2005). It remains unclear, however, whether the current recordings were, indeed, from true astrocytes or from NG2-glia, which display a much more 'excitable' behaviour.

The $Ca^{2+}$-dependent $K^+$ channels ($K_{Ca}$), although being members of the $K_v$ superfamily, have a dual gating mechanism, being controlled by both membrane voltage and cytosolic $Ca^{2+}$ concentration, whereby $Ca^{2+}$ binding to the intracellular portion of the channel is required for its activation. Three types of $K_{Ca}$ can be distinguished by their biophysical properties (BK, IK and SK), and glia express both BK and SK. BK channels are strongly voltage-dependent and sensitive to micromolar calcium, whereas SK are weakly voltage-dependent and sensitive to nanomolar calcium. $K_{Ca}$ currents have been found in cultured astrocytes (Quandt & MacVicar, 1986) and in freshly isolated neocortical astrocytes; in the latter, the currents were mediated by $K_{Ca}3.1$ (SK) channels (Longden *et al.*, 2011).

The functional role of outwardly rectifying $K^+$ channels in astrocytes remains unclear, because these cells rarely experience depolarisations above $-40\,mV$, which is a threshold for activation of $K_v$ channels. They may, however, be activated when extracellular potassium concentration or neurotransmitter levels are elevated sufficiently to depolarise the cell membrane. There is also evidence that $K_v$ channels are involved in regulation of astroglial proliferation.

**(ii)  Voltage-operated sodium channels (Na$_v$)** *Voltage-operated sodium channels* have been detected at both mRNA and protein levels in many types of astroglial cells, including those from retinal hippocampus, cortex and spinal cord (Black & Waxman, 1996; Verkhratsky & Steinhauser, 2000). Early studies detected TTX-sensitive and TTX-resistant voltage-activated $Na^+$ currents in cultured astrocytes from hippocampus, spinal cord and optic nerve (Olsen & Sontheimer, 2005). mRNA encoding $Na_v1.1$, $Na_v1.2$ and $Na_v1.3$ channels was detected in cultured spinal cord astrocytes, although only $Na_v1.2$ channels were detected immunohistochemically in the same astrocytes *in situ*. There are also unconfirmed reports that astrocytes express $Na_v1.6$ channels (see Olsen & Sontheimer, 2005) for relevant references). Many of the early studies, however, could have been done on NG2-glia, which express $Na_v$ and could have been mistaken for astrocytes.

The molecular structure and biophysical properties of $Na_V$ channels studied in astrocytes are similar to those present in neurones or muscle cells. The main difference is the channel density: glial cells have about one $Na_V$ channel per $10\,\mu m^2$, whereas their density in neurones can reach $1,000–10,000$ per $1\,\mu m^2$. The role of $Na_V$ channels in glia remains unclear. Interestingly, glial progenitor cells may have a much higher density of $Na_V$, and similarly very high densities of $Na_V$ were found in tumours of glial origin, suggesting that $Na_V$ channels are involved in the control of glial cell proliferation, differentiation and/or migration. There is some evidence that astroglial expression of $Na_V$ channels can be substantially up-regulated in pathological conditions, for example in multiple sclerosis and in ischaemic insults (Black *et al.*, 2010).

**(iii)  Calcium channels**  There is little evidence for functional expression of *voltage-operated $Ca^{2+}$ channels* (VOCCs) in astrocytes *in situ/in vivo*. Calcium channels have been identified in cultured astrocytes which expressed mRNA for L- ($Ca_V1.2$), N- ($Ca_V2.2$), P/Q- ($Ca_V2.1$), R- ($Ca_V2.3$) and T- ($Ca_V3.1$) types of calcium channels. Similarly, voltage-activated $Ca^{2+}$ currents and associated $[Ca^{2+}]_i$ transients have been detected in cultured astrocytes (see Parpura *et al.*, 2011; Verkhratsky & Steinhauser, 2000 and references therein). In cultured astroglia, induction of VOCCs expression often requires trophic manipulations – for example, incubation with dibutyryl-cyclic adenosine monophosphate, or co-culturing with neurones, or by acute oxidative stress (Parpura *et al.*, 2011).

Voltage-activated $Ca^{2+}$ currents reported for immature hippocampal astrocytes in brain slices (Akopian *et al.*, 1996) most likely represented recordings from then unidentifiable NG2-glia. In astrocytes in slices from the ventrobasal thalamus, VOCCs were considered to participate in spontaneous $[Ca^{2+}]_i$ oscillations, since the latter were inhibited by nifedipine and enhanced by Bay K8644 (Parri & Crunelli, 2003). Immunoreactivity for N ($Ca_V2.2$) and R ($Ca_V2.3$) channels subtypes was detected in pituicytes (hypophyseal astrocytes) *in situ*, and water deprivation for 24 hours induced a significant increase in immunoreactivity of L ($Ca_V1.2$)-type channels in these cells (Wang *et al.*, 2009). These observations, however, remain sporadic. As a rule, mature astroglial cells *in situ* do not demonstrate measurable voltage-operated $Ca^{2+}$ currents. There are some indications about up-regulation of L- and P/Q- channels in cells undergoing reactive astrogliosis in status epilepticus (see Parpura *et al.*, 2011; Verkhratsky *et al.*, 2012b for further details).

**(iv)  Transient receptor potential or TRP channels**  TRP channels belong to a highly diverse multigene class of ion channels represented by 28 members (Nilius & Owsianik, 2011), some of which are present in astroglia. Astrocytes express several members of the TRPC (canonical) subfamily (Parpura *et al.*, 2011), which are involved in a store-operated $Ca^{2+}$ entry (see below).

**(v)  Anion/chloride channels**  Anion channels belong to a rather diverse class of ion channels. This class comprises several families of *CFTR (cystic fibrosis* *transmembrane conductance regulator) channels, CLC (9-gene family of chloride channels), bestrophins, and anoctamins.* In addition to these main families, there are ligand-activated Cl⁻ channels (discussed in the section dedicated to GABA/-glycine receptors), *intracellular chloride channels of CLIC family, Ca²⁺-activated Cl⁻ channels*, and so-called *Tweety Cl⁻ channels*, initially found in *Drosophila* (Duran *et al.*, 2010). There is also evidence that pannexin-1 may form an anion channel (Ma *et al.*, 2012).

These channels have little in common and do not display many similarities with cation channels. All are, in fact, non-selective anion channels. In physiological conditions, however, Cl⁻ is the main current carrier, simply because its concentration is much higher than any other anion. To make things more confusing, some of the solute transporters (most notably glutamate transporters) can have a permeation pathway for Cl⁻, and many members of Cl⁻ channel families act as transmembrane transporters. As has been already mentioned, astrocytes have high intercellular Cl⁻ concentration, and therefore Cl⁻ currents activated at physiological potentials are always inward (i.e. Cl⁻ leaks out of the cell) and depolarising, in contrast to mature neurones, in which Cl⁻ currents usually trigger hyperpolarisation (and thus inhibition of electrical excitability).

Anion channels in astrocytes are rather poorly characterised, although they are likely to be directly involved in astroglial volume regulation. Several types of Cl⁻ channels have been detected in cultured astrocytes, including CLC-1, CLC-2 and CLC-3. Similarly, cultured astrocytes expressed Cl⁻ currents activated by depolarisation, although the resting Cl⁻ permeability of astroglial cells is quite small. Immunoreactivity for CLC-2 channels was detected in astrocytes *in situ*, and in CLC-2 knockout mice astrocytes lacked hyperpolarisation-activated Cd²⁺-sensitive Cl⁻ currents (see Kimelberg *et al.*, 2006 for details and references).

Most astrocytes express *volume-regulated anion channels or VRACs* (which have several names and are also known as volume-sensitive outwardly rectifying, VSOR, Cl⁻ channels or volume-sensitive organic anion channels, VSOAC). These channels are activated upon osmotic stress and are critical for volume regulation in astroglial cells, manifested, in particular, by regulatory volume decrease (RVD). The molecular identity of these channels remains unknown. An important role of anion channels is connected with their permeability to relatively large anions, such as glutamate and ATP and, consequently, these anion channels can be involved in release of these neurotransmitters from astrocytes (see below).

**(vi)  Aquaporins**  Astrocytes abundantly express *aquaporins, or water channels* (which are also permeable to some other molecules, e.g. glycerol and urea). Aquaporins (AQPs) are represented by an extended family which comprises 11 members in mammals (AQP0 to AQP10) and >150 members in other vertebrates, invertebrates, plants and bacteria. Aquaporins are constructed from four subunits which always assemble in homomeric fashion.

There are two subfamilies of aquaporins in mammals: the true aquaporins, i.e. water channels (AQP0,1,2,4,5,6); and aquaglyceroporins, channels which are permeable for water and glycerol (AQP3,7,9). AQP8 is classified as a metazoan aquaporin.

Aquaporins are concentrated on astroglial perivascular endfeet, where AQP4 are co-localised with $K_{ir}4.1$ and are involved in CNS water homeostasis. In the hypothalamus and in osmosensory areas of the subfornical organ, tanycytes exclusively express AQP9 (and do not possess AQP4), which may be involved in regulation of systemic water homeostasis.

## 4.5.3 Receptors to neurotransmitters and neuromodulators

Glial cells are capable of expressing the same extended variety of receptors as neurones, which allows glia to sense information delivered by neurotransmitters released during synaptic transmission. Glia, similar to neurones, are endowed with both ionotropic and metabotropic receptors, and the main classes of glial neurotransmitter receptors are summarised in Table 4.2 and Figure 4.11.

Probably the first experimental evidence demonstrating the effect of neurotransmitters on membrane potential of neuroglial cells was obtained during intracellular microelectrode recordings from pericruciate cortical cells of anesthetised cats. These were blind recordings, which clearly distinguished between electrically excitable neurones and electrically passive or 'unresponsive' cells, which were neuroglia. Many of these glial cells responded by depolarisation to iontophoretic injections of γ-aminobutyric acid (GABA), and acetylcholine (ACh) (Krnjevic & Schwartz, 1967). In these early studies, the involvement of specific receptors was not considered, and it was suggested that GABA and ACh effects were mediated through modulation of active transport. Similarly, microelectrode recordings from organotypic cultures prepared from medulla oblongata, pons and spinal cord found that inhibitory amino acids GABA, glycine, β-alanine and taurine depolarised astrocytes, although this action was also believed to be indirect and associated with release of $K^+$ from adjacent neurones (Hosli et al., 1981).

In 1984, however, direct electrophysiological recordings from purified astroglial cell cultures demonstrated that excitatory and inhibitory amino acids aspartate, glutamate, GABA and glycine directly depolarised astrocytes (Bowman & Kimelberg, 1984; Kettenmann et al., 1984). The absence of neurones in these cultures excluded $K^+$ efflux and led to the realisation that astrocytes express neurotransmitter receptors. Cultured astrocytes were subsequently found to be responsive to almost every neuroactive agent presented to them (Figure 4.10; (Finkbeiner, 1993; Verkhratsky & Kettenmann, 1996; von Blankenfeld & Kettenmann, 1991) for early studies). This promiscuity of cultured glia towards various ligands is generally regarded as a drawback and, in this respect, cultured neuroglial

**Table 4.2** Astroglial receptors to neurotransmitters and neuromodulators

| Receptor type | Properties/physiological effect | Localisation *in situ*/ |
|---|---|---|
| *Ionotropic receptors* | | |
| Glutamate AMPA receptors | $Na^+/K^+$ channels<br>$Na^+/K^+/Ca^{2+}$ channels. receptors lacking GluA2 subunit have some $Ca^{2+}$ permeability ($P_{Ca}/P_{monovalent} \approx 1$)<br>Activation triggers cell depolarisation and some $Ca^{2+}$ influx | Ubiquitous (hippocampus, cortex, cerebellum, white matter)<br>Bergmann glial cells, immature astrocytes |
| Glutamate NMDA receptors | $Na^+/K^+/Ca^{2+}$ channels<br>Activation triggers current, cell depolarisation and $Ca^{2+}$ entry.<br>Astroglial receptors display weak $Mg^{2+}$ block and intermediate $Ca^{2+}$ permeability ($P_{Ca}/P_{monovalent} \approx 3$) | Cortex, spinal cord |
| GABA_A receptors | $Cl^-$ channel<br>Activation triggers $Cl^-$ efflux and cell depolarisation | Ubiquitous (hippocampus, cortex, cerebellum, optic nerve, spinal cord, pituitary gland) |
| P2X (ATP) Purinoreceptors | $Na^+/K^+/Ca^{2+}$ channels<br>Activation triggers cationic current, cell depolarisation and cause $Ca^{2+}$ entry<br>$Ca^{2+}$ permeability of P2X_{1/5} receptors is: $P_{Ca}/P_{monovalent} \approx 2$<br>$Ca^{2+}$ permeability of P2X_7 receptors depends on the pore formation and can be very high ($P_{Ca}/P_{monovalent} > 10$) | Functional P2X_{1/5} receptors are present in cortex<br>Functional P2X_7 receptors are reported in cortex, in hippocampus and in retina |
| Glycine receptors | $Cl^-$ channel<br>Activation triggers $Cl^-$ efflux and cell depolarisation | Spinal cord |
| Nicotinic cholinoreceptors nAChR | $Na^+/K^+/Ca^{2+}$ channels<br>contains $\alpha 7$ subunit which confers high $Ca^{2+}$ permeability ($P_{Ca}/P_{monovalent} \approx 6$) | Hippocampus, cultured astrocytes |
| *Metabotropic receptors* | | |
| Glutamate receptors (mGluRs) | Group I (mGluR1,5) control PLC, InsP_3 production and $Ca^{2+}$ release from the ER<br>Group II (mGluR2,3) and Group III (mGluR4,6,7) control synthesis of cAMP | Ubiquitous |
| GABA_B receptors | Control PLC, InsP_3 production and $Ca^{2+}$ release from the ER | Hippocampus |

**Table 4.2** (*Continued*)

| Receptor type | Properties/physiological effect | Localisation *in situ*/ |
|---|---|---|
| Adenosine receptors $A_1$, $A_{2A}$, $A_{2B}$, $A_3$ | $A_1$ receptors control PLC, $InsP_3$ production and $Ca^{2+}$ release from the ER<br><br>$A_2$ receptors increase cAMP | Hippocampus, cortex |
| P2Y (ATP) Purinoreceptors | Control PLC, $InsP_3$ production and $Ca^{2+}$ release from the ER | Ubiquitous |
| Adrenergic receptors $\alpha_1 AR$, $\alpha_2 AR$ | Control PLC, $InsP_3$ production and $Ca^{2+}$ release from the ER | Hippocampus, Bergmann glial cells |
| $\beta_1 AR$, $\beta_1 AR$ | Control glial cell proliferation and astrogliosis; $\beta_2 AR$ are up-regulated in pathology | Cortex, optic nerve |
| Muscarinic cholinoreceptors mAChR $M_1$–$M_5$ | Control PLC, $InsP_3$ production and $Ca^{2+}$ release from the ER | Hippocampus, amygdala |
| Oxytocin and vasopressin receptors | Control PLC, $InsP_3$ production and $Ca^{2+}$ release from the ER; may regulate water channel (aquaporin) | Hypothalamus, other brain regions(?) |
| Vasoactive Intestinal Polypeptide receptors (VIPR 1,2,3) | Control PLC, $InsP_3$ production and $Ca^{2+}$ release from the ER; may regulate energy metabolism, expression of glutamate transporters, induce release of cytokines and promote proliferation | Supraoptic nucleus; other brain regions(?) |
| Serotonin receptors 5-$HT_{1A}$, 5-$HT_{2A}$, 5-$HT_{5A}$ | Increase in cAMP, energy metabolism | ? |
| Angiotentsin receptors $AT_1$, $AT_2$ | Control PLC, $InsP_3$ production and $Ca^{2+}$ release from the ER | White matter (optic nerve, corpus callosum, white mater tracts in cerebellum and subcortical areas) |
| Bradykinin receptors $B_1$, $B_2$ | Control PLC, $InsP_3$ production and $Ca^{2+}$ release from the ER | ? |
| Thyrotropin-releasing hormone receptors, $TRH_1$ | ? | Spinal cord |
| Opioid receptors, $\mu$, $\delta$, $\kappa$ | Inhibition of DNA synthesis, proliferation and growth, inhibition of cAMP production. | Hippocampus |
| Histamine receptors, $H_1$ | Control PLC, $InsP_3$ production and $Ca^{2+}$ release from the ER | Hippocampus, cerebellum |
| $H_2$ | Control synthesis of cAMP | |
| Dopamine receptors $D_1$–$D_5$ | Control synthesis of cAMP; Control PLC, $InsP_3$ production and $Ca^{2+}$ release from the ER | Substantia nigra, basal ganglia |

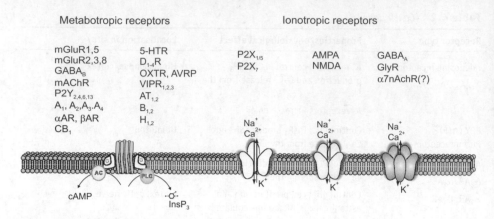

**Figure 4.11** Receptors to neurotransmitters and neuromodulators in astroglia. For abbreviations, see text and Table 4.2.

cells are very poor models of glia *in vivo*, both morphologically and functionally. Nonetheless, these early experiments were fundamentally important because they showed beyond any doubt that neuroglia are endowed with the molecular machinery to participate in chemical transmission in neural networks.

The receptor patterns expressed by astrocytes *in situ* are very different than *in vitro*, as the complement of receptors is quite restrictive, depending on the brain region. Usually, the modality of neurotransmitter receptors expressed by astroglia matches that of their neuronal neighbours and is most likely controlled by the local neurotransmitter environment (see (Verkhratsky, 2010; Verkhratsky *et al.*, 1998 for references and detailed discussion). For example (see Figure 4.12), Bergmann glial cells express receptors that exactly match the modality of receptors expressed by its neuronal neighbour, the Purkinje neurone. In both cells, the repertoire of receptors is optimised to sense neurotransmitters released by neuronal afferents, which form synapses on this neurone-glial unit. Indeed, Bergman glial cells and their intimate associates, Purkinje neurones, express receptors for adrenalin, histamine, glutamate, GABA and adenosine 5'-triphosphate (ATP), these receptors being congruent to the neurotransmitters released in this anatomical region.

Receptor expression can be even more spatially segregated – the same Bergmann glial cells specifically concentrate receptors for GABA in the membranes surrounding inhibitory synapses signalling to Purkinje neurones. Similarly, astrocytes express glycine receptors only in the spinal cord, where glycine acts as a main inhibitory mediator, whereas astroglial expression of dopamine receptors is restricted to basal ganglia, which have prominent dopaminergic transmission, and astroglial expression of serotonin receptors is restricted to areas contacting serotonergic terminals. Therefore, the expression of specific receptors is selectively regulated, which makes astrocytes perceptive towards chemical signals specific for each particular region of the brain.

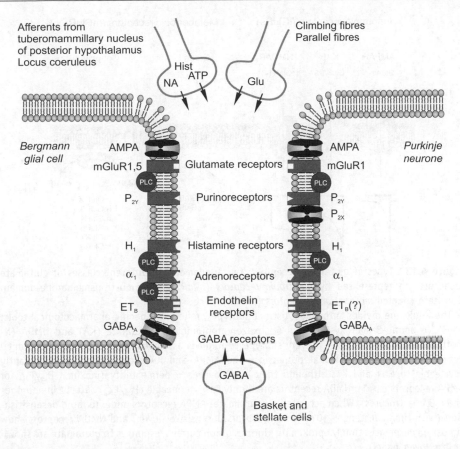

**Figure 4.12** Receptors expressed in Bergman glial cells *in situ* are limited to those specific to neurotransmitters released in their vicinity. Reproduced with permission from Verkhratsky et al., 1998.

**(i)  Glutamate receptors**  The excitatory action of glutamate in the CNS was identified in the 1950s (Hayashi, 1954). Soon, it become generally acknowledged that glutamate is the main excitatory neurotransmitter in the mammalian brain, and that glutamate-mediated intercellular transmission is primarily responsible for higher brain functions such as learning, memory and cognition (Watkins & Evans, 1981).

*Ionotropic glutamate receptors (iGluRs)* are abundantly expressed in astroglial cells throughout the CNS. Classically, iGluRs are subdivided into three major classes (Figure 4.13), which differ in molecular structure, pharmacology and biophysical properties. The first class is represented by *AMPA-type receptors*, so called because they are specifically activated by α-amino-3-hydroxy-5-methyl-4-isoxazolepropionate (AMPA). The AMPA receptors are assembled from four subunits, GluA1 to GluA4 (according to the current IUPHAR classification (see www.iuphar-db.org); also known as GluR1–4 or GluR A–D), which form cation channels permeable to $Na^+$ and $K^+$. When the GluA2 subunit is missing from the

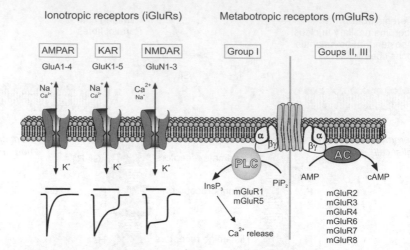

**Figure 4.13** Types of glutamate receptors; two fundamentally different classes of glutamate receptors are represented by *ionotropic receptors* (*iGluR*) and seven-transmembrane-domain G-protein-coupled *metabotropic receptors* (*mGluR*).

The iGluRs are divided into three distinct subtypes, reflecting specific pharmacological tools: AMPA ($\alpha$-amino-3-hydroxy-5-methyl-4-isoxazolepropionic acid), kainate (KA) and NMDA (N-methyl-D-aspartate) receptors. Every subtype of iGluR is assembled from four subunits, which determines receptor functional properties. The AMPA and KA receptors are predominantly permeable to $Na^+$ and $K^+$, although they may have $Ca^{2+}$ permeability (maximal $P_{Ca}/P_{Na}$ for AMPA receptors is $\approx 1$); NMDA receptors are highly $Ca^{2+}$ permeable ($P_{Ca}/P_{Na} \approx 10$–11 in neurones and $\approx 3$ in astrocytes). When activated by glutamate, AMPA receptors undergo rapid desensitisation (with time constant 2–10 ms), KA receptors desensitise slower, and NMDA receptors show almost no desensitisation (approximate kinetics of ion current responses to glutamate are shown on the lower panel).

The mGluR-mediated intracellular second messenger signalling cascades represented by the $InsP_3$/DAG cascade (mGluRs of Group I, linked to PLC) and cAMP cascade (mGluRs of Groups II and III, linked to AC).

assembly, the cation channel is also permeable to $Ca^{2+}$ ions. Glutamate rapidly opens AMPA receptors and, in the presence of agonist, they undergo swift desensitisation – i.e. membrane responses mediated through AMPA receptors are fast and are fully inactivated within $\approx 100$ ms. AMPA receptors are present in astroglial cells in most CNS regions, such as cortex, hippocampus, cerebellum, corpus callosum, retina and spinal cord (Seifert & Steinhauser, 2001).

All four main subunits of AMPA receptors are expressed in astrocytes, although their combinations are different in cells from different brain regions. Hippocampal astrocytes express all four subunits, with predominance of GluA2 and GluA4 subunits, which is reflected by their electrophysiology (linear I-V relation and very low $Ca^{2+}$ permeability). In spinal cord astroglia, GluA4 immunostaining was specifically concentrated in the perivascular processes, while the somata were positive for GluA2/3 subunits (see Lalo *et al.*, 2011b; Seifert & Steinhauser, 2001 for details). In cortical astrocytes, the GluA1 and GluA4 subunits are most abundant. Bergmann glial cell AMPA receptors lack the GluA2 subunit, which underlies their double-rectifying I-V relationships and $Ca^{2+}$ permeability ($P_{Ca}$/P-monovalent ≈ 1). At the same time, astrocytes from the rat supraoptic nucleus do not express functional iGluR (Israel *et al.*, 2003).

Functional expression of the second class of iGluR, the *kainate receptors*, has not been detected in astrocytes, although immunoreactivity for GluK1, 2, 3 and 5 subunits (formerly known as GluR5–7 and KA2 subunits) has been found in astrocytes from corpus callosum.

The presence of the third class of iGluR, the *NMDA receptors*, in astroglia has been confirmed only recently. Indeed, for a long time the general belief regarded NMDA receptors as specifically neuronal. This was mainly because of strong $Mg^{2+}$ block characteristic of NMDA receptors. At hyperpolarised membrane potentials, $Mg^{2+}$ binds to the receptor and precludes its activation by glutamate. Only after depolarisation to ≈−40 mV can the $Mg^{2+}$ block be removed and NMDA receptors become sensitive to glutamate. It was for a long time assumed that astrocytes, being generally unable to depolarise because of their electrical inexcitability, cannot produce conditions pertinent for NMDA receptor activation.

The expression of NMDA receptors in astrocytes *in situ* was initially detected by immunocytochemistry and mRNA analysis (Conti *et al.*, 1996; Schipke *et al.*, 2001). mRNA specific for GluN1, GluN2A and GluN2B (formerly known as NR1, NR2A and NR2 subunits) have been detected in cortical astrocytes and in cerebellar Bergmann glial cells, whereas the immunoreactivity for these same subunits has been observed in the distal processes of cortical astrocytes. In human foetal cultured astrocytes, all seven NMDA receptor subunits (GluN1, 2A-D and GluN3A,B) were detected at mRNA and protein levels (Lee *et al.*, 2010a).

In physiological experiments, NMDA-induced membrane currents and $Ca^{2+}$ signals were characterised in astrocytes from cortex, spinal cord and in some hippocampal astrocytes (see (see Verkhratsky & Kirchhoff, 2007 for comprehensive review). These initial experiments, however, could not unequivocally attribute these responses to direct activation of astroglial NMDA receptors. For example, NMDA-induced $[Ca^{2+}]_i$ responses observed in hippocampal slices were sensitive to tetrodotoxin, thus indicating indirect mechanisms most likely associated with neuronal activation. Furthermore, astrocytes acutely isolated from hippocampi failed to respond to direct NMDA application, and NMDA-induced currents measured from Bergmann glial cells had rather uncharacteristic properties, in that they reversed at −40 mV, were insensitive to glycine and had no $Ca^{2+}$ permeability (see Verkhratsky & Kirchhoff, 2007 and references therein).

Compelling evidence for astroglial expression of NMDA receptors was found in cortical astrocytes. NMDA applied to astrocytes mechano-dissociated from mouse somato-sensory cortex induced cationic currents. These currents were positively modulated by glycine and blocked by specific NMDA receptor antagonists MK-801 and D-2-amino-phosphonopentanoic acid (D-AP5). Application of glutamate to the same cells triggered a biphasic current, the components of which had a distinct pharmacological profile. The fast component was inhibited by AMPA receptor blocker 6-cyano-7-nitroquinoxaline-2,3-dione (CNQX), whereas the slow component was sensitive to D-AP5 and MK801. Subsequent evidence for the expression of $Ca^{2+}$-permeable NMDA receptors in a sub-population of cortical astrocytes came from $Ca^{2+}$-imaging experiments on acute slices (see Lalo *et al.*, 2011b for references).

Astroglial NMDA receptors differ from neuronal ones in several fundamental properties. First and foremost, glial NMDA receptors are much less susceptible to $Mg^{2+}$ block. In astrocytes held at $-80\,mV$, the NMDA-evoked currents were not affected by extracellular $Mg^{2+}$ and the $Mg^{2+}$ block required stronger hyperpolarisation, being fully developed at $-120\,mV$ (Palygin *et al.*, 2011). Incidentally, a similar weak $Mg^{2+}$ block was observed in oligodendrocytes, where both NMDA-induced currents and NMDA-triggered $[Ca^{2+}]_i$ transients were readily recorded at physiological concentrations of $Mg^{2+}$ (see, for example, Karadottir *et al.*, 2005). The absence of $Mg^{2+}$ block therefore seems to be idiosyncratic for neuroglial NMDA receptors, and it permits their activation at the negative membrane potentials characteristic of glia.

Second, NMDA receptors in astroglia had a substantially lower $Ca^{2+}$ permeability compared to the neuronal receptors: the $P_{Ca}/P_{monovalent}$ for NMDA receptors expressed in astrocytes was determined at $\approx 3$, whereas neuronal NMDA receptors have a permeability ratio of $Ca^{2+}$ to monovalent cations of $\approx 10$ (Palygin *et al.*, 2010).

Third, astroglial NMDA receptors have a specific pharmacology, being rather sensitive to memantine and the GluNR2C/D subunit-selective antagonist UBP141 (Palygin *et al.*, 2011). These properties allow some deduction of the molecular composition of glial NMDA receptors. The low $Mg^{2+}$ sensitivity may result, for example, from a specific expression of GluN3 NMDA receptor subunits, because it is known that incorporation of this subunit into dimeric GluN1/GluN3 or tri-heteromeric GluN1/2/3 receptors confers low sensitivity to $Mg^{2+}$-block. The dimeric GluN1/GluN3 receptors, however, are resistant to broad NMDA receptor agonists D-AP5 and MK-801. At the same time, astroglial NMDA receptor-mediated currents are effectively inhibited by D-AP5 and MK-801, indicating the presence of GluN2 subunits, which is also consistent with their sensitivity to UBP141. Therefore, the most probable composition of astroglial NMDA receptors is the heteromeric assembly of two GluN1, one GluN2 and one GluN3 subunits (see Lalo *et al.*, 2011b for further details).

Astrocytes throughout the brain typically express *metabotropic glutamate receptors (mGluRs)* that belong to seven-transmembrane-domain (7TM) receptors. The mGluRs are represented by three groups associated with distinct intracellular signalling pathways (Figure 4.13). The Group I receptors (mGluR1 and mGluR5) are positively coupled to phospholipase C, and their activation increases the intracellular concentration of $InsP_3$, which subsequently triggers $Ca^{2+}$ release from the endoplasmic reticulum (ER) store. The remaining mGluR subtypes, which belong to Group II (mGluR2, mGluR3) and Group III (mGluR4, mGluR6–8) are coupled to adenylate cyclase and regulate intracellular levels of cAMP. Astroglial cells predominantly express mGluR1, mGluR3 and mGluR5 (i.e. Group I and II), and hence glutamate triggers glial $Ca^{2+}$ signals and regulates cAMP-dependent reactions, such as inhibition of $K^+$ currents, swelling, proliferation and regulation of expression of glutamate transporters.

**(ii)   Purinoceptors**   The purinergic signalling system that utilises extracellular purines (most notably ATP and adenosine) and pyrimidines as signalling molecules, has several unique features. First and foremost, it is literally omnipresent, being operative in virtually all tissues and cell types. Second, it is unusually widely distributed among living forms, being detected in plants, fungi, protozoa and animals, indicating ancient phylogenetic roots. Third, in contrast to the majority of transmitter systems, purinergic transmission does not have anatomical segregation (for a comprehensive overview of purinergic signalling and its evolution see Burnstock *et al.*, 2010; Burnstock *et al.*, 2011; Burnstock & Verkhratsky, 2009).

Purinergic signalling mechanisms are abundantly present in the brain (Abbracchio *et al.*, 2009). In physiological conditions, the principal purinergic transmitter ATP is released from both neurones and neuroglia via multiple mechanisms, which include $Ca^{2+}$-regulated exocytosis, release from lysosomes and diffusion through plasmalemmal channels (mechanisms of neurotransmitter release from astroglia will be discussed in detail in subsequent sections). The purinergic signalling system is particularly important for neuroglia, because all types of glial cells, whether of ectodermal/neural origin (astrocytes, oligodendrocytes and NG2-glia) or of mesodermal origin (microglia), express purinoceptors which control many of their vital functions (see Verkhratsky *et al.*, 2009 for overview). In addition, ATP is massively released from damaged cells, being a universal 'danger' signal that is specifically important for controlling many defensive reactions associated with neuroglial activation and, particularly, with astrogliosis.

The physiological impact of purinergic signalling is inherently complex, due to interconversion of nucleosides (e.g. adenosine and guanosine) and nucleotides (e.g. ATP and GTP or corresponding dinucleotides) and their differential actions of various receptors. For example, ATP, once released to the extracellular space, is rapidly degraded by membrane-bound ecto-nucleotidases, thus producing a trail of derivatives such as ADP, AMP and adenosine which, in turn, activate different plasma membrane receptors, quite often with opposite actions. Moreover, there is a cross-talk between purinoceptors and other receptors systems such as glutamate, GABA and serotonin receptors.

The broad class of purinoceptors is represented by molecules sensing various purinergic nucleotides, which are commonly present in the brain interstitium. Generally, purinoceptors are divided into *adenosine receptors* (also known as P1) and ATP or *P2 receptors* of the *P2X (ionotropic) and P2Y (metabotropic)* subtypes (Figure 4.14). All glial cell types have been shown to express at least one type of purinoceptor.

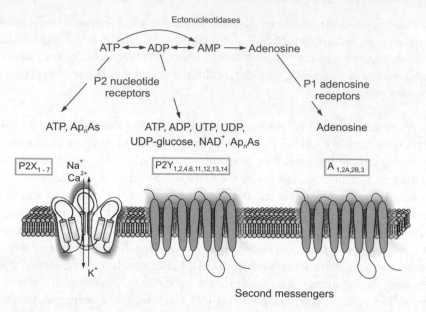

**Figure 4.14** Classes of purinoceptors. ATP, after being released from neurones and glia, is rapidly degrading by ectonucleotidases into ADP, AMP and adenosine, which act on P1 metabotropic adenosine receptors, P2X ionotropic and P2Y metabotropic nucleotide receptors.

*Adenosine (P1) receptors* are classical 7-TM metabotropic receptors coupled to several families of $G_i$ and $G_o$ proteins. Four types of adenosine receptors ($A_1$, $A_{2A}$, $A_{2B}$ and $A_3$) with distinct pharmacological and functional properties, have been cloned and characterised. As a rule, the $A_1$ and $A_3$ receptors exert an inhibitory effect on adenyl cyclase (mediated through $G_{i/o}$ proteins). In addition, activation of $A_1$ and $A_3$ receptors stimulates $K^+$ channels and reduces voltage-dependent $Ca^{2+}$ currents. The $A_{2A}$ receptors activate cyclic AMP (cAMP) production via $G_s$ (or $G_{olf}$ in striatal neurones) proteins. $A_{2B}$ receptors couple to many G proteins, including $G_s$, $G_q$ and $G_{12}$, and also stimulate cAMP production. $A_1$ and $A_3$ receptors also regulate phospholipase C (PLC), and thus $InsP_3$ synthesis. In some cells, $A_1$ receptors are reported to activate $K^+$ and/or $Ca^{2+}$ channels (Burnstock *et al.*, 2011 and references therein).

All four types of adenosine receptors ($A_1$, $A_{2A}$, $A_{2B}$ and $A_3$) are expressed in astroglial cells, as has been shown both *in vitro* and *in vivo*, and are involved in regulation of many glial functions (comprehensively reviewed by Boison *et al.*, 2010; Dare *et al.*, 2007; Verkhratsky *et al.*, 2009). For example, $A_1$ and $A_3$ receptors inhibit, whereas $A_2$ receptors stimulate, glial proliferation. In addition, stimulation of adenosine receptors may regulate expression of glutamate transporters, sensitivity of cells to glutamate, etc.

There is quite a degree of heterogeneity in expression of adenosine receptors and in their action. Adenosine often induces astroglial $Ca^{2+}$ signalling, although the receptors involved differ between different preparations. In cultured cortical astrocytes, and in astrocytes in olfactory bulb slices, for example, adenosine triggers $Ca^{2+}$ signals, mediated through $A_{2A}$ receptors; whereas in cultured astrocytes from neonatal forebrain, similar $Ca^{2+}$ signals are mediated by $A_1$ receptors. In primary cultures from the whole mouse brain, $A_3$ receptors mediate $Ca^{2+}$ signalling in $\approx 85$ per cent of astrocytes. Numerous experiments demonstrated that adenosine modulates $Ca^{2+}$ signals induced by activation of other metabotropic receptors, such as mGluRs, P2Y purinoceptors and muscarinic ACh receptors. In different experiments, this modulation was mediated by either $A_1$ or $A_{2A}$ receptors. These diverse findings most likely result from culture-associated remodelling of astroglial receptor expression.

Various types of brain insults are associated with massive release of ATP and adenosine from stressed cells. Overall, the adenosine concentrations in injured brain interstitium can reach up to 50 μM (see Dale & Frenguelli, 2009 for a comprehensive review). In general, adenosine exerts a neuroprotective action on the brain tissue, and astroglial $A_{2A}$ receptors have complex actions on neuronal survival, being involved in neuroprotection and regulation of cell death, whereas astroglial $A_3$ receptors are involved in regulation of chemokine release and neuroprotection. Additionally, $A_{2A}$ receptors can promote astrogliosis in various neuropathologies and have glio-protective actions in conditions of ischaemia and glucose deprivation.

Astroglial adenosine receptors also modulate their uptake of glutamate, whereby activation of $A_{2A}$ receptors in hippocampal astrocytes reduced glutamate uptake via inhibition of GLT-1 transporter and resulted in glutamate release from astrocytes through $[Ca^{2+}]_i$ and a protein kinase A-dependent pathway. This, in turn, potentiates neuronal activity in the hippocampus due to an increase in glutamate concentration in the synaptic zones (Li et al., 2001; Nishizaki et al., 2002).

The P2Y metabotropic purinoceptors (Figure 4.14) are abundantly expressed in the majority of astrocytes, both in vitro and in situ (Burnstock et al., 2011; Verkhratsky et al., 2009). The most abundant receptor types are represented by $P2Y_1$, $P2Y_2$ and $P2Y_6$ receptors. Functionally, the P2Y receptors are positively coupled to PLC and their activation triggers cytoplasmic $Ca^{2+}$ signals and intercellular $Ca^{2+}$ waves. These $Ca^{2+}$ signals have been characterised in astrocytes from most brain regions in cultures and in brain slices. For example, the P2Y receptor-mediated $Ca^{2+}$ signalling was observed in astrocytes from the stratum radiatum region of mouse hippocampus, in mouse olfactory bulb, in Bergmann glial cells in cerebellum, in retinal Müller cells, in astrocytes from optic nerve, etc.

The activation of P2Y receptors results in a transient increase in cytosolic $Ca^{2+}$ that can last for seconds to minutes. These $Ca^{2+}$ signals do not require extracellular $Ca^{2+}$, and they are sensitive to inhibitors of ER $Ca^{2+}$ pumps (thaspigargin and cyclopiazonic acid) and $InsP_3$ receptors (heparin). $P2Y_1$ and $P2Y_2$ receptors play the major role in generation and maintenance of propagating $Ca^{2+}$ waves in astrocytes in hippocampus and spinal cord (see Verkhratsky et al., 2009, 1998 for review). P2Y receptors can also be coupled to various intracellular signalling cascades, which regulate both physiological and pathophysiological astroglial reactions (Figure 4.15).

Importantly, stimulation of P2Y receptors triggers release of neurotransmitters from astroglia. For example, ATP stimulation of cultured astrocytes triggers release of ATP and glutamate, as well as release of TNF-α, prostaglandins, etc. P2Y receptors also stimulate mobilisation of arachidonic acid and eicosanoid production

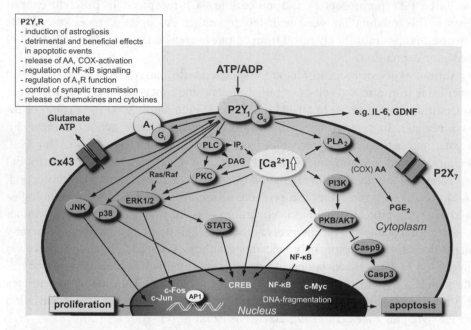

**Figure 4.15**   Schematic illustration of examples of signal transduction pathways in astroglial cells following P2Y$_1$ receptor activation.

Stimulation of P2Y$_1$ receptors leads to the activation of phospholipases A2 and C (PLA2, C) and protein kinase C (PKC), as well as an increase in intracellular calcium ([Ca$^{2+}$]$_i$). The activation of P2Y$_1$ receptors also results in the induction of second messenger and enzyme cascades, e.g. activation of the mitogen-activated protein kinase (MAPK) pathway proteins (ERK1/2), p38 MAPK, c-Jun N-terminal kinase (JNK), and PI3K/Akt activation. P2Y$_1$ receptor-mediated signal transducer and activator of transcription 3 (STAT3) signalling may play a role in astrocyte proliferation and reactive astrogliosis. P2Y$_1$ receptor activation is also involved in the activation of caspase (Casp) cascades and the release of arachidonic acid and increase in prostaglandin E2 (PGE2) levels. In addition, P2Y$_1$ receptor activation induces the activity of transcription factors such as nuclear factor κB (NF-κB), cyclic element-binding protein (CREB), activator protein (AP-1) (which up-regulate the expression of proinflammatory early response genes, e.g. c-Fos, c-Jun, c-Myc). Interaction between adenosine A$_1$ and P2Y$_1$ receptors may alter the nucleotide signalling cascades. Modulation of astrocytic P2Y$_1$ receptors by the C-terminal domain of the gap junction protein connexin43 (Cx43) appears to be involved in release of ATP and glutamate. The present data suggest that astroglial P2Y$_1$ receptor stimulation is associated with neurological disorders leading to neuroinflammation, and apoptosis.

The inset summarizes examples of P2Y$_1$ receptor-mediated effects in astrocytes.

in cultured astroglia, an effect which depends on synergy between P2Y-mediated $[Ca^{2+}]_i$ elevation and direct coupling of a subset of P2Y receptors with PLA2.

Stimulation of metabotropic P2Y receptors increases synthesis of prostaglandins and brain-derived neurotrophic factors. For example, $P2Y_4$ receptors regulate expression and release of glycoprotein thrombospondin (TSP)-1, which is a potent stimulator of synaptogenesis. In astroglial cultures, activation of $P2Y_2/P2Y_4$ receptors triggers release of NO, which in turn suppresses synaptic activity in neurones co-cultured with astroglia.

Finally, P2Y receptors exert multiple trophic effects on astrocytes. For example, exposure of astroglial cultures to purines promotes astroglial differentiation and growth of their processes, and P2Y receptors also mediate effects of ATP on morphological differentiation in development (Verkhratsky et al., 2009 and references therein).

*Ionotropic P2X purinoceptors* are classical ligand-gated cation channels (Figure 4.14), formed by homo- or hetero-trimeric expression of seven distinct subunits, classified $P2X_1$ to $P2X_7$ according to historical order of cloning (Burnstock et al., 2010; North, 2002). In physiological conditions, activation of P2X receptors results in depolarising currents carried mainly by $Na^+$ and $Ca^{2+}$ ions. The $Ca^{2+}$ permeability of P2X receptors is determined by subunit composition and can vary widely, the $P_{Ca}/P_{monovalent}$ being between 1 and 10 for different receptors and cell types (Lalo et al., 2011c; Verkhratsky et al., 2012a).

mRNA and proteins for almost all P2X subunits have been detected in astroglia; for example, the $P2X_{1,2,3,4,6,7}$ were identified in hippocampal astroglia, $P2X_2$, $P2X_3$ and $P2X_4$ were detected by immunostaining in astrocytes in nucleus accumbens, $P2X_1$ and $P2X_2$ receptors were found in astrocytes from cerebellum and spinal cord, while $P2X_4$ receptors were localised in the astroglia from the brainstem (Verkhratsky et al., 2009).

Much less is known about functional expression of P2X receptors in astroglia. P2X receptor-mediated currents were observed in early experiments on cultured astrocytes (Walz et al., 1994). In experiments *in situ*, functional expression of a rather peculiar receptor type, the heteromeric $P2X_{1/5}$ receptor, was detected in cortical astrocytes (see Lalo et al., 2011c for details). Heteromeric $P2X_{1/5}$ receptors are extraordinarily sensitive to ATP, with a threshold for activation lying at $\approx 1$ nM and $EC_{50}$ of $\approx 50$ nM ATP. These astroglial receptors have little desensitisation and are moderately $Ca^{2+}$ permeable ($P_{Ca}/P_{monovalent} \approx 2.2$). $P2X_{1/5}$ receptors contribute to electrical and $Ca^{2+}$ signals triggered in cortical astrocytes by stimulation of neuronal inputs, indicating their activation by synaptically released ATP. Arguably, these highly sensitive purinoceptors allow astrocytes to monitor low ATP concentrations, which can be indicative of physiological synaptic transmission.

Astrocytes throughout the brain also express functional $P2X_7$ receptors (see Illes et al., 2012 for details). These receptors are the most unusual members of the P2X family, in that they are activated by rather high ($>1$ mM) concentrations of ATP and, upon prolonged stimulation, the $P2X_7$ receptors form a high-permeability pore that allows the passage of cations and anions with molecular weights of up to 1000 Da. The nature of the pore remains unresolved, and it may reflect either dilation of the channel itself (which is characteristic of a number of P2X receptors, in addition to the $P2X_7$ subtype, albeit to a much lesser extent), or be associated with a secondary activation of auxiliary channel pore-forming proteins such as connexons.

The sensitivity of $P2X_7$ receptors to ATP greatly increases in divalent-free extracellular solutions. The dilated pore of $P2X_7$ receptors displays high $Ca^{2+}$ permeability and may form a pathway for release of neurotransmitters, most notably ATP and glutamate. Activation of $P2X_7$ receptors is associated with neuro-pathology, as they are involved in initiation of apoptosis, and they may act as 'emergency' receptors aimed at restraining the excessive astrogliosis triggered by brain injuries (Franke *et al.*, 2012).

In addition, $P2X_7$ receptors are coupled to a wide range of intracellular signalling pathways (Figure 4.16), such as processing and release of interleukin-1$\beta$, and cytoskeletal changes. This most likely results from interactions between the unusually long C-terminus of the receptor with multiple proteins, including enzymatic and signalling cascades, including extracellular signal-regulated protein kinases (ERKs), serine-thereonine kinase Akt (Akt), c-Jun N terminal kinases (JNKs), and p38 kinase. The activation of $P2X_7$ receptors also increases protein tyrosine phosphorylation, ultimately leading to mitogen-activated protein kinase (MAPK) pathway activation. Finally, $P2X_7$ receptors display significant polymor-phism ($\approx 32$ single nucleotide polymorphisms have been identified), which includes gain or loss of function variants that are implicated in the pathogenesis of various diseases, such as bipolar disorder and multiple sclerosis.

**(iii)   γ-aminobutyiric acid receptors (GABA) receptors**   Astrocytes in various brain regions (spinal cord, hippocampus, optic nerve, retina and cerebellum) express *GABA_A receptors* (Figure 4.17). Molecularly, these receptors are the same as neuronal ones, being in essence ligand-gated $Cl^-$ channels. Functionally, however, there is a remarkable difference, because (as has been mentioned previously) glial cells contain much more $Cl^-$ than mature neurones (35 mM vs. $\approx 3$–5 mM), and therefore the equilibrium potential for $Cl^-$ is about $-40$ mV, whereas in neurones it lies somewhere near $-70$ mV. As a consequence, activation of $GABA_A$ receptors in astrocytes triggers efflux of $Cl^-$ ions and cell depolarisation.

Activation of $GABA_A$ receptors also inhibits astroglial $K^+$ channels, thus facilitating depolarisation. There is evidence that $GABA_A$ receptors concentrate in the perisynaptic processes facing inhibitory GABA-ergic neuronal terminals. Astrocytes also express metabotropic $GABA_B$ receptors that are activated in response to GABA release from neuronal terminals in hippocampus, and these astroglial $GABA_B$ receptors are involved in a specific form of synaptic plasticity known as heterosynaptic depression (see Velez-Fort *et al.*, 2012 for references).

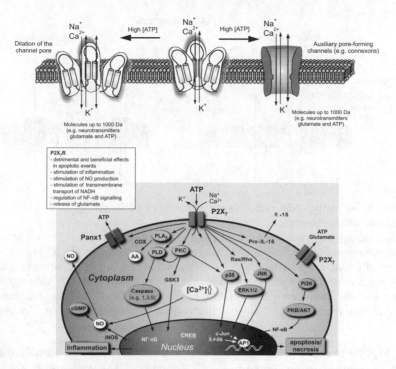

**Figure 4.16**  Signalling through P2X$_7$ receptors.

*Top panel:* prolonged activation of P2X$_7$ receptors by high (>1 mM) ATP concentrations results in formation of a transmembrane pore, permeable to relatively large molecules with molecular weights of up to 1000 Da. The nature of the pore remains unresolved, and it may reflect either dilation of the channel itself or be associated with a secondary activation of auxiliary channel pore-forming proteins such as connexons.

*Bottom panel:* Schematic illustration of examples of signal transduction pathways in astroglial cells following P2X$_7$ receptors activation. Activated P2X$_7$ receptors are permeable for Na$^+$, K$^+$ and Ca$^{2+}$, as well as (upon pore formation) larger molecules. Activation of P2X$_7$ receptors triggers the efflux of K$^+$ from cells and activates IL-1 converting enzyme, leading to cleavage of pro-IL-1β to mature IL-1β, which is released from the cell. Many events downstream of P2X$_7$ receptors activation are dependent on extracellular Ca$^{2+}$ influx. Stimulation of ionotropic P2X$_7$ receptors leads to activation of phospholipases A2 and D (PLA2, D) and protein kinase C (PKC), resulting, for example, in the activation of glycogen synthase kinase 3 (GSK3) or the activation of caspase cascades. Furthermore, the induction of second messenger and enzyme cascades promotes activation of mitogen-activated protein kinase (MAPK) pathway proteins (ERK1/2), p38 MAPK, and c-*Jun* N-terminal kinase (JNK), as well as PI3K/Akt activation. The activity of transcription factors, such as nuclear factor κB (NF-κB), cyclic element-binding protein (CREB) and activator protein (AP-1) are also up-regulated, leading to the expression of proinflammatory genes such as cyclooxygenase-2 (COX-2) or inducible nitric oxide oxidase (iNOS); these in turn, cause the production of arachidonic acid (AA) or nitric oxide (NO), respectively. Finally, ATP and glutamate can be released though P2X$_7$-receptors coupled hemichannels or through the receptor pore. The present data suggest that astroglial P2X$_7$ receptor stimulation is associated with neurological disorders, leading to neuroinflammation and apoptosis.

The inset summarizes examples of P2X$_7$ receptors-mediated effects in astrocytes.

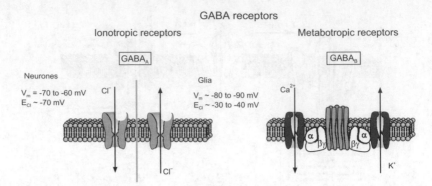

**Figure 4.17** Astroglial GABA receptors are represented by ionotropic GABA$_A$ receptors and metabotropic GABA$_B$ receptors.

GABA$_A$ receptors are ligand-gated Cl$^-$ channels, and on their activation Cl$^-$ moves according to the electrochemical gradient; in neurones, the equilibrium potential for Cl$^-$ ($E_{Cl}$) is $-70$ mV, and activation of GABA$_A$ receptors results in Cl$^-$ influx and hyperpolarisation, whereas glia have a strongly negative resting membrane potential ($V_m$) and high intracellular Cl$^-$ concentration ($E_{Cl}$ of $-30$ to $-40$ mV), so that activation of GABA$_A$ receptors results in Cl$^-$ efflux and depolarization. GABA$_B$ receptors are coupled to G proteins that control opening of K$^+$ and Ca$^{2+}$ channels.

**(iv)  Glycine receptors**  Glycine receptors in astroglia are functionally similar to GABA$_A$ receptors, being ligand-gated Cl$^-$ channels. These receptors are specifically expressed in spinal cord astrocytes, which reflects the anatomical segregation of glycinergic transmission to the spinal cord. Activation of glycine receptors causes efflux of Cl$^-$ and astrocyte depolarisation.

**(v)  Acetylcholine receptors**  Functional *nicotinic (ionotropic) ACh receptors* have been found in cultured astrocytes and in astrocytes in hippocampal slices (Sharma & Vijayaraghavan, 2001; Shen & Yakel, 2012). These receptors contain the $\alpha 7$ subunit (being therefore of neuronal type), which confers significant Ca$^{2+}$ permeability ($P_{Ca}/P_{monovalent} \approx 6$). As a result, activation of nicotinic ACh receptors triggers Ca$^{2+}$ signals in astroglial cells, both *in vitro* and *in situ*. Astroglia also express metabotropic *muscarinic ACh receptors*, all five subtypes of which (M1–M5 receptors) have been found in cultured astrocytes. Muscarinic ACh receptors are coupled with InsP$_3$ production, and thus stimulate Ca$^{2+}$ release from the intracellular stores. Stimulation of cholinergic neuronal inputs in hippocampus triggers Ca$^{2+}$ signals in astrocytes through muscarinic receptors; this type of signal is involved in regulation of ACh-dependent synaptic plasticity in the hippocampus (Navarrete *et al.*, 2012). Similarly, muscarinic ACh receptors initiate Ca$^{2+}$ signals in hypothalamic tanycytes.

**(vi)  Adrenergic receptors**  Astrocytes in culture and in brain slices express both $\alpha$- ($\alpha$-AR) and $\beta$- ($\beta$-AR) adrenergic receptors. The $\alpha_1$AR are coupled to phospholipase C, and their activation results in formation of InsP$_3$ and subsequent Ca$^{2+}$

release from the ER. These receptors can be stimulated by synaptically released noradrenaline, which, for example was found in Bergmann glial cells in cerebellum. Both $\alpha$ and $\beta$ adrenoceptors mediate astroglial activation *in vivo* following stimulation of locus coeruleus, which sends adrenergic projections around the brain (Bekar *et al.*, 2008). The $\alpha_2$-ARs are present in hippocampal astrocytes, being concentrated on their perisynaptic processes. The $\beta$-AR, and especially $\beta_2$-AR, are related to astrogliosis and are up-regulated in pathological conditions. This up-regulation seems to be functionally relevant, as pharmacological inhibition of $\beta_2$AR affects scar formation. Astroglial $\beta_1$AR are also connected with glycogen synthesis and may mediate cyclic AMP-dependent inhibition of astrocytic $K^+$ channels.

**(vii) Serotonin receptors** Several subtypes of *serotonin or 5-hydroxytryptamine (5-HT) receptors*, including $5\text{-HT}_{1A}$, $5\text{-HT}_{2A}$, $5\text{-HT}_{2B}$ and $5\text{-HT}_{5A}$ receptors, have been identified in astrocytes in cultures, in freshly isolated cells and in brain tissues. The physiological role of these receptors in astrocytes remains largely unknown. Some of the 5-HT receptors are related to neuropathology – for example, astroglial $5\text{-HT}_{5A}$ receptors are up-regulated in reactive astrocytes and in schizophrenia.

**(viii) Histamine receptors** The $H_1$, $H_2$ and $H_3$ histamine receptors, which all represent $G_s/G_q$-protein coupled 7-TM metabotropic receptors, have been found in astrocytes in cultures and *in situ*. $H_1$ and $H_2$ receptors are coupled to the $InsP_3/Ca^{2+}$ release signalling pathway, and their stimulation has been shown to induce $Ca^{2+}$ signals and $[Ca^{2+}]_i$ oscillations in cultured astrocytes, in astrocytes in hippocampal slices, and in Bergmann glial cells in cerebellar slices. Activation of $H_1$ receptors has been reported to increase breakdown of glycogen.

**(ix) Cannabinoid receptors** Cannabinoid receptors of $CB_1$ type have been identified in cultured astrocytes and in astrocytes in brain tissue. These receptors (see Stella, 2010 for comprehensive recent review) are coupled to $G_{o/i}$ proteins, and they mainly regulate astroglial metabolism and have general anti-inflammatory actions, negatively regulating production and secretion of astroglial pro-inflammatory factors. The $CB_1$ receptors are preferentially expressed in perivascular astrocytes, and have been suggested to regulate astroglia-dependent neuronal metabolic support. Stimulation of $CB_1$ receptors also triggers astroglial $Ca^{2+}$ signals, which may be involved in synaptic potentiation in hippocampus (Navarrete & Araque, 2010).

**(x) Neuropeptide receptors** Astrocytes in cultures and *in situ* express a wide variety of neuropeptide receptors, which include receptors to somatostatin, vasoactive intestinal peptide (VIP), tachykinines, oxytocin and vasopressin, calcitonin, glucagon, bradykinin, angiotensin II, atrial natriuretic peptide, opioid peptides, neuropeptide Y, endothelin and many more (see, e.g., Deschepper, 1998). These

receptors control multiple intracellular signalling cascades that regulate many
aspects of astroglial functional responses, e.g. uptake of glucose and neurotransmitters, morphological plasticity, gap junctional permeability, etc. For example,
activation of astroglial endothelin receptors ($ET_A$ and $ET_B$) decreases expression of
gap junctions and therefore inhibits coupling in the astroglial networks. ET
receptors are also linked to astroglial $Ca^{2+}$ signalling through $InsP_3$.

**(xi)  Cytokine and chemokine receptors**  Astroglial cells express various combinations of cytokine and chemokine receptors which, in general, control their
proliferation, growth and metabolism. These receptors are involved in numerous
pathological reactions. The cytokine receptors are represented by two types – type I
and type II receptors – which are activated by interferons and interleukins (IL-2, 4,
6, 10, 12, 15 and 21). The signalling pathways triggered by activation of these
receptors involve the Janus kinases (JAKs) which, in turn, control numerous
secondary signal transduction proteins, such as Signal Transducers and Activators
of Transcription (STATs). The latter, after being phosphorylated by JAKs, translocate into the nucleus, where they initiate transcription of various genes, generally
known as cytokine responsive genes (Figure 4.18).

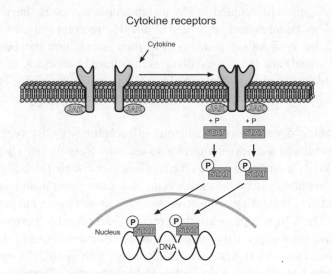

**Figure 4.18**   Cytokine receptors.
   There are many cytokine receptors, but the most common are associated with the Janus
kinase/signal transducer and activator of transcription (JAK/STAT) pathway. Binding of cytokines
to the receptor initiates receptor oligomerisation and phosphorylation by closely associated JAKs.
The phosphorylated receptor becomes a docking site for STAT proteins, which are also phosphorylated by JAKs. Phosphorylated STATs dissociate from the receptors, dimerise and are translocated to the nucleus, where they interact with DNA, hence regulating transcription of genes.

Redrawn from Wessman and Benveniste, 2005.

The second main signalling pathway controlled by cytokines is represented by tumour necrosis factor (TNF) receptors of the TNFRI and TNFRII families, present in all types of glial cells. Activation of TNF receptors regulates activity of JAKs and also utilises the activation of intracellular transcription factor NF-κB.

Astrocytes also express a variety of chemokine receptors. The chemokines are small signalling molecules (8–14 kDa) which regulate cell migration. Chemokine receptors (designated as CCR1–9 and CXCRs) belong to classic seven-transmembrane-domain metabotropic receptors coupled with G proteins which, in turn, control activation of PLC and phosphatidylinositol-3-OH-kinase (PI3K). Further signalling proceeds through either InsP$_3$, which activates Ca$^{2+}$ release from the ER, or through DAG, which activates protein kinase C (PKC). Activation of chemokine receptors may also activate JAK/STAT and NF-κB pathways.

**(xii) Complement receptors** The complement system is one of the key parts of immune responses, components of which are also present in the CNS. In particular, the complement anaphylotoxines C3a and C5a are released in the brain at sites of complement activation. Both astrocytes and microglial cells express C3a and C5a receptors, which control Ca$^{2+}$ release from the ER stores via the InsP$_3$-dependent pathway. Expression of C3a and C5a receptors may be up regulated during inflammation.

**(xiii) Platelet-activating factor receptors** Platelet-activating factor (PAF) is a potent biological mediator; it activates platelets and has various effects on other tissues, including the CNS, where it is involved in regulation of neuronal plasticity, inflammation, apoptosis, etc. The PAF receptors have been identified in cultured astrocytes, and activation of these receptors may induce the release of prostaglandins and mediate cell death.

**(xiv) Thrombin receptors** Thrombin (or factor IIa) is a serine-protease which is involved in cleaving fibrinogen, a central event in the coagulation cascade. Additionally, thrombin triggers various responses in both peripheral tissues and neural cells. In particular, thrombin is suspected to cause severe damage to neural cells and to act as a link between injury, haemostasis and inflammation. The thrombin receptors belong to a family of *protease-activated receptors* (*PAR*) that includes four members, PAR-1 to PAR-4, out of which thrombin activates the PAR1, PAR3 and PAR4 receptors, while PAR2 receptors are sensitive to trypsin or trypsin-like substrate preference proteases. The PAR1 and PAR2 receptors have been found in cultured astrocytes and are implicated in initiation and/or regulation of reactive astrogliosis. These receptors are also believed to regulate release of ATP and glutamate, as well as some chemokines from astroglia.

**(xv) Ephrin receptors** The ephrin B (EphB) receptors are tyrosine kinases, which are activated following binding to the membrane-associated ephrin ligands, generally responsible for contact-dependent cell to cell communication. The EphB receptors have been identified in astrocytes in hippocampus and other brain regions, where they negatively regulate expression of glutamate transporters GLT1 and GLAST. In cultured astrocytes, activation of EphB receptors has been found to increase synthesis and release of the neuromodulator D-serine. These findings suggest that EphB receptors may be involved in synaptic plasticity (see Murai & Pasquale, 2011, for details).

**(xvi)  Succinate receptors**  Specific receptors to extracellular succinate, which is a part of the citric acid cycle and a general metabolite, have been found in astrocytes from nucleus accumbens. These receptors belong to the 7-TM metabotropic family, and the astroglial type most likely is represented by succinate receptor 1 or SUCNR1/GPCR91. Activation of this receptor by exogenous succinate triggers $Ca^{2+}$ signalling (by activation of $Ca^{2+}$ release from the ER) in a subpopulation of nucleus accumbens astrocytes (Molnar *et al.*, 2011).

## 4.5.4  Astroglial membrane transporters

Members of the extended class of molecules that reside in the cellular membranes and provide for specific transport of substances across these membranes are generally classified as membrane transporters. These are very many, and the human genome contains $\approx 1,020$ genes encoding membrane transporters, which generally are sub-classified into secondary transporters, ion and water channels, and ATP-dependent transporters (Figure 4.19). Of these, the largest group ($\approx 44$ per cent) is

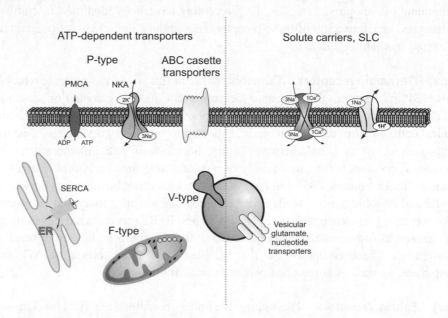

**Figure 4.19**  Classification of membrane transporters (see text for further explanations).

represented by secondary transporters, so named because transport of their preferred substances is coupled to movement of other solutes down the electrochemical gradients; these gradients act as a form of pre-accumulated energy. The ATP-dependent transporters directly utilise ATP to fuel their activities. The membrane transporters are particularly important for astrocytes because, as CNS homeostatic cells, they control movements of a great deal of various substances, including ions, neurotransmitters and metabolic substrates. As a result, astrocytes express a huge variety of transporters, which will be overviewed below.

**(i)  ATP-dependent transporters**  These are grouped into four main classes which include the ion-pumps of *P-type, F-type and V-type* and *ATP-binding cassette (ABC) transporters* that translocate various substrates such as sugars, peptides, polysaccharides, proteins and also ions. Astrocytes contain several P-type ion pumps. These pumps are tetramers, being composed of two $\alpha$ and two $\beta$ subunits; the $\alpha$ subunit contains the ATP-binding/phosphorylation site. The most characterised P-type astroglial ATP-dependent transporter is the *sodium-potassium pump or $Na^+/K^+$ ATPase (NKA)*; in astroglia it is mostly composed of $\alpha2$ subunits. The NKA extrudes $Na^+$ to the extracellular space, while delivering $K^+$ to the cytosol. An $\alpha2$ subtype of NKA co-localises with the $Na^+/Ca^{2+}$ exchanger in astrocytes at plasma membrane-ER junctions – a site of presumed 'sodium micro-domains' (Lencesova *et al.*, 2004), which will be discussed in depth later in the context of astroglial $Na^+$ signalling.

The continuous NKA-dependent maintenance of the $Na^+$ gradient is a major ATP expenditure in astrocytes. Astroglial plasma membrane also contains ATP-dependent $Ca^{2+}$ pumps or *plasmalemmal $Ca^{2+}$ ATPases (PMCAs)*, which extrude excess of $Ca^{2+}$ into the extracellular space, thus maintaining cell $Ca^{2+}$ homeostasis.

The intracellular endomembrane of the endoplasmic reticulum contains another subfamily of $Ca^{2+}$ pumps known as *Sarco(Endo)Plasmic Reticulum $Ca^{2+}$ATP-ases or SERCAs*. The SERCA pumps are responsible for $Ca^{2+}$ accumulation into the lumen of the endoplasmic reticulum, and are therefore critical for intracellular $Ca^{2+}$ release.

The *F-type* and *V-type ion pumps* are involved in proton transport. The V-type pumps are present in lysosomes and have been found in astrocytes, where they provide for an acidic intralysosmal environment. In addition, astrocytes contain neurotransmitter vesicles that express V-type $H^+$ pumps, which provide the $H^+$ gradient needed for accumulation of glutamate and ATP into these vesicles. The F-type pumps are ubiquitously present in mitochondria, where they provide for ATP synthesis.

The *ABC transporters* represent an extended superfamily of ATP-dependent transporters, of which more than 100 members are known (Hartz & Bauer, 2011). These pumps are sub-classified into five groups (from A to G) and are expressed throughout the CNS. In particular, ABC transporters are fundamental for transport of many substances across the blood-brain barrier. Astrocytes express several types of ABC transporters, mostly of group A, although their functions remain generally unknown.

**(ii)  Secondary transporters**   These are mostly represented by solute carrier or SLC transporters which are represented by ≈378 members divided into 51 different families according to their structural similarities and preferred substrates (Hediger *et al.*, 2004; Ren *et al.*, 2007; see www.bioparadigms.org/slc/menu.asp). Most of the SLC transporters move two solutes across the plasma membrane, either in the same direction (symports) or in opposite directions (antiports). Astrocytes express multiple SLC transporters (see Featherstone, 2011, for a recent comprehensive review), the most important of which are described below.

- *Glutamate transporters* (see Danbolt, 2001; Eulenburg & Gomeza, 2010 and references therein), belong to the SLC1 superfamily and are represented by *Excitatory Amino Acid Transporters 1–5* (EAAT1/SLC1A3, EAAT2/SLC1A2, EAAT3/SLC1A1, EAAT4/SLC1A6 and EAAT5/SLC1A7). Astrocytes specifically express EAAT-1 and EAAT-2 transporters, which, in rodents, are designated as glutamate/aspartate transporter (GLAST) and glutamate transporter-1 (GLT-1). Glutamate is a monovalent anion at physiological pH, and transport of a single molecule requires influx of three $Na^+$ ions and efflux of one $K^+$ ion down their concentration gradients. In addition, glutamate brings one more $H^+$ ion into the cell. The net influx of cations manifests the electrogenic effect of glutamate transporters, which appears in the form of an inward current. Sodium influx associated with glutamate transport may increase intracellular $Na^+$ concentration by tens of mM.

- *GABA transporters* (*GAT*). Four GATs are known and are represented by GAT-1/SLC6A1, GAT-2/SLC6A11, GAT-3/SLC6A12 and betaine/GABA transporter-1, BGT-1/SLC6A13. Astrocytes predominantly express GAT-3 (see Conti *et al.*, 2004 for review). GATs mediate the symport of one uncharged GABA molecule, two $Na^+$ ions and one $Cl^-$ ion (Attwell *et al.*, 1993). Similar to EAATs, GABA uptake via GATs is an electrogenic process, which is manifested by an inward current, and activation of GATs can elevate $[Na^+]_i$ by up to ≈5–7 mM (Eulenburg & Gomeza, 2010; Kirischuk *et al.*, 2012).

- *Glycine transporters* (*GlyT*). Astrocytes in hippocampus, cortex, cerebellum, brain stem and spinal cord express (more or less specifically) the glycine transporter GlyT1/ SLC6A9. GlyT1 transports glycine, together with $2Na^+$ and $1~Cl^-$ (Eulenburg & Gomeza, 2010). These transporters are important for maintaining extracellular glycine homeostasis, and their genetic ablation triggers respiratory abnormalities and early death (Gomeza *et al.*, 2003).

- *Sodium-calcium exchanger,* or *NCX*. NCX belong to the SLC8 family (Lytton, 2007) and is represented by three gene products, NCX1/SLC8A1,

NCX2/SLC8A2 and NCX3/SLC8A3, all of which are expressed in astroglia (Kirischuk *et al.*, 2012). The NCX exchanges $2Na^+$ for 1 $Ca^{2+}$ and, according to the thermodynamics, may operate in both forward ($Ca^{2+}$ extrusion associated with $Na^+$ influx) and reverse ($Ca^{2+}$ entry associated with $Na^+$ extrusion) modes. The switch between forward/reverse operational modes is controlled by $Na^+$ and $Ca^{2+}$ transmembrane ion gradients and the level of membrane potential. Depolarisation and increased intracellular $Na^+$ concentration favours reverse mode of NCX.

Incidentally, another version of the $Na^+/Ca^{2+}$ exchanger, the $K^+$-dependent NCX (the NCKX/SLC24 exchangers), although being expressed in the brain, are exclusively present in neurones, and have not been detected in astrocytes (Altimimi & Schnetkamp, 2007). *The mitochondrial $Na^+/Ca^{2+}$ exchanger, or NCXL*, transports $Na^+$ into and $Ca^+$ out of the mitochondrial matrix, and is present in astrocytes.

- *Sodium-proton exchanger, or* NHE. The $Na^+/H^+$ exchangers (plasmalemmal and intracellular) are ubiquitous for all lifeforms (Brett *et al.*, 2005). In mammals, the NHE pumps protons into the cells, utilising the transmembrane $Na^+$ gradient to counteract alkalisation of the cytoplasm. There are at least eight genes (NHE1-8/SLC9A1-A8) encoding this exchanger in human genome. Astrocytes express NHE, although their intracellular pH is less dominated by it due to the presence of sodium bicarbonate co-transporter.

- *Sodium-bicarbonate co transporter, NBC* (which in humans is encoded by SLC4A5 gene), is involved in pH homeostasis by providing for transmembrane translocation of bicarbonate (Deitmer & Rose, 2010). The NBC is electrogenic, with stoichiometry of 1 $Na^+$: 2 or 3 $HCO_3^-$; NBC is expressed in astroglia, with higher expression levels in grey matter astrocytes and in Bergmann glia (Schmitt *et al.*, 2000).

- *Sodium-potassium chloride co-transporter, NKCC1.* The $Na^+$-$K^+$-$Cl^-$ cotransporter 1 (encoded by SLC12A2 gene) contributes to the regulation of extracellular $K^+$ homeostasis in the CNS. It electroneutrally transports $Na^+$, $K^+$, and $Cl^-$ ions into and out of cells with a stoichiometry of 1 $Na^+$: 1$K^+$: 2$Cl^-$. Based on their pharmacological sensitivity to furosemide or bumetanide, NKCC1 has been shown to functionally operate in cultured astrocytes and in astrocytes from the rat optic nerve. In the latter preparation, its expression was also confirmed by immunostaining (MacVicar *et al.*, 2002).

- Vesicular transporters for *glutamate (VGluT/SLC17A6-8)* and for *nucleotides (VNUT/SLC17A9)* are present in astroglial cells, where they mediate accumulation of glutamate and ATP into vesicles that underlie $Ca^{2+}$-regulatied exocytosis of neurotransmitters from astrocytes (see Sreedharan *et al.*, 2010 for detailed review).

- Another functionally important family of transporters is represented by the *monocarboxylate transporters (SLC16 family)*. Astrocytes use *monocarboxylate transporter 1 (SLC16A1)* to release lactate that is subsequently used by neurones as an energy substrate.

- Astrocytes also specifically express *sodium coupled neutral amino acid transporters SN1/SNAT3/SLC38A3 and SN2/SNAT5/SLC38A5*, which mediate glutamine efflux from astroglia and thus are critically important for the glutamate-glutamine and GABA-glutamine shuttle (see Section 4.5.9).

## 4.5.5  Calcium signalling in astroglia

Despite a common ontogenetic origin, neurones and astroglia are fundamentally different in their excitability. Neuronal excitability, which is generally defined as electrical excitability, is determined by the existence of a specific complement of voltage-operated ion channels ($Na^+$ channels, $K^+$ channels and, to a lesser extent, $Ca^{2+}$ channels) in the plasmalemma. Depolarisation of the neuronal plasma membrane (resulting from a sensory or synaptic input) to a certain threshold activates these channels, which in turn generate regenerative action potentials that propagate mainly along the axon. Astrocytes are electrically non-excitable and unable to generate plasmalemmal action potentials, due to a very low density of voltage-operated channels in their plasma membrane. Nevertheless, glial cells are excitable in the sense of responding actively to information from their surroundings. One of the principal mechanisms used by astroglia as a substrate of their excitability is $Ca^{2+}$ signalling, the main principles of which were discussed in Chapter 2.

**(i)  Endoplasmic reticulum provides for $Ca^{2+}$ excitability of astrocytes**  Astroglial $Ca^{2+}$ excitability is almost exclusively controlled by receptors to neurotransmitters and neurohormones. The main route for astroglial responses to chemical stimulation is associated with $Ca^{2+}$ release from the endoplasmic reticulum (ER) $Ca^{2+}$ store. The ER is highly developed in astrocytes; the intricate network of microtubulae and cisternae that constitutes the ER forms the nuclear envelope, occupies the cell body and penetrates into cell processes (Figure 4.20).

Regenerative opening of ER $Ca^{2+}$ channels creates a propagating wave of endomembrane excitation, and subsequent activation of SERCA pumps terminates the $Ca^{2+}$ signal. The intra-ER $Ca^{2+}$ concentration in glial cells varies between 100–300 μM, thus being lower compared to neurones, where intra-ER free $Ca^{2+}$ reaches 300–800 μM. Numerous experiments on neuroglial cells *in vitro*, *in situ* and *in vivo* have identified expression of multiple metabotropic receptors that, when activated by physiological stimulation, trigger production of inositol 1,4,5-trisphosphate ($InsP_3$) and subsequent $InsP_3$-induced $Ca^{2+}$ release from the ER.

Generally, $Ca^{2+}$ signals induced by activation of metabotropic receptors (most notably by ATP and glutamate) share a similar set of properties. These $[Ca^{2+}]_i$

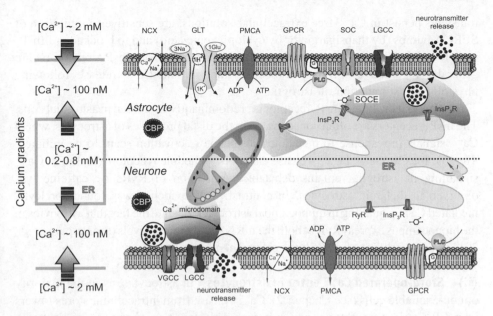

**Figure 4.20**   Calcium signalling cascades in neurones and glia.

The force driving calcium signalling is formed by $Ca^{2+}$ concentration gradients, which in turn are created by energy-dependent $Ca^{2+}$ transport across cellular membranes. Physiological stimulation opens plasmalemmal or intracellular $Ca^{2+}$ channels, thus creating $Ca^{2+}$ fluxes affecting $[Ca^{2+}]$ in various intracellular compartments. In neural cells, calcium signalling events occur either in the form of localised $[Ca^{2+}]_i$ microdomains or as global $[Ca^{2+}]_i$ elevation. The $Ca^{2+}$ microdomains regulate various localised functional responses, being primarily responsible for the release of neuro- and gliotransmitters. Conceptually, neuronal $Ca^{2+}$ signals mainly rely on $Ca^{2+}$ entry via voltage- and ligand-gated plasmalemmal $Ca^{2+}$ channels; this $Ca^{2+}$ entry creates short-lived $[Ca^{2+}]_i$ microdomains, which determine fast and focal neurotransmitter release from the synaptic terminals. In glial cells, $Ca^{2+}$ signals are usually initiated by $Ca^{2+}$ release from the ER that create more widespread and longer-lasting $[Ca^{2+}]_i$ elevation, thus determining slower and more sustained release of gliotransmitters. The domains of elevated $[Ca^{2+}]_i$ are sensed by mitochondria, which are able to accumulate $Ca^{2+}$ via uniporters. Mitochondrial $Ca^{2+}$ entry acts as the main link between neural cells, activity and energy production, by regulating mitochondrial electron transport and ATP synthesis.

The $Ca^{2+}$ signalling cascades are tightly integrated in the overall cellular homeostatic system. In astrocytes, in particular, the sodium-calcium exchanger is co-localised with $Na^+$-dependent glutamate transporters. This arrangement allows rapid reversal of the transporter in response to $[Na^+]_i$ elevation associated with glutamate transport, which (i) maintains $Na^+$ gradients needed for glutamate transporter function and (ii) creates local $Ca^{2+}$ signals by $Ca^{2+}$ entry through the exchanger.

*Abbreviations*: CBP – $Ca^{2+}$-binding protein; ER – endoplasmic reticulum; GLT – glutamate transporter; GPCR – G-protein coupled receptor; $InsP_3R$ – inositol(1,4,5)triphosphate receptor; LGCC – ligand-gated $Ca^{2+}$ channel; NCX – sodium-calcium exchanger; PMCA – plasmalemmal $Ca^{2+}$ ATP-ase; RyR – ryanodine receptor; SERCA – sarco(endo)plasmic reticulum $Ca^{2+}$ ATP-ase; SOC – store-operated $Ca^{2+}$ channel; VGCC – voltage-operated $Ca^{2+}$ channel; 'Maxi' channel – high-permeability plasma-lemmal channels (such as connexins or pannexins or $P2X_7$ receptors or volume-regulated anion channels) which can act as a pathway for non-exocytotic gliotransmitter release. The role of $Ca^{2+}$ signals in controlling the activation and permeability status of these channels remains unknown.

transients persist in $Ca^{2+}$-free extracellular solutions, are sensitive to inhibition of SERCA pumps (by thapsigargin or by cyclopiazonic acid) and to blockade of $InsP_3$ receptors by intracellular administration of heparin. The $InsP_3$ receptors are generally regarded as primary molecules that initiate $Ca^{2+}$ release following physiological stimulation of astroglia.

It seems that the type 2 $InsP_3$ receptor is predominantly expressed in astroglial cells. The $InsP_3$ receptors are often concentrated in the distal processes of astrocytes, where $Ca^{2+}$ signals in response to metabotropic receptor activation seem to be initiated. The role for $Ca^{2+}$-gated $Ca^{2+}$ release channels/ryanodine receptors (RyRs) in $Ca^{2+}$ signalling in astroglia remains debatable. Activation of RyRs by caffeine was observed in thalamic astrocytes. In contrast, little evidence was found for RyR-mediated $Ca^{2+}$ signalling in hippocampal astrocytes, despite the fact that astrocytes in the hippocampus express RyR at both the mRNA and protein levels (see Parpura *et al.*, 2011; Verkhratsky *et al.*, 2012b for comprehensive review).

**(ii)  Store-operated $Ca^{2+}$ entry in astrocytes**  In astrocytes, as in the majority of non-excitable cells (see Chapter 2), $Ca^{2+}$ release from intracellular stores lowers intra-ER $Ca^{2+}$ concentration, which in turn activates store-operated $Ca^{2+}$ entry or SOCE. Astroglial SOCE has been characterised in numerous experiments both *in vitro* and *in situ*, and is mediated through TRP channels. Astrocytes (both freshly isolated and in culture) were found to express canonical type TRP (TRPC) channels assembled from an obligatory TRPC1 combined with ancillary TRPC4 and/or TRPC5 proteins (Malarkey *et al.*, 2008; Parpura *et al.*, 2011). Down-regulation of expression of TRPC1 channel by antisense knock-down, or its inhibition by a blocking antibody directed at an epitope in the pore-forming region of the TRPC1 protein, significantly suppresses SOCE in cultured astrocytes.

The classical $Ca^{2+}$-release activated $Ca^{2+}$ channels (CRACs), which produce $Ca^{2+}$-release activated $Ca^{2+}$ currents ($I_{CRAC}$) in many non-excitable cells (see Chapter 2), have not been detected in astrocytes. Although there are certain similarities in the pharmacological profiles of SOCE in astroglia and in the rat basophilic leukaemia cell line, which express the CRAC mechanism, the Orai and STIM1 proteins, which underlie CRAC channel functional activity, have only been found in an astroglial cell line; their expression in astrocytes *in situ* has not been indentified. Therefore, TRPC channels are likely candidates for SOCE in astroglial cells.

**(iii)  Ionotropic $Ca^{2+}$ permeable receptors in astrocytes**  $Ca^{2+}$ entry pathways in mature glial cells are represented by several types of $Ca^{2+}$-permeable ligand-gated channels. As has been already discussed above, astrocytes express several types of ionotropic receptors with $Ca^{2+}$ permeability, which are mainly represented by AMPA and NMDA glutamate receptors, together with $P2X_{1/5}$ and $P2X_7$ purinoceptors. These receptors, when activated by synaptically released neurotransmitter, can generate $Ca^{2+}$ signals in astrocytes in brain slices (Palygin *et al.*, 2010).

**(iv)   Sodium/calcium exchanger in astroglial Ca$^{2+}$ signalling**   Another molecular pathway for plasmalemmal Ca$^{2+}$ fluxes in astroglia is represented by Na$^+$/Ca$^{2+}$ exchangers. NCX-mediated Ca$^{2+}$ fluxes in both forward and reverse modes have been found in astrocytes in culture and in brain slices.

The interplay between Ca$^{2+}$ release, Ca$^{2+}$ reuptake into the ER, Ca$^{2+}$ entry/efflux through store-operated channels, ionotropic receptors, NCX and plasmalemmal Ca$^{2+}$ pumps determines the shape of the resulting Ca$^{2+}$ signal, which may vary from a rapid and transient peak-like response, through [Ca$^{2+}$]$_i$ elevations lasting up to hundreds of seconds with a clear plateau, to Ca$^{2+}$ oscillations. These kinetically different [Ca$^{2+}$]$_i$ changes underlie the temporal coding of the Ca$^{2+}$ signal, whereas [Ca$^{2+}$]$_i$ oscillations are responsible for frequency coding of the Ca$^{2+}$ signal.

**(v)   Mitochondria in astroglial Ca$^{2+}$ signalling**   Mitochondria play a dual role in astroglial Ca$^{2+}$ signalling, acting both as a Ca$^{2+}$ buffer and as a Ca$^{2+}$ source. Inhibition of the mitochondrial uniporter by Ruthenium 360, and hence blockade of mitochondrial Ca$^{2+}$ sequestration, has been shown to increase the amplitude of mechanically-stimulated [Ca$^{2+}$]$_i$ transients in cultured astrocytes. Conversely, limiting mitochondrial Ca$^{2+}$ release by inhibiting the mitochondrial Na$^+$/Ca$^{2+}$ exchanger with 7-chloro-5-(2-chlorophenyl)-1,5-dihydro-4,1-benzothiazepin-2 (3H)-one (CGP37157), reduces mechanically-induced [Ca$^{2+}$]$_i$ increase. Similar attenuation of astroglial Ca$^{2+}$ signalling can be achieved by an inhibition of the mitochondrial transition permeability pore (MPTP), a high conductance channel whose transient openings may underlie rapid Ca$^{2+}$ removal from mitochondria. Inhibition of MPTP opening with cyclosporin A reduced astroglial [Ca$^{2+}$]$_i$ transients (Reyes & Parpura, 2008).

**(vi)   Calcium waves in astrocytes**   In physiological conditions, glia are stimulated by relatively brief and local exposures to neurotransmitters. This local stimulation produces similarly localised events of Ca$^{2+}$ release through InsP$_3$R, yet these highly localised events may give rise to a propagating signal that will swamp the whole cell. Importantly, in glial cells – and particularly in astrocytes – propagation of these Ca$^{2+}$ waves is not limited by cellular borders, and instead can cross the intercellular boundaries to spread over a relatively long distance through the astrocytic syncytium.

*Intracellular Ca$^{2+}$ waves* occur because of a special property of the ER membrane, which, similar to the plasmalemma of excitable cells, is able to convert a local supra-threshold response into a propagating wave of excitation. The Ca$^{2+}$ sensitivity of InsP$_3$R and RyR is what makes the ER membrane an excitable medium. A focal Ca$^{2+}$ release, induced by a localised elevation of InsP$_3$, recruits neighbouring channels, which not only amplifies the initial Ca$^{2+}$ release event but also creates a propagating wave of Ca$^{2+}$ release along the ER membrane (Figure 4.21). This simple mechanism underlies the propagation of Ca$^{2+}$ signals in almost all types of non-excitable cell. It is important to remember that the Ca$^{2+}$

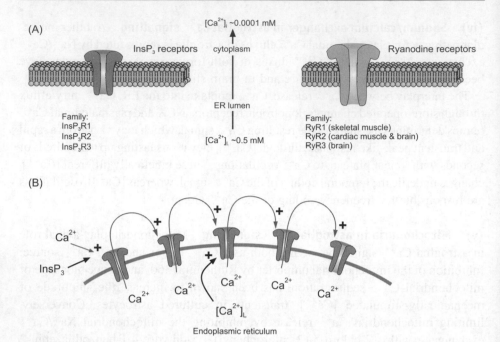

**Figure 4.21** Mechanisms of propagating waves of calcium release from the endoplasmic reticulum.

A. Intracellular $Ca^{2+}$ release channels are represented by two families: $InsP_3$-gated $Ca^{2+}$ channels or $InsP_3$ receptors ($InsP_3R$), and $Ca^{2+}$-gated $Ca^{2+}$ channels, or Ryanodine receptors (RyR).

B. Mechanism of propagating intracellular $Ca^{2+}$ waves is determined by the $Ca^{2+}$ sensitivity of both $InsP_3R$ and RyR; local increases in $[Ca^{2+}]_i$ activate neighbouring channels and produce a propagating wave of excitation of ER-resident $Ca^{2+}$ release channels.

wave is not a propagating wave of $Ca^{2+}$ ions themselves, because the movement of $Ca^{2+}$ ions is severely restricted by cytoplasmic $Ca^{2+}$ buffering. Instead, the $Ca^{2+}$ wave results from a propagating wave of elementary $Ca^{2+}$ release events associated with the opening of $Ca^{2+}$ release channels through the endomembrane.

*Intercellular $Ca^{2+}$ waves in astroglial networks:* the intercellular $Ca^{2+}$ waves that propagate between astrocytes were, for the first time, discovered in confluent astroglial cell cultures. In these experiments, cultured astrocytes were focally stimulated with glutamate, and this local stimulation triggered an initial $Ca^{2+}$ rise in several cells, which subsequently spread through the whole culture. The propagating $Ca^{2+}$ waves had a complex path, crossing cell borders without delay and travelling through the cells with a velocity of $\approx15$–$20$ $\mu m/s$ (Cornell Bell *et al.*, 1990). The intercellular $Ca^{2+}$ waves in cultured astroglia could also be evoked by focal mechanical stimulation, although these waves were somewhat different in that they demonstrated delay at cell borders (Charles *et al.*, 1991).

These observations were soon confirmed by several groups, and it was also discovered that the propagation of astroglial $Ca^{2+}$ waves ultimately requires functional ER $Ca^{2+}$ stores; $Ca^{2+}$ waves are completely blocked either by inhibition of SERCA-mediated ER $Ca^{2+}$ accumulation (exposure to thapsigargin or cyclopiazonic acid) or by inhibition of PLC with the specific inhibitor U73122.

Subsequently, propagating $Ca^{2+}$ waves were discovered in astrocytes in organo-typic and acute slices from hippocampus and corpus callosum. Propagating $Ca^{2+}$ waves were also observed in acutely isolated preparations of retina (Newman & Zahs, 1997), where they could be elicited by focal applications of ATP, carbachol or phenylephrine (incidentally, glutamate was inactive, once more indicating functional heterogeneity of astrocytes). Retinal $Ca^{2+}$ waves propagated at the speed of $\approx 25$ μm/s and were completely blocked by thapsigargin (for detailed overview of $Ca^{2+}$ waves and relevant references, see Scemes & Giaume, 2006).

The extent, and even physiological existence, of propagated astroglial $Ca^{2+}$ waves *in vivo* is yet to be fully characterised. In several imaging experiments of rodent brain, astroglial $Ca^{2+}$ waves appeared to be restricted to individual astrocytes or to a limited number of adjacent cells, without much spreading to neighbouring regions. Similarly, stimulation of sensory inputs (e.g. mechanical displacement of whiskers in mice) induced $Ca^{2+}$ signals in astrocytes in the barrel cortex, but these signals were confined to single cells and did not produce propagating $Ca^{2+}$ waves (Wang *et al.*, 2006). Likewise, in the visual cortex of ferrets, sensory stimulation induced $Ca^{2+}$ responses in individual astrocytes but did not trigger $Ca^{2+}$ waves (Schummers *et al.*, 2008).

At the same time, synchronised propagating $Ca^{2+}$ waves that rapidly engulf hundreds (if not thousands) of astrocytes have been recorded *in vivo* in mouse hippocampus and neocortex (Kuga *et al.*, 2011). These $Ca^{2+}$ waves, which the authors of the study called '*glissandi*'[1], embraced almost all astrocytes in the entire CA1 region and spread with a velocity of $\approx 60$ μm/s, thus being much faster compared to $Ca^{2+}$ waves observed in culture and in slice preparations. These hippocampal glissandi were blocked by tetrodotoxin (which inhibits action poten-tials in neurones) and were sensitive to inhibitors of gap junctions and purinocep-tors. Inhibition by tetrodotoxin is somewhat suspicious, indicating a primary role for electrical activity of neuronal networks in this phenomenon. Propagating $Ca^{2+}$ waves were also observed in cortical astrocytes imaged *in vivo* in response to focal application of α/β-adrenoceptors agonists (Bekar *et al.*, 2008).

There are several distinct mechanisms that may generate propagating $Ca^{2+}$ waves in astroglial networks (see schemes on Figure 4.22), which include:

1. direct intercellular diffusion of InsP$_3$ via gap junctions;

2. regenerative release of a diffusible extracellular messenger (e.g. ATP) trigger-ing metabotropic receptor-mediated $Ca^{2+}$ release in neighbouring cells;

---

[1] *Glissandi* is plural from *glissando*, which means a rapid series of ascending or descending notes on the musical scale. The authors probably tried to stress the speed and uni-directional character of these $Ca^{2+}$ waves.

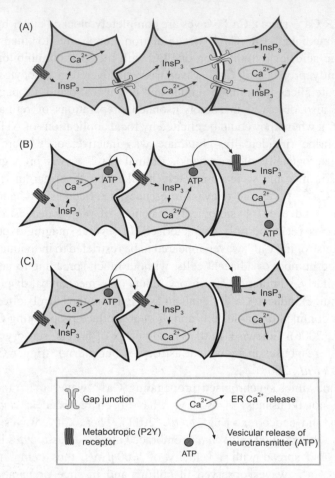

**Figure 4.22** Mechanisms of generation of propagating intercellular $Ca^{2+}$ waves.

Propagation of inter-glial $Ca^{2+}$ waves can be supported by several distinct mechanisms, which can operate separately or in combination:

A.  $Ca^{2+}$ waves can be maintained by diffusion of $InsP_3$ through the gap junction and secondary initiation of $InsP_3$-induced $Ca^{2+}$ release.

B.  $Ca^{2+}$ waves can be maintained by regenerative $Ca^{2+}$-dependent release of 'gliotransmitters' (see Figure 5.14) acting on neighbouring cells through extracellular diffusion.

C.  $Ca^{2+}$ waves can result from a focal release of 'gliotransmitter', which then diffuses over a long distance.

3. diffusion of an extracellular messenger after release from a single cell;

4. any combination of the above.

Historically, the first mechanism to be described was the diffusion of InsP$_3$ through gap junctions. The role for gap junctions in $Ca^{2+}$ wave propagation was suggested following the observation that wave propagation was blocked by broad spectrum gap junction inhibitors, such as octanol and halothane. Subsequently, it was shown that in C6 gliomas intercellular $Ca^{2+}$ waves could be generated only in cultures transfected with gap junction-forming proteins – connexins. Importantly, the gap junction-mediated connectivity that controls the extent of propagation and direction of astroglial $Ca^{2+}$ waves can be regulated by neuronal firing and various neurotransmitters (Giaume & McCarthy, 1996). In addition, the gap junctional communication pathway strictly depends on the anatomical segregation of astroglial syncytia networks, which will be dealt with in detail below.

The second and third mechanisms involve extracellular diffusion of transmitters (usually ATP or glutamate) released by astrocytes. This was initially discovered *in vitro* in confluent astroglial cultures. In these cultures, a cell-free line was mechanically drawn and the $Ca^{2+}$ wave was shown to jump over this cell-free gap of up to 120 μm in width, thus suggesting the role of a diffusable extracellular messenger (Hassinger *et al.*, 1997). This mechanism was subsequently confirmed and it was found that transmitters can be released from astroglia either through $Ca^{2+}$-regulated exocytosis or through diffusion via plasmalemmal pores associated with unpaired connexin hemichannels or ATP-permeable anion channels (Anderson *et al.*, 2004; Arcuino *et al.*, 2002).

These main mechanisms of $Ca^{2+}$ wave propagation may co-exist, or may be differentially employed in astroglial syncytia in different brain regions. In neocortex, for example, propagating astroglial $Ca^{2+}$ waves ultimately depend on the expression of Cx43, as genetic deletion of this protein results in the complete disappearance of astroglial $Ca^{2+}$ waves. In contrast, the spread of $Ca^{2+}$ waves in hippocampus and corpus callosum relies primarily on release of ATP and subsequent activation of metabotropic P2Y receptors (Haas *et al.*, 2006). In the retina, gap junctions propagate $Ca^{2+}$ wave between astrocytes, while ATP release mediates $Ca^{2+}$ waves between astrocytes and Müller cells (Newman & Zahs, 1997).

In conclusion, intercellular $Ca^{2+}$ waves provide astrocytes with the means for long-distance communication. Thus, astrocytes are 'excitable', but signal propagation is fundamentally different from that in neurones. In neurones, the substrate for excitability is the plasma membrane, which generates a rapidly (milliseconds) propagating wave of openings/closures of $Na^+/K^+$ channels (propagating action potential). In contrast, the substrate for excitability in astrocytes is the intracellular ER membrane, which generates a much slower (seconds to minutes) propagating wave of openings/closures of $Ca^{2+}$ channels.

## 4.5.6   Sodium signalling in astrocytes

Intracellular fluctuations in concentrations of sodium ions ($[Na^+]_i$), which frequently occur in physiologically stimulated astrocytes, may also serve a signalling function and translate extracellular events (e.g. increase in extracellular glutamate) into various astroglial functional responses. Sodium ions enter the astroglial cytoplasm through channels, exchangers and transporters. In particular, ionotropic receptors expressed in astrocytes in a physiological context mainly generate $Na^+$ currents. This reflects the much higher concentration of $Na^+$ in the extracellular space. Some astrocytes (e.g. those located in subfornical organ, which are involved in systemic $Na^+$ homeostasis, as discussed below) express specific sodium channels activated by extracellular $Na^+$ concentration ($Na_x$ channels; Shimizu *et al.*, 2007). Finally, astrocytes express Epithelial Sodium Channel (ENaC), proton-activated Acid Sensing Ion Channels (ASIC) and several types of transient receptor potential (TRP) channels, which all can generate substantial $Na^+$ influx in physiological conditions (Kirischuk *et al.*, 2012).

Many types of plasmalemmal transporters ($Na^+/K^+$ ATPase, $Na^+/HCO_3^-$ cotransporter (NBC), $Na^+/H^+$ exchanger (NHE), $Na^+/K^+/Cl^-$ cotransporter 1 (NKCC1) and $Na^+/Ca^{2+}$ exchanger (NCX)) also generate substantial $Na^+$ fluxes. In addition, $Na^+$ influx into astrocytes is mediated by $Na^+$-dependent neurotransmitter transporters. The glutamate transporters EAAT1 and EAAT2, and GABA transporters GAT-1 and GAT-3, are activated during synaptic transmission and generate substantial $Na^+$ inward currents.

Importantly, morphological studies have demonstrated that neurotransmitter receptors (e.g. NMDA receptors), NCX, $Na^+/K^+$ ATPase and glutamate/GABA transporters are concentrated and co-localised in astroglial perisynaptic processes, thereby being strategically placed for sensing synaptic events.

Stimulation of astrocytes in cultures and *in situ* by neurotransmitters may increase $[Na^+]_i$ by 10–20 mM. Similarly, electrical stimulation of neuronal afferents induce a $[Na^+]_i$ rise in astrocytes. This is mainly mediated by activation of glutamate and/or GABA transporters (Deitmer & Rose, 2010; Kirischuk *et al.*, 2012). The astroglial $[Na^+]_i$ increases may also form propagating $[Na^+]_i$ waves, which spread through many cells and are mediated by $Na^+$ diffusion through gap junctions formed by connexins Cx30 and Cx43 (Langer *et al.*, 2012).

As has been already mentioned, the resting cytosolic $Na^+$ concentration ($[Na^+]_i$) in astrocytes is generally higher compared to neurones. For example, the resting $[Na^+]_i$ in cultured hippocampal astrocytes has been determined at 15–17 mM, which is about two times higher when compared to neurones. This high resting $[Na^+]_i$ sets the reversal potential for the $Na^+$ dependent transporters; for example, the reversal potential for NCX and GABA transporters is close to the astroglial resting potential, so that even relatively small depolarisations or increases in $[Na^+]_i$ turn them into the reverse mode, thus initiating $Ca^{2+}$ influx or GABA efflux.

It has become obvious recently that activity-dependent fluctuations in astroglial $[Na^+]_i$ regulate numerous pathways directly involved in astroglial homeostatic responses and, therefore, in astroglial-neuronal communications. Many membrane transporters are affected by changing the transmembrane $Na^+$ gradient and, hence, their appropriate reversal potentials (see Figure 4.23).

First, fluctuations in $[Na^+]_i$ affect homeostasis of several neurotransmitters (most notably glutamate, GABA and glycine). Astroglial glutamate uptake though EAAT1/2 is driven by the transmembrane $Na^+$ gradient, which dynamically controls functional activity of the glutamate transporter. Increases in $[Na^+]_i$ at the very peak of glutamatergic synaptic transmission events reduce glutamate uptake, thus transiently increasing the effective glutamate concentration in the synaptic cleft. In addition, $[Na^+]_i$ regulates the efficacy of glutamate to glutamine conversion through direct action on glutamine synthetase, and subsequent export of glutamine from astrocytes to neurones is also mediated through sodium-coupled neutral amino acid transporter SNAT3/SLC38A3. Similarly, $[Na^+]_i$ regulates and even directs movements of GABA and glycine, and raised $[Na^+]_i$ stimulates the release of both neurotransmitters.

Second, by controlling forward/reverse mode of NCX, $[Na^+]_i$ controls $Ca^{2+}$ influx and may contribute to the generation of rapid localised $[Ca^{2+}]_i$ increases. These $[Ca^{2+}]_i$ microdomains can be important for localised astroglial responses, such as activation of exocytosis.

Third, $[Na^+]_i$ fluctuations control the activity of many ion transporters involved in control of CNS ion homeostasis. For example, $[Na^+]_i$ may regulate $K^+$ buffering through affecting $Na^+/K^+$ ATPase and $Na^+/K^+/Cl^-$ co-transporter NKCC1. Changes in $[Na^+]_i$ also directly modulate $H^+/OH^-/HCO_3^-$ transport systems, which are fundamental for pH homeostasis, both intra- and extracellular. By regulating these many ion transporters, $[Na^+]_i$ is also involved in regulation of astroglial cell volume.

Fourth, $[Na^+]_i$ regulates another fundamental function of astroglia – that is, providing the metabolic substrate (lactate) to neurones. Indeed, $[Na^+]_i$-dependent activation of the $Na^+/K^+$ ATPase initiates the astrocyte-neurone lactate shuttle, which represents a mechanism for activity-dependent neuronal metabolic support and will be discussed in detail in following sections. Furthermore, $[Na^+]_i$ may regulate the monocarboxylase transporter 2, which exports lactate to the extracellular space, where from where it is taken up by neurones.

All in all, dynamic changes in $[Na^+]_i$ regulate numerous astroglial responses and can represent an additional mechanism for rapid neurone-glial signalling, especially at the single synapse level.

## 4.5.7  Release of neurotransmitters and neuromodulators from astroglia

The discovery of neurotransmitter release from astroglia has been of fundamental importance to our views on the role of these cells in the nervous system. Indeed, this implies a more active role for astroglial networks in the CNS, since they are capable

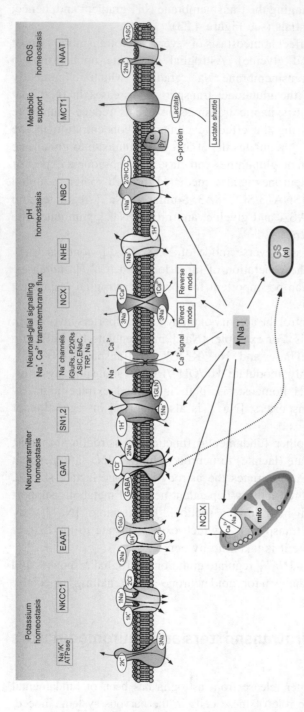

**Figure 4.23**  Molecules of Na$^+$ homeostasis and targets of Na$^+$ signalling in astroglia.

Schematic diagram showing receptors and transporters involved in and sensitive to changes in [Na$^+$]$_i$ and their relations to main homeostatic functions of astroglia.

Abbreviations: ASIC – acid sensing ion channels; EAAT – excitatory amino acid transporters; ENaC – epithelial sodium channels; GAT – GABA transporters; GS – glutamine synthetase, iGluRs – ionotropic glutamate receptors; mito – mitochondrion; Na$_x$ – Na$^+$ channels activated by extracellular Na$^+$; NAAT – Na$^+$-dependent ascorbic acid transporter; NBC – Na$^+$/HCO$_3^-$ (sodium bicarbonate) co-transporter; NCX – Na$^+$/Ca$^{2+}$ exchanger; NCLX – mitochondrial Na$^+$/Ca$^{2+}$ exchanger; NHE – Na$^+$/H$^+$ exchanger; NKCC1 – Na$^+$/K$^+$/Cl$^-$ cotransporter; MCT1 – monocarboxylase transporter 1; P2XRs – ionotropic purinoceptors; SN1.2 – sodium-coupled neutral amino acid transporters which underlie exit of glutamine; TRP – transient receptor potential channels.

Reproduced, with permission, from Kirischuk, S. et al. (2012) Sodium dynamics: another key to astroglial excitability? Trends in Neurosciences 35:8, pp. 497-498. © Elsevier.

of receiving information from neurones via expression of neurotransmitter receptors, converting this information into an alternative form of long-range excitability, in the form of $Ca^{2+}$ waves, and finally releasing extracellular signalling molecules. The concept of regulated neurotransmitter release from astrocytes is generally known as *gliotransmission*, and the released substances are referred to as *gliotransmitters*.

These definitions, however, require certain care and can even be somewhat misleading. Astrocytes are shown to release several classical neurotransmitters and neuromodulators, such as glutamate, ATP, GABA, D-serine, taurine or atrial natriuretic peptide (ANP). All of these substances are equally released by neurones. Arguably, there is only one specific neuromodulator released by astroglia, namely kynurenic acid (Wu *et al.*, 2007), which seems to be produced specifically in astrocytes and acts as an inhibitor of NMDA and nicotinic ACh receptors. The physiological relevance and mechanisms of action of astroglia-derived kynurenic acid remain unknown.

Hence, it seems more natural to define molecules responsible for chemical transmission between neural cells (and astrocytes *are* neural cells) as neurotransmitters and neuromodulators, which can, however, mediate *homocellular* signalling *(neurone to neurone, or astrocyte to astrocyte)* and *heterocellular* signalling *(neurone to astrocyte and other cells, or astrocyte to neurone and other cells)*.

The first experimental evidence for the release of neurotransmitter from glial cells came from the peripheral nervous system in desheathed superior cervical ganglia, in which satellite glial cells were observed to accumulate and release GABA via specific transporter systems. In 1990, the reversed glutamate-transporter current was detected in cultured retinal Müller glial cells subjected to depolarisation and intracellular perfusion with high concentrations of glutamate (up to 100 mM) and $Na^+$ (also up to 100 mM) (Szatkowski *et al.*, 1990). In the same year, the release of glutamate, aspartate and taurine was directly detected in cultured astrocytes in response to hypo-osmotic shock; all of these amino acids diffused from astrocytes through volume-activated anion channels (Kimelberg *et al.*, 1990). In subsequent years, the ability of astroglia to release neuroactive molecules was confirmed in many experiments in different preparations (for references and detailed overview, see Malarkey & Parpura, 2008; Volterra & Meldolesi, 2005).

In general, astrocytes release neurotransmitters by several different mechanisms, which can broadly be divided into exocytotic release, diffusional release through plasmalemmal pores, or transporter mediated release (Figure 4.24).

**(i)  Exocytotic release of neurotransmitters from astrocytes**  Despite the fact that a role for astroglia as brain secretory cells had already been suggested at the beginning of 20th century by Jean Nargeotte and Hans Held (see Chapter 1), for many decades, exocytotic release of neurotransmitters was believed to occur exclusively from neurones. Exocytotic release of glutamate from cultured astrocytes was discovered in 1994 by Vladimir Parpura, Philipp Haydon and their associates (Figure 4.25; Parpura *et al.*, 1994), and has been corroborated by many experiments performed since (see Parpura & Zorec, 2010; Zorec *et al.*, 2012 for details).

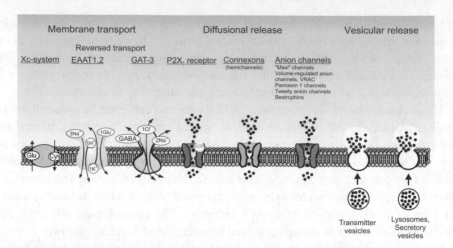

**Figure 4.24**  Major pathways for neurotransmitter release from astrocytes.

Abbreviations: Xc system – cystine-glutamate exchanger; EAAT1,2 – excitatory amino acid transporters type 1 and 2; GAT-3 – GABA transporter type 3.

Reproduced with permission from Verkhratsky et al., 2012.

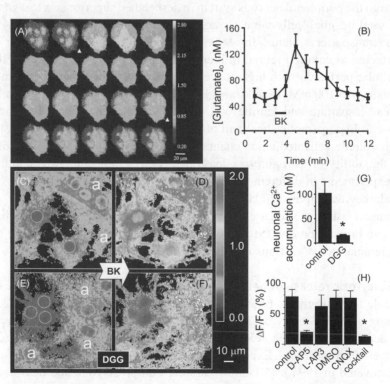

**Figure 4.25**  The first experimental evidence for glutamate-mediated astrocyte-neurone signalling. (*Continued on next page*)

Exocytotic or vesicular release is an evolutionary conserved mechanism that is accomplished through complex machinery, associated with vesicles and pre-synaptic membranes, which includes morphologically defined vesicles, vesicular transporters that allow concentration of neurotransmitters within the vesicular lumen, and numerous proteins providing for excitation-secretion coupling.

The morphological element of regulated exocytosis is represented by secretory vesicles. Several types of such vesicles have been found in astrocytes. Generally, astroglial vesicles vary in size (between 30–700 nm), with the majority of vesicles

---

**Figure 4.25 (*Continued*)**

A. Bradykinin (BK) causes $[Ca^{2+}]_i$ elevations in cultured astrocytes originating from visual cortex (A), and also stimulates glutamate release from these cells (B).

   A: $Ca^{2+}$ levels in astrocytes were monitored using a $Ca^{2+}$ indicator fura-2. Images were acquired 5 seconds apart, with sequence staring from top left corner and ending at the bottom right corner. BK was added to astrocytes (top arrowhead) and washed away after 65 seconds (bottom arrowhead), causing transient $[Ca^{2+}]_i$ elevations in these cells. Colour scale is a pseudocolour representation shown in the form of the ratio of fura-2 emission at 510 nm due to sequential excitation at 350 and 380 nm. Astrocytic resting $[Ca^{2+}]_i$ was ≈100 nM, while the peak response was up to ≈1 μM.

B. BK causes release of glutamate from astrocytes. The superfusate from astrocytes was collected at 1-minute intervals and levels of extracellular glutamate were measured using high-performance liquid chromatography.

C–H. Bradykinin causes a glutamate-mediated accumulation of internal $Ca^{2+}$ in neurones co-cultured with astrocytes from visual cortex. The $[Ca^{2+}]_i$ in neurones (dotted circles in C and E) and astrocytes (a in C and E) was monitored using fura-2. C. Mixed culture at rest.

D. Application of BK caused an elevation in $[Ca^{2+}]_i$ in astrocytes and neurones.

E. However, when co-cultures were bathed in the broad spectrum glutamate receptor (GluR) antagonist, D-glutamylglycine (DGG), application of BK did not significantly alter neuronal $[Ca^{2+}]_i$ calcium levels, even though BK elevated the astrocytic $[Ca^{2+}]_i$.

F. Colour scale as in A.

G. The mean BK-evoked internal $Ca^{2+}$ accumulations (peak value subtracted from resting) in neurones are shown (in control and when pre-incubated with DGG). BK elevated neuronal $[Ca^{2+}]_i$ when neurones were co-cultured with astrocytes, and DGG blocked this response.

H. GluR pharmacology was studied using confocal microscopy and the $Ca^{2+}$ indicator fluo-3. BK-induced elevations of internal $Ca^{2+}$ in neurones were reduced by N-methyl D-aspartate receptor antagonist D-2-amino-phosphonopentanoic acid (D-AP5), but not by an α-amino-3-hydroxy-5-methyl-isoxazole propionate (AMPA) receptor antagonist 6-cyano-7-nitroquinoxaline-2,3-dione (CNQX) or a metabotropic GluR antagonist 2-amino-3-phosphonopropionic acid (L-AP3). Cocktail contained all three GluR inhibitors. Dimethyl sulphoxide (DMSO) is a carrier for CNQX.

*Significant at $p < 0.01$. Points and bars in B, G and H indicate means ± s.e.m.

being electron-lucent (clear). A subpopulation of dense core vesicles with diameters ≈115 nm were shown to contain the secretory peptide secretogranin II and ATP. About 85 per cent of all vesicles in astrocytes contained glutamate (as judged by specific expression of vesicular glutamate transporter), which probably was co-stored with ATP. Several techniques using, for example, immunocytochemistry, recycling dye FM1-43, or total internal reflection microscopy, confirmed size heterogeneity of glutamatergic vesicles, which are represented by several sub-population with diameters 30–50 nm and 300–400 nm.

Astroglial secretory vesicles express the major vesicular transporters responsible for accumulation of neurotransmitters (Figure 4.26). Astroglial vesicles possess the vacuolar V-type proton ATPase (V-ATPase). This $H^+$-ATPase pumps protons into the vesicular lumen, thus creating a high concentration of $H^+$ inside the secretory vesicle, which makes its interior more positive than the cytosol. The electro-chemical gradient drives uptake of neurotransmitters mediated by specific trans-porters. Astrocytes express all three types of vesicular glutamate transporters VGLUT1, 2 and 3 and nucleotide transporter VNUT, which transports ATP.

Astrocytes also express the set of proteins directly involved in the fusion of vesicles with the plasma membrane (Figure 4.27). This secretory process is generally believed to be mediated by the core complex containing the soluble N-ethyl

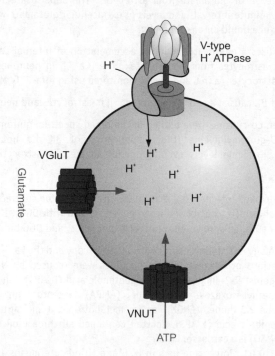

**Figure 4.26** Accumulation of neurotransmitters into vesicles. Glutamate is transported by vesicular glutamate transporters 1–3 (VGluT/SLC17A6-8), and ATP by Vesicular Nucleotide Transporter VNUT (SLC17A9). Both types of transporters utilise proton electrochemical gradient created by proton pump or Vacuolar-type $H^+$-ATPase.

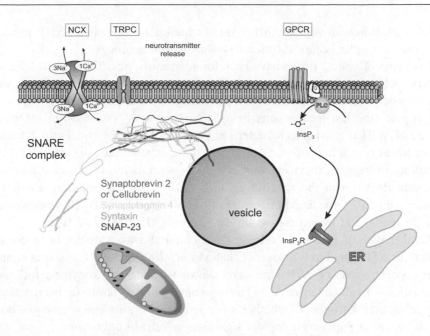

**Figure 4.27** Ca$^{2+}$-dependent vesicular release of gliotransmitters from astrocytes.
Cytosolic Ca$^{2+}$ signal in the astrocyte cytoplasm is sufficient and necessary to cause vesicular fusions and release of neurotransmitter(s). The process of vesicular fusions requires the ternary SNARE complex, consisting of: (i) synaptobrevin 2 and/or cellubrevin located at the vesicular membrane; (ii) synaptotagmin 4; and (iii) the binary cis complex pre- formed at the plasma membrane and composed of syntaxin and synaptosome-associated protein of 23 kDa SNAP-23. (Full colour version in plate section.)

maleimide-sensitive fusion protein attachment protein receptors (SNAREs), including synaptobrevin 2 (also referred to as vesicle-associated membrane protein 2, VAMP2), synaptosome-associated protein of 25 kDa (SNAP25) and syntaxin. Until recently, a view of the SNARE complex formation implied that a preassembled syntaxin 1-SNAP25 intermediate binary *cis* complex located at the plasma membrane interacts with the vesicular synaptobrevin to form the core SNARE complex, a process that eventually leads to vesicular and plasma membrane fusion.

Numerous biochemical studies have demonstrated that astrocytes express key secretory proteins of the core SNARE complex, including synaptobrevin 2, its homologue cellubrevin, syntaxin (isoforms 1, 2 and 4) and synaptosome-associated protein of 23 kDa SNAP-23. Astrocytes also express synaptotagmin 4, but they are devoid of synaptotagmin 1, which acts as the Ca$^{2+}$ sensor in neurones, and the identity of the Ca$^{2+}$ sensor for regulated exocytosis in astrocytes remains unknown.

Functionally, the process of astroglial exocytosis was confirmed by electro-physiological monitoring of quantal release of glutamate or ATP using so-called 'sniffer' cells (i.e. cells containing specific receptors which were placed very close to the membrane of astrocytes and employed as biosensors), fluorescent microscopy for ATP and glutamate, and amperometric measurements. Astroglial exocytosis was also confirmed by measurements of membrane capacitance, which increases following fusion with vesicles. All of these experiments demonstrated that exocytosis from astroglia occurs 100 times slower than in neurones.

Two types of vesicle fusion have been found in astrocytes. These are full fusion, when vesicles completely integrate with the plasma membrane, and transient fusion, where vesicles remain attached to the plasma membrane and transiently open the fusion pore (the last mechanisms being also known as 'kiss-and-run'). Quantal release of ATP has also been characterised in freshly isolated cortical astrocytes and in astrocytes *in situ* in neocortical slices. In these experiments, the astroglial $Ca^{2+}$ signalling to trigger exocytosis was evoked by stimulation of protease activated receptors PAP-1 with the specific agonist TLLFR; this stimulation resulted in appearance of P2X-mediated miniature currents in sniffer cells (P2X$_2$ expressing HEK293 cells) and in cortical pyramidal neurones (Lalo *et al.*, 2011c).

Another type of exocytotic release from cultured astrocytes has been demonstrated for ATP stored in lysosomes (Zhang *et al.*, 2007). These lysosomes contain high concentrations of ATP and were shown to undergo exocytosis following stimulation with glutamate or ATP. The lysosomal pathway has so far been detected only in cultured astroglia, so whether it is operational *in situ*, and what could be its physiological or pathophysiological significance, remain unknown.

The main event triggering astroglial exocytosis is the cytoplasmic $Ca^{2+}$ signals associated with both intracellular $Ca^{2+}$ release and $Ca^{2+}$ entry through plasmalemmal channels (ionotropic receptors and TRP channels) or NCX operating in the reverse mode. Pharmacological manipulations with all these pathways have been shown to interfere with vesicular release of neurotransmitters from astrocytes (see Parpura *et al.*, 2011 for details). The existence of these multiple pathways may provide for plasticity of astroglial neurotransmitter release tailored to a specific physiological context.

### (ii)    Diffusional release of neurotransmitters from astrocytes

The diffusion pathway is generally associated with the release of negatively charged transmitters such as glutamate, ATP and GABA. The cytoplasm of astrocytes contains high concentrations of these molecules, which provide a gradient for their diffusion out of the cells. This concentration difference is maximal for ATP; the cytosolic ATP concentration reaches levels of >5 mM, whereas the extracellular concentration is maintained at a low nM level by constant ectonucleotidase-catalysed ATP degradation. The intracellular concentration of GABA in astrocytes can reach 2 mM, compared to ≈200 nM in the ECS. Cytosolic glutamate levels are relatively low, in a range of 0.5–1 mM, because of the high activity of glutamine synthetase, but this is substantially higher than the extracellular concentration of glutamate, which is maintained low (at ≈25 nM) by the activity of powerful plasmalemmal glutamate transporters.

All neurotransmitters mentioned above are weak acids and, therefore, they permeate various anion channels, many of which are expressed in neuroglia (Fields, 2011). First, there are so-called '*maxi*' $Cl^-$ *channels* that are activated by mechanical stimulation, such as cell swelling (Sabirov & Okada, 2009); both glutamate and ATP have been reported to permeate through these channels. Second, neurotransmitters can be exported from astrocytes through *volume-regulated anion channels* (*VRACs; also known as volume-sensitive outwardly rectifying, VSOR Cl⁻ channels*), which are ubiquitously expressed in mammalian tissues (Nilius *et al.*, 1997), as virtually every cell type responds to osmotic shock with activation of these channels. VRAC channels have a large pore diameter ($\approx 0.7$ nm) and can be permeable to various organic anions, including ATP and glutamate. Activation of VRAC channels in cultured astrocytes by bradykinin triggers release of glutamate.

The extended family of *bestrophins*, which are also anion channels, can be involved in release of neurotransmitters. Activation of Bestrophin 1, for example, has been shown to mediate release of GABA from astrocytes in cerebellum (Lee *et al.*, 2010b). ATP can also be released from different types of non-excitable cells via the *cystic fibrosis transmembrane conductance regulator* (*CFTR*) anion channels, although the expression and functional role of CFTR in astroglia remains uncharacterised. *Pannexin 1*, which recently has been shown to form anion channels (Ma *et al.*, 2012) can also provide for release of neurotransmitters, most notably ATP, from astrocytes.

The second class of channels involved in diffusional neurotransmitter release from astrocytes is represented by unpaired connexons or 'hemichannels'. These are halves of gap junctional channels (see above), which reside in the plasma membrane outside of gap junctional plaques, and which can be activated by a variety of extra- and intracellular cues, including changes in $Ca^{2+}$ concentration, by different kinases, phosphatases or calmodulin, etc. (Decrock *et al.*, 2011). These connexon channels are permeable to ATP and glutamate and have been shown to mediate the release of the latter in astroglial cells in culture and probably *in situ* (Spray *et al.*, 2006; Ye *et al.*, 2003).

Neurotransmitters can also exit astrocytes through the pores associated with overstimulation of P2X₇ receptors (as discussed above). ATP release through the P2X₇ pore was initially identified in cells transfected with P2X₇ receptors and membrane-tagged luciferase; stimulation of these cells with 2′(3′)-O-(4-benzoyl-benzoyl) adenosine 5′-triphosphate (Bz-ATP) was observed to trigger massive release of ATP, with concentrations reaching $\approx 250$ μM near the plasma membrane (Pellegatti *et al.*, 2005). P2X₇ mediated release of ATP and glutamate was found in astroglial cell lines and in primary cultured astrocytes from spinal cord and cortex (see Verkhratsky *et al.*, 2012c for further details).

### (iii) Transporter-mediated neurotransmitter release from astrocytes

Neurotransmitters can also be released from astrocytes through the reverse operation of plasmalemmal transporters. This type of release in physiological conditions is most likely restricted to GABA and, possibly, glycine. The reversal potential of astroglial GABA transporter GAT-3 is set very close to the resting membrane potential, and even relatively small depolarisations or rises in the intracellular $Na^+$ concentration can switch this transporter into the reverse mode, triggering release of GABA into the extracellular space. This type of astroglial GABA release has, for example, been identified in the neocortex (see Kirischuk *et al.*, 2012 for details). Reversal of glutamate transporters in physiological conditions seems to be very unlikely. The reversal potential of glutamate transporters lies at a very positive value ($>+40$ mV), and its reversal requires a simultaneous increase in cytosolic $Na^+$ and glutamate concentrations, substantial cell depolarisation and an increase in extracellular $K^+$ concentration. Such conditions may possibly occur only in pathological states.

Glutamate, however, can be released from astroglial cells via normal operation of the cystine-glutamate exchanger, represented by $Na^+$-dependent $X_{AG^-}$ and $Na^+$-independent $X_c$ systems. Astrocytes express most of the brain cystine-glutamate exchanger, and these transporters provide astrocytes with cystine, which is critical for glutathione metabolism. Astroglial release of glutamate mediated through cystine-glutamate exchange was reported to be associated with the modulation of synaptic transmission and the expression of animal behaviour related to addiction (see Parpura & Zorec, 2010 for review).

**(iv)  Astrocytes as a main source of adenosine in the CNS**  Fluctuations in the levels of adenosine in the CNS are fundamentally important for multiple aspects of CNS signalling, including general inhibition of neuronal signalling, anti-inflammatory protection, sleep and circadian rhythms. In particular, adenosine provides for pre-synaptic inhibition, because most of pre-synaptic terminals express $A_1$ adenosine receptors that tune down synaptic release of neurotransmitters. Astrocytes are most likely the main source of adenosine in the CNS through tonic release of ATP, which subsequently catabolises to adenosine through ecto-nucleotidases ubiquitously present in the nervous tissue. The primary role of astrocytes in setting the adenosine tone has been demonstrated in experiments on transgenic mice that express a dominant-negative SNARE domain selectively in astrocytes. In these animals, there was complete loss of the adenosine $A_1R$-mediated tonic inhibition of synaptic transmission, indicating that astrocytes do, indeed, act as the main source of adenosine (Boison *et al.*, 2010).

**(v)  Physiological role of astroglial release of neurotransmitters**  The question of how neurotransmitters released from astroglia affect information processing in the CNS remains open. The appealing hypothesis that these neurotransmitters can participate in the regulation of ongoing neuronal transmission, and may even participate in synaptic events, has been extensively tested in the last decade. Results of this testing remain controversial. First and foremost, astrocytes do not demonstrate preferred zones of higher concentration of neurotransmitter-containing vesicles, which are characteristic for pre-synaptic terminals. If anything, the vesicles are rather homogeneously spread through astroglial cells. Second, astroglial vesicular release is substantially slower in comparison to neuronal exocytosis. Therefore, it well might be that neurotransmitters and neuromodulators released from astrocytes exert a more global action, modulating synaptic fields rather than intervening in elementary synaptic events. This question, nonetheless, needs a great deal of further investigation.

# 4.6   Functions of astroglia

Astroglial functions are many. Generally, they perform every known housekeeping and homeostatic function in the CNS: they provide structural support and define brain architecture; they establish a link between brain parenchyma and vasculature; and they are indispensable for neurogenesis and development of the nervous system. Conceptually, astroglial functions can be divided into several important groups, as presented in Table 4.3.

**Table 4.3**   Functions of astrocytes

| | |
|---|---|
| Development of the CNS | Neurogenesis |
| | Neural cell migration and formation of the layered grey matter |
| | Synaptogenesis |
| Structural support | Parcelling of the grey matter though the process of 'tiling' |
| | Delineation of *pia mater* and the vessels by perivascular glia |
| | Formation of neuro-vascular unit |
| Barrier function | Regulation of formation and permeability of blood-brain and CSF-brain barriers |
| | Formation of glial-vascular interface |
| Homeostatic function | Control over extracellular $K^+$ homeostasis through local and spatial buffering |
| | Control over extracellular pH |
| | Regulation of water transport |
| | Removal of neurotransmitters from extracellular space |
| Metabolic support | Uptake of glucose; deposition of glycogen |
| | Providing energy substrate lactate to neurones in activity-dependent manner |
| Synaptic transmission | Regulation of synapse maintenance and assisting in synaptic pruning |
| | Providing glutamate for glutamatergic transmission (through *de novo* synthesis and glutamate-glutamine shuttle) |
| | Regulating synaptic plasticity |
| | Integrating synaptic fields |
| | Providing humoral regulation of neuronal networks through secretion of neurotransmitters and neuromodulators |
| Regulation of blood flow | Regulate local blood supply (functional hyperaemia) through secretion of vasoconstrictors or vasodilators |
| Higher brain functions | Chemoception – regulation of body $Na^+$ homeostasis |
| | Chemoception – regulation of $CO_2$ and ventilatory behaviour |
| | Sleep |
| | Memory and learning |
| Brain defence, neuroprotection and post-injury remodelling | Isomorphic and anysomorphic reactive astrogliosis |
| | Scar formation |
| | Catabolising ammonia in the brain |
| | Immune responses and secretion of pro-inflammatory factors (cytokines, chemokines and immune modulators) |

## 4.6.1    Developmental function: neurogenesis and gliogenesis

(i)   **Embryonic neurogenesis and gliogenesis**    All neural cells (i.e. neurones and macroglia) are of ectodermal origin and derive from the neuroepithelium, which forms the neural tube. These *neuroepithelial cells* are pluripotent in a sense that their progeny may differentiate into neurones or macroglial cells with equal probability, and therefore the neuroepithelial cells may be defined as true *neural stem cells*. These neural progenitors either directly produce neurones and glia, or give rise to neuronal or glial precursor cells ('*neuroblasts*' and '*glioblasts*', respectively), which subsequently differentiate into neurones or macroglial cells.

For many years, it was believed that the neuroblasts and glioblasts (or spongioblasts, as the latter were once called) separate very early in development, and that they form two distinct and non-interchangeable pools committed, respectively, to producing strictly neuronal or strictly glial lineages. It was also taken more or less for granted that the pool of precursor cells is fully depleted around birth, and that neurogenesis is totally absent in the mature brain. Recently, however, this paradigm has been challenged, as it appears that neuronal and glial lineages are much more closely related than was previously thought, and the mature brain still has numerous stem cells, which may provide for neuronal replacement. Moreover, it turns out that neural stem cells have many properties of astroglia (see Kriegstein & Alvarez-Buylla, 2009 for comprehensive review).

The modern scheme of neural cell development is illustrated in Figure 4.28. At the origin of all neural cell lineages lie pluripotent neural stem cells in the form of *neuroepithelial cells*. Morphologically, neuroepithelial cells appear as elongated cells extending between the two surfaces (ventricular and pial) of the neural tube. Very early in development (around embryonic day 9–10 in the mouse, which is when neurogenesis begins), the neuroepithelial cells convert into *radial glial cells* (Rakic, 2003). These cells maintain the overall morphology of neuroepithelial cells, in that their processes contact both pial and ventricular surfaces while their cell bodies stay in the ventricular zone. At the same time, radial glial cells acquire glial markers, such as astroglia-specific glutamate transporters, brain lipid-binding protein and Tenascin C.

These radial glial cells are the central element in subsequent neurogenesis, because they act as the main neural progenitors during development, giving rise to neurones, astrocytes, oligodendrocytes and ependymal cells. Radial glia can generate neural cells through either asymmetric division, which directly produces neurones, or through generation of several *intermediate progenitor cells,* which are more or less restricted in their potency to either neuronal, oligodendroglial or astroglial progenitors (*nIPCs, oIPCs* and *aIPCs* respectively).

Several pools of intermediate progenitors, with full or partial commitments to a particular lineage, co-exist during development. Asymmetric division produces daughter cells without much affecting the mother cell. The processes of

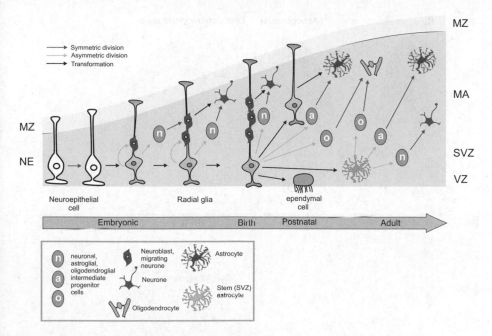

**Figure 4.28** Embryonic development of neural cells.

Neuroepithelial cells are omnipotent neural stem cells; in very early development, they multiply through symmetric division and some of them may divide asymmetrically to generate the first neurones. At later stages, neuroepithelial cells convert into radial glial cells. Radial glia divide asymmetrically to generate neurones and intermediate progenitor cells for neuronal, astroglial and oligodendroglial lineages. At the end of embryonic development, radial glia convert into astrocytes and also into ependymal cells. Some radial glia continue to act as neural progenitors in the neonatal period. A subpopulation of radial glial cells converts into adult stem or SVZ astrocytes, which act as a neural stem cells in the adult brain.

Abbreviations: MA – mantle; MZ – marginal zone; NE – neuroepithelium; SVZ – subventricular zone; VZ – ventricular zone.

Redrawn from Kriegstein & Alvarez-Buylla, 2009. (Full colour version in plate section.)

asymmetrically dividing radial glia stay put in their appropriate places, and asymmetric division does not affect migration of neurones along the cell process, which is already in progress. Already from the very early developmental stages, radial glial cells become functionally heterogeneous, in that they produce subsets of rather distinct neuronal types. The process of neurogenesis is regulated by $Ca^{2+}$ waves spontaneously occurring in radial glial cells; these waves require $InsP_3$ diffusion through gap junctions, together with ATP release and activation of $P2Y_1$ receptors (Weissman *et al.*, 2004).

The newly generated neurones migrate through the neural tube using processes of radial glial cells as guides, which results in an increase in thickness of the neural tissue and eventual formation of layers. This also triggers progressive elongation of the processes of radial glia and up-regulation of their (glia-specific) cytoskeletal proteins such as GFAP and vimentin. Gliogenesis starts later in development; the first cells to be

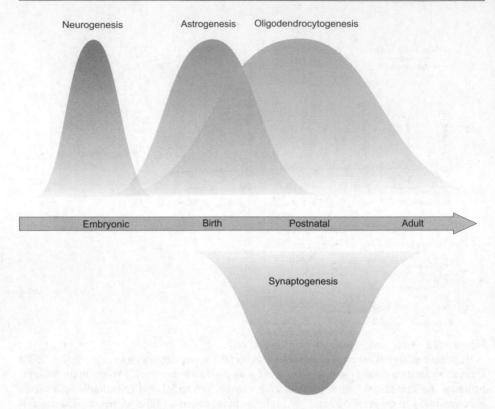

**Figure 4.29** Time course of neural cell development. Note that the wave of synaptogenesis immediately follows the massive appearance of astrocytes.

massively generated are neurones, the second are astrocytes and the third oligodendrocytes, the latter process extending well into the postnatal period (Figure 4.29).

Astrogenesis occurs from both radial glia and from committed precursors. Radial glial cells generate astrocytes through asymmetric division and, at the end of the neuronal migration period, radial glia retract processes and convert into parenchymal astrocytes (the process was originally described by Ramón y Cajal; see Chapter 1). In addition, neonatal astrocytes retain proliferative capabilities and are involved in astrogenesis (See chapter 3). In mammals, radial-like specialised glia remain in the adulthood only in several brain regions (e.g. Bergmann glia in cerebellum and Müller glia in retina). In the subventricular zone, the radial glial cells convert into astrocytes that retain stem cell properties throughout the life-span (see below). The proportion of the final population of astrocytes derived from radial glia and glial precursors depends on the region of the CNS. The majority of oligodendrocytes originate from intermediate precursor cells that populate specific sites in the brain and spinal cord.

**(ii)   Neurogenesis and gliogenesis in the adult brain**   In many vertebrates, neurogenesis persists in adulthood throughout the CNS (for a detailed account, see

Alvarez-Buylla & Lim, 2004; Nottebohm, 2004). For example, new neurones are continuously born in the ventricular zone in birds, after which they migrate through the whole telencephalon; the neural progenitors in birds are radial glia (Alvarez-Buylla *et al.*, 1990). Lizards can very effectively regenerate the retina and spinal cord.

Neurogenesis is generally present throughout life in most poikilotherms; similarly to birds, the radial glia act as neural stem cells. In primates, including humans, neurogenesis in the adult is restricted to the hippocampus and subventricular zone (SVZ), known as *neurogenic niches*. In the SVZ, new cells are primarily born in the walls of the lateral ventricles, and these newly born neurones migrate to the olfactory bulb to replace interneurones. In the hippocampus, neurogenesis mainly occurs in the subgranular layer of the dentate gyrus; these newly produced neurones stay in hippocampus, and some of them integrate into existing neuronal networks.

In both locations, the stem elements that produce neurones are astroglia (Doetsch *et al.*, 1999). These 'stem' astrocytes have the morphology, physiology and biochemical/immunological markers characteristic for astrocytes. They express GFAP, form vascular endfeet, have negative resting membrane potentials, are nonexcitable, and predominantly express $K^+$ channels.

'Stem' astrocytes differ from 'classical' mature astrocytes by specific expression of the protein nestin (a marker for neural stem cells), and some of them form cilia. In the subvetricular zone, the stem astrocytes are also known as 'B cells', and these give rise to 'C cells', which are actively proliferating intermediate precursors. The 'C cells' in their turn generate neuroblasts, known also as 'A cells' (Kriegstein & Alvarez-Buylla, 2009). 'Stem' astrocytes residing in the hippocampus and subventricular zone are multipotent, as they give birth to both neurones and glia; the production of glia or neurones is under control of numerous chemical factors (Figure 4.30). Another neurogenic niche in the mammalian brain can be associated with a subset of hypothalamic astrocytes, the tanycytes, which can generate hypothalamic regulatory neurones (Lee *et al.*, 2012).

In the adult brain, in contrast to neurogenesis, gliogenesis appears to occur everywhere. New glial cells are born locally, and the locality also mainly determines the type of glial cell produced. In the subcortical white matter, most of the newly produced glial cells are oligodendrocytes, whereas, in the spinal cord, both astrocytes and oligodendrocytes are produced roughly in the same quantities.

## 4.6.2  Neuronal guidance

The vertebrate brain develops from the embryonic neuroectoderm, which lies above the notochord and gives rise to the entire nervous system. The notochord induces neuroectodermal cells to generate neural stem cells and form the neural plate which, in turn, forms the neural tube, from which the brain and spinal cord are derived. The neural stem cells and intermediate progenitors of the neural tube give rise to both neurones and glia in response to multiple inductive signals produced by the

| Factors favouring gliogenesis | Factors favouring neurogenesis |
|---|---|
| Fibroblast growth factor 2<br>Bone morphogenetic protein<br>Notch<br>Platelet-derived growth factor<br>Neuregulins<br>Unmyelinated axons | Epidermal growth factor 2<br>Transforming growth factor α<br>Vascular endothelial growth factor<br>Insulin-like growth factor 1<br>Platelet-derived growth factor<br>Activated astrocytes |

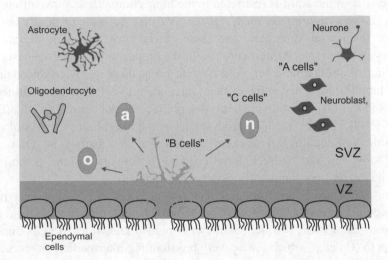

**Figure 4.30** Adult neurogenesis. The SVZ stem astrocytes (also known as 'B cells') act as pluripotent neural progenitor cells, generating committed neuronal, astroglial, and oligodendroglial precursors (also known as 'C cells'); neuronal precursors transform into young neurones (or 'A cells'), which subsequently migrate to the olfactory bulb or hippocampus, where they can convert into mature neurones.

SVZ – subventricular zone; VZ – ventricular zone.

notochord, floor plate, roof plate, dorsal ectoderm and somites (e.g. retinoic acid, fibroblast growth factor, bone morphogenetic proteins, etc.). Inductive signals regulate transcription factors and gene expression, including the homeobox (Hox) genes, which influence the development of the neural tube into the major brain regions, namely the forebrain (prosencephalon), midbrain (mesencephalon) and hindbrain (rhombencephalon). The first neural cells to develop are radial glia. After this, neuroblasts in the ventricular zone (VZ) and subventricular zone (SVZ) immediately surrounding the lumen of the neural tube have to migrate to their final destinations and give rise to the enormously diverse range of neurones found in the adult brain (Figure 4.31).

An important function of foetal radial glial cells is to provide the scaffolding along which these neural precursors migrate (Figure 4.31; see also Kriegstein & Alvarez-Buylla, 2009; Rakic, 2003). Not all neurones migrate along radial glia, but

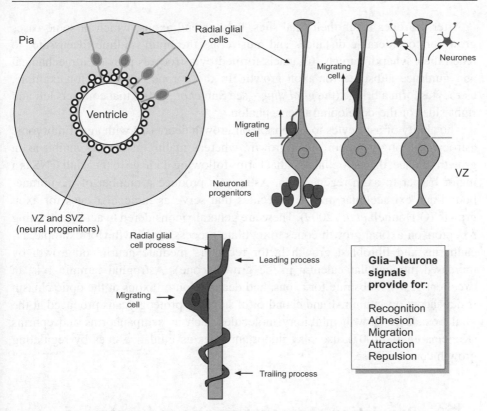

**Figure 4.31** Radial glial cells form a scaffold that assists neuronal migration in the developing nervous system. Radial glial cells extend their processes from the ventricular zone (VZ) and subventricular zone (SVZ), where neural progenitors reside, towards the pia. Neuronal precursors attach to the radial glial cells and migrate along their processes towards their final destination. Numerous reciprocal factors released by both neurones and glia regulate the processes of mutual recognition, attraction, adhesion, migration and final repulsion.

it is always the case where neurones are organised in layers, such as in the cerebellum, hippocampus, cerebral cortex and spinal cord.

In the cerebral cortex, for example, bipolar postmitotic neurones migrate several millimetres from the ventricular zone to the pia along the processes of radial glia; the cerebral cortex is formed inside out, whereby the innermost layers are formed first and the superficial layers are formed later by neurones that migrate through the older cells. In the cerebellum, granule cells migrate along Bergmann glia, which are derived from radial glia. Migration depends on recognition, adhesion and neurone-glial interactions, which are under the influence of cell membrane bound molecules, and diffusible and extracellular matrix molecules. Although the specific signals are not fully resolved, they include laminin-integrin interactions and neuregulin, which is expressed by migrating neurones and interacts with glial epidermal growth factor (ErbB) receptors. Subsequently, foetal radial glia disappear and transform into astrocytes.

After neurones reach their final sites, they extend axons, which in some cases grow for considerable distances and must cross the brain midline (decussate) to reach their synaptic targets. Channels formed by astrocytes provide a mechanical and guidance substrate for axon growth. In the corpus callosum, for example, astrocytes form a bridge (the *glial sling* – see Shu *et al.*, 2003) that connects left and right sides of the developing telencephalon.

The ability of astrocytes to support axon growth decreases with age. Embryonic astrocytes strongly support axon growth, whereas mature astrocytes inhibit axon growth – hence, the astroglial scar that forms following damage to the adult CNS is a major barrier to axon regeneration. Astrocytes produce a number of membrane-bound and extracellular matrix molecules that serve as molecular cues for axon growth (O'Donnell *et al.*, 2009). These are generally considered to act by activating receptors on axonal growth cones to regulate process outgrowth (for example, N-cadherins and fibroblast growth factor receptors mediate neurite outgrowth by increased intracellular calcium in the growth cone). Astroglial laminin-1 is an excellent growth substrate for axons, and decussation of axons at the optic chiasm is dependent on laminin-1 and chondroitin sulphate proteoglycans produced at the glial boundary. Growth inhibitory molecules such as sempaphorins and ephrins (Koncina *et al.*, 2007) also play important roles as guidance cues by regulating growth cone collapse.

## 4.6.3   Regulation of synaptogenesis and control of synaptic maintenance and elimination

The living brain constantly remodels and modifies its cellular networks. Throughout life, synapses continuously appear, strengthen, weaken or die (Kelsch *et al.*, 2010; Waites *et al.*, 2005). These processes underlie the adaptation of the brain to the constantly changing external environment and, in particular, represent what we know as learning and memory. For many years, the process of synaptogenesis, maintenance and elimination of the synaptic contacts was considered to be solely neuronal responsibility; only very recently it has become apparent that glial cells (astrocytes in the CNS and Schwann cells in the PNS) control the birth, life and death of synapses formed in neuronal networks (Figure 4.32; for references and further details, see Eroglu & Barres, 2010; Pfrieger, 2010).

In general, the life cycle of the synapse proceeds through several stages:

1.  formation of an initial contact between pre-synaptic terminal and post-synaptic neurone;

2.  maturation of the synapse, when it acquires its specific properties, in particular the neurotransmitter(s) modality;

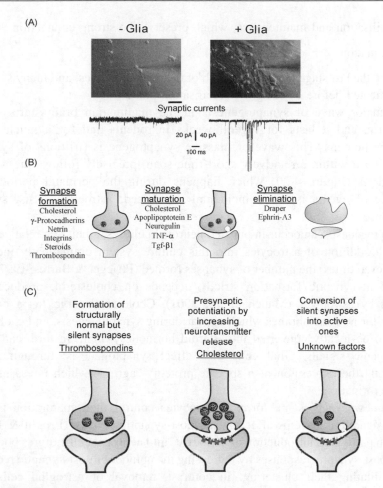

**Figure 4.32**  Astroglia control synaptogenesis.

A.  The critical role of astrocytes was initially identified *in vitro*. It turned out that without glia, neurones in culture form only a very few synapses, whilst addition of glia significantly increases the number of synapses formed (about seven times).

B.  The formation and maturation of synapses is regulated by many factors released from astrocytes that include, for example, cholesterol, integrins, neuregulin, etc. Astrocytes also control synapse elimination, which occurs quite often when unused synaptic contacts have to be pruned. Importantly, astrocytes may also limit the number of synapses that appear on a given neurone, as astroglial membranes ensheathing the neurolemma prevent the formation of new synaptic contacts.

C.  Astrocytes also control the functional status of synapses that have been already formed. For example, thrombospondins secreted from astroglia favour formation of structurally normal, but silent synapses. Cholesterol, released from astrocytes, boosts pre-synaptic potentiation by increasing neurotransmitter release. Some other, yet unknown, factors of astroglial origin convert silent synapses into active ones.

Reproduced, with permission, from Pfrieger & Barres 1997 (A); redrawn from Pfrieger 2010 (B); Redrawn from Eroglu & Barres 2010 (C).

3.  stabilisation and maintenance, which preserve the strong connections; and

4.  elimination.

In fact, the last stage may follow each of the preceding ones, and many synapses are eliminated before entering the stabilisation phase.

The major wave of synaptogenesis in the mammalian brain starts shortly after birth, and it lasts for several weeks in rodents and for a much longer period in humans. This wave of massive synaptogenesis (trillions of synapses have to form within a relatively short time span) precisely follows the wave of astrogenesis (Figure 4.29) which happens during the perinatal period. This sequence of events is not coincidental as, indeed, astrocytes assist synapse appearance.

Synaptogenesis can occur in purified neuronal cultures, albeit at a relatively low rate, and addition of astrocytes into this culture system dramatically increases (about seven times) the number of synapses formed (Pfrieger & Barres, 1997). This increase in synaptic formation strictly depends on cholesterol, produced and secreted by astrocytes (Mauch *et al.*, 2001). Cholesterol serves as a building material for new membranes which appear during synaptogenesis, and cholesterol may also be locally converted into steroid hormones which, in turn, can act as synaptogenic signals. Glial cells also affect synaptogenesis, through signals influencing the expression of a specific protein – agrin – which is essential for synapse formation.

After new synapses are formed, astrocytes control their maturation through several signalling systems affecting the post-synaptic density (Eroglu & Barres, 2010). In particular, introduction of astrocytes into neuronal cell cultures boosts the size of post-synaptic responses by increasing the number of post-synaptic receptors and facilitating their clustering. In contrast, removal of astroglial cells from neuronal cultures decreases the number of synapses.

In part, these effects are mediated by several soluble factors released by astrocytes, although direct contact between glial and neuronal membranes also exerts a clear influence (of yet unidentified nature) on synapse maturation. Several distinct soluble factors have been identified that are released by glial cells and affect synapse maturation. One of them is tumour necrosis factor α (TNFα), which regulates the insertion of glutamate receptors into post-synaptic membranes; another is activity-dependent neurotrophic factor (ADNF) which, after being secreted by astrocytes, increases the density of NMDA receptors in the membrane of neighbouring post-synaptic neurones. In chick retina, Müller glial cells control the expression of M2 muscarinic ACh receptors in retinal neurones through a hitherto unidentified protein.

Astrocytes may also limit the number of synapses that appear on a given neurone, as astroglial membranes ensheathing the neurolemma prevent the formation of new synaptic contacts. Astroglial cells can also be involved in the elimination of synapses in the CNS, the process which underlies the final tuning and plasticity of the neuronal inputs. This may be achieved by secretion of certain factors or proteolytic enzymes, which demolish the extracellular matrix and reduce the stability of the synaptic contact. Subsequently, astroglial processes may enter the synaptic cleft and literally close and substitute the synapse.

## 4.6.4 Structural function: astrocytes define the micro-architecture of the grey matter and create neurovascular units

Protoplasmic astrocytes in the grey matter of the brain and of the spinal cord are organised in a very particular way, with each astrocyte controlling its own three-dimensional anatomical territory (Figure 4.33; Bushong *et al.*, 2002; Nedergaard *et al.*, 2003). These anatomical territories are called *astroglial domains*. Astroglial domains are regularly spaced and parcel the grey matter into relatively independent three-dimensional fields which are morphologically defined by the arborisation of individual astrocytes. The process of grey matter parcelling starts in late embryo-genesis and has been termed *tiling*. The overlap between territories of neighbouring astroglial cells is minimal and it does not exceed five per cent, i.e. astrocytes contact each other only by the most distal processes. These distal processes, however, contain most of the gap junctional plaques and are thus responsible for astroglial coupling.

Astrocytic processes show a very high degree of morphological plasticity. Many processes send very fine expansions, the lamellopodia and filopodia, which contact synaptic regions, and these lamellopodia and filopodia are motile, expanding and shrinking at a speed of several μm per minute. The lamellopodia show gliding movements along neuronal surfaces, and filopodia are able to protrude rapidly towards, or retract from, the adjacent neuronal membranes or synaptic structures.

Using clearly delineated anatomical territories, astrocytes divide the whole of grey matter (both in the brain and in the spinal cord) into separate domains, the elements of which (neurones, synaptic terminals and blood vessels) are integrated via the processes of protoplasmic astrocytes. Membranes of a single astrocyte may cover about 100,000 synapses present in its domain in rodents, and up to two million in humans. The astrocytic processes provide for local signalling within the domain, as their membranes that contact neurones, synapses and blood vessels are packed with receptors which sense the ongoing activity. Signals activated by glial receptors may propagate through the astrocyte cytoplasm, thus integrating distant parts of the domain. Importantly, the processes of the same astrocyte are often directly coupled via reflexive gap junctions, which establish diffusion shortcuts, allowing the local metabolic signals to spread rapidly through these processes, bypassing the soma.

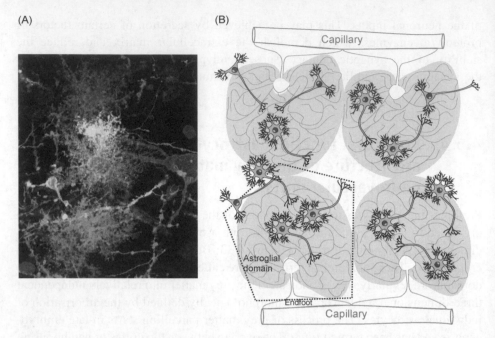

**Figure 4.33**  Astrocytic domains form the micro-architecture of grey matter.

A.  Each single astrocyte occupies a well-defined territory; astroglial contacts occur only through distal processes and, overall, the overlap between astrocyte territories does not exceed 3– 5 per cent. Images show neighbouring hippocampal astrocytes stained with different fluorescent dyes.

B.  Schematic representation of astrocytic domains, which are organised in rows along the vessels, the latter typically being positioned in the narrow interface between astrocytes.

(A) Kindly provided by Professor Maiken Nedergaard, Rochester University. (Full colour version in plate section.)

Astrocytes form two interfaces within their domains, with neuronal membranes and blood vessels, the latter being almost completely plastered by astroglial endfeet. These two interfaces within the astroglial domain form a morphological basis for a *neuro-vascular unit,* which is central for neuro-vascular coupling and neuronal metabolic support, as will be discussed in detail below.

## 4.6.5   Structural function: astrocytes and the brain-blood barrier

The central nervous system is separated from the rest of the body by a system of barriers, which act as a fundamental part of the CNS homeostatic system that dynamically denies or permits and regulates molecular exchange between the blood and the nervous tissue. The brain tissue is separated from blood by three barrier systems:

1.  The *choroid plexus blood-cerebrospinal fluid (CSF) barrier* in the ventricles of the brain, formed by tight junctions between the choroid plexus cells, which also produce the CSF.

2.  The *arachnoid blood-CSF barrier*, separating the subarachnoid CSF from the blood and formed by tight junctions between the cells of the arachnoid mater surrounding the brain.

3.  The *blood-brain barrier* (*BBB*) between the intracerebral blood vessels and the brain parenchyma, formed by tight junctions between the endothelial cells of the blood vessels and the surrounding astroglial endfeet.

The barrier between the blood and the brain was discovered by Paul Ehrlich, who, when doing his doctoral studies, realised that injection of soluble dyes into the bloodstream stains all organs and systems but the brain and the spinal cord (Ehrlich, 1885). In fact, Erlich was not certain about the barrier; he considered that either nervous tissue is somehow averse to staining by the dyes he was using, or that the vascular walls in the brain had smaller pores compared to those in peripheral tissues.

The concept of a barrier to dyes was introduced by Erlich's pupil Edwin Goldmann, who did the alternative experiment by injecting the soluble dye trypan blue into the cerebrospinal fluid (Goldmann, 1913). In this instance, the dye stained the nervous tissue but failed to penetrate into the circulation. As a result, Goldman introduced a concept of tissue border membrane, or *physiologische Grenzmembran*, which shields the brain and the placenta from the circulation. The term 'blood-brain barrier' (or BBB) (*bluthirnschranke*) is usually credited to Max Lewandowsky, who found that strychnine and potassium ferrocyanate, when injected directly into the nervous tissue, were 100 times more potent then when applied through the bloodstream. This observation led him to suggest that the wall of brain capillaries blocked transport of certain molecules (Lewandowsky, 1900).

The blood-brain barrier exists throughout the brain, with the exception of circumventricular organs, neurohypophysis, pineal gland, subfornical organ and lamina terminalis, which are involved in neurosecretion and regulation of the endocrine and autonomic systems. In these parts of the brain, capillary walls are fenestrated, which allows the free exchange of large metabolites and hormones between the blood and the CNS. A permeability barrier formed by tight junctions between the cells lining the brain ventricles prevents leakage of these chemicals into the CSF and the rest of the brain tissue. In addition, junctional complexes between astrocyte endfeet that form the subpial glial limiting membranes, and between ependymal cells lining the brain ventricles, restrict the movement of large solutes between the brain tissue and the subarachnoid CSF and the ventricular CSF, respectively.

The endothelial cells that line CNS blood vessels differ from those outside the nervous system, which determines the fundamental differences in the features of brain and non-brain capillaries (Figure 4.34).

The endothelial cells in brain capillaries form numerous tight junctions which effectively prevent paracellular transport of macromolecules or invasion of blood cells. The tight junctions are complex structures (Figure 4.35) which include several proteins represented by junctional adhesion molecule JAM-1 (a 40 kDa member of the immunoglobulin G superfamily that participates in the attachment of adjacent cell membranes), occludin (a 60–56 kDa protein that spans through the intercellular cleft) and the claudins (an extended family of relatively small proteins of 20–24 kDa which also occupy the intercellular cleft).

The development of an endothelial blood-brain barrier is a relatively late evolutionary acquisition (Figure 4.36). The ancestral blood-brain barrier that appeared in the invertebrates is formed exclusively by astrocytes (Bundgaard & Abbott, 2008) which cover the vascular walls and provide for selective molecular transport. The glial barrier is also present in elasmobranch fishes (such as sharks), where the barrier is formed by astroglial endfeet; sometimes the astrocytes completely

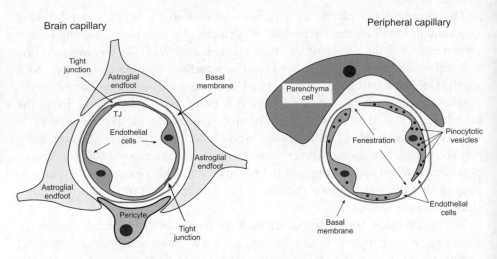

**Figure 4.34**   General structure of brain and peripheral capillaries.

The scheme shows a cross-section of brain (CNS) and peripheral (systemic) capillaries. The endothelial cells of the brain capillary are sealed by tight junctions (TJ), which are the physical substrate of the blood-brain barrier and almost completely restrict diffusion of solutes between the blood and brain; hence, all solutes must pass through the endothelial cell. Astroglial endfeet completely ensheath CNS capillaries and are important for induction and maintenance of blood-brain barrier properties and ion and water transport. In contrast, in peripheral blood vessels, the intercellular junctions between endothelial cells are open and often fenestrated, and endothelial cells contain pinocytic vesicles, which are absent from most brain capillaries.

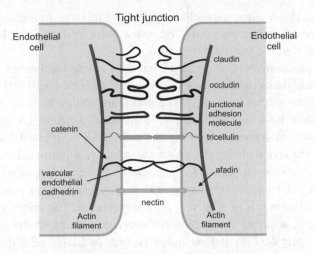

**Figure 4.35** Structure of tight junction.

enwrap vessels, making them endocellular capillaries. The first evolutionary shift of barrier function to muscle cells and pericytes occurred in cephalopods, but without phylogenetic consequences. In high vertebrates, the barrier function is fully shifted to endothelial cells.

In contrast, in non-neural capillaries the endothelial cells do not form continuous tight junctions (Figure 4.34), but the intercellular junctions are freely permeable to most solutes and, in some cases, capillaries have relatively large passages known as

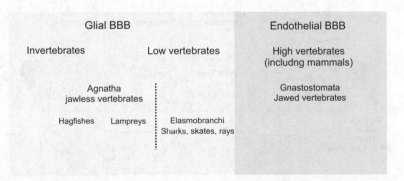

**Figure 4.36** Evolutionary transition from glial to endothelial blood-brain barrier.
In insects, the barrier is made by perineural glia, sheath glia and fenestrated glia. In cephalopods, the barrier is made at the level of pericytes and smooth muscle cells. In the Elasmobranch fish, the barrier is formed by perivascular glial endfeet, or else vessels are completely surrounded by astroglia (endocellular capillaries).

fenestrations. These allow paracellular diffusion of large molecular weight molecules and provide, when necessary, the pathway for infiltration of blood cells (i.e.
macrophages) into the surrounding tissue.

The tight junctions between endothelial cells create the barrier between brain
parenchyma and the circulation, essentially forming a sealed wall to the movement of
even the smallest solutes (e.g. ions). The main function of this barrier is, indeed, to
isolate the brain from the blood and to provide a substrate for the brain's own
homeostatic system. Almost everything that must cross the blood-brain barrier has to
pass through the endothelial cells, which are selectively permeable to allow energy
substrates and other essentials to enter the brain tissue, and metabolites to exit.

The paracellular aqueous pathway, which may carry some ions through tight
junctions, exists, but it is of relatively little importance. The selective permeability
of the barrier is achieved by specific transporters residing in the endothelial cell
membrane (Figure 4.37; for details and references on BBB, see Abbott *et al.*, 2010,
2006; Hawkins & Davis, 2005; Sa-Pereira *et al.*, 2012). These transporters are many
and include:

1.  the energy-dependent ABC cassette transporters, which excrete xenobiotics
    (this mainly determines the impermeability of the blood-brain barrier to many
    drugs, such as antibiotics, cytostatics, etc.);

2.  amino acid transporters;

3.  glucose transporter of GLUT1 type;

4.  multiple ion exchangers and solute carriers.

Many biologically active substances (for example catecholamines) cannot enter
the brain precisely because the endothelial cells do not have the relevant

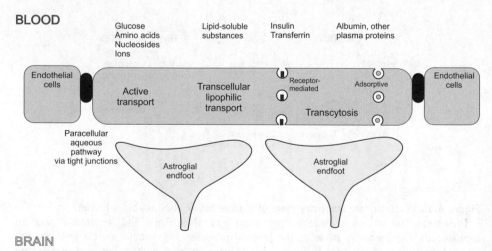

**Figure 4.37**  Mechanisms of transport through blood-brain barrier. See text for explanation.

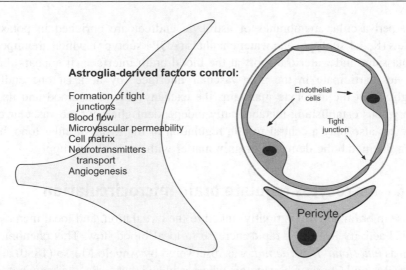

**Astroglia-derived factors control:**

Formation of tight
  junctions
Blood flow
Microvascular permeability
Cell matrix
Neurotransmitters
  transport
Angiogenesis

Endothelial cells

Tight junction

Pericyte

**Figure 4.38** Astroglia secrete factors controlling formation, maintenance and function of the blood-brain barrier.

transporters. In addition, substances can be transported through endothelial cells through transcytosis, in which molecules either (i) bind to receptors and are subsequently internalised in endosomes which undergo transcellular transport, or (ii) are directly absorbed by the endosomes. Lipid soluble substances travel through the transcellular lipophilic route.

From the brain side, the anatomical substrate of the blood-brain barrier is created by astroglial endfeet which closely enwrap the capillary wall (Figure 4.38). The presence of an astroglial compartment around the blood vessels is of paramount importance for modifying the endothelial cells, as astrocytes release several regulatory factors (such as transforming growth factor α, TGFα, and glial-derived neurotrophic factor, GDNF), which induce the formation of tight junctions between endothelial cells and stimulate the polarisation of their luminal and basal cell membranes (with respect to expression of various ion channels and proteins involved in transport across the blood-brain barrier). The endothelial cells, in turn, also signal to astrocytes, in particular through leukaemia-inhibitory factor (LIF), which promotes astrocyte maturation. Contacts between astroglial endfeet and the endothelial cells also regulate expression of receptors and ion channels (especially aquaporins and $K^+$ channels) in the glial membrane.

Astrocytes are not very much involved in blood-brain barrier function *per se* (which is determined largely by the endothelial cells), but astrocytes are important in the regulation of the blood-brain interface as a whole. Astrocyte endfeet membranes are enriched with numerous receptors, transporters and channels which mediate glial-endothelial communication and regulate exchange through the glial-vascular interface. In particular, endfeet are endowed with glucose transporters, which facilitate glucose uptake and its distribution to neurones (see below).

The perivascular membranes of astrocyte endfeet are enriched in potassium channels ($K_{ir}4.1$ subtype) and water channels (AQP4 subtype), which are important for potassium and water transport at the blood-brain interface. It appears that all astrocytes participate in the glial-vascular interface (by at least one endfoot), through which the astrocyte maintains the exchange between blood and its own territory, thus establishing metabolically independent glia-neurone-vascular units. Astrocytes also play a central role in regulation of the local vascular tone, hence linking the metabolic demands of grey matter with local blood supply.

## 4.6.6   Astrocytes regulate brain microcirculation

Increase in brain activity is tightly linked to the circulation, and local increases in neuronal activity triggers a rapid increase in local blood flow. This phenomenon, known as *functional hyperaemia*, was discovered by Angelo Mosso (1880) and by Charles Roy and Charles Sherrington, who postulated that ' . . . *the brain possesses an intrinsic mechanism by which its vascular supply can be varied locally in correspondence with local variations of functional activity*' (Roy & Sherrington, 1890). Furthermore, Roy and Sherrington suggested the involvement of '*chemical products of cerebral metabolism ... cause variations of caliber of the cerebral vessels*'.

Functional hyperaemia is a local phenomenon, as vasodilatation occurs in small vessels within $\approx$200–250 µm from the site of increased neuronal activity. Mechanisms of functional hyperaemia remained enigmatic for a long time, and several hypotheses have highlighted the role of local release of vasoactive factors, local innervation or activation of nitric oxide synthase and generation of nitric oxide.

The brain is one of the most vascularised organs of the human body (Figure 4.39). The brain vasculature occupies $\approx$ 25 per cent of the total brain volume, the total length of capillaries is $\approx$650 km and their total surface area is $\approx$12 m$^2$ (Zlokovic & Apuzzo, 1998). This massive system accommodates $\approx$1 litre/min of blood circulation in adult humans. The pial arteries, which run along the brain surface, are separated from the organ parenchyma by a so-called *Virchow-Robin space*, which is, in essence, a tunnel filled with interstitial fluid that surrounds the artery penetrating into the brain (see Iadecola, 2004; Peters *et al.*, 1991 for anatomy and functional details).

When arterioles penetrate deeper into the parenchyma, this space disappears and the outer walls of the vessels (formed by basement membrane) become completely enwrapped by astroglial endfeet (Figure 4.39). The diameter of arteries and arterioles is controlled by contraction/relaxation of smooth muscle cells. Capillaries do not possess myocytes, and their diameter is controlled by pericytes, which are also capable of contractile activity. The dilation/constriction of arteries is mainly controlled by endothelial cells that release several types of vasoconstrictors (endothelin and the endothelium-derived constrictor factor) and vasodilators (nitric

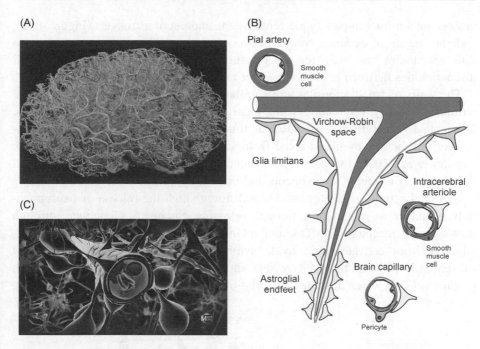

**Figure 4.39** Astroglia and brain vessels.

A. Blood vessels in human brain. A plastic emulsion was injected into the brain vessels and brain parenchymal tissue was dissolved.

B. Artistic impression of astroglial endfeet covering brain capillary.

C. Astrocytes and brain vessels. Pial arteries are in contact with the glia limitans, which envelops the brain surface. Penetrating arterioles and capillaries are surrounded by astrocytic endfeet. Diameter of pial arteries and arterioles is controlled by smooth muscle cell layer, whereas diameter of capillaries is regulated by pericytes.

Reproduced with permission from Zlokovic & Apuzzo, 1998 (A); from Wikipedia: http://en. wikipedia.org/wiki/File:Blood_Brain_Barriere.jpg (B); redrawn based on Iadecola, 2004; Iadecola & Nedergaard, 2007. (Full colour version in plate section.)

oxide (NO), prostacyclin, carbon monoxide and the endothelium-derived hyperpolarising factor), which are released in response to activation of terminal innervating arteries, or in response to shear stress following changes in intravascular blood pressure and rate of blood flow (Faraci & Heistad, 1998).

Pial arteries are innervated by perivascular nerves, which not only signal to endothelial cells but release numerous vasoactive factors on their own accord (vasodilators: NO, acetylcholine, vasoactive intestinal polypeptide (VIP), calcitonin gene-related peptide, substance P and cholecystokinin neurokinin A; vasoconstrictors: noradrenaline, neuropeptide Y and serotonin).

The functional hyperaemia that couples neuronal activity with vessel diameter is executed mostly at the level of terminal arterioles and capillaries. The walls of these vessels are almost completely plastered by the endfeet of astrocytes (Figure 4.39), and the degree of coverage varies between 80 and 100 per cent, according to different studies and brain regions (Mathiisen *et al.*, 2010). Even those small discontinuities between astroglial endfeet are filled with processes of microglia.

The walls of small arterioles and capillaries are also in contact with neuronal terminals, usually originating from local interneurones or intrinsic neurones. Conceptually, therefore, local vascular tone can be controlled either by neuronal-derived factors, by glia-derived factors or by both (see Attwell *et al.*, 2010; Gordon *et al.*, 2008; Iadecola, 2004; Iadecola & Nedergaard, 2007 for detailed description of concepts, experiments and critical appraisal of the data).

Neuronal activity regulates local blood flow though the release of neurotransmitters and, most importantly, through releasing glutamate. Glutamate, through post-synaptic receptors (NMDA and mGluRs), triggers neuronal $Ca^{2+}$ signals, which in turn activate nitric oxide synthase, which produces NO. The NO subsequently diffuses to blood vessels and activates guanylate synthase, which produces cGMP, which mediates vasodilation. In parallel, a rise in neuronal $[Ca^{2+}]_i$

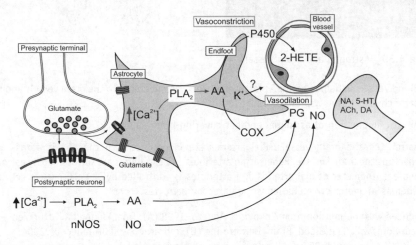

**Figure 4.40** Regulation of local blood flow in the brain.

The vascular tone is controlled by neurone- and astroglial-derived factors. Activation of glutamate receptors in the post-synaptic neurone triggers elevation in $[Ca^{2+}]_i$ which stimulates production of NO by neuronal NO synthase and arachidonic acid by phospholipase A2. Terminals of perivascular neurones localised close to the brain vasculature release neurotransmitters (acetylcholine, ACh, noradrenaline, NA, dopamine DA, serotonin, 5-HT), which may regulate smooth muscle contraction.

Astrocytes couple neuronal activity with local circulation by releasing vasoconstrictors and vasodilators. Glutamate released at synapses during increased neuronal activity triggers calcium signals in perisynaptic astrocytic processes. Calcium signals propagate through the astroglial cell (and astroglial syncytium) to reach the perivascular endfoot, where $Ca^{2+}$ triggers the release of arachidonic acid (AA). Depending on the brain region and local enzymatic systems, AA can be converted to vasodilatatory prostaglandins (PG) by cyclo-oxygenase (COX), or to a vasoconstrictive agent, 20 hydroxyeicosatetraenois acid (2-HETE), by a cytochrome P450 epoxygenase of the arteriole smooth muscle.

may stimulate production of arachydonic acid by phospholipase $A_2$ ($PLA_2$), which, when converted to prostaglandins, acts as a powerful vasodilator (Figure 4.40).

An alternative pathway, centred on astroglia, has been identified relatively recently (Mulligan & MacVicar, 2004; Takano *et al.*, 2006; Zonta *et al.*, 2003). The notion that astroglial cells provide a metabolic connection between neurones and blood vessels was initially made by Camillo Golgi in the 1870s, and direct control over the diameter of the brain vessels by astrocytes was suggested also by Ramón y Cajal (1895; and see Chapter 1). The mechanisms of this control were identified using *in situ* and *in vivo* imaging techniques, which demonstrated that glutamate, released during neuronal activity, acts on astroglial receptors and induces astroglial $Ca^{2+}$ signals. These enter endfeet and initiate the release of vasoactive substances, which in turn affect the tone of small arterioles and/or capillaries enwrapped by these endfeet (Figure 4.40). Inhibition of astroglial $Ca^{2+}$ signalling inhibits the functional link between neuronal activation and changes in vascular tone.

In fact, astrocytes are able to provide dual control over the neighbouring blood vessels; they may either induce vasodilatation or vasoconstriction. Both effects begin with $Ca^{2+}$ elevation in the endfeet and the release of arachidonic acid (AA). The latter can be transformed into prostaglandin derivatives by cyclo-oxygenase (COX), which can be blocked by aspirin; these derivatives of AA effectively relax the vascular muscle cells and cause vasodilatation and increased blood flow. Alternatively, AA can be converted into the vasoconstrictive agent 20 hydroxyei-cosatetraenois acid (2-HETE) by a cytochrome 450 enzyme residing in the arteriole smooth muscle. Additionally, astrocytes can affect blood vessel tone by releasing $K^+$ from the endfeet (see $K^+$ buffering below). Local increases in $K^+$ can hyper-polarise smooth muscle cells, thus limiting activation of $Ca^{2+}$ channels and hence $Ca^{2+}$ influx, therefore promoting dilation of the vessel. This possibility, however, has not been confirmed in direct experiments.

Of course, in a textbook dedicated to glia, we are somewhat biased, yet one should not underestimate the importance of neural control over blood circulation. The brain blood vessels are innervated by a complex network of perivascular neurones, terminals of which are localised in close proximity to smooth muscle cells of brain arteries and arterioles. This innervation is certainly instrumental for regulation of brain circulation.

All in all, functional hyperaemia is most likely controlled by both neuronal and astroglial pathways. Which one dominates? This remains an open question, and may vary between brain regions and physiological context.

## 4.6.7 Brain energetics and neuronal metabolic support

The brain is the human body's most energy-demanding organ. In its resting state, the brain, which represents only two per cent of total body mass, consumes $\approx 20$ per cent of all energy produced by the body and needs about ten per cent of the total cardiac output. Most of this energy is spent on restoration of transmembrane ion gradients (because every action potential drives sodium ions into the cytosol and potassium into the extracellular space, and all these ions must be returned to their original position). The most energy-dependent part of the neurone is the synapse, where most of the ion displacements occur. The synapse consumes ≈75 per cent of all energy of the individual neurone (Figure 4.41; Magistretti, 2009). This is quite understandable because, in both neuronal somata and axons, ion movements occur in very restricted parts of the plasmalemma. In axons, this happens only at the initial segment (axon hillock) and nodes of Ranvier, whereas most of the somatic plasmalemma is non-excitable, being represented by post-synaptic densities.

The brain produces energy by oxidising glucose, which the brain receives with oxygen from the blood supply. Glucose is transported across the blood-brain barrier

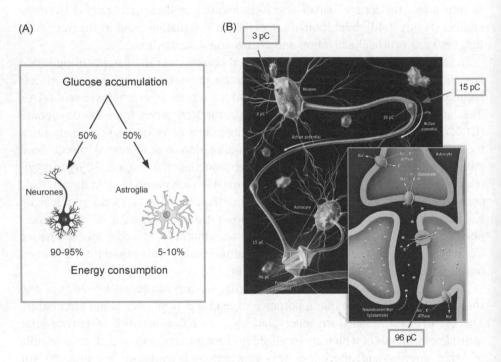

**Figure 4.41**  Fundamentals of brain energetics.

A.  Glucose distribution and energy consumption by neurones and astroglia.

B.  Energy consumed in a mammalian hippocampal neurone is in proportion to the charge transfer that produces different potentials (values for charge transfer are shown in pC, picocoulombs) along the axon, dendrites, and across the synapse. The charge transfer involved in restoration of ion balance in post-synaptic terminals is about six times greater than that underlying action potentials (96 pC versus 15 pC, respectively), with marginal contributions by dendritic action potentials (3 pC) and depolarisation of pre-synaptic terminals (1 pC; see the figure). Thus, post-synaptic potentials dominate the energy requirements for neuronal signalling (Alle *et al.*, 2009; Magistretti, 2009).

Reproduced with permission from Magistretti 2009. (Full colour version in plate section.)

via glucose transporter type 1 (GLUT1), which is expressed in endothelial cells forming the capillary walls. Following transport across the blood-brain barrier, glucose is released into the extracellular space and is accumulated by neural cells via plasmalemmal glucose transporters; neurones predominantly express GLUT3, whereas astrocytes possess GLUT1.

Upon entering the cells, glucose is oxidised through glycolysis and the tricarboxylic acid cycle (TCA or Krebs cycle), which are central steps in energy production. Neurones account for about 90 per cent of brain energy consumption and glial cells are responsible for the remaining 10 per cent. As has been already discussed, neurones require a continuous supply of energy to fuel their $Na^+$-$K^+$-ATPases ($Na^+$-$K^+$ pumps), which are constantly active to maintain ion gradients across neuronal cell membranes in the face of the continuous ionic fluxes during synaptic activity and action potential propagation. However, monitoring the distribution of glucose in the brain tissue has demonstrated that it is accumulated more or less equally by neurones and astroglial cells.

This implies the involvement of an intermediate product of glucose utilisation, which is produced by astrocytes and subsequently transported to neurones. Furthermore, the utilisation of glucose by the brain strongly depends on neural activity, a process that can be readily demonstrated by functional brain imaging (e.g. positron emission tomography, PET). It turns out that astrocytes are ideally situated and have the biochemical machinery to provide metabolic support for neurones via the so-called '*astrocyte-neurone lactate shuttle*', the concept introduced by Pierre Magistretti and Luc Pellerin (Pellerin & Magistretti, 1994; for a review of the history and current state of the ANLS as the astrocyte-neurone lactate shuttle become generally known, see Belanger *et al.*, 2011; Pellerin & Magistretti, 2012).

Astrocytes do, indeed, occupy a strategic position for regulation of brain energetics, which was already recognised by Camillo Gilgo and William Lloyd Andriezen (See Chapter 1). Indeed, perivascular astroglial processes and, specifically, their endfeet, are particularly rich in astroglial glucose transporters GLUT1, making endfeet a 'privileged' glucose uptake site. Astrocytes are the only cells in the brain able to synthesise glycogen, and this acts as an energy reserve. Astroglial processes cover neuronal membranes and synaptic structures that allow redistribution of energy substrates in an activity-dependent way.

Astroglial biochemical processing of glucose takes a specific route, known as aerobic glycolysis, by which glucose is converted into pyruvate and then into lactate in the presence of oxygen; the latter step is catalysed by lactate dehydrogenase type 5 (LDH5), which is exclusively expressed in astrocytes. Aerobic glycolysis in astroglial cells is closely linked to their ability to accumulate and process glutamate.

The major fraction of glutamate released during synaptic activity is accumulated by perisynaptic astrocytes via $Na^+$-dependent glutamate transporters (see section 4.5.12). Glutamate accumulation into the astrocyte leads to an increase in cytosolic $Na^+$ concentration, which in turn activates the $Na^+$-$K^+$ ATPase ($Na^+$-$K^+$ pumps), which expels the excess $Na^+$ into the extracellular space. Activation of $Na^+$-$K^+$

ATPase stimulates phosphoglycerate kinase (PGK) and triggers aerobic glycolysis, which produces lactate.

Lactate is then released into the extracellular space and is taken up by neurones by two transporters, monocarboxylase transporter 1 and 2 (MCT-1 and 2). MCT-2 is predominantly expressed by neurones, MCT-1 by astrocytes. Once transported into the neurone, lactate is converted into pyruvate by lactate dehydrogenase type 1 (LDH1), which is expressed in neurones, as well as other lactate-consuming tissues. Pyruvate enters the TCA cycle and is utilised to produce energy (Figure 4.42).

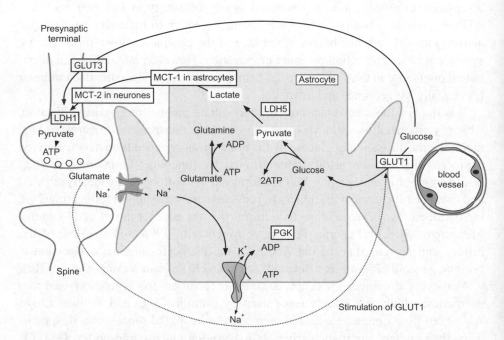

**Figure 4.42**  The 'astrocyte–neuronal lactate shuttle' – a mechanism by which astrocytes can provide an energy substrate to active neurones.

The scheme shows biochemical and physiological pathways that have been demonstrated in astrocytes and neurones. Astrocytes take up glucose via GLUT1. Glutamate released during neuronal activity is taken up by astrocytes though $Na^+$-dependent glutamate transporter. This results in an increase in cytoplasmic sodium concentration, which stimulates $Na^+/K^+$ ATPase; the latter consumes ATP and activates phosphoglycerate kinase, which stimulates aerobic glycolysis that produces pyruvate and, subsequently lactate, the latter reaction being catalysed by lactatede hydrogenase type 5. Lactate is then released into the extracellular space and is taken up by neurones via two transporters, monocarboxylase transporter 1 and 2 (MCT-1 and 2). MCT-2 is predominantly expressed by neurones, MCT-1 by astrocytes. Once transported into the neurone, lactate is converted into pyruvate by lactate dehydrogenase type 1, which is expressed in neurones (as well as in many other lactate-consuming tissues). Pyruvate enters the TCA cycle and is utilised to produce energy.

Abbreviations: GLUT1 – astroglial glucose transporter type 1; GLUT3 – neuronal glucose transporter type 3; LDH1 and LDH5 – lactatede hydrogenase type 1 and 5; MCT-1 and MCT-2 – monocarboxylase transporters 1 and 2; PGK – phosphoglycerate kinase.

Thus, glutamate released in the course of synaptic transmission acts as a specific signal on astrocytes to increase their delivery of an energy supply to active neurones. Every molecule of glutamate taken up by the astrocyte brings with it three $Na^+$ ions. This activates $Na^+/K^+$ ATPase and aerobic glycolysis, which produces two molecules of ATP and two molecules of lactate from one molecule of glucose. The ATP so produced is consumed by $Na^+/K^+$ ATPase (one ATP molecule for expelling the three $Na^+$ ions accumulated from glutamate transport), and by glutamine synthetase (one ATP molecule is needed for conversion of one molecule of the accumulated glutamate into one molecule of glutamine). The resulting two molecules of lactate are transported to the neurone, where each lactate molecule, being processed through the TCA cycle, delivers 17 molecules of ATP.

This process of activity-induced astrocyte-neurone lactate shuttle is further assisted by stimulation of astroglial glucose transporters by glutamate, which rapidly (in $\approx 10$ seconds) induces a 2–3 fold increase in astrocyte GLUT1-mediated glucose uptake. Feeding neurones with astroglia-derived lactate is critical for higher cognitive functions of the brain; inhibition of astroglial lactate transport disrupts long-term potentiation, memory formation and causes amnesia, but all of these impairments can be rescued by exogeneous lactate (Suzuki *et al.*, 2011). The astrocyte-neurone lactate shuttle supports not only neurones, but also other types of neural cells. For example, in the white matter, the astroglia-derived lactate is critical for metabolic support of oligodendrocytes.

Finally, neuronal energetics is further supported by *astroglial metabolic networks*. Both glucose and its derivatives can travel through astroglial syncytia through Cx43 and/or Cx30 formed gap junctions (Rouach *et al.*, 2008). This syncytial transport of energy substrates is regulated by neuronal synaptic activity most likely through activation of astroglial AMPA receptors. Such metabolic networking becomes critical in conditions of local glucose deprivation, when astrocytes are capable of sustaining synaptic transmission only when gap junctions remain operative.

It has to be noted that the astrocyte-lactate shuttle concept is not universally accepted. There are a number of contradictory views, the most extravagant of which suggests that glucose in the brain is metabolised chiefly by neurones, and that neurones also appear as a main exporter of lactate, which subsequently is taken up and utilised by astrocytes. This hypothesis is known as *neurone-astrocyte lactate shuttle* or NALS (Mangia *et al.*, 2011; Simpson *et al.*, 2007). Nonetheless, taking the currently accumulated experimental knowledge, the astrocyte neuronal shuttle concept seems, at least from the point of view of the authors of this book, more elaborated and more credible.

Besides providing for the activity-dependent nourishment of neurones through the glucose-lactate shuttle, astrocytes also contain the brain reserve energy system. This system relies upon glycogen which, in the brain, is present almost exclusively in astroglial cells. Glycogen is mobilised and turned into glucose upon intensive stimulation of the CNS. Subsequently, the glucose so produced can be used by neurones (through the lactate shuttle), or by astrocytes themselves to meet high energy demands in response to intensive synaptic activity.

## 4.6.8 Astroglia and neuroimaging

Several neuroimaging techniques are based on recording the levels of brain metabolism. Positron emission tomography (PET) visualises changes in glucose utilisation and oxygen consumption; functional magnetic resonance imaging (fMRI) monitors the degree of blood oxygenation; magnetic resonance spectroscopy (MRS) records changes in concentrations of certain metabolic substrates, such as glucose and lactate. The cellular origin of neuroimaging signals is, surprisingly, yet to be identified. It is, however, perfectly reasonable to suggest that a substantial part of these signals comes from astroglia. Indeed, an increase in uptake of $^{18}$fluorodeoxyglucose ($^{18}$FDG), regarded as a sign of higher neuronal activity as visualised by PET, can be considered to be an astroglial signal.

## 4.6.9 Ion homeostasis in the extracellular space

Maintenance of the extracellular ion composition is of paramount importance for brain function, because every shift in ion concentrations profoundly affects the membrane properties of nerve cells and, hence, their excitability. Brain extracellular space contains high amounts of $Na^+$ ($[Na^+]_o \approx 130\,mM$) and $Cl^-$ ($[Cl^-]_o \approx 100\,mM$), whereas it is rather low in $K^+$ ($[K^+]_o \approx 2–2.5\,mM$). This is reversed inside the nerve cells, as the cytosol of most neurones is rich in $K^+$ ($[K^+]_i \approx 100–140\,mM$) and poor in $Na^+$ ($[Na^+]_i \approx <10\,mM$); glial cells have similar $[K^+]_i$ to neurones and about 2 times more $[Na^+]_i$.

The intracellular chloride concentration is, as a rule, low in neurones ($[Cl]_{i-} \approx 2–10\,mM$) and is relatively high in glial cells ($[Cl]_{i-} \approx 30–60\,mM$), due to $Cl^-$ influx in exchange for $Na^+$ and $K^+$ by the $Na^+/K^+/Cl^-$ transporters. The extracellular concentration of another important cation, $Ca^{2+}$, is relatively low in the extracellular space ($[Ca^{2+}]_o \approx 1.5–2\,mM$), but nevertheless it is still about 20,000 times lower in the cytosol ($[Ca^{2+}]_i \approx 0.0001\,mM$).

These transmembrane ion gradients, together with selective plasmalemmal ion channels, form the basis for generation and maintenance of the resting membrane potential and underlie neuronal excitability. The safeguarding of transmembrane ion gradients is the task of numerous ion-transporting systems, which allow ion movements either by diffusion (ion channels) or at the expense of energy (ion pumps and exchangers), as was discussed previously in section 4.4.4.

**(i)  Astrocytes and extracellular potassium homeostasis**  Apart from preserving their own transmembrane ion homeostasis, astroglial cells are specifically involved in the maintenance of extracellular ion concentrations. The critical role for astrocytes in maintaining extracellular $K^+$ homeostasis in the CNS was proposed in 1965 by Leif Hertz (Hertz, 1965). As neuronal activity is inevitably associated with influx of $Na^+$ and $Ca^{2+}$ (depolarisation) and efflux of $K^+$ (repolarisation), the extracellular concentrations of these ions vary.

The relative variations are especially high for $K^+$, due to a low $[K^+]_o$ and a very limited volume of the CNS extracellular space (i.e. even a relatively modest amount of $K^+$ released by neurones can rather substantially affect the extracellular $K^+$ concentration). If the $K^+$ released during action potential propagation were allowed to accumulate in the extracellular space, this would cause neuronal depolarisation. Small increases in $[K^+]_o$ would increase neuronal excitability by bringing their membrane potential closer to the action potential threshold, would slow down action potential repolarisation and would affect synaptic release of neurotransmitters. If $[K^+]_o$ rises sufficiently to depolarise the neurones past the threshold for $Na^+$ channel activation, neurones become non-excitable, because $Na^+$ channels become inactivated and there is a conduction block. Astrocytes help prevent the accumulation of extracellular $K^+$, thereby stabilising neuronal activity.

During intense (but still physiological) neuronal activity, the extracellular potassium concentration may rise almost two-fold, from 2–2.5 mM to 4–4.2 mM. Such an increase can be observed, for example, in the cat spinal cord during rhythmic and repetitive flexion/extension of the knee joint. As a rule, however, during regular physiological activity in the CNS, the $[K^+]_o$ rarely increases by more than 0.2– 0.4 mM. Nonetheless, locally, in tiny microdomains (e.g. in narrow clefts between neuronal and astroglial membranes in perisynaptic areas), $[K^+]_o$ may transiently attain much higher levels.

The relatively small rises in $[K^+]_o$ accompanying physiological neuronal activity indicate that powerful mechanisms controlling extracellular potassium are in operation. Disruption of these mechanisms, which do occur in pathology, results in a profound $[K^+]_o$ dyshomeostasis; during epileptic seizures, for example, $[K^+]_o$ may reach 10–12 mM, while during brain ischaemia and spreading depression, $[K^+]_o$ can transiently peak at 50–60 mM (see Kofuji & Newman, 2004; Olsen & Sontheimer, 2008 for overview of $K^+$ buffering).

The major system which removes $K^+$ from the extracellular space is located in astrocytes and is represented by *local $K^+$uptake* and *$K^+$spatial buffering*. *Local $K^+$uptake* occurs in the individual cells and is mediated by diffusion through $K^+$ channels and $K^+$ uptake mediated by exchangers and transporters (Figure 4.43). Diffusional local $K^+$ uptake occurs though inward rectifying $K_{ir}4.1$ channels abundantly expressed in astrocytes.

The resting membrane potential ($V_m$) of astrocytes ($\approx -90$ mV) is determined almost exclusively by the high $K^+$ permeability of their plasmalemma associated with $K_{ir}4.1$ channels; the astrocytic $V_m$, therefore, is very close to the $K^+$ equilibrium potential, $E_K$. Increases in $[K^+]_o$ would instantly shift the $E_K$ towards depolarisation, which would generate an inflow of $K^+$ ions (as the $V_m < E_K$). However, this inward $K^+$ current rapidly depolarises the membrane and, soon, $V_m$ becomes equal to $E_K$ and $K^+$ influx ceases.

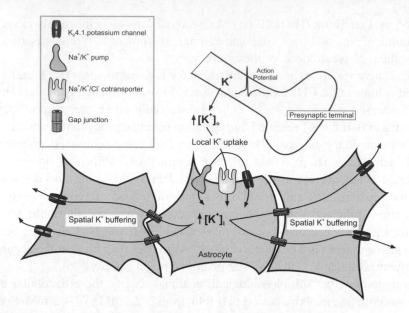

**Figure 4.43**   Astrocytes control extracellular potassium homeostasis.

Potassium is released into the extracellular space during neuronal activity ($K^+$ efflux underlies the recovery phase – repolarisation – of the action potential).

Buffering of extracellular potassium occurs through astroglial inward rectifier potassium channels $K_{ir}4.1$, $Na^+/K^+$ ATPase and $K^+/Na^+/Cl^-$ co-transporters, which all provide for local potassium buffering. Astrocytes take up excess of $K^+$, redistribute the $K^+$ through the astroglial syncytium via gap junctions (spatial potassium buffering) and release $K^+$ through $K_{ir}4.1$ distantly. See the text for further details.

A substantial part of local $K^+$ uptake is mediated by $Na^+/K^+$ pumps and $Na^+/K^+/Cl^-$ transporters. The $Na^+/K^+$ pump expels $Na^+$ out of the cell and brings $K^+$ into it. The glial $Na^+/K^+$ pumps are specifically designed for the removal of $K^+$ from the extracellular space when $[K^+]_o$ is increased, as they saturate at around 10–15 mM $[K^+]_o$; in contrast, neuronal $Na^+/K^+$ pumps are fully saturated already at 3 mM $[K^+]_o$.

The activity of $K^+$ transport by astroglial $Na^+/K^+$ pumps is regulated by cytoplasmic $Ca^{2+}$ and $Na^+$. For example, astroglial $Ca^{2+}$ signals trigger $Na^+$ entry through reversed $Na^+/Ca^{2+}$ exchanger, and resulting increase in $[Na^+]_i$ stimulates $K^+$ uptake (Wang *et al.*, 2012). Similar stimulation can occur in response to astroglial $Na^+$ fluctuations.

Uptake of $K^+$ is also assisted by $Na^+/K^+/Cl^-$ cotransport via several SLC transporters, in which $Cl^-$ influx balances $K^+$ entry. However, the capacity for local $K^+$ uptake is rather limited, because it is accompanied by an overall increase in intracellular $K^+$ concentration; water follows and enters the cells, resulting in their swelling. The operational co-existence of several molecularly distinct pathways for $K^+$ uptake in astroglia serves as a safety factor; to affect astroglial $K^+$ buffering, at least two of these pathways have to be blocked.

A much more powerful and widespread mechanism for the removal of excess extracellular $K^+$ is *spatial buffering*, a model proposed by Richard Orkand and Wolfgang Walz in the early 1980s (Orkand, 1980; Walz, 1982). According to this concept, $K^+$ ions entering a single cell are redistributed throughout the glial syncytium by intercellular $K^+$ currents through gap junctions. After this spatial redistribution, $K^+$ ions are expelled into either the interstitium or the perivascular space, where they are removed into the blood. In spatial $K^+$ buffering, the $K^+$ ions are transported across the plasma membranes using $K_{ir}4.1$ channels, exchangers and $Na^+/K^+$ pumps. Local $K^+$ entry depolarises the cell, which creates an electrical and chemical gradient between this cell and neighbouring astrocytes connected via gap junctions. This provides the force for $K^+$ ions to diffuse into the syncytium, preventing local membrane depolarisation (thus maintaining $K^+$ influx) and dispersing $K^+$ ions through many cells, so that the actual elevation in cytoplasmic $K^+$ concentration is minimal (Figure 4.43).

The principal $K^+$ channels responsible for spatial buffering are inwardly rectifying channels of $K_{ir}4.1$ type. These channels are only mildly rectifying, i.e. they allow both inward and outward $K^+$ movements at the resting membrane potential levels. This is important, as $K^+$ is finally expelled from the glial syncytium also though the $K_{ir}4.1$ channels. Another important feature of $K_{ir}$ channels is that their conductance is directly regulated by the $[K^+]_o$ levels; the conductance increases as a square root of increase in $[K^+]_o$. In other words, local increases in $[K^+]_o$ augments the rate of $K^+$ accumulation of glial cells.

The $K_{ir}4.1$ channels are clustered in perisynaptic processes of astroglial cells and in their endfeet (where the density of $K_{ir}$ channels can be up to ten times larger that in the rest of the cell membrane). This peculiar distribution facilitates $K^+$ uptake around areas of neuronal activity and $K^+$ extrusion directly into the vicinity of blood vessels.

Sometimes, $K^+$ spatial buffering may take place within the confines of an individual glial cell. A particular example of this process, known as *$K^+$ siphoning*, was described in retinal Müller cells by Eric Newman in the 1980s (Newman *et al.*, 1984; Figure 4.44). Müller cells have contacts with virtually all the cellular elements of the retina. The main endfoot of the Müller cell closely apposes the vitreous space, whereas the apical part projects into the subretinal space. Müller cells also send perivascular processes which enwrap retinal capillaries. Importantly, the endfoot and perivascular processes contain very high densities of $K_{ir}4.1$ channels.

Potassium buffering mediated by Müller cells occurs primarily in the inner plexiform layer of the retina, which contains most of the retinal synapses. The $K^+$ ions released during synaptic activity enter the cytosol of the glial cell, through which they are rapidly equilibrated. Subsequently, the excess potassium is expelled into the vitreous humour, through $K_{ir}$ channels located in the endfoot, or into the perivascular space, through $K_{ir}$ channels located in perivascular processes. Some of the $K^+$ ions may also be released through apical processes, where light induces a decrease in $[K^+]_o$ in the subretinal space.

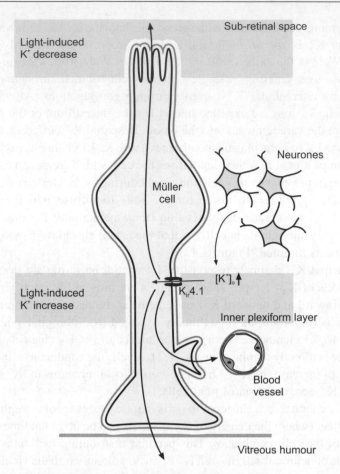

**Figure 4.44** 'Potassium siphoning' in retinal Müller glial cell.

Potassium buffering in the retina is provided by Müller glial cells. $K^+$ ions enter (mainly through $K_{ir}4.1$ channels) the cytosol of the Müller cell in the inner plexiform layer. $K^+$ then equilibrates within the glial cytosol, and excess $K^+$ is expelled through $K_{ir}4.1$ channels located in the end-foot into the vitreous humour, or through $K_{ir}$ channels located in perivascular processes into the perivascular space. Some of the $K^+$ ions may be also released through apical processes, where light induces a decrease in $[K^+]_o$ in the subretinal space. The same process of $K^+$ siphoning can occur in astrocytes, taking up $K^+$ via their perisynaptic or perinodal processes and releasing $K^+$ via their perivascular endfeet.

**(ii)  Astrocytes and chloride homeostasis**  Astrocytes contribute to overall chloride homeostasis by activation of anion channels. As the cytosolic concentration of $Cl^-$ in astroglial cells is high, opening of anion channels will cause $Cl^-$ efflux. This efflux is activated during hypo-osmotic stress. Alternatively, astrocytes can accumulate chloride by $Na^+/K^+/2Cl^-$ cotransporter.

**(iii)  Astrocytes and extracellular $Ca^{2+}$**  Calcium concentration in small extracellular compartments, and particularly in perisynaptic compartments, may fluctuate rather substantially, as $Ca^{2+}$ is accumulated by neurones when the invading action potential activates $Ca^{2+}$ channels. The actual $[Ca^{2+}]_o$ can decrease below 1 mM, which may affect generation of $Ca^{2+}$ signals in the terminal and, hence, neurotransmission (Rusakov & Fine, 2003).

Incidentally the lowering of extracellular $Ca^{2+}$ concentration to $\approx 0.5$ mM triggers $Ca^{2+}$ signalling in astrocytes (Zanotti & Charles, 1997), which originates from $InsP_3$-driven intracellular $Ca^{2+}$ release from the ER stores. The actual mechanisms of this response remain rather unclear but it may, in principle, help restore $[Ca^{2+}]_o$, as $Ca^{2+}$ can leave the astrocyte through either plasmalemmal $Ca^{2+}$ pumps or sodium-calcium exchangers. Extracellular $Ca^{2+}$ concentration may plunge much deeper (to 0.01–0.1 mM) under ischaemic conditions, which in turn can initiate seizures (see Chapter 10).

**(iv)  Astrocytes and regulation of pH**    The pH in both the extracellular space and the cytoplasm of neural cells is the subject of tight control by numerous buffering systems. The extracellular pH ($pH_o$) varies between 7.1 and 7.3, whereas intracellular pH in both neurones and glia lies in a range of 6.8–7.5. This means that the concentration of free protons, $H^+$, is quite low, being somewhere around 50 nM in the extracellular milieu and 30–160 nM in the cytosol of neural cells.

Maintenance of extracellular pH is physiologically important, as even small fluctuations of $pH_o$ may significantly affect synaptic transmission and neuronal excitability. Lowering of pH below 7.0, for example, almost completely inhibits NMDA receptors. In addition, acidification of the extracellular space can activate proton-sensitive cationic channels (known as ASICs – Acid-Sensitive Ion Channels) present in many types of neurones.

Neurones and neuronal terminals are the main source of protons in the brain. Neurones, as the main consumers of energy, produce $CO_2$, which is an end product of oxidative metabolism. The $CO_2$, by reacting with water, produces protons:

$$CO_2 + H_2O \leftrightarrow H_2CO_3 \leftrightarrow HCO_3^- + H^+$$

Furthermore, protons are released in the course of synaptic transmission, since the contents of synaptic vesicles are acidic (pH $\approx 5.6$). These changes, at least in part, are counterbalanced by bicarbonate (through the sodium bicarbonate co-transporter NBC) and proton transporters (by the sodium-proton exchanger, NHE) present in astroglial cells (for a comprehensive review and appropriate references see Deitmer & Rose, 1996, 2010). Particularly important is the $Na^+/HCO_3^-$ cotransporter (NBC), which can operate in both directions, either supplying $HCO_3^-$ or removing it from the extracellular space also. NBC is present in all types of glia; it transports 1 $Na^+$ ion in exchange for two or three $HCO_3^-$, being therefore electrogenic, and it can be readily reversed, depending on membrane potential and intracellular $Na^+$ concentration. The NBC is very sensitive to bicarbonate levels, being active at $[HCO_3^-]$ as low as 0.3 mM. It provides the main buffering capacity for the astroglial cytosol.

Astrocytes participate in setting extracellular proton concentration in several ways. First, astrocytes release $H^+$, together with lactate, via the MCT-1 transporter. Lactate/$H^+$ transport can be coordinated with movements of bicarbonate by NBC, which reportedly may facilitate lactate release. Second, astrocytes remove $H^+$ from the extracellular space by glutamate transporters that co-transport glutamate with three $Na^+$ and one $H^+$. All of these carriers are controlled by transmembrane ion gradients and can operate in forward and reverse modes.

**(v)  Astrocytes and zinc homeostasis**   Zinc ions are involved in the regulation of numerous enzymatic processes in eukaryotic cells, which have developed a sophisticated machinery for $Zn^{2+}$ homeostasis. In the CNS, $Zn^{2+}$ is mainly released from glutamatergic synapses and interacts with plasmalemmal receptors and post-synaptic compartments. $Zn^{2+}$ is transported through the plasma membranes via dedicated transporters (ZnTs/SLC30 and ZIPs/SLC39), which generally mediate $Zn^{2+}$ efflux into the extracellular space or $Zn^{2+}$ accumulation into intracellular organelles or synaptic vesicles. Zinc can also permeate through cation channels. Some astrocytes (in particular, Bergmann glial cells) express high densities of ZnTs, although the precise role of astroglia in $Zn^{2+}$ homeostasis and potential signalling is in need of characterisation (for available data and relevant references, see Sekler & Silverman, 2012).

## 4.6.10   Astrocytes and homeostasis of reactive oxygen species

Astroglia represent the main cellular component of anti-oxidative defence of the brain. First, astrocytes are the producers of glutathione, which is one of the major scavengers of ROS. Astrocytes produce glutathione from cystine, which they accumulate from the extracellular space through the cystine-glutamate exchanger. Cystine is reduced to cysteine, which is converted to γ-glutamylcysteine and subsequently to glutathione.

Neurones lack the ability to synthesise glutathione directly, because they cannot reduce cystine to cysteine. They therefore utilise astroglia-derived glutathione. Astrocytes are also critical for maintaining another anti-oxidant system associated with ascorbic acid (vitamin C). Ascorbic acid is a potent antioxidant which, upon reacting with ROS, transforms into its oxidised form, or dehydroascorbic acid, which is a highly neurotoxic compound. Neurones release dehydroascorbic acid, which is accumulated into astrocytes through a $Na^+$-dependent electrogenic co-transporter that transports one ascorbic acid anion, together with two $Na^+$ cations. This is a powerful system, which may bring the intracellular level of ascorbic acid in astrocytes *in vitro* up to 8 mM. Inside astrocytes, dehydroascorbic acid is converted to ascorbate, which is then released into extracellular space, ready for the next cycle of ROS scavenging.

## 4.6.11   Water homeostasis and regulation of the extracellular space volume

**(i)   Regulation of water homeostasis**   Astrocytes regulate water exchange between blood and brain and within the brain compartments, through specific expression of water channels aquaporins (see section 4.4.2). Astrocytes specifically express AQP4 (which is also the main AQP channel of the CNS). AQP4 channels are specifically concentrated in the astroglial perivascular and subpial endfeet, where the density of channels is about ten times higher then in the rest of the plasma membrane; AQP4 channels are also present in perisynaptic processes (Figure 4.45).

The AQP4 channels in the endfeet are co-localised with $K_{ir}4.1$ channels, and both channels are anchored to the endfeet region via a dystrophin/$\alpha$-syntrophin complex containing a PDZ domain. In the plasma membrane, AQP4 is organised in regular structures called orthogonal arrays of particles (Wolburg *et al.*, 2011). This close co-localisation of AQP4 and $K_{ir}4.1$ channels is functionally important because of the tight coupling of the $K^+$ and water movements (Amiry-Moghaddam & Ottersen, 2003); disruption of water transport affects $K^+$ clearing by spatial buffering through glial syncytia.

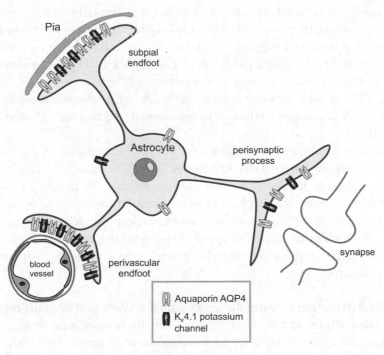

**Figure 4.45**   Distribution of aquaporin AQP4 channels and their co-localisation with $K_{ir}4.1$ potassium channels in perivascular and subpial endfeet and perisynaptic processes.

On a systemic level, water homeostasis in the brain is controlled by several neuropeptides, produced and released by neurosecretory cells. These peptides are vasopressin, atrial natriuretic peptide (ANP or atriopeptin), angiotensinogen and angiotensin.

Vasopressin increases water content in the brain by increasing the water permeability of astrocytes. This effect is mediated through astroglial vasopressin $V_1$ receptors that control intracellular $Ca^{2+}$ release. The effects of vasopressin are antagonised by ANP, which itself is produced by astrocytes. ANP is accumulated into vesicles resembling secretory granules and is released through $Ca^{2+}$-dependent exocytosis.

Water homeostasis is also controlled by the renin-angiotensin system, which is present in the brain. This system converts angiotensinogen into angiotensin II, which acts as a potent hormone regulating fluid homeostasis and blood pressure. Astrocytes are the main source of brain angiotensinogen, which is present in astroglial cells in all brain regions. How and where angiotensinogen is converted into angiotensin II remains unknown, although many astrocytes express functional angiotensin II receptors of the $AT_1$ type, and activation of these receptors causes intracellular $Ca^{2+}$ release and secretion of prostacyclin from a subpopulation of astrocytes in the cerebellum and medulla.

**(ii)   Regulatory volume decrease in astrocytes**   Astrocytes are also able to sense changes in extracellular osmolarity. When the osmolarity of the extracellular milieu is decreased (hypo-osmotic stress), astrocytes rapidly swell. This swelling is followed by a so-called regulatory volume decrease (RVD), which corrects the initial increase in cell volume (Kimelberg *et al.*, 1992). RVD is a complex process which involves extrusion of intracellular osmotically active substances, including $K^+$ and $Cl^-$, as well as some organic molecules (e.g. organic amines). Hypo-osmotic shock also triggers efflux of neurotransmitters glutamate, glycine, taurine and GABA.

The precise mechanisms of RVD are not yet fully understood. A particular role may be played by volume (swell)-activated $K^+$ and $Cl^-$ channels, and the latter may also be permeable to glutamate and taurine. Release of taurine is especially important in the osmosensitive regions of the brain. In conditions of hypo-osmotic stress, astrocytes in the supra-optic nucleus and in circumventricular organs release taurine, which activates glycine receptors of osmosensitive neurones. Rapid volume changes in astrocytes can significantly influence the volume fluctuations of the extracellular space.

**(iii)   Redistribution of water during neuronal activity and dynamic regulation of the extracellular space**   High synaptic activity is associated with a transient decrease in the extracellular space surrounding active synapses. This is physiologically important, as local restriction of the extracellular space modulates the efficacy of synaptic transmission by:

1. increasing the local concentration of neurotransmitter; and

2. limiting the spillover of the transmitter from the synaptic cleft.

This local shrinkage of the extracellular space following neuronal activity is regulated by water transport across astroglial membranes and water redistribution through the glial syncytium. Water accumulated at the site of high neuronal activity is released distantly, which causes an increase in extracellular volume. Such coordinated changes in extracellular volume have been directly observed, for example, in the cortex, where stimulation of neuronal afferents causes a local decrease in extracellular volume in layer IV and a simultaneous increase in the extracellular space in layer I. These changes in extracellular volume are directly coupled to the astroglial syncytium, as they can be eliminated following uncoupling of the glial cells by pharmacological inhibition of gap junctions.

This redistribution of water during neuronal activity is mediated through aquaporins (Haj-Yasein *et al.*, 2012; Nagelhus *et al.*, 2004). Synaptic activity causes local elevations of extracellular concentrations of glutamate, $K^+$ and $CO_2$. Glutamate and $K^+$ are accumulated by astrocytes through glutamate transporters, $K_{ir}4.1$ channels and $K^+$ transporters, whereas $CO_2$ is transported into the astrocyte by $Na^+/HCO_3^-$ co-transport. These events increase local osmotic pressure at the astrocyte membrane, which favours water intake through the aquaporins, and the removal of extracellular water leads to shrinkage of the extracellular space. Locally accumulated water is redistributed through the astroglial network and is extruded distantly (also through aquaporins), thereby increasing the extracellular volume at the site of efflux (Figure 4.46).

This scheme of water redistribution following neuronal activity is equivalent to that of spatial $K^+$ buffering, further illustrating the tight coordination between water and $K^+$ transport across astroglial membranes.

## 4.6.12 Neurotransmitter homeostasis

Astroglia, through specific expression of transporters and enzymatic cascades, are fundamental for controlling homeostasis of several key neurotransmitters in the CNS – most notably glutamate, GABA and adenosine. Astrocytes remove neurotransmitters from the extracellular cleft, thus terminating synaptic transmission and preventing possible toxicity. Furthermore, astrocytes catabolise these neurotransmitters into inert intermediates, which are then returned to neurones to be transformed into active molecules, thus maintaining synaptic transmission.

**(i) Astroglia control glutamate homeostasis and glutamatergic transmission in the CNS** Glutamic acid, commonly known as glutamate, is an amino acid that is ubiquitously present in cells, tissues and organs. In the CNS, glutamate also serves as the main excitatory neurotransmitter, which is exocytotically released

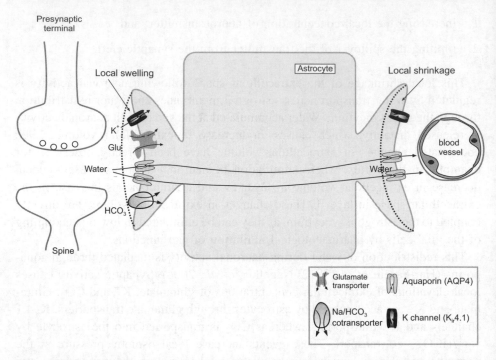

**Figure 4.46** Water transport and neuronal-activity-dependent regulation of extracellular volume by astrocytes.

Synaptic activity causes a local elevation in the concentrations of extracellular glutamate, $K^+$ and $CO_2$. Glutamate and $K^+$ are accumulated by astrocytes via glutamate transporters and $K_{ir}4.1$ channels, respectively, whereas $CO_2$ enters the cell in the form of $HCO_3^-$ via $Na^+/HCO_3^-$ cotransporter. These events increase local osmotic pressure within the astrocyte, which favours water influx through aquaporins, resulting in local swelling of the astrocyte processes and shrinkage of the extracellular space. Locally accumulated water is redistributed through the astroglial network and can be extruded distantly, e.g. at blood vessels (also through aquaporins), resulting in local shrinkage of the astrocyte processes, and therefore increasing the extracellular volume near the site of efflux.

from presynaptic terminals. This imposes severe restrictions on the brain glutamate homeostatic system, which must:

1.  prevent contamination by non-synaptically released glutamate;

2.  allow rapid removal of glutamate from the synaptic cleft; and

3.  provide the means for rapid replenishment of the glutamate-releasable pool.

There is also an important biochemical restriction. Neurones are incapable of *de novo* synthesis of glutamate, whereas astrocytes can synthesise it from glucose as a by-product of the tricarboxylic acid cycle, using a specific enzyme pyruvate carboxylase which is expressed only in astroglia (Hertz *et al.*, 1999). Neurones synthesise glutamate from glutamine, the source of which is the blood (glutamine is taken up across the blood-brain barrier) and astrocytes (via the glutamate-glutamine shuttle, as described below). Furthermore, background extracellular glutamate concentration must always be kept very low, as glutamate in excess is highly neurotoxic. Precise regulation of extracellular concentration of glutamate is, therefore, of paramount importance for brain function.

The first cornerstone of glutamate homeostasis is laid by the blood-brain barrier, which does not allow glutamate from the circulation to enter the CNS; consequently, all glutamate in the brain must be synthesised *within* the brain from glutamine, which is taken up by facilitated transport from plasma by the blood-brain barrier, via the L1 neutral amino acid transporter. A second important part of the glutamate homeostatic system is created by the specific morphological organisation of glutamatergic synapses, which are often completely enclosed by the membrane of astrocytic perisynaptic processes. Such an organisation prevents glutamate from spilling over from the synaptic cleft and contaminating nearby synapses. Third, glutamate in the synaptic cleft is removed very rapidly by glutamate transporters, which are mostly located in astroglial membranes or, to a considerably lesser extent, in the postsynaptic neuronal membrane. The pre-synaptic terminal is devoid of glutamate transporters.

Astroglial cells represent the main sink of glutamate in the brain (Figure 4.47; see Danbolt, 2001; Eulenburg & Gomeza, 2010 for a comprehensive review).

From the bulk of glutamate released during synaptic transmission, about 20 per cent is accumulated into post-synaptic neurones and the remaining 80 per cent is taken up by perisynaptic astrocytes. Thus, synaptic transmission is associated with a

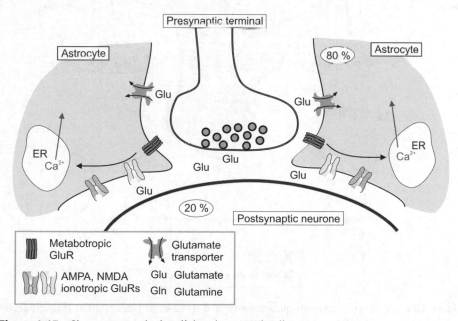

**Figure 4.47** Glutamate uptake by glial and neuronal cells.
Glutamate released during synaptic activity is removed from the cleft by glutamate transporters. About 80 per cent of glutamate is accumulated by astrocytes and ≈20 per cent by postsynaptic neurones. Pre-synaptic terminals do not accumulate glutamate.

continuous one-directional flow of glutamate into astroglial cells. Obviously, such a process would eventually deplete the pool of releasable neurotransmitter, so astrocytes therefore have a special system for recovering glutamate to the pre-synaptic terminal. After being accumulated by astrocytes, glutamate is converted into glutamine, which astrocytes release into the extracellular space for subsequent uptake into presynaptic neurones – the so-called *glutamate-glutamine shuttle* (Figure 4.48). As glutamine is physiologically inactive, its appearance in the extracellular milieu is harmless.

Conversion of glutamate to glutamine is catalysed by glutamine synthetase (highly expressed by astrocytes and used as their specific marker) and requires energy (one ATP molecule per conversion). Glutamine synthetase is, additionally, a key enzyme of nitrogen metabolism because it utilises ammonia, which is the end product of amino acid degradation (in fact, astrocytes utilise the ammonia produced by neurones when they convert glutamine back to glutamate).

Transport of glutamine from astrocytes and into neurones is mediated by two cell-segregated families of amino acid transporters. Astrocytes express the system N transport (represented by $Na^+/H^+$ dependent sodium coupled neutral amino acid transporters SN1/SNAT3/SLC38A3 and SN2/SNAT5/SLC38A5), which mediate

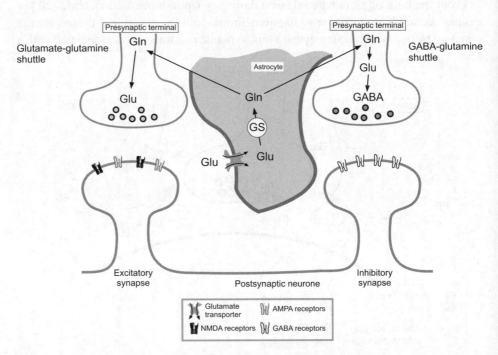

**Figure 4.48** Astrocytes maintain glutamatergic and GABA-ergic transmissions through gluta-mate-glutamine and GABA-glutamine shuttle.

After entering the astrocyte, glutamate is converted into glutamine, which is then transported back to the presynaptic terminals, where it is converted into glutamate in excitatory synapses and into GABA in inhibitory synapses; subsequently, these neurotransmitters are accumulated into synaptic vesicles. This recycling of glutamate by astrocytes is known as the glutamate-glutamine shuttle.

glutamine efflux from astroglial compartments. These transporters can be reversed (e.g. by $[Na^+]_i$ fluctuations), even in physiological conditions, thus controlling overall glutamine movements. Neurones specifically express the system A glutamine transporters (the sodium coupled neutral amino acid transporters ATA1/SNAT1/SLC38A1 and ATA2/SNAT2/SLC38A2), which act as influx transporters, mediating glutamine accumulation into the neuronal compartment (Edwards, 2007).

When glutamine enters the presynaptic neurone, it is hydrolysed to glutamate. This process, which is assisted by phosphate-activated glutaminase, does not require energy. The newly synthesised glutamate is concentrated in synaptic vesicles, endowed with specific vesicular glutamate transporters. This is the endpoint for the glutamate-glutamine shuttle, which allows for sustained glutamatergic synaptic transmission.

How rapidly is the neuronal glutamate pool depleted in conditions of ceased supply of glutamine? This varies widely between different brain regions. Glutamate-dependent memory formation in chicks is inhibited five minutes after blockade of the astroglial TCA cycle, whereas, in the retina, the response to light vanishes two minutes after inhibition of astroglial glutamine synthase; in the hippocampus, however, glutamatergic activity can be sustained for some hours after termination of glutamine supply.

Astroglial glutamate uptake is also fundamentally important in preventing excitotoxic accumulation of high glutamate levels in the extracellular space. The removal of astrocytes from neuronal glial co-cultures, for example, greatly increases neuronal vulnerability and amplifies neuronal death

**(ii) Astroglia and GABA-ergic transmission** Astrocytes are critically important for the maintenance of inhibitory transmission in the brain, which is mediated by GABA. First, astrocytes participate in removal of GABA from the synaptic cleft by glutamate transporters GAT-3 (main astroglial subtype) and GAT-1. Second, and even probably more important, GABA in neuronal terminals is synthesised from glutamate, which, in turn, arrives from the astroglial glutamate-glutamine shuttle. Inhibition of the shuttle, which, for inhibitory neurones, is often referred to as *GABA-glutamine shuttle* (Figure 4.48), rapidly decreases neuronal GABA production, depletes pre-synaptic GABA, and thus reduces inhibitory transmission (Ortinski *et al.*, 2010).

Third, astrocytes can release GABA either through anion channels or through reversed GABA transport. Astrocytes are fully equipped with GABA metabolising enzymes, which include the GABA synthesising enzyme GAD 67 and the GABA catabolising enzyme GABA-T. The cytosolic concentration of GABA in astroglial cells can be quite high, approaching $\approx 2.5$ mM (Lee *et al.*, 2011). The reversal potential of astroglial GABA transporters lies very close to astroglial resting membrane potential and, hence, even small depolarisations favour GABA efflux. In addition, GABA transport is directly controlled by $Na^+$ concentration inside astrocytes (see Section 4.4.6), and an increase in $[Na^+]_i$ also favours reversal of

GABA transporters. Diffusional release of GABA via anion channels of the Bestrophin 1 subfamily has been identified in cerebellar astrocytes (Lee *et al.*, 2010b). Astroglial release of GABA can contribute to tonic inhibition in the CNS.

**(iii)  Astroglia and adenosine homeostasis**   Physiological levels of adenosine in the CNS are generally regulated by the astroglial adenosine cycle (reviewed in Boison *et al.*, 2010). Astrocytes constitutively release ATP via several mechanisms (exocytosis and diffusion through plasmalemmal channels, as discussed above) and ATP, in turn, is degraded to adenosine by ecto-nucleotidases. Adenosine is taken up into the astrocytes by two equilibrium transporters and one $Na^+$-dependent concentration transporter. Subsequently, adenosine is catabolised intracellularly by adenosine kinase (Figure 4.49).

Adenosine kinase, which is the main determinant of adenosine metabolism in the CNS, is predominantly expressed in astrocytes. Various experimental interventions aimed at adenosine kinase substantially affect CNS levels of adenosine. For example, genetic ablation of the enzyme *in vitro* promotes adenosine release from astrocytes. Overexpression of adenosine kinase induces seizures because of lowered adenosine levels and decreased pre-synaptic inhibition. Conversely, pharmacological blockade of adenosine kinase reduces seizures in epileptic animal models because of increased adenosine concentration and increased pre-synaptic inhibition.

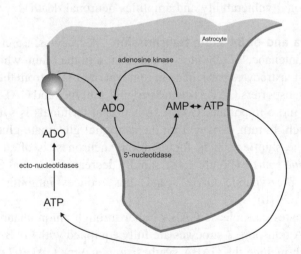

**Figure 4.49**   The levels of adenosine in the CNS are regulated by an astrocyte-based adenosine-cycle. ATP in the extracellular space is rapidly degraded by ecto-nucleotidases into adenosine (ADO), which is accumulated into astrocytes by nucleotide transporters. Inside the astrocytes, adenosine levels are controlled by the astroglia-specific enzyme adenosine kinase, which is part of an adenosine/AMP cycle. Even relatively small changes in the activity of adenosine kinase result in large changes in adenosine concentrations. Adenosine kinase is, therefore, regarded as a metabolic reuptake system for adenosine (Boison et al., 2010).

As a result, astroglia-localised adenosine kinase acts as a dynamic controller of adenosine levels in the CNS. This is a vital function because of the omnipresence of adenosine receptors in neural cells and their role in tonic inhibition. Transgenic deletion of adenosine kinase is lethal. Moreover, the enzyme is strictly conserved evolutionarily and there are no known mutations of it, most likely because sporadic mutations are inconsistent with life.

## 4.6.13 Astroglia in synaptic transmission

### (i) The astroglial synaptic compartment: concept of the tripartite synapse
In the grey matter, astrocytes are closely associated with neuronal membranes and, specifically, with synaptic regions, so that in many cases astroglial membranes completely or partially enwrap pre-synaptic terminals as well as post-synaptic structures. In the hippocampus, for example, about 60 per cent of all axon-dendritic synapses are surrounded by astroglial membranes. These astrocyte-synapse contacts show peculiar specificity; astroglial membranes enwrap about 80 per cent of large perforated synapses (which are probably the most functionally active), whereas only about half of small (known as macular) synapses are covered by glial membranes. In the cerebellum, glial-synaptic relations are even more intimate, as nearly all of the synapses formed by parallel fibres on the dendrites of Purkinje neurones are covered by the membranes of Bergmann glial cells; each individual Bergmann cell enwraps between 2,000 and 8,000 synaptic contacts.

The astroglial terminal structures that cover synapses have a rather complex morphology. Bergmann glial cells, for example, send specialised appendages, which cover several synapses and form a relatively independent compartment (Figure 4.50). This coverage is quite intimate, as the distance between glial membranes and synaptic structures in the cerebellum and hippocampus is as close as 1 μm.

The very intimate morphological apposition of astrocytes and synaptic structures allows the former to be exposed to the neurotransmitters released from the synaptic terminals. Functionally, the processes of astroglial cells are endowed with neurotransmitter receptors and most importantly, the modalities of receptors expressed by astroglial membranes precisely match the neurotransmitters released at the synapses they cover. In this respect, astrocytes have a complement of receptors very similar to that of their neuronal neighbour (see also Section 4.4.3). In the cerebellum, for example, the Purkinje neurone/Bergmann glia pair receives several synaptic inputs, which use as neurotransmitters glutamate, ATP, noradrenalin, histamine and GABA; both neurones and glial cells express receptors specific for these substances (see Figure 4.12). In the cortex, both pyramidal neurones and neighbouring astroglial cells express glutamate and purinoceptors, whereas, in the basal ganglia, neurones and astrocytes are sensitive to dopamine. In the ability to sense neurotransmitter release, therefore, the astroglial cell closely resembles the post-synaptic neurone.

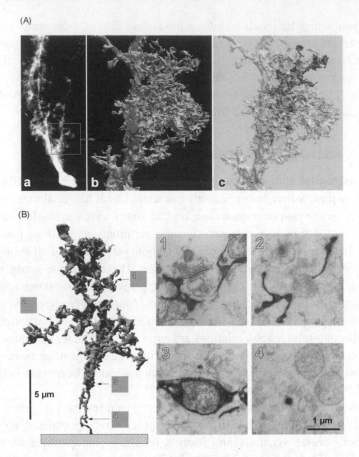

**Figure 4.50**  Close morphological contacts between Bergmann glial cells and Purkinje neurones in the cerebellum.

A.  Ultrastructure of a Bergmann glial cell.
   (a) Fluorescence light micrograph of a dye-injected Bergmann glial cell process; the red square (20 × 20 μm) corresponds to the portion that was reconstructed from consecutive ultrathin sections, shown on (b) and (c).
   (b) One of the lateral appendages, arising directly from the primary process of the Bergmann glial cell.
   (c) The same structure as shown in (b), but with one of the appendages marked by blue. This labelled structure is shown in isolation and at higher magnification in B.

B.  Left panel shows a three-dimensional reconstruction of an appendage (same as shown in A(c), extending from the process of the Bergmann glial cell. Electron micrographs of four sections contributing to the reconstruction (designated 1–4) are shown on the right; glial compartments appear black (from the injected dye). The location of these sections in the reconstruction is indicated by the labelled arrows.
   (1) Region directly contacting synapses.
   (2) Glial compartments without direct synaptic contacts.
   (3) Bulging glial structure containing a mitochondrion.
   (4) The stalk of the appendage. Note how completely the glial membranes enwrap the synaptic terminal in panel (1).

Modified and reproduced with permission from Grosche *et al.*, 1999. (Full colour version in plate section.)

The close morphological relations between astrocytes and synapses, as well as functional expression of relevant receptors in the astroglial cells, were synthesised into the concept of a *synaptic triad* (Kettenmann *et al.*, 1996), which subsequently developed into the *tripartite synapse* (Araque *et al.*, 1999; Halassa *et al.*, 2007a; Perea *et al.*, 2009). According to this concept, synapses are built from three equally important parts, the pre-synaptic terminal, the post-synaptic neuronal membrane and the surrounding astrocyte (Figure 4.51). Neurotransmitter released from the pre-synaptic terminal activates receptors in both the post-synaptic neuronal membrane and the perisynaptic astroglial membranes. This results in the generation of a post-synaptic potential in the neurone and a $Ca^{2+}$ signal in the astrocyte. The latter may propagate through the astroglial cell body or through the astrocytic syncytium; this $Ca^{2+}$ signal is assumed to trigger release of neurotransmitters from astrocytes, which in turn will signal onto both pre- and post-synaptic neuronal membranes.

Neurotransmitter-mediated signalling between neurones and astroglia has been firmly established in many experiments both *in situ* and *in vivo*, which demonstrate that electrical stimulation of neuronal inputs trigger $[Ca^{2+}]_i$ transients in astrocytes. Similarly, stimulation of sensory inputs evokes $[Ca^{2+}]_i$ responses in astroglia in the intact brain. Astrocytes are able to distinguish the intensity of neuronal activity. Astroglial $Ca^{2+}$ oscillations induced by neuronal stimulation are frequency encoded, the frequency increasing following an increase in synaptic activity. For example, astrocytes in the hippocampus are able to follow the frequency of stimulation of neuronal afferents (Carmignoto, 2000).

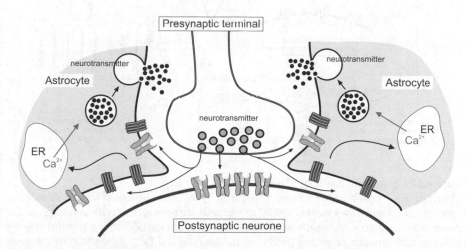

**Figure 4.51** The tripartite synapse.

The concept of the tripartite synapse assumes that it is constructed from a pre-synaptic terminal, the post-synaptic neuronal membrane and surrounding astrocyte processes. The neurotransmitter released from the pre-synaptic terminal interacts with specific receptors located in both the post-synaptic neuronal membrane and in the astroglial membrane. This triggers astroglial $Ca^{2+}$ signals, which induce the release of neurotransmitters from astrocytes that signal back to neuronal compartment.

The low frequency stimulation of neuronal fibres (the so-called Schaffer collaterals, through which neurones in the CA3 area are synaptically connected with neurones in the CA1 region) do not evoke any responses in astrocytes surrounding the synaptic terminals. High frequency stimulation, however, evoke repetitive $Ca^{2+}$ signals in astrocytes, and the frequency of astroglial $[Ca^{2+}]_i$ elevations is directly dependent on the frequency or intensity of stimulation – increases in either lead to a more frequent astrocytic response.

Importantly, the $Ca^{2+}$ responses in astrocytic processes are asynchronous, indicating the existence of relatively isolated compartments, able to follow activation of single synapses or small groups of synapses surrounded by a particular process. Similar to neurones, astrocytes also display cellular memory; periods of intense synaptic stimulation induce a long-lasting potentiation of the frequency of the subsequent responses (Figure 4.52). This phenomenon, indeed, resembles the long-term potentiation of synaptic activity in neurones, in which intense synaptic stimulation induces a

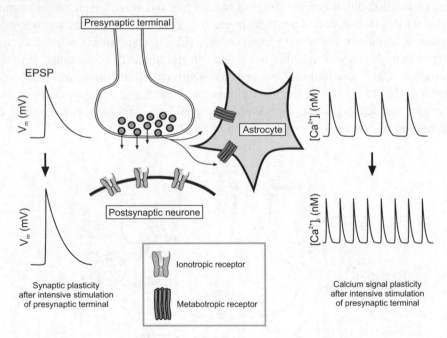

**Figure 4.52**  Long-term plasticity of astroglial $Ca^{2+}$ signals.
Astroglial $Ca^{2+}$ signals undergo a long-term plasticity following periods of intense stimulation of pre-synaptic inputs, in a manner similar to neuronal post-synaptic electrical responses. The scheme shows a central glutamatergic synapse. Electrical stimulation of the terminal triggers excitatory post-synaptic potentials (EPSPs) in the neurone and $Ca^{2+}$ signals in glial processes surrounding the synapse. Intense stimulation of synaptic inputs results in a long-term increase in the amplitude of the EPSP in the post-synaptic neurone (the phenomenon known as long-term potentiation, LTP), and in astrocytes this results in a long-term increase in the frequency of glial $Ca^{2+}$ responses.

Modified and redrawn from Carmignoto, 2000.

long-lasting increase in the amplitude of post-synaptic potentials. The only difference between neurones and glia is in the parameter under regulation; in neurones, this is the amplitude of the response, whereas in astrocytes it is the frequency.

Glial calcium responses can also be spatially compartmentalised. For example, in the cerebellum, fine processes of Bergmann glia enwrap synaptic terminals formed by parallel fibres on dendrites of Purkinje neurones. Stimulation of these parallel fibres results in highly localised $Ca^{2+}$ signals in the processes of Bergmann glial cells (Figure 4.53), indicating the existence of relatively independent signalling microdomains which can be individually activated by release of neurotransmitter from closely associated synaptic terminals.

The glial-neuronal signalling mediated through neurotransmitters released by astrocytes is more controversial. Astroglial release of neurotransmitters *in vitro* is established, yet whether this release can directly influence synaptic events and provide for rapid regulation of synaptic transmission in the living brain remains less clear. This controversy is well documented, and the reader is referred to several recent papers that summarise the data in favour of astrocytic transmitter release and synaptic modulation (Halassa & Haydon, 2010; Volterra & Meldolesi, 2005), or provide evidence against it (Agulhon *et al.*, 2008), or are sceptical (Hamilton & Attwell, 2010; Nedergaard & Verkhratsky, 2012).

**(ii)  The astroglial synaptic compartment: concept of the astroglial cradle** Astroglial perisynaptic membranes in the CNS serve another set of very important functions providing for functional isolation and maintenance of synaptic transmission through local homeostatic support. This role is synthesised in the *astroglial cradle* model (Figure 4.54; Nedergaard & Verkhratsky, 2012). First and foremost, astrocytes, through their exceptionally developed perisynaptic processes, contact and enwrap tens and hundreds of thousands of synapses residing in astroglial territorial domains. This provides the physical separation of synapses in the CNS that shields them from neurotransmitter interference from nearby synapses, thus preserving spatial and temporal selectivity of synaptic inputs. In addition to a physical barrier, astroglial membranes contain high densities of neurotransmitter (glutamate, GABA glycine, adenosine) transporters, which complements and reinforces physical barriers by further limiting transmitter spillover and extrasynaptic neurotransmission.

The astroglial compartment is critical for the maintenance of synaptic transmission through controlling ion homeostasis in the cleft, through providing the energy substrate lactate to the active synapses and through supplying pre-synaptic terminals with glutamine for replenishing neurotransmitters in the vesicles. The regulatory function of astroglial membranes also depends on the glial syncytia; disruption of the latter by genetic deletion of gap junctions, for example, affects synaptic transmission tone in the hippocampus through compromised ion and neurotransmitter homeostasis. All in all, astrocytes truly nurture synapses in many different ways that are critically important for maintaining normal synaptic transmission.

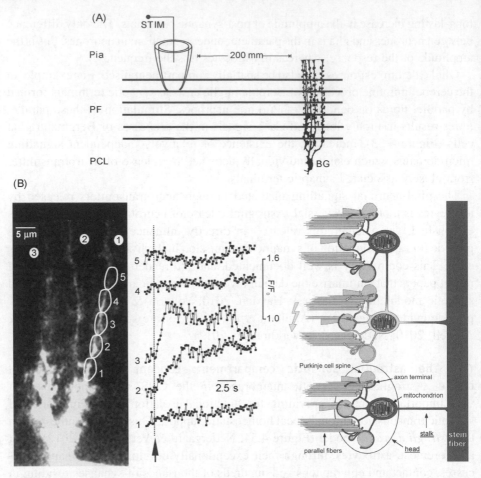

**Figure 4.53**  Localised intracellular $Ca^{2+}$ signals in processes of Bergmann glial cells in response to synaptic activity.

A.  Experimental protocol. Parallel fibres (PF) were stimulated via a pipette connected to a stimulator (STIM), while calcium-dependent fluorescence responses were recorded in a Bergmann glial cell (BG); PCL, Purkinje cell layer.

B.  The left panel shows a confocal fluorescence intensity image of a patch-clamped Bergmann glial cell dialysed with a calcium-sensitive dye (Oregon green 488 BAPTA-1). Three processes were distinguished (indicated as 1–3). Calcium signals in response to PF stimulation were measured independently in each process. The responding process (1) was subdivided into five regions of interest (marked 1–5), in which calcium signals were measured separately (middle panel: time of PF stimulation marked by an arrow and a dotted line).

C.  Schematic representation of a Bergmann glial microdomain. The basic components of the microdomain – the stalk and the 'head' – are shown together with their relationships to the neighbouring neuronal elements. Stimulation of several closely positioned parallel fibres may activate a single microdomain, inducing both membrane currents and local $Ca^{2+}$ signals.

Modified and reproduced with permission from Grosche et al., 1999.

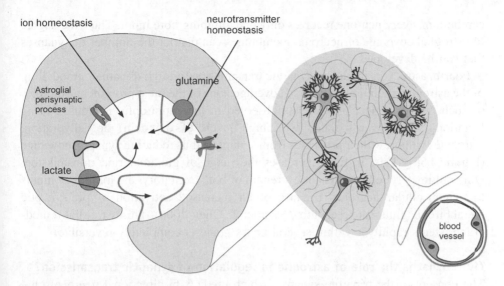

ion homeostasis

neurotransmitter
homeostasis

glutamine

Astroglial
perisynaptic
process

lactate

blood
vessel

**Figure 4.54**  Astroglial cradle.
In the 'astroglial cradle' model, the main function of perisynaptic glial processes is to isolate and support the function of individual synapses, thus ensuring the spatial specificity and optimal function of synaptic transmissions (Nedergaard & Verkhratsky, 2012).

**(iii)   Morphological plasticity of the astroglial synaptic compartment**   Astrocytes are highly morphologically plastic *in vitro* and *in situ*; they are constantly changing their volume and remodelling their processes. This morphological plasticity can be executed at several levels that affect the synaptic coverage and influence synaptic transmission, which is very much in agreement with the concept of an astroglial cradle. First, astrocytes dynamically regulate the volume of the synaptic cleft by concerted movements of solutes and water (see section 4.5.10). These changes can affect the concentration of neurotransmitters in the cleft, hence affecting the time course of synaptic events.

Second, astroglial processes can be instrumental in the formation of synapses and correct placement of pre- and post-synaptic membranes. As has been described above, astroglial processes send highly motile filopodia-like processes (Hirrlinger *et al.*, 2004), the movements of which are coordinated with the appearance and remodelling of dendritic spines (Haber *et al.*, 2006).

Third, astrocytes are fundamental for the synaptogenesis and maturation of synapses (see section 4.5.1). These are not only confined to the developing brain, but proceed throughout the life-span. Astrocytes are required for the generation and stabilisation of dendritic spines, and dynamically regulate their morphology. In addition, astroglial membranes may determine the number of synapses that can be formed on the neuronal surface. Retraction of Bergmann glial processes from Purkinje neurones in genetically modified mice, in which astrocytes express $Ca^{2+}$ impermeable AMPA glutamate receptors (Iino *et al.*, 2001), causes multiple innervation of Purkinje neurones with climbing fibres, whereas in normal cerebellum, every neurone receives only one climbing fibre input. Thus, the degree of astroglial coverage of neuronal membranes can restrict the number of synapses that can be developed.

Fourth, astrocytes modulate synaptic transmission through dynamic remodelling of the astroglial membrane synaptic coverage. One of the most prominent examples of such morphological plasticity is observed in the supra-optic nucleus. During lactation (which is associated with high levels of oxytocin) or dehydration, astrocytes withdraw their processes from synapses, thus reducing synaptic coverage (Figure 4.55). This, in turn, increases the range of glutamatergic transmission, which ultimately reduces synaptic strength of both excitatory and inhibitory inputs to magnocellular neurones because of an increased activation of pre-synaptic metabotropic glutamate receptors (Panatier & Oliet, 2006). This astroglial remodelling occurs rapidly – within several hours – and is completely reversible.

### (iv)  What is the role of astroglia in regulation of synaptic transmission?

The concept of the tripartite synapse, which predicts bi-directional neuronal glial communication at the synaptic level, remains under debate. Conceptually, there are several main problems with direct involvement of astrocytes in synaptic transmission:

- First, it seems unlikely that neurotransmitters originating from astrocytes have immediate access to the post-synaptic density; there are no indications that astroglia-derived neurotransmitters can trigger post-synaptic excitatory potentials.

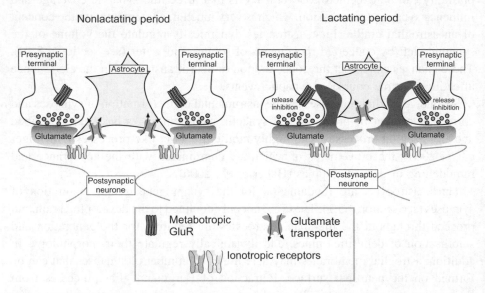

**Figure 4.55**  Morphological plasticity of astroglia in hypothalamus. Upon lactation astrocyte processes shrink, thus allowing more glutamate in the synaptic cleft, thereby strengthening synaptic transmission (Panatier and Oliet, 2006).

- Second, several observations that reduction in astroglial synaptic coverage generally increases synaptic strength clearly indicate the absence of an apparent role for glia-derived transmitters (see the previous section on morphological plasticity for details).

- Third, in different experiments, astroglial $Ca^{2+}$ signals, which are central to the concept of 'gliotransmission' and direct modulation of synapses through $Ca^{2+}$-regulated exocytosis of neurotransmitters from astroglia, have been observed to cause either inhibition or potentiation, or to have no effect on both excitatory and inhibitory transmission.

- Fourth, astroglia-specific interference with $Ca^{2+}$ signalling machinery seems not to induce any apparent changes in synaptic transmission.

At the same time, astrocytes obviously affect synaptic transmission in many ways, and regulate numerous aspects of synaptic morphology and function:

- First, they modulate synaptic strength by controlling the concentration of neurotransmitter in the cleft via glial transporters. This is the case for most synapses that use amino acid neurotransmitters, such as glutamate, GABA and monoamines, where astrocytes express specific transporters, depending on the synapse. Alternative mechanisms of affecting neurotransmitter concentration exist in central cholinergic synapses. Astrocytes covering these synapses are able to synthesise and release the acetylcholine binding protein (AChBP), which is structurally similar to the nicotinic cholinoreceptor and has a high-affinity binding site for ACh. Extensive stimulation of cholinergic terminals enhances the release of AChBP, which enters the synaptic cleft, binds ACh and effectively lowers the concentration of the latter, thus attenuating the synaptic strength.

- Second, astrocytes control the volume of the extracellular space and neurotransmitters and ion concentration in the cleft, thus defining synaptic strength.

- Third, astrocytes provide synapses with neurotransmitter precursors and with energy substrates, both of these processes being rather critical for normal synaptic transmission. Furthermore, lactate secreted by astrocytes can also carry signalling function by, for example, regulating neuronal ATP-dependent channels.

- Fourth, astrocytes determine synaptic formation and maintenance, thus regulating long-lasting synaptic plasticity.

It seems plausible that glial networks interact with neuronal networks through many mechanisms, of which glial release of neurotransmitters may not be the only one and may not be the most important. The role of astrocytes in synaptic transmission is unlikely to be executed through local exocytotic release of neurotransmitters that modulate the function of a single or few synapses within a short time scale. Rather, the role of astrocytes is more global, with astroglia being responsible for tonic and long-lasting modulation of neural networks and larger synaptic fields. In this long-lasting regulation, the exocytotic release of neuro-transmitters and neuromodulators can certainly be involved, by providing some sort of local hormonal effects. At the same time, neurotransmitter release from astroglia can also be highly heterogeneous, depending on brain region and specific function (e.g. as takes place in astrocytes involved in chemoception).

## 4.6.14   Astroglia and central chemoception of pH and $CO_2$

Preservation of $CO_2$ and pH homeostasis in the body is of vital importance and pH and $CO_2$ homeostasis is regulated by numerous systems. The $CO_2$ levels are regulated by systemic responses controlling respiration. The level of $CO_2$ in the arterial blood is monitored by chemosensors located in the carotid and aortic bodies and in dedicated regions of the CNS. The central chemosensors, localised mainly in the lower brainstem, take the leading role in regulation of respiration, as up to 80 per cent of the ventilatory response is controlled by them.

It has been generally accepted that chemosensors are localised in specialised neurones in the medulla oblongata and pons. Recent studies, however, highlighted the central role of astrocytes in central chemoception (Gourine & Kasparov, 2011; Gourine et al., 2010; Gourine et al., 2009; Huckstepp et al., 2010).

Astroglial cells localised in brainstem chemosensing areas are highly sensitive to physiological fluctuations of pH and $pCO_2$, mediated at least in part through heteromeric $K_{ir}4.1/5.1$ channels. Even a small decrease in pH initiates astroglial $Ca^{2+}$ signals, which trigger the release of ATP. ATP, in turn, induces propagating $Ca^{2+}$ waves through ventral medullary astroglial syncytia and stimulates respiratory neurones and rhythm-generating respiratory circuits that control the ventilatory response (Figure 4.56). Similar astroglial release of ATP is produced by increases in $pCO_2$. Importantly, pH-sensitive and $CO_2$-sensitive ATP release occur indepen-dently using distinct mechanisms – $Ca^{2+}$-regulated exocytosis in the case of pH, and diffusional ATP release through connexon hemichannels in the case of $CO_2$. Chemosensing is idiosyncratic to astrocytes from brainstem, as astroglial cells from other brain regions do not possess such a capability.

## 4.6.15   Astrocytes in regulation of systemic sodium homeostasis

The input signals for body sodium homeostatic systems are located in the circum-ventricular organs which surround the ventricles. These areas are not covered by blood-brain or CSF-brain barriers, so the cells in these regions can directly monitor chemical concentrations in the blood. In particular, these organs act as 'salt sensors', and increases in $Na^+$ concentration in blood plasma or in CSF modulate the activity

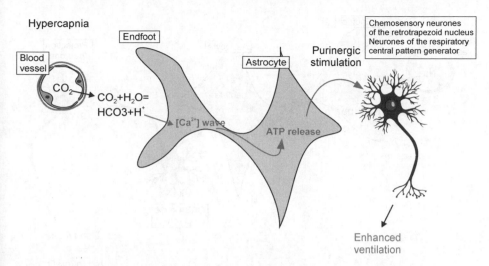

**Figure 4.56** Astrocytes as chemosensors: role in systemic pH and $CO_2$ homeostasis.

of circumventricular neurones. These neurones, in turn, send many projections to other regions of the brain, through which they regulate $Na^+$ homeostatic systemic responses, such as avoidance of dietary NaCl and increase in $Na^+$ excretion through kidneys (Skott, 2003).

The molecular nature of salt sensing was identified only recently, and it appears to be mediated through astrocytes. Astrocytes and ependymal cells located in circumventricular organs (and in particular in the subfornical organ) specifically express a peculiar channel known as $Na_x$. This channel is a distant relative of voltage-operated $Na^+$ channels, and it is activated by an increase in concentration of extracellular $Na^+$. Genetic deletion of this type of channel alters $Na^+$-aversive behaviours following $Na^+$ overload (achieved by dehydration or injection of $Na^+$ hypertonic solution). Increased plasma $Na^+$ concentration above 150 mM activates astroglial $Na_x$ channels that lead to an increase in cytosolic $Na^+$ concentration (see Figure 4.57 and Shimizu *et al.*, 2007). This, in turn, activates $Na^+/K^+$ ATPase, which (as has been already discussed in Section 4.5.7) stimulates glycolysis and lactate production.

Lactate released by astrocytes is supplied to neighbouring GABA-ergic neurones, which increase their production of ATP. Increased ATP, in turn, shuts down neuronal ATP-sensitive $K^+$ channels, which results in neuronal depolarisation, hence increasing activity. GABA-ergic neurones subsequently signal to other neurones in circumventricular organs, which initiates $Na^+$ homeostatic behaviour.

## 4.6.16 Astroglia and glucose sensing

Astrocytes are involved in central glucose sensing. Inhibition of astroglial glutamine synthetase, for example, alters responses of hypothalamic and brainstem

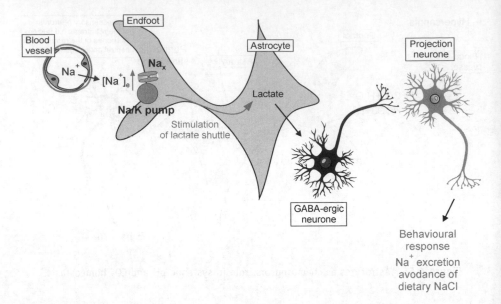

**Figure 4.57**  Astrocytes as chemosensors: role in systemic sodium homeostasis.

'glucosesensitive' neurones, which are manifested by altered insulin secretion (Guillod-Maximin *et al.*, 2004). Astrocytes also regulate the activity of hypo-thalamic orexin neurones (which produce orexin, the neurohormone involved in regulation of arousal and food intake) through the lactate shuttle and ATP-sensitive $K^+$ channels (Parsons & Hirasawa, 2010).

Tanycytes (hypothalamic astrocytes) can sense glucose directly. Application of glucose to tanycytes triggers $Ca^{2+}$ signals, which in turn trigger release of ATP that amplifies the initial $Ca^{2+}$ response and triggers $Ca^{2+}$ waves in the tanycyte layer. Tanycyte-derived ATP possibly also signals to glucose-sensing neurones of the hypothalamic nuclei. The mechanism of glucose action on tanycytes remains unresolved, and may involve either reversal of NCX (due to $[Na^+]_i$ increase associated with glucose transport by $Na^+$-dependent transporters), or direct activation of specific (and as yet unknown) G-protein coupled receptors by glucose, with secondary $[Ca^{2+}]_i$ elevation and ATP release (Frayling *et al.*, 2011).

## 4.6.17  Astroglia and circadian rhythms

In mammals, circadian rhythms are controlled by a specific pacemaker associated with a tightly coupled neuronal network of about 20,000 neurones localised in the suprachiasmatic nuclei (SCN) within the anterior hypothalamus. The clock is controlled by light stimuli, which reset the periodic activation of various clock genes and respective proteins. These proteins are expressed in both neurones and astroglia residing in the SCN (for more details in glial involvement in circadian rhythms see, for example, Jackson, 2011). The clock genes have also been identified in glial cells from the circadian oscillator ($\approx$150 cells) in Drosophila fly.

The clock genes in astrocytes show rhythmic regulation of expression; this rhythmicity is sustained for a while even in cultures, but gradually subsides. The glial rhythms can be restored by co-culturing with SCN neurones (indicating the importance of neuronal input), or by incubation of glial cultures with $Ca^{2+}$ ionophore, or with the stimulator of cAMP synthesis forskolin.

*In situ*, astroglia in the SCN display rhythmic morphological changes, changing from stellate to more protoplasmic-like during the day/night cycle. This is paralleled by changes in expression of GFAP and glutamate transporters, and it coincides with day/night changes in glial coverage of synapses in the SCN – glial coverage is higher at night than during the day. Incidentally, this coincides with day/night changes in the synaptic densities; the number of synapses on SCN neurones may increase by about 30 per cent during the day, which may be related somehow to decreased glial coverage.

The day/night change in astroglial morphology has also been found in some other brain areas. For example, the surface area of astrocytes surrounding gonadotropin-releasing hormone (GnRH) neuronal cell bodies of the organum vasculosum of the lamina terminalis (OVLT) and the medial preoptic nucleus (MPN) are largest in the mornings, which may somehow be connected with reproductive behaviour.

Astrocytes are also in possession of neurone-independent circadian rhythmicity in ATP release. In astrocytes cultured from the SCN, ATP release peaks during dark periods of the cycle (which, for nocturnal rodents, corresponds to the peak of activity). The rhythmicity of astroglial ATP release persists even in constant darkness, indicating some intrinsic regulatory clock.

## 4.6.18 Astroglia and sleep

The fundamental role of astroglia in regulation of sleep/wakefulness, suggested in 1895 by Ramón y Cajal (see Chapter 1), has been confirmed recently, mostly by the efforts of Philipp Haydon and his colleagues (Florian *et al.*, 2011; Halassa *et al.*, 2009). The astroglial regulation of sleep is achieved through fluctuations in adenosine levels in the CNS, of which astrocytes, as was described above, are the main regulators. Sleep is generally controlled by the circadian clock and by the so-called sleep homeostat – the system that integrates the length of wakefulness and increases the drive to sleep.

The sleep homeostat turns out to be critically dependent on adenosine. During wakefulness, the level of adenosine in the CNS gradually increases, and this promotes sleep (Schmitt *et al.*, 2012). However, when sleeping, the CNS levels of adenosine decrease, which resets the sleep homeostat. Adenosine accumulation in the CNS is, in turn, regulated by astrocytes, and genetic deletion of SNARE proteins responsible for exocytotic release of ATP (the main source of adenosine) significantly reduces the accumulation of sleep drive.

## 4.6.19   Astroglia and control of reproduction

Reproduction in mammals is regulated by a highly coordinated release of luteinising hormone and follicle-stimulating hormone that are, in their turn, controlled by gonadotropin-releasing hormone (GnRH) secreted by specific gonadotropin-releasing hormone neurones in the hypothalamus. Functional activity of these neurones is, to a significant extent, controlled by hypothalamic astrocytes. The latter synthesise and secrete neuromodulators such as prostaglandin 2, growth factors and neuro-steroids (e.g. 3α-hydroxy-5α-pregnane-20-one), which all stimulate GnRH neuro-secretion. In addition, hypothalamic astrocytes regulate synaptic plasticity in the hypothalamus through extension and retraction of perisynaptic processes; this form of plasticity modulates the activity status of GnRH neurones.

Astroglia-dependent regulation of synaptic plasticity in the hypothalamus is controlled by the levels of 17β-estradiol, which is the key factor triggering GnRH release and hypophysal secretion of luteinising and follicle-stimulating hormones. Astrocytes therefore may represent a mechanistic link between plasma levels of 17β-estradiol and pulsative secretion of gonadotropin hormones (see Dhandapani *et al.*, 2003 for detailed overview).

## 4.6.20   Müller glial cells as light guides in retina

A rather unusual function was recently discovered for retinal Müller cells by Andreas Reichenbach and his colleagues (Franze *et al.*, 2007). These cells, besides performing many normal astroglial functions associated with controlling homeostasis in the retinal tissue, act as light guides facilitating transmission of photons through the retina to the photoreceptors. It is well known from anatomical studies that, in vertebrates, the retina is inverted in respect to the light path. Indeed, light must travel through all the thickness of retina (which comprise many different cells with different reflective/absorbing properties) before reaching the photoreceptors. It turned out in this study that the Müller cells, which span the whole thickness of retina and are oriented along the direction of the light path, act as single-cell optical fibres that convey light directly to photoreceptors with minimal distortion or loss of photons (Figure 4.58). Every mammalian Müller cell is coupled to one cone photoreceptor cell (responsible for sharp sight under daylight conditions, i.e. photopic vision) and with several (≈10 in humans) rod photoreceptor cells.

## 4.6.21   Astroglia in ageing

The human brain is arguably the most age-resistant organ of the body. Adulthood coincides with the rather rapid deterioration of functional performance of most

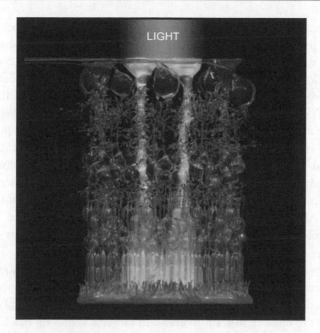

**Figure 4.58** Müller cells as light guides. Shown as an artistic impression; the light penetrates the retina using Müller glial cells as guides.
  Artwork courtesy of Dr. Jens Grosche, Leipzig University. (Full colour version in plate section.)

peripheral systems, and athletes in their mid-40s rarely win competitions associated with excessive physical feats. In contrast, human cognitive performance attains its peak in middle age (reflecting, of course long-lasting processes of gaining experience and wisdom) and stays mostly unaffected well into late adulthood. Nonetheless, senescence represents the main risk factor for neurodegenerative diseases, and is often associated with age-dependent decline in cognitive functions in advanced years. The remarkable resistance of the brain to ageing most likely reflects its high plastic potential, which can compensate for functional decline and, arguably, is also associated with the potency of homeostatic regulation directly connected with neuroglia.

Normal ageing is not associated with substantial changes in the numbers of neurones and glia. Age-dependent changes in astrocytes have been studied relatively little and the data describing astroglia in aged brains are scarce and controversial. There is a general consensus that overall levels of GFAP expression are increased in the aged brain, which is considered to be a sign of reactive astrogliosis. Nonetheless, these changes can be region-, species- and age-specific. For example, in rat retinal preparations, ageing was associated with a decrease in the total number of astrocytes, and with an increase in the proportion of cells with gliotic morphology.

Conversely, a rather significant (by one third) increase in the number of astrocytes was observed in hippocampus of female B57 mice. A similar age-dependent increase in astrocytes was found in CA1 hippocampal area and in frontal cortex of male Sprague-Dawley rats; this was accompanied with hypertrophic remodelling that was more prominent in the cortex. An increase of about 20 per cent in the number of astrocytes was detected in parietal cortex and dentate gyrus of old Wistar rats.

No change in the number of astroglial profiles was found in the primary visual cortex of old rhesus monkeys, and similarly the quantity of astrocytes in human neocortex did not change with age. However, significant increases in GFAP expression and astroglial hypertrophy were detected in the white matter of senescent monkeys brain, hinting at specific age-dependent alterations in axonal connectivity in the CNS. All in all, not much is known about astroglia in aged human brain (for further references, see Cotrina & Nedergaard, 2002; Mansour *et al.*, 2008; Pakkenberg *et al.*, 2003; Verkhratsky *et al.*, 2010).

Our own observations (Rodrigues & Verkhratsky, unpublished) shows that, while GFAP-positive astroglial profiles are increased in the ageing hippocampus, there is an age-dependent decrease in GFAP immunoreactivity in entorhinal cortex. In the human brain, the most significant increase in GFAP expression has been observed in the hippocampus, with a less obvious change in the cortical structures. Even less is known about age-associated changes in glial physiology. The overall density of neurotransmitter receptors in the cortex seems to diminish in old mice (Lalo *et al.*, 2011a), although the functional consequences remain unknown.

## 4.6.22   Astrocytes as a cellular substrate of memory and consciousness?

Contemporary neuroscience regards neuronal networks, and neuronal networks only, as the substrate of memory and consciousness. More than that, current understanding, in essence, denies the existence of special cells or cellular groups which can be the residence of memory, consciousness and/or other high cognitive functions. At the same time, information processing (as we portray it, based on current knowledge) in the neuronal networks relies entirely on a simple binary code, which might not necessarily offer a sufficient level of sophistication to explain how the human brain thinks and becomes self-aware.

In contrast, the astroglial syncytium allows much more diverse routes for informational exchange (as intracellular volume transmission allows passage of many important molecules within the connected astroglial network). Astrocytes divide the space of the grey matter into individual domains, where all neuronal and non-neuronal elements are controlled by a single astroglial cell. By extensive contacts with synaptic membranes belonging to these domains, every astrocyte can integrate all the information flowing though neuronal networks, and is capable of regulating these neuronal networks through the release of neurotransmitters, regulation of the extracellular environment and by affecting neuronal metabolism.

The individual microdomains are further integrated through intercellular contacts which multiply the processing capabilities.

As a result, it is entirely possible (and conceptually simpler) to conceive how astrocytes may provide the substrate for memory and cognition, whereas neurones are specialised to serve as the transducers of information between different brain regions and between the brain and the rest of the body. Will such an 'astrocentric' theory stand the scrutiny of experimental testing? This has to be seen in the future.

## 4.7   Concluding remarks

Astrocytes are the main homeostatic cells in the CNS, and they have multiple functions regulating all aspects of CNS homeostasis. These include neurogenesis and nervous system development, control of ion and neurotransmitter homeostasis, regulation of brain metabolic support, systemic homeostatic reactions, etc. Astrocytes are fully integrated into the brain cellular circuitry and are an indispensable part of neural networks. Conceptually, neurones and astroglia are equally important for the neural circuitry; their functions are congruent and complementary.

However, a fundamental question remains. Do astrocytes participate in higher brain functions and are they directly involved in information processing?

## References

Abbott NJ, Ronnback L, Hansson E. (2006). Astrocyte-endothelial interactions at the blood-brain barrier. *Nature Reviews Neuroscience* **7**(1), 41–53.

Abbott NJ, Patabendige AA, Dolman DE, Yusof SR, Begley DJ. (2010). Structure and function of the blood-brain barrier. *Neurobiology of Disease* **37**(1), 13–25.

Abbracchio MP, Burnstock G, Verkhratsky A, Zimmermann H. (2009). Purinergic signalling in the nervous system: an overview. *Trends In Neurosciences* **32**(1), 19–29.

Agulhon C, Petravicz J, McMullen AB, Sweger EJ, Minton SK, Taves SR, Casper KB, Fiacco TA, McCarthy KD. (2008). What is the role of astrocyte calcium in neurophysiology? *Neuron* **59**(6), 932–46.

Akopian G, Kressin K, Derouiche A, Steinhauser C. (1996). Identified glial cells in the early postnatal mouse hippocampus display different types of $Ca^{2+}$ currents. *Glia* **17**(3), 181–94.

Alle H, Roth A, Geiger JR. (2009). Energy-efficient action potentials in hippocampal mossy fibers. *Science* **325**(5946), 1405–8.

Altimimi HF, Schnetkamp P.P. (2007). $Na^+/Ca^{2+}$-$K^+$ exchangers (NCKX): functional properties and physiological roles. *Channels (Austin)* **1**(2), 62–9.

Alvarez-Buylla A, Lim DA. (2004). For the long run: maintaining germinal niches in the adult brain. *Neuron* **41**(5), 683–6.

Alvarez-Buylla A, Theelen M, Nottebohm F. (1990). Proliferation "hot spots" in adult avian ventricular zone reveal radial cell division. *Neuron* **5**(1), 101–9.

Amiry-Moghaddam M, Ottersen OP. (2003). The molecular basis of water transport in the brain. *Nature Reviews Neuroscience* **4**(12), 991–1001.

Anderson CM, Bergher JP, Swanson RA. (2004). ATP-induced ATP release from astrocytes. *Journal of Neurochemistry* **88**(1), 246–56.

Appaix F, Girod S, Boisseau S, Romer J, Vial JC, Albrieux M, Maurin M, Depaulis A, Guillemain I, van der Sanden B. (2012). Specific *in vivo* staining of astrocytes in the whole brain after intravenous injection of sulforhodamine dyes. *PLoS One* **7**(4), e35169.

Araque A, Parpura V, Sanzgiri RP, Haydon PG. (1999). Tripartite synapses: glia, the unacknowledged partner. *Trends In Neurosciences* **22**(5), 208–15.

Arcuino G, Lin JH, Takano T, Liu C, Jiang L, Gao Q, Kang J, Nedergaard M. (2002). Intercellular calcium signaling mediated by point-source burst release of ATP. *Proceedings of The National Academy Of Sciences Of The United States Of America* **99**(15), 9840–5.

Attwell D, Barbour B, Szatkowski M. (1993). Nonvesicular release of neurotransmitter. *Neuron* **11**(3), 401–7.

Attwell D, Buchan AM, Charpak S, Lauritzen M, Macvicar BA, Newman EA. (2010). Glial and neuronal control of brain blood flow. *Nature* **468**(7321), 232–43.

Bekar LK, He W, Nedergaard M. (2008). Locus coeruleus alpha-adrenergic-mediated activation of cortical astrocytes *in vivo*. *Cerebral Cortex* **18**(12), 2789–95.

Belanger M, Allaman I, Magistretti PJ. (2011). Brain energy metabolism: focus on astrocyte-neuron metabolic cooperation. *Cell Metabolism* **14**(6), 724–38.

Black JA, Waxman SG. (1996). Sodium channel expression: a dynamic process in neurons and non-neuronal cells. *Developmental Neuroscience* **18**(3), 139–52.

Black JA, Newcombe J, Waxman SG. (2010). Astrocytes within multiple sclerosis lesions upregulate sodium channel Nav1.5. *Brain* **133**(Pt 3), 835–46.

Boison D, Chen JF, Fredholm BB. (2010). Adenosine signaling and function in glial cells. *Cell Death & Differentiation* **17**(7), 1071–82.

Bolton S, Greenwood K, Hamilton N, Butt AM. (2006). Regulation of the astrocyte resting membrane potential by cyclic AMP and protein kinase A. *Glia* **54**(4), 316–28.

Bonfanti L, Poulain DA, Theodosis DT. (1993). Radial glia-like cells in the supraoptic nucleus of the adult rat. *Journal of Neuroendocrinology* **5**(1), 1–5.

Bosco D, Haefliger JA, Meda P. (2011). Connexins: key mediators of endocrine function. *Physiological Reviews* **91**(4), 1393–445.

Bowman CL, Kimelberg HK. (1984). Excitatory amino acids directly depolarize rat brain astrocytes in primary culture. *Nature* **311**(5987), 656–9.

Brett CL, Donowitz M, Rao R. (2005). Evolutionary origins of eukaryotic sodium/proton exchangers. *American Journal of Physiology. Cell Physiology* **288**(2), C223–39.

Brisset AC, Isakson BE, Kwak BR. (2009). Connexins in vascular physiology and pathology. *Antioxidants and Redox Signaling* **11**(2), 267–82.

Bundgaard M, Abbott NJ. (2008). All vertebrates started out with a glial blood-brain barrier 4-500 million years ago. *Glia* **56**(7), 699–708.

Burnstock G, Verkhratsky A. (2009). Evolutionary origins of the purinergic signalling system. *Acta Physiologica (Oxford)* **195**(4), 415–47.

Burnstock G, Fredholm BB, North RA, Verkhratsky A. (2010). The birth and postnatal development of purinergic signalling. *Acta Physiologica (Oxford)* **199**(2), 93–147.

Burnstock G, Fredholm BB, Verkhratsky A. (2011). Adenosine and ATP receptors in the brain. *Current Topics in Medicinal Chemistry* **11**(8), 973–1011.

Bushong EA, Martone ME, Jones YZ, Ellisman MH. (2002). Protoplasmic astrocytes in CA1 stratum radiatum occupy separate anatomical domains. *Journal of Neuroscience* **22**(1), 183–92.

Butt AM, Kalsi A. (2006). Inwardly rectifying potassium channels (Kir) in central nervous system glia: a special role for Kir4.1 in glial functions. *Journal of Cellular and Molecular Medicine* **10**(1), 33–44.

Butt AM, Colquhoun K, Tutton M, Berry M. (1994). Three-dimensional morphology of astrocytes and oligodendrocytes in the intact mouse optic nerve. *Journal of Neurocytology* **23**(8), 469–85.

Carmignoto G. (2000). Reciprocal communication systems between astrocytes and neurones. *Progress In Neurobiology* **62**(6), 561–81.

Chan-Palay V, Palay SL. (1972). The form of velate astrocytes in the cerebellar cortex of monkey and rat: high voltage electron microscopy of rapid Golgi preparations. *Zeitschrift fur Anatomie und Entwicklungsgeschichte* **138**(1), 1–19.

Charles AC, Merrill JE, Dirksen ER, Sanderson MJ. (1991). Intercellular signaling in glial cells: calcium waves and oscillations in response to mechanical stimulation and glutamate. *Neuron* **6**, 983–992.

Colombo JA, Reisin HD. (2004). Interlaminar astroglia of the cerebral cortex: a marker of the primate brain. *Brain Research* **1006**(1), 126–31.

Colombo JA, Fuchs E, Hartig W, Marotte LR, Puissant V. (2000). "Rodent-like" and "primate-like" types of astroglial architecture in the adult cerebral cortex of mammals: a comparative study. *Anatomy and Embryology* **201**(2), 111–20.

Colombo JA, Reisin HD, Miguel-Hidalgo JJ, Rajkowska G. (2006). Cerebral cortex astroglia and the brain of a genius: a propos of A. Einstein's. *Brain Research Reviews* **52**(2), 257–63.

Conti F, DeBiasi S, Minelli A, Melone M. (1996). Expression of NR1 and NR2A/B subunits of the NMDA receptor in cortical astrocytes. *Glia* **17**(3), 254–8.

Conti F, Minelli A, Melone M. (2004). GABA transporters in the mammalian cerebral cortex: localization, development and pathological implications. *Brain Research Reviews* **45**(3), 196–212.

Cornell Bell AH, Finkbeiner SM, Cooper MS, Smith SJ. (1990). Glutamate induces calcium waves in cultured astrocytes: long- range glial signaling. *Science* **247**, 470–473.

Cotrina ML, Nedergaard M. (2002). Astrocytes in the aging brain. *Journal of Neuroscience Research* **67**(1), 1–10.

Dale N, Frenguelli BG. (2009). Release of adenosine and ATP during ischemia and epilepsy. *Current Neuropharmacology* **7**(3), 160–79.

Danbolt NC. (2001). Glutamate uptake. *Progress In Neurobiology* **65**, 1–105.

Dare E, Schulte G, Karovic O, Hammarberg C, Fredholm BB. (2007). Modulation of glial cell functions by adenosine receptors. *Physiology and Behavior* **92**(1–2), 15–20.

Decrock E, Vinken M, Bol M, D'Herde K, Rogiers V, Vandenabeele P, Krysko DV, Bultynck G, Leybaert L. (2011). Calcium and connexin-based intercellular communication, a deadly catch? *Cell Calcium* **50**(3), 310–21.

Deitmer JW, Rose CR. (1996). pH regulation and proton signalling by glial cells. *Progress In Neurobiology* **48**(2), 73–103.

Deitmer JW, Rose CR. (2010). Ion changes and signalling in perisynaptic glia. *Brain Research Reviews* **63**(1–2), 113–29.

Dermietzel R, Spray DC. (1998). From neuro-glue ('Nervenkitt') to glia: a prologue. *Glia* **24**(1), 1–7.

Dermietzel R, Hwang TK, Spray DS. (1990). The gap junction family: structure, function and chemistry. *Anatomy and Embryology* **182**(6), 517–28.

Deschepper CF. (1998). Peptide receptors on astrocytes. *Frontiers In Neuroendocrinology* **19**(1), 20–46.

Dhandapani KM, Mahesh VB, Brann DW. (2003). Astrocytes and brain function: implications for reproduction. *Experimental Biology and Medicine (Maywood, NJ)* **228**(3), 253–60.

Doetsch F, Caille I, Lim DA, Garcia-Verdugo JM, Alvarez-Buylla A. (1999). Subventricular zone astrocytes are neural stem cells in the adult mammalian brain. *Cell* **97**(6), 703–16.

Duran C, Thompson CH, Xiao Q, Hartzell HC. (2010). Chloride channels: often enigmatic, rarely predictable. *Annual Review of Physiology* **72**, 95–121.

Edwards RH. (2007). The neurotransmitter cycle and quantal size. *Neuron* **55**(6), 835–58.

Ehrlich P. (1885). *Das sauerstufbudurfnis des organismus, in Eine Farbenanalytische Studie.* Berlin: Hirschwald.

Emsley JG, Macklis JD. (2006). Astroglial heterogeneity closely reflects the neuronal-defined anatomy of the adult murine CNS. *Neuron Glia Biology* **2**(3), 175–186.

Eroglu C, Barres BA. (2010). Regulation of synaptic connectivity by glia. *Nature* **468**(7321), 223–31.

Eulenburg V, Gomeza J. (2010). Neurotransmitter transporters expressed in glial cells as regulators of synapse function. *Brain Research Reviews* **63**(1–2), 103–12.

Faraci FM, Heistad DD. (1998). Regulation of the cerebral circulation: role of endothelium and potassium channels. *Physiological Reviews* **78**(1), 53–97.

Featherstone DE. (2011). Glial solute carrier transporters in Drosophila and mice. *Glia* **59**(9), 1351–63.

Feig SL, Haberly LB. (2011). Surface-associated astrocytes, not endfeet, form the glia limitans in posterior piriform cortex and have a spatially distributed, not a domain, organization. *Journal of Comparative Neurology* **519**(10), 1952–69.

Fields RD. (2011). Nonsynaptic and nonvesicular ATP release from neurons and relevance to neuron-glia signaling. *Seminars in Cell and Developmental Biology* **22**(2), 214–9.

Finkbeiner SM. (1993). Glial calcium. *Glia* **9**(2), 83–104.

Florian C, Vecsey CG, Halassa MM, Haydon PG, Abel T. (2011). Astrocyte-derived adenosine and A1 receptor activity contribute to sleep loss-induced deficits in hippocampal synaptic plasticity and memory in mice. *Journal of Neuroscience* **31**(19), 6956–62.

Franke H, Verkhratsky A, Burnstock G, Illes P. (2012). Pathophysiology of astroglial purinergic signalling. *Purinergic Signalling* in press.

Franze K, Grosche J, Skatchkov SN, Schinkinger S, Foja C, Schild D, Uckermann O, Travis K, Reichenbach A, Guck J. (2007). Muller cells are living optical fibers in the vertebrate retina. *Proceedings of The National Academy Of Sciences Of The United States Of America* **104**(20), 8287–92.

Frayling C, Britton R, Dale N. (2011). ATP-mediated glucosensing by hypothalamic tanycytes. *Journal of Physiology* **589**(Pt 9), 2275–86.

Giaume C, Koulakoff A, Roux L, Holcman D, Rouach N. (2010). Astroglial networks: a step further in neuroglial and gliovascular interactions. *Nature Reviews Neuroscience* **11**(2), 87–99.

Giaume C, Liu X. (2011). From a glial syncytium to a more restricted and specific glial networking. *Journal of Physiology* Paris.

Giaume C, McCarthy KD. (1996). Control of gap-junctional communication in astrocytic networks. *Trends In Neurosciences* **19**(8), 319–25.

Goldmann EE. (1913). Vitalfarbung am zentralnervensystem. *Abhandl Konigl preuss Akad Wiss* **1**, 1–60.

Gomeza J, Hulsmann S, Ohno K, Eulenburg V, Szoke K, Richter D, Betz H. (2003). Inactivation of the glycine transporter 1 gene discloses vital role of glial glycine uptake in glycinergic inhibition. *Neuron* **40**(4), 785–96.

Gordon GR, Choi HB, Rungta RL, Ellis-Davies GC, MacVicar BA. (2008). Brain metabolism dictates the polarity of astrocyte control over arterioles. *Nature* **456**(7223), 745–9.

Gourine AV, Kasparov S. (2011). Astrocytes as brain interoceptors. *Experimental Physiology* **96**(4), 411–6.

Gourine AV, Wood JD, Burnstock G. (2009). Purinergic signalling in autonomic control. *Trends In Neurosciences* **32**(5), 241–8.

Gourine AV, Kasymov V, Marina N, Tang F, Figueiredo MF, Lane S, Teschemacher AG, Spyer KM, Deisseroth K, Kasparov S. (2010). Astrocytes control breathing through pH-dependent release of ATP. *Science* **329**(5991), 571–5.

Grosche J, Matyash V, Moller T, Verkhratsky A, Reichenbach A, Kettenmann H. (1999). Microdomains for neuron-glia interaction: parallel fiber signaling to Bergmann glial cells. *Nature Neuroscience* **2**(2), 139–43.

Guillod-Maximin E, Lorsignol A, Alquier T, Penicaud L. (2004). Acute intracarotid glucose injection towards the brain induces specific c-fos activation in hypothalamic nuclei: involvement of astrocytes in cerebral glucose-sensing in rats. *Journal of Neuroendocrinology* **16**(5), 464–71.

Haas B, Schipke CG, Peters O, Sohl G, Willecke K, Kettenmann H. (2006). Activity-dependent ATP-waves in the mouse neocortex are independent from astrocytic calcium waves. *Cerebral Cortex* **16**(2), 237–46.

Haber M, Zhou L, Murai KK. (2006). Cooperative astrocyte and dendritic spine dynamics at hippocampal excitatory synapses. *Journal of Neuroscience* **26**(35), 8881–91.

Haj-Yasein NN, Jensen V, Ostby I, Omholt SW, Voipio J, Kaila K, Ottersen OP, Hvalby O, Nagelhus EA. (2012). Aquaporin-4 regulates extracellular space volume dynamics during high-frequency synaptic stimulation: A gene deletion study in mouse hippocampus. *Glia* **60**(6), 867–74.

Halassa MM, Haydon PG. (2010). Integrated brain circuits: astrocytic networks modulate neuronal activity and behavior. *Annual Review of Physiology* **72**, 335–55.

Halassa MM, Fellin T, Haydon PG. (2007a). The tripartite synapse: roles for gliotransmission in health and disease. *Trends in Molecular Medicine* **13**(2), 54–63.

Halassa MM, Fellin T, Takano H, Dong JH, Haydon PG. (2007b). Synaptic islands defined by the territory of a single astrocyte. *Journal of Neuroscience* **27**(24), 6473–7.

Halassa MM, Florian C, Fellin T, Munoz JR, Lee SY, Abel T, Haydon PG, Frank MG. (2009). Astrocytic modulation of sleep homeostasis and cognitive consequences of sleep loss. *Neuron* **61**(2), 213–9.

Hamilton NB, Attwell D. (2010). Do astrocytes really exocytose neurotransmitters? *Nature Reviews Neuroscience* **11**(4), 227–38.

Hanner F, Sorensen CM, Holstein-Rathlou NH, Peti-Peterdi J. (2010). Connexins and the kidney. *American Journal of Physiology – Regulatory, Integrative and Comparative Physiology* **298**(5), R1143–55.

Hartel K, Singaravelu K, Kaiser M, Neusch C, Hulsmann S, Deitmer JW. (2007). Calcium influx mediated by the inwardly rectifying $K^+$ channel $K_{ir}4.1$ (KCNJ10) at low external $K^+$ concentration. *Cell Calcium* **42**(3), 271–80.

Hartz AM, Bauer B. (2011). ABC transporters in the CNS – an inventory. *Current Pharmaceutical Biotechnology* **12**(4), 656–73.

Hassinger TD, Guthrie PB, Atkinson PB, Bennet MVL, Kater SB. (1997). An extracellular signaling component in propagation of astrocytic calcium waves. *Proceedings of The National Academy Of Sciences Of The United States Of America* **93**, 13268–13273.

Hatton GI. (1988). Pituicytes, glia and control of terminal secretion. *Journal of Experimental Biology* **139**, 67–79.

Hawkins BT, Davis TP. (2005). The blood-brain barrier/neurovascular unit in health and disease. *Pharmacological Reviews* **57**(2), 173–85.

Hayashi T. (1954). Effects of sodium glutamate on the nervous system. *Keio Journal of Medicine* **3**, 192–193.

Hediger MA, Romero MF, Peng JB, Rolfs A, Takanaga H, Bruford EA. (2004). The ABCs of solute carriers: physiological, pathological and therapeutic implications of human membrane transport proteinsIntroduction. *Pflugers Archiv* **447**(5), 465–8.

Hertz L. (1965). Possible role of neuroglia: a potassium-mediated neuronal-neuroglial-neuronal impulse transmission system. *Nature* **206**(989), 1091–4.

Hertz L, Dringen R, Schousboe A, Robinson SR. (1999). Astrocytes: glutamate producers for neurons. *Journal of Neuroscience Research* **57**(4), 417–28.

Hirrlinger J, Hulsmann S, Kirchhoff F. (2004). Astroglial processes show spontaneous motility at active synaptic terminals *in situ*. *European Journal of Neuroscience* **20**(8), 2235–9.

Hirrlinger PG, Scheller A, Braun C, Quintela-Schneider M, Fuss B, Hirrlinger J, Kirchhoff F. (2005). Expression of reef coral fluorescent proteins in the central nervous system of transgenic mice. *Molecular and Cellular Neurosciences* **30**(3), 291–303.

Hosli L, Hosli E, Andres PF, Landolt H. (1981). Evidence that the depolarization of glial cells by inhibitory amino acids is caused by an efflux of $K^+$ from neurones. *Experimental Brain Research* **42**(1), 43–8.

Huckstepp RT, id Bihi R, Eason R, Spyer KM, Dicke N, Willecke K, Marina N, Gourine AV, Dale N. (2010). Connexin hemichannel-mediated $CO_2$-dependent release of ATP in the medulla oblongata contributes to central respiratory chemosensitivity. *Journal of Physiology* **588**(Pt 20), 3901–20.

Iadecola C. (2004). Neurovascular regulation in the normal brain and in Alzheimer's disease. *Nature Reviews Neuroscience* **5**(5), 347–60.

Iadecola C, Nedergaard M. (2007). Glial regulation of the cerebral microvasculature. *Nature Neuroscience* **10**(11), 1369–76.

Iino M, Goto K, Kakegawa W, Okado H, Sudo M, Ishiuchi S, Miwa A, Takayasu Y, Saito I, Tsuzuki K and others. (2001). Glia-synapse interaction through $Ca^{2+}$-permeable AMPA receptors in Bergmann glia. *Science* **292**(5518), 926–9.

Illes P, Verkhratsky A, Burnstock G, Franke H. (2012). P2X Receptors and Their Roles in Astroglia in the Central and Peripheral Nervous System. *Neuroscientist*.

Israel JM, Schipke CG, Ohlemeyer C, Theodosis DT, Kettenmann H. (2003). GABAA receptor-expressing astrocytes in the supraoptic nucleus lack glutamate uptake and receptor currents. *Glia* **44**(2), 102–10.

Jackson FR. (2011). Glial cell modulation of circadian rhythms. *Glia* **59**(9), 1341–50.

Karadottir R, Cavelier P, Bergersen LH, Attwell D. (2005). NMDA receptors are expressed in oligodendrocytes and activated in ischaemia. *Nature* **438**(7071), 1162–6.

Kelsch W, Sim S, Lois C. (2010). Watching synaptogenesis in the adult brain. *Annual Review of Neuroscience* **33**, 131–49.

Kettenmann H. (1990). Chloride channels and carriers in cultured glial cells? In: Alvarez-Leefmans F, Russel JM. (eds.). *Chloride channels and carriers in nerve, muscle, and glial cells*, pp. 193–208. New York: Plenum.

Kettenmann H, Backus KH, Schachner M. (1984). Aspartate, glutamate and gamma-aminobutyric acid depolarize cultured astrocytes. *Neuroscience Letters* **52**(1–2), 25–9.

Kettenmann H, Faissner A, Trotter J. (1996). Neuron-glia interactions in homeostasis and degeneration. In: Greger R, Windhort U. (eds.). *Comprehensive human physiology*, pp. 533–543. Berlin, Heidelberg: Springer Verlag.

Kimelberg HK. (2004). The problem of astrocyte identity. *Neurochemistry International* **45**(2–3), 191–202.

Kimelberg HK. (2009). Astrocyte heterogeneity or homogeneity? In: Parpura V, Haydon PG. (eds.). *Astrocytes in (Patho)Physiology of the Nervous System*, pp. 1–25. NY: Springer.

Kimelberg HK. (2010). Functions of mature mammalian astrocytes: a current view. *Neuroscientist* **16**(1), 79–106.

Kimelberg HK, Goderie SK, Higman S, Pang S, Waniewski RA. (1990). Swelling-induced release of glutamate, aspartate, and taurine from astrocyte cultures. *Journal of Neuroscience* **10**(5), 1583–91.

Kimelberg HK, Sankar P, O'Connor ER, Jalonen T, Goderie SK. (1992). Functional consequences of astrocytic swelling. *Progress In Brain Research* **94**, 57–68.

Kimelberg HK, Macvicar BA, Sontheimer H. (2006). Anion channels in astrocytes: biophysics, pharmacology, and function. *Glia* **54**(7), 747–57.

Kirischuk S, Verkhratsky A. (1996). $[Ca^{2+}]_i$ recordings from neural cells in acutely isolated cerebellar slices employing differential loading of the membrane-permeant form of the calcium indicator fura-2. *Pflugers Archiv* **431**(6), 977–83.

Kirischuk S, Parpura V, Verkhratsky A. (2012). Sodium dynamics: another key to astroglial excitability? *Trends In Neurosciences* **35**(8), 497–506.

Kjenseth A, Fykerud T, Rivedal E, Leithe E. (2010). Regulation of gap junction intercellular communication by the ubiquitin system. *Cellular Signalling* **22**(9), 1267–73.

Kofuji P, Newman EA. (2004). Potassium buffering in the central nervous system. *Neuroscience* **129**(4), 1045–56.

Koncina E, Roth L, Gonthier B, Bagnard D. (2007). Role of semaphorins during axon growth and guidance. *Advances In Experimental Medicine and Biology* **621**, 50–64.

Kriegstein A, Alvarez-Buylla A. (2009). The glial nature of embryonic and adult neural stem cells. *Annual Review of Neuroscience* **32**, 149–84.

Krnjevic K, Schwartz S. (1967). Some properties of unresponsive cells in the cerebral cortex. *Experimental Brain Research* **3**(4), 306–19.

Kuga N, Sasaki T, Takahara Y, Matsuki N, Ikegaya Y. (2011). Large-scale calcium waves traveling through astrocytic networks *in vivo*. *Journal of Neuroscience* **31**(7), 2607–14.

Lalo U, Palygin O, North RA, Verkhratsky A, Pankratov Y. (2011a). Age-dependent remodelling of ionotropic signalling in cortical astroglia. *Aging Cell* **10**(3), 392–402.

Lalo U, Pankratov Y, Parpura V, Verkhratsky A. (2011b). Ionotropic receptors in neuronal-astroglial signalling: what is the role of "excitable" molecules in non-excitable cells. *Biochimica Et Biophysica Acta* **1813**(5), 992–1002.

Lalo U, Verkhratsky A, Pankratov Y. (2011c). Ionotropic ATP receptors in neuronal-glial communication. *Seminars in Cell and Developmental Biology* **22**(2), 220–8.

Langer J, Stephan J, Theis M, Rose CR. (2012). Gap junctions mediate intercellular spread of sodium between hippocampal astrocytes *in situ*. *Glia* **60**(2), 239–52.

Lee DA, Bedont JL, Pak T, Wang H, Song J, Miranda-Angulo A, Takiar V, Charubhumi V, Balordi F, Takebayashi H and others. (2012). Tanycytes of the hypothalamic median eminence form a diet-responsive neurogenic niche. *Nature Neuroscience* **15**(5), 700–2.

Lee M, McGeer EG, McGeer PL. (2011). Mechanisms of GABA release from human astrocytes. *Glia* **59**(11), 1600–11.

Lee MC, Ting KK, Adams S, Brew BJ, Chung R, Guillemin GJ. (2010a). Characterisation of the expression of NMDA receptors in human astrocytes. *PLoS One* **5**(11), e14123.

Lee S, Yoon BE, Berglund K, Oh SJ, Park H, Shin HS, Augustine GJ, Lee CJ. (2010b). Channel-mediated tonic GABA release from glia. *Science* **330**(6005), 790–6.

Lencesova L, O'Neill A, Resneck WG, Bloch RJ, Blaustein MP. (2004). Plasma membrane-cytoskeleton-endoplasmic reticulum complexes in neurons and astrocytes. *Journal of Biological Chemistry* **279**(4), 2885–93.

Lewandowsky M. (1900). Zur lehre von der cerebrospinalflussigkeit. *Z Klin Med* **40**, 480–494.

Li XX, Nomura T, Aihara H, Nishizaki T. (2001). Adenosine enhances glial glutamate efflux via A2a adenosine receptors. *Life Sciences* **68**(12), 1343–50.

Longden TA, Dunn KM, Draheim HJ, Nelson MT, Weston AH, Edwards G. (2011). Intermediate-conductance calcium-activated potassium channels participate in neurovascular coupling. *British Journal of Pharmacology* **164**(3), 922–33.

Lu Z. (2004). Mechanism of rectification in inward-rectifier K+ channels. *Annual Review of Physiology* **66**, 103–29.

Lytton J. (2007). Na$^+$/Ca$^{2+}$ exchangers: three mammalian gene families control Ca$^{2+}$ transport. *Biochemical Journal* **406**(3), 365–82.

Ma W, Compan V, Zheng W, Martin E, North RA, Verkhratsky A, Surprenant A. (2012). Pannexin 1 forms an anion-selective channel. *Pflugers Archiv* **463**(4), 585–92.

MacVicar BA, Feighan D, Brown A, Ransom B. (2002). Intrinsic optical signals in the rat optic nerve: role for K$^+$ uptake via NKCC1 and swelling of astrocytes. *Glia* **37**(2), 114–23.

Magistretti PJ. (2009). Neuroscience. Low-cost travel in neurons. *Science* **325**(5946), 1349–51.

Malarkey EB, Parpura V. (2008). Mechanisms of glutamate release from astrocytes. *Neurochemistry International* **52**(1–2), 142–54.

Malarkey EB, Ni Y, Parpura V. (2008). Ca$^{2+}$ entry through TRPC1 channels contributes to intracellular Ca$^{2+}$ dynamics and consequent glutamate release from rat astrocytes. *Glia* **56**(8), 821–35.

Mangia S, DiNuzzo M, Giove F, Carruthers A, Simpson IA, Vannucci SJ. (2011). Response to 'comment on recent modeling studies of astrocyte-neuron metabolic interactions': much ado about nothing. *Journal of Cerebral Blood Flow and Metabolism* **31**(6), 1346–53.

Mansour H, Chamberlain CG, Weible MW, 2nd, Hughes S, Chu Y, Chan-Ling T. (2008). Aging-related changes in astrocytes in the rat retina: imbalance between cell proliferation and cell death reduces astrocyte availability. *Aging Cell* **7**(4), 526–40.

Mathiisen TM, Lehre KP, Danbolt NC, Ottersen OP. (2010). The perivascular astroglial sheath provides a complete covering of the brain microvessels: an electron microscopic 3D reconstruction. *Glia* **58**(9), 1094–103.

Matyash V, Kettenmann H. (2010). Heterogeneity in astrocyte morphology and physiology. *Brain Research Reviews* **63**(1–2), 2–10.

Mauch DH, Nagler K, Schumacher S, Goritz C, Muller EC, Otto A, Pfrieger FW. (2001). CNS synaptogenesis promoted by glia-derived cholesterol. *Science* **294**(5545), 1354–7.

McKhann GM, 2nd, D'Ambrosio R, Janigro D. (1997). Heterogeneity of astrocyte resting membrane potentials and intercellular coupling revealed by whole-cell and gramicidin-perforated patch recordings from cultured neocortical and hippocampal slice astrocytes. *Journal of Neuroscience* **17**(18), 6850–63.

Molnar T, Dobolyi A, Nyitrai G, Barabas P, Heja L, Emri Z, Palkovits M, Kardos J. (2011). Calcium signals in the nucleus accumbens: Activation of astrocytes by ATP and succinate. *BMC Neuroscience* **12**, 96.

Mosso A. (1880). Sulla circolazione del sangue nel cervello dell'uomo. *Mem Real Acc Lincei* **5**, 237–358.

Mugnaini E. (1986). Cell junctions of astrocytes, ependymal and related cells in the mammal central nervous system, with emphasis on the hypothesis of a generalized syncytium of supporting cells. In: Federoff S, Vernadakis A, (eds.). *Astrocytes*, pp. 329–371. New York: Academic Press.

Mulligan SJ, MacVicar BA. (2004). Calcium transients in astrocyte endfeet cause cerebrovascular constrictions. *Nature* **431**(7005), 195–9.

Murai KK, Pasquale EB. (2011). Eph receptors and ephrins in neuron-astrocyte communication at synapses. *Glia* **59**(11), 1567–78.

Nagelhus EA, Mathiisen TM, Ottersen OP. (2004). Aquaporin-4 in the central nervous system: cellular and subcellular distribution and coexpression with KIR4.1. *Neuroscience* **129**(4), 905–13.

Nagy JI, Rash JE. (2000). Connexins and gap junctions of astrocytes and oligodendrocytes in the CNS. *Brain Research Brain Research Reviews* **32**(1), 29–44.

Navarrete M, Araque A. (2010). Endocannabinoids potentiate synaptic transmission through stimulation of astrocytes. *Neuron* **68**(1), 113–26.

Navarrete M, Perea G, Fernandez de Sevilla D, Gomez-Gonzalo M, Nunez A, Martin ED, Araque A. (2012). Astrocytes mediate *in vivo* cholinergic-induced synaptic plasticity. *PLoS Biology* **10**(2), e1001259.

Nedergaard M, Verkhratsky A. (2012). Artifact versus reality: How astrocytes contribute to synaptic events? *Glia* **60**(7), 1013–1023.

Nedergaard M, Ransom B, Goldman SA. (2003). New roles for astrocytes: redefining the functional architecture of the brain. *Trends In Neurosciences* **26**(10), 523–30.

Nedergaard M, Rodriguez JJ, Verkhratsky A. (2010). Glial calcium and diseases of the nervous system. *Cell Calcium* **47**(2), 140–9.

Newman EA, Zahs KR. (1997). Calcium waves in retinal glial cells. *Science* **275**, 844–847.

Newman EA, Frambach DA, Odette LL. (1984). Control of extracellular potassium levels by retinal glial cell K+ siphoning. *Science* **225**(4667), 1174–5.

Nickel R, Forge A. (2008). Gap junctions and connexins in the inner ear: their roles in homeostasis and deafness. *Current Opinion in Otolaryngology & Head and Neck Surgery* **16**(5), 452–7.

Nilius B, Owsianik G. (2011). The transient receptor potential family of ion channels. *Genome Biology* **12**(3), 218.

Nilius B, Eggermont J, Voets T, Buyse G, Manolopoulos V, Droogmans G. (1997). Properties of volume-regulated anion channels in mammalian cells. *Progress In Biophysics and Molecular Biology* **68**(1), 69–119.

Nimmerjahn A, Kirchhoff F, Kerr JN, Helmchen F. (2004). Sulforhodamine 101 as a specific marker of astroglia in the neocortex *in vivo*. *Nature Methods* **1**(1), 31–7.

Nimmerjahn A, Mukamel EA, Schnitzer MJ. (2009). Motor behavior activates Bergmann glial networks. *Neuron* **62**(3), 400–12.

Nishizaki T, Nagai K, Nomura T, Tada H, Kanno T, Tozaki H, Li XX, Kondoh T, Kodama N, Takahashi E *et al.* (2002). A new neuromodulatory pathway with a glial contribution mediated via A(2a) adenosine receptors. *Glia* **39**(2), 133–47.

Nolte C, Matyash M, Pivneva T, Schipke CG, Ohlemeyer C, Hanisch UK, Kirchhoff F, Kettenmann H. (2001). GFAP promoter-controlled EGFP-expressing transgenic mice: a tool to visualize astrocytes and astrogliosis in living brain tissue. *Glia* **33**(1), 72–86.

North RA. (2002). Molecular physiology of P2X receptors. *Physiological Reviews* **82**(4), 1013–67.

Nottebohm F. (2004). The road we travelled: discovery, choreography, and significance of brain replaceable neurons. *Annals of The New York Academy Of Sciences* **1016**, 628–58.

O'Donnell M, Chance RK, Bashaw GJ. (2009). Axon growth and guidance: receptor regulation and signal transduction. *Annual Review of Neuroscience* **32**, 383–412.

Oberheim NA, Wang X, Goldman S, Nedergaard M. (2006). Astrocytic complexity distinguishes the human brain. *Trends In Neurosciences* **29**(10), 547–53.

Oberheim NA, Takano T, Han X, He W, Lin JH, Wang F, Xu Q, Wyatt JD, Pilcher W, Ojemann JG and others. (2009). Uniquely hominid features of adult human astrocytes. *Journal of Neuroscience* **29**(10), 3276–87.

Oberheim NA, Goldman SA, Nedergaard M. (2012). Heterogeneity of astrocytic form and function. *Methods In Molecular Biology* **814**, 23–45.

Olabarria M, Noristani HN, Verkhratsky A, Rodriguez JJ. (2011). Age-dependent decrease in glutamine synthetase expression in the hippocampal astroglia of the triple transgenic Alzheimer's disease mouse model: mechanism for deficient glutamatergic transmission? *Molecular Neurodegeneration* **6**, 55.

Olsen ML, Campbell SL, Sontheimer H. (2007). Differential distribution of Kir4.1 in spinal cord astrocytes suggests regional differences in K+ homeostasis. *Journal of Neurophysiology* **98**(2), 786–93.

Olsen ML, Sontheimer H. (2005). Voltage-activated ion channels in glial cells. In: Kettenmann H, Ransom BR. (eds.). *Neuroglia*, pp. 112–130. Oxford: Oxford University Press.

Olsen ML, Sontheimer H. (2008). Functional implications for Kir4.1 channels in glial biology: from K+ buffering to cell differentiation. *Journal of Neurochemistry* **107**(3), 589–601.

Orkand RK. (1980). Extracellular potassium accumulation in the nervous system. *Federation Proceedings* **39**(5), 1515–8.

Ortinski PI, Dong J, Mungenast A, Yue C, Takano H, Watson DJ, Haydon PG, Coulter DA. (2010). Selective induction of astrocytic gliosis generates deficits in neuronal inhibition. *Nature Neuroscience* **13**(5), 584–91.

Pakkenberg B, Pelvig D, Marner L, Bundgaard MJ, Gundersen HJ, Nyengaard JR, Regeur L. (2003). Aging and the human neocortex. *Experimental Gerontology* **38**(1–2), 95–9.

Palygin O, Lalo U, Pankratov Y. (2011). Distinct pharmacological and functional properties of NMDA receptors in mouse cortical astrocytes. *British Journal of Pharmacology*.

Palygin O, Lalo U, Verkhratsky A, Pankratov Y. (2010). Ionotropic NMDA and P2X1/5 receptors mediate synaptically induced $Ca^{2+}$ signalling in cortical astrocytes. *Cell Calcium* **48**(4), 225–31.

Panatier A, Oliet SH. (2006). Neuron-glia interactions in the hypothalamus. *Neuron Glia Biology* **2**(1), 51–8.

Parpura V, Zorec R. (2010). Gliotransmission: Exocytotic release from astrocytes. *Brain Research Reviews* **63**(1–2), 83–92.

Parpura V, Basarsky TA, Liu F, Jeftinija K, Jeftinija S, Haydon PG. (1994). Glutamate-mediated astrocyte-neuron signalling. *Nature* **369**(6483), 744–7.

Parpura V, Grubisic V, Verkhratsky A. (2011). $Ca^{2+}$ sources for the exocytotic release of glutamate from astrocytes. *Biochimica Et Biophysica Acta* **1813**(5), 984–91.

Parri HR, Crunelli V. (2003). The role of $Ca^{2+}$ in the generation of spontaneous astrocytic $Ca^{2+}$ oscillations. *Neuroscience* **120**(4), 979–92.

Parsons MP, Hirasawa M. (2010). ATP-sensitive potassium channel-mediated lactate effect on orexin neurons: implications for brain energetics during arousal. *Journal of Neuroscience* **30**(24), 8061–70.

Pellegatti P, Falzoni S, Pinton P, Rizzuto R, Di Virgilio F. (2005). A novel recombinant plasma membrane-targeted luciferase reveals a new pathway for ATP secretion. *Molecular Biology of The Cell* **16**(8), 3659–65.

Pellerin L, Magistretti PJ. (1994). Glutamate uptake into astrocytes stimulates aerobic glycolysis: a mechanism coupling neuronal activity to glucose utilization. *Proceedings of The National Academy Of Sciences Of The United States Of America* **91**(22), 10625–9.

Pellerin L, Magistretti PJ. (2012). Sweet sixteen for ANLS. *Journal of Cerebral Blood Flow and Metabolism* E-pub ahead of print, doi: 10.1038/jcbfm.2011.149.

Perea G, Navarrete M, Araque A. (2009). Tripartite synapses: astrocytes process and control synaptic information. *Trends In Neurosciences* **32**(8), 421–31.

Peters A, Palay S, Webster HD. (1991). *The Fine Structure of the Nervous System*. New York: Oxford University Press.

Peters NS. (2006). Gap junctions: clarifying the complexities of connexins and conduction. *Circulation Research* **99**(11), 1156–8.

Pfrieger FW. (2010). Role of glial cells in the formation and maintenance of synapses. *Brain Research Reviews* **63**(1–2), 39–46.

Pfrieger FW, Barres BA. (1997). Synaptic efficacy enhanced by glial cells *in vitro*. *Science* **277**(5332), 1684–7.

Quandt FN, MacVicar BA. (1986). Calcium activated potassium channels in cultured astrocytes. *Neuroscience* **19**(1), 29–41.

Rakic P. (2003). Elusive radial glial cells: historical and evolutionary perspective. *Glia* **43**(1), 19–32.

Ramón y Cajal S. (1895). *Algunas conjeturas sobre el mechanismoanatomico de la ideacion, asociacion y atencion*: Imprenta y Libreria de Nicolas Moya.

Rechenbach A, Wolburg H (2005) Astrocytes and ependymal glia, In: Kettenmann H, Ransom BR. (eds.). *Neuroglia*, p. 20. OUP.

Ren Q, Chen K, Paulsen IT. (2007). TransportDB: a comprehensive database resource for cytoplasmic membrane transport systems and outer membrane channels. *Nucleic Acids Research* **35**(Database issue), D274–9.

Retzius G. (1894). *Biologishe Untersuchungen. Neue Folge*, Vol VI. Mit 32 Tafeln. jena – Stockholm: Von Gustav Fischer.

Reyes RC, Parpura V. (2008). Mitochondria modulate $Ca^{2+}$-dependent glutamate release from rat cortical astrocytes. *Journal of Neuroscience* **28**(39), 9682–91.

Rodriguez EM, Blazquez JL, Pastor FE, Pelaez B, Pena P, Peruzzo B, Amat P. (2005). Hypothalamic tanycytes: a key component of brain-endocrine interaction. *International Review of Cytology* **247**, 89–164.

Rosso L, Mienville JM. (2009). Pituicyte modulation of neurohormone output. *Glia* **57**(3), 235–43.

Rouach N, Koulakoff A, Abudara V, Willecke K, Giaume C. (2008). Astroglial metabolic networks sustain hippocampal synaptic transmission. *Science* **322**(5907), 1551–5.

Roy CS, Sherrington CS. (1890). On the regulation of the blood-supply of the brain. *Journal of Physiology (London)* **11**, 85–108.

Rusakov DA, Fine A. (2003). Extracellular $Ca^{2+}$ depletion contributes to fast activity-dependent modulation of synaptic transmission in the brain. *Neuron* **37**(2), 287–97.

Sa-Pereira I, Brites D, Brito MA. (2012). Neurovascular unit: a focus on pericytes. *Molecular Neurobiology* **45**(2), 327–47.

Sabirov RZ, Okada Y. (2009). The maxi-anion channel: a classical channel playing novel roles through an unidentified molecular entity. *Journal of Physiological Sciences* **59**(1), 3–21.

Saez JC, Berthoud VM, Branes MC, Martinez AD, Beyer EC. (2003). Plasma membrane channels formed by connexins: their regulation and functions. *Physiological Reviews* **83**(4), 1359–400.

Scemes E, Giaume C. (2006). Astrocyte calcium waves: what they are and what they do. *Glia* **54**(7), 716–25.

Schipke CG, Ohlemeyer C, Matyash M, Nolte C, Kettenmann H, Kirchhoff F. (2001). Astrocytes of the mouse neocortex express functional N-methyl-D-aspartate receptors. *The FASEB Journal* **15**(7), 1270–2.

Schmitt BM, Berger UV, Douglas RM, Bevensee MO, Hediger MA, Haddad GG, Boron WF. (2000). Na/HCO$_3$ cotransporters in rat brain: expression in glia, neurons, and choroid plexus. *Journal of Neuroscience* **20**(18), 6839–48.

Schmitt LI, Sims RE, Dale N, Haydon PG. (2012). Wakefulness affects synaptic and network activity by increasing extracellular astrocyte-derived adenosine. *Journal of Neuroscience* **32**(13), 4417–25.

Schummers J, Yu H, Sur M. (2008). Tuned responses of astrocytes and their influence on hemodynamic signals in the visual cortex. *Science* **320**(5883), 1638–43.

Seifert G, Huttmann K, Binder DK, Hartmann C, Wyczynski A, Neusch C, Steinhauser C. (2009). Analysis of astroglial K+ channel expression in the developing hippocampus reveals a predominant role of the Kir4.1 subunit. *Journal of Neuroscience* **29**(23), 7474–88.

Seifert G, Steinhauser C. (2001). Ionotropic glutamate receptors in astrocytes. *Progress In Brain Research* **132**, 287–99.

Sekler I, Silverman WF. (2012). Zinc homeostasis and signaling in glia. *Glia* **60**(6), 843–50.

Sharma G, Vijayaraghavan S. (2001). Nicotinic cholinergic signaling in hippocampal astrocytes involves calcium-induced calcium release from intracellular stores. *Proceedings of The National Academy Of Sciences Of The United States Of America* **98**(7), 4148–53.

Shen JX, Yakel JL. (2012). Functional alpha7 Nicotinic ACh Receptors on Astrocytes in Rat Hippocampal CA1 Slices. *Journal of Molecular Neuroscience* doi: 10.1007/s12031-012-9719-3.

Shimizu H, Watanabe E, Hiyama TY, Nagakura A, Fujikawa A, Okado H, Yanagawa Y, Obata K, Noda M. (2007). Glial $Na_x$ channels control lactate signaling to neurons for brain $[Na^+]$ sensing. *Neuron* **54**(1), 59–72.

Shu T, Li Y, Keller A, Richards LJ. (2003). The glial sling is a migratory population of developing neurons. *Development* **130**(13), 2929–37.

Simpson IA, Carruthers A, Vannucci SJ. (2007). Supply and demand in cerebral energy metabolism: the role of nutrient transporters. *Journal of Cerebral Blood Flow and Metabolism* **27**(11), 1766–91.

Skott O. (2003). Body sodium and volume homeostasis. *American Journal of Physiology – Regulatory, Integrative and Comparative Physiology* **285**(1), R14–8.

Sontheimer H, Trotter J, Schachner M, Kettenmann H. (1989). Channel expression correlates with differentiation stage during the development of oligodendrocytes from their precursor cells in culture. *Neuron* **2**(2), 1135–45.

Spray DC, Ye ZC, Ransom BR. (2006). Functional connexin "hemichannels": a critical appraisal. *Glia* **54**(7), 758–73.

Sreedharan S, Shaik JH, Olszewski PK, Levine AS, Schioth HB, Fredriksson R. (2010). Glutamate, aspartate and nucleotide transporters in the SLC17 family form four main phylogenetic clusters: evolution and tissue expression. *BMC Genomics* **11**, 17.

Stella N. (2010). Cannabinoid and cannabinoid-like receptors in microglia, astrocytes, and astrocytomas. *Glia* **58**(9), 1017–30.

Suzuki A, Stern SA, Bozdagi O, Huntley GW, Walker RH, Magistretti PJ, Alberini CM. (2011). Astrocyte-neuron lactate transport is required for long-term memory formation. *Cell* **144**(5), 810–23.

Szatkowski M, Barbour B, Attwell D. (1990). Non-vesicular release of glutamate from glial cells by reversed electrogenic glutamate uptake. *Nature* **348**(6300), 443–6.

Takano T, Tian GF, Peng W, Lou N, Libionka W, Han X, Nedergaard M. (2006). Astrocyte-mediated control of cerebral blood flow. *Nature Neuroscience* **9**(2), 260–7.

Theis M, Sohl G, Eiberger J, Willecke K. (2005). Emerging complexities in identity and function of glial connexins. *Trends In Neurosciences* **28**(4), 188–95.

Thompson RJ, Macvicar BA. (2008). Connexin and pannexin hemichannels of neurons and astrocytes. *Channels (Austin)* **2**(2), 81–6.

Velez-Fort M, Audinat E, Angulo MC. (2012). Central Role of GABA in Neuron-Glia Interactions. *Neuroscientist* doi: 10.1177/1073858411403317.

Verkhratsky A. (2010). Physiology of neuronal-glial networking. *Neurochemistry International* **57**(4), 332–43.

Verkhratsky A, Kettenmann H. (1996). Calcium signalling in glial cells. *Trends In Neurosciences* **19**(8), 346–52.

Verkhratsky A, Kirchhoff F. (2007). NMDA receptors in glia. *Neuroscientist* **13**(1), 28–37.

Verkhratsky A, Steinhauser C. (2000). Ion channels in glial cells. *Brain Research Brain Research Reviews* **32**(2–3), 380–412.

Verkhratsky A, Orkand RK, Kettenmann H. (1998). Glial calcium: homeostasis and signaling function. *Physiological Reviews* **78**(1), 99–141.

Verkhratsky A, Krishtal OA, Burnstock G. (2009). Purinoceptors on neuroglia. *Molecular Neurobiology* **39**(3), 190–208.

Verkhratsky A, Olabarria M, Noristani HN, Yeh CY, Rodriguez JJ. (2010). Astrocytes in Alzheimer's disease. *Neurotherapeutics* **7**(4), 399–412.

Verkhratsky A, Parpura V, Rodriguez JJ. (2011). Where the thoughts dwell: the physiology of neuronal-glial "diffuse neural net". *Brain Research Reviews* **66**(1–2), 133–51.

Verkhratsky A, Pankratov Y, Lalo U, Nedergaard M. (2012a). P2X receptors in neuroglia. *WIREs Membrane Transport and Signaling* **1**, 151–161.

Verkhratsky A, Rodriguez JJ, Parpura V. (2012b). Calcium signalling in astroglia. *Molecular and Cellular Endocrinology* **353**(1–2), 45–56.

Verkhratsky A, Rodriguez JJ, Parpura V. (2012c). Neurotransmitters and integration in neuronal-astroglial networks. *Neurochemical Research*.

Volterra A, Meldolesi J. (2005). Astrocytes, from brain glue to communication elements: the revolution continues. *Nature Reviews Neuroscience* **6**(8), 626–40.

von Blankenfeld G, Kettenmann H. (1991). Glutamate and GABA receptors in vertebrate glial cells. *Molecular Neurobiology* **5**(1), 31–43.

Waites CL, Craig AM, Garner CC. (2005). Mechanisms of vertebrate synaptogenesis. *Annual Review of Neuroscience* **28**, 251–74.

Walz W. (1982). Do neuronal signals regulate potassium flow in glial cells? Evidence from an invertebrate central nervous system. *Journal of Neuroscience Research* **7**(1), 71–9.

Walz W, Gimpl G, Ohlemeyer C, Kettenmann H. (1994). Extracellular ATP-induced currents in astrocytes: involvement of a cation channel. *Journal of Neuroscience Research* **38**(1), 12–8.

Wang D, Yan B, Rajapaksha WR, Fisher TE. (2009). The expression of voltage-operated $Ca^{2+}$ channels in pituicytes and the up-regulation of L-type $Ca^{2+}$ channels during water deprivation. *Journal of Neuroendocrinology* **21**(10), 858–66.

Wang DD, Bordey A. (2008). The astrocyte odyssey. *Progress In Neurobiology* **86**(4), 342–67.

Wang F, Smith NA, Xu Q, Fujita T, Baba A, Matsuda T, Takano T, Bekar L, Nedergaard M. (2012). Astrocytes modulate neural network activity by $Ca^{2+}$-dependent uptake of extracellular k+. *Science Signaling* **5**(218), ra26.

Wang X, Lou N, Xu Q, Tian GF, Peng WG, Han X, Kang J, Takano T, Nedergaard M. (2006). Astrocytic $Ca^{2+}$ signaling evoked by sensory stimulation *in vivo*. *Nature Neuroscience* **9**(6), 816–23.

Watkins JC, Evans RH. (1981). Excitatory amino acid transmitters. *Annual Review of Pharmacology and Toxicology* **21**, 165–204.

Weissman TA, Riquelme PA, Ivic L, Flint AC, Kriegstein AR. (2004). Calcium waves propagate through radial glial cells and modulate proliferation in the developing neocortex. *Neuron* **43**(5), 647–61.

Wessman DR, Benveniste EN. (2005). Cytokine and chemokine receptors and signaling. In: Kettenmann H, Ransom BR. (eds.). *Neuroglia*, pp. 146–162. Oxford: Oxford University Press.

Wilhelmsson U, Bushong EA, Price DL, Smarr BL, Phung V, Terada M, Ellisman MH, Pekny M. (2006). Redefining the concept of reactive astrocytes as cells that remain within their unique domains upon reaction to injury. *Proceedings of The National Academy Of Sciences Of The United States Of America* **103**(46), 17513–8.

Wolburg H, Wolburg-Buchholz K, Fallier-Becker P, Noell S, Mack AF. (2011). Structure and functions of aquaporin-4-based orthogonal arrays of particles. *International Review of Cell and Molecular Biology* **287**, 1–41.

Wu HQ, Rassoulpour A, Schwarcz R. (2007). Kynurenic acid leads, dopamine follows: a new case of volume transmission in the brain? *Journal of Neural Transmission* **114**(1), 33–41.

Ye ZC, Wyeth MS, Baltan-Tekkok S, Ransom BR. (2003). Functional hemichannels in astrocytes: a novel mechanism of glutamate release. *Journal of Neuroscience* **23**(9), 3588–96.

Zanotti S, Charles A. (1997). Extracellular calcium sensing by glial cells: low extracellular calcium induces intracellular calcium release and intercellular signaling. *Journal of Neurochemistry* **69**(2), 594–602.

Zhang Y, Barres BA. (2010). Astrocyte heterogeneity: an underappreciated topic in neurobiology. *Current Opinion In Neurobiology* **20**(5), 588–94.

Zhang Z, Chen G, Zhou W, Song A, Xu T, Luo Q, Wang W, Gu XS, Duan S. (2007). Regulated ATP release from astrocytes through lysosome exocytosis. *Nature Cell Biology* **9**(8), 945–53.

Zhou M, Xu G, Xie M, Zhang X, Schools GP, Ma L, Kimelberg HK, Chen H. (2009). TWIK-1 and TREK-1 are potassium channels contributing significantly to astrocyte passive conductance in rat hippocampal slices. *Journal of Neuroscience* **29**(26), 8551–64.

Zlokovic BV, Apuzzo ML. (1998). Strategies to circumvent vascular barriers of the central nervous system. *Neurosurgery* **43**(4), 877–8.

Zonta M, Angulo MC, Gobbo S, Rosengarten B, Hossmann KA, Pozzan T, Carmignoto G. (2003). Neuron-to-astrocyte signaling is central to the dynamic control of brain microcirculation. *Nature Neuroscience* **6**(1), 43–50.

Zorec R, Araque A, Carmignoto G, Haydon PG, Verkhratsky A, Parpura V. (2012). Astroglial excitability and gliotransmission: an appraisal of $Ca^{2+}$ as a signalling route. *ASN Neuro* **4**(2).

# 5
# Oligodendrocytes

*Glial Physiology and Pathophysiology*, First Edition. Alexei Verkhratsky and Arthur Butt.
© 2013 by John Wiley & Sons, Ltd. Published 2013 by John Wiley & Sons, Ltd.

Oligodendrocytes are evolutionarily specialised to form the insulating myelin sheaths around CNS axons (see Chapter 3), performing the same function as Schwann cells in the PNS (see Chapter 7). The myelin sheath is a fatty insulating layer that provides for the rapid conduction of nerve impulses. The myelinating function of oligodendrocytes was proposed by Del Rio Hortega (Penfield, 1932), and the cellular connection between oligodendrocytes and myelin sheaths was finally demonstrated by EM (Bunge, 1968; Hirano, 1968; Peters, 1964). Myelin sheaths are extraordinary expansions of the glial cell membrane, and it is the primary function of oligodendrocytes and Schwann cells to produce this remarkable living structure continuously.

The fundamental structure and function of myelin is the same in the CNS and PNS, but there are important differences between oligodendrocytes and Schwann cells and in the biochemistry of CNS and PNS myelin. Oligodendrocytes or Schwann cells, and the axons they myelinate, are entirely interdependent functional units, governed by intimate interactions between the glial and neural elements. Oligodendrocytes differentiate from oligodendrocyte progenitor cells (OPCs) in response to multiple intrinsic and extrinsic factors, including interactions with axon-derived factors that drive maturation of the oligodendrocyte-axon unit. This practically symbiotic relationship is essential for the normal development and functioning of the nervous system, as shown devastatingly by demyelinating diseases (see Chapter 10).

This chapter will deal with the myelinating function and development of oligodendrocytes. In addition, oligodendrocytes express a wide range of ion channels, receptors and other proteins, through which they interact dynamically with their environment, and we will highlight their roles in normal oligodendrocyte physiology.

# 5.1   Oligodendrocyte anatomy

## 5.1.1   The generalised structure of a myelinating oligodendrocyte

*Oligodendrocyte units* myelinate up to 30 axons within a relatively short distance of the cell body (Figure 5.1A; Butt & Ransom, 1989; Ransom *et al.*, 1991). Longitudinally along the length of an axon, myelin sheaths are interrupted by nodes of Ranvier, the highly specialised region of myelinated axons where action potentials are generated. The myelinated segments between nodes are called internodes, and these are connected to the cell body by a process that contacts each internodal myelin sheath (or myelin segment) at its approximate midpoint, giving the oligodendrocyte a symmetrical appearance (Figure 5.1B, C).

Ultrastructurally, oligodendrocyte somata have generally round, dark nuclei, which are surrounded by dark cytoplasm containing granular endoplasmic reticulum, polyribosomes, short mitochondria and Golgi apparatus – the machinery for myelin production (Figure 5.1D; Sandell & Peters, 2003). The nuclei contain dense patches of chromatin and clumps of chromatin beneath the nuclear envelope, an indication of the high degree of epigenetic regulation in oligodendrocytes. Chromatin is composed of histones, which provide epigenetic control of gene expression by regulating transcript levels, independently of changes in DNA sequence (Yu *et al.*, 2010; see Section 5.4.3).

The myelin sheath itself is seen in transverse EM section as concentric layers or lamellae wrapped around the axon (Figure 5.1E, F). If unwrapped, the myelin sheath would be a large trapezoid expansion of the glial cell membrane, in which the cytoplasm is extruded to form compacted myelin, except for a cytoplasmic ridge that extends around the compacted myelin sheet (Figure 5.1C). The cytoplasmic ridges form the inner and outer myelin tongue processes or mesaxons seen in EM profiles, and the compacted myelin is formed by the phospholipid bilayers, fused at their intracellular faces to form the major dense line, and at their extracellular faces to form the intraperiod line (Figure 5.1E, F).

The lateral cytoplasmic ridges of the myelin sheath stack upon each other to produce the paranodal loops at nodes of Ranvier (Figure 5.1G). The paranodal loops form complex axoglial adhesion junctions seen as *transverse bands* in EM, which involve a neurofascin-155 (NF155)-Caspr-Contactin axoglial adhesion complex, and are important in the separation of ion channels at nodes of Ranvier (see Section 5.2.2).

Intracellular dye-filling has enabled visualisation of the cytoplasmic compartments in oligodendrocytes and myelin (Figure 5.1A). The inner and outer tongue processes 'corkscrew' around the axon and form cytoplasmic networks (reticulations) within the compacted myelin sheath that include Schmidt-Lanterman incisures (Berry *et al.*, 1995; Ransom *et al.*, 1991; Velumian *et al.*, 2011). These provide cytoplasmic access to the compacted myelin, and the entire cytoplasmic ridge is attached to the cell body via a connecting process that provides the channel by

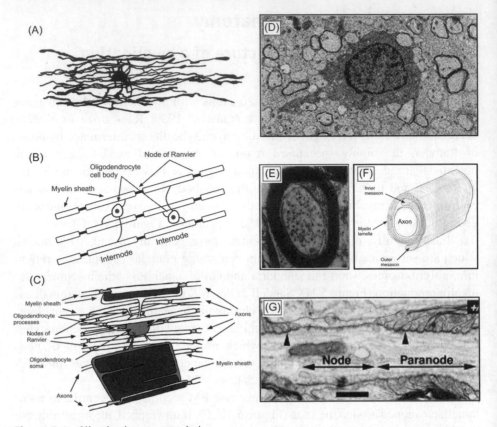

**Figure 5.1**  Oligodendrocyte morphology.

A–C.  Three-dimensional oligodendrocyte morphology, illustrated by *camera lucida* drawing of dye-filled oligodendrocyte (A) and diagrammatic representation. Based on data from Butt et al. (1994). (B), illustrating the centrally located cell body and fine processes connecting parallel arrays of up to 30 myelin sheaths.

  C.  If the myelin sheath could be unravelled, it would appear as a large, trapezoid sheet of compacted myelin surrounded by a cytoplasmic ridge that is continuous with the cytoplasm of the cell body.

D–G.  Oligodendrocyte ultrastructural morphology, illustrated by EM of cell body and its myelinated axons (D), the myelin sheath in transverse profile, (E) diagrammatic representation of the concentric lamellae wrapped around the axons, (F) and a longitudinal section through the node of Ranvier, illustrating the paranodal loops.

(D) kindly provided by Klaus Armen-Nave, (F) from  Padovani-Claudio et al. (2006), and (G) from Thaxton et al. (2011), with permissions.

which the constituents of myelin are transported to the sheath from the cell body, where they are manufactured (see Section 5.2.5). It takes over an hour for small (<500 Da) molecules to diffuse from the cell body through the cytoplamsic compartments of the whole myelin sheet (Velumian *et al.*, 2011).

## 5.1.2 Subtypes of myelinating oligodendrocytes

Oligodendrocytes types I-IV were described originally by Del Rio Hortega (Penfield, 1932), who classified them based on the shape and size of their somata, the number of their cellular processes and the size of the axons they myelinate, as well as their location and age of development (Figure 5.2). Over the ensuing century, the diversity of oligodendrocyte morphology was confirmed by histochemistry, EM, immunolabelling, intracellular dye injection, and then by expression of oligodendrocyte specific reporter genes (Berry *et al.*, 1995; Bjartmar *et al.*,

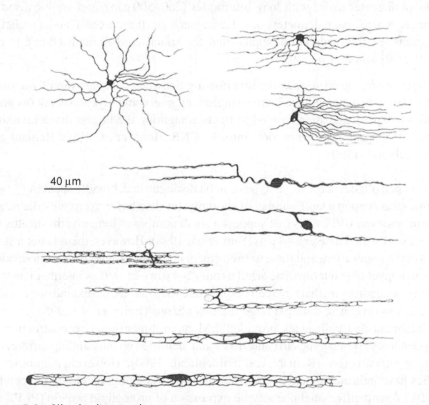

**Figure 5.2** Oligodendrocyte phenotypes.
*Camera lucida* drawings of oligodendrocytes type I–IV taken from Golgi stained spinal cord of the toad. Cells are arranged to show the variation in the orientation of their processes, and intermediate forms between the main phenotypes. The large calibre sheaths of types III and IV oligodendrocytes have fine reticulae.

Reproduced, with permission, from Stensaas LJ, Stensaas SS. 1968. Astrocytic neuroglial cells, oligodendrocytes and microgliacytes in the spinal cord of the toad. I. Light microscopy. Z Zellforsch Mikrosk Anat 84(4):473–89 © Springer Publishing.

1994; Butt *et al.*, 1998; Murtie *et al.*, 2007; Remahl & Hildebrand, 1990; Stensaas & Stensaas, 1968; Weruaga-Prieto *et al.*, 1996).

- *Type I oligodendrocytes* have small rounded somata, are most numerous in the cortex and grey matter and have a complex process arborisation, with fine branching process that myelinate 30 or more small diameter axons with short internodes that pass in multiple directions (Murtie *et al.*, 2007).

- *Type II units* are similar to type I, but have parallel arrays of intermediate length internodes (100–250 μm), and are most common in white matter, such as the corpus callosum, optic nerve, cerebellum and spinal cord (Butt *et al.*, 1994; Weruaga-Prieto *et al.*, 1996).

- *Type III oligodendrocytes* have larger irregular cell bodies, with one or more thick primary processes that rarely branch and myelinate a small number of large diameter axons with long internodes (250–500 μm), and are localised to areas where axon diameters are large, such as the cerebral and cerebellar peduncles, the medulla oblongata, and the spinal cord funiculi (Berry *et al.*, 1995; Bjartmar *et al.*, 1994).

- *Type IV oligodendrocytes*, like myelinating Schwann cells, are directly applied to a large diameter axon to form a single long internodal myelin sheath (as great as 1,000 μm), and are restricted to tracts containing the largest diameter axons near the entrance of nerve roots into the CNS (Berry *et al.*, 1995; Remahl and Hildebrand, 1990).

Two main oligodendrocyte subtypes can be distinguished, broadly speaking – type I/II units that support a large number of short myelin sheaths for axons with diameters $\leq 2$ μm, and type III/IV units that support a small number of long myelin sheaths for larger axons with diameters $\geq 4$ μm (Butt *et al.*, 1998). However, there is not a strict phenotypic segregation, and there are intermediate forms of type II/III oligodendrocytes that myelinate intermediate sized axons (2–4 μm), as well as intermediate type III/IV oligodendrocytes that have cell bodies attached to axons, but extend one or more processes to myelinate multiple large diameter axons (Berry *et al.*, 1995).

Hildebrand and colleagues provided EM three-dimensional reconstruction of oligodendrocyte phenotypes I/II and III/IV and identified no outstanding differences in their ultrastructure (Remahl and Hildebrand, 1990). However, a number of studies have indicated biochemical differences between oligodendrocyte types I/II and III/IV, with differential phenotypic expression of proteolipid protein (PLP), the small isoform of myelin associated glycoprotein (S-MAG), carbonic anhydrase II (CAII) and the microtubule associated protein (MAP) tau (Butt & Berry, 2000; Song *et al.*, 2001). These biochemical differences may underlie the greater susceptibility of type I/II oligodendrocytes to a range of pathologies compared to type III/IV oligodendrocytes (Hildebrand *et al.*, 1993).

Developmentally, the appearance of oligodendrocyte phenotypes is related to the size of the axons they myelinate, whereby large diameter fibres develop earlier than small diameter fibres and are myelinated by type III/IV oligodendrocytes that differentiate embryonically, while small diameter fibres are myelinated later in development, by type I/II oligodendrocytes that differentiate perinatally in rodents (Butt *et al.*, 1997; Hildebrand *et al.*, 1993).

Early and late developing oligodendrocytes arise from different ventral and dorsal sources, respectively (see Section 5.4.1). Early ventral specification of OPCs is dependent on sonic hedgehog (Shh), whereas late dorsal specification is independent of Shh and dependent on fibroblast growth factor 2 (FGF2) and other signalling pathways (see Section 5.4.2). It is possible that these factors help to determine the phenotypic divergence of oligodendrocyte subtypes. However, there are no evident phenotypic or physiological differences between early and late developing OPCs, and they do not appear to be inherently programmed to myelinate a specific size of axon (Almeida *et al.*, 2011; Butt *et al.*, 1999; Fanarraga *et al.*, 1998; Tripathi *et al.*, 2011). It appears that axon growth and oligodendrocyte phenotype divergence are interdependent, but it is not known how these are regulated by local axoglial signals (see Section 5.4.4).

Remyelination results in aberrant axon-myelin sheath relations, following demy-elination in diseases such as MS, or as a part of natural age-related degenerative changes. Myelin dysfunction is also implicated in schizophrenia and bipolar dis-order (Fields, 2008b). Remyelinated axons have much thinner myelin sheaths and shorter internodes than those established during normal development, indicating that local axoglial signals that regulate myelin growth within oligodendrocyte units are defective (see Section 5.4.4). The consequence is much less efficient neural transmission, underlying the neurological deficits in demyelinating diseases, as well as age-related cognitive decline. Understanding the factors that control oligoden-drocyte phenotypic characteristics is important, therefore, since they determine the speed of conduction within oligodendrocyte-axon units and, hence, the massive computing power and higher cognitive functions of the brain.

## 5.1.3 Non-myelinating oligodendrocytes

In addition to myelinating oligodendrocytes, there are two significant populations of non-myelinating oligodendrocyte lineage cells in the CNS – NG2-glia (adult OPCs) and *perineuronal* or *satellite* oligodendrocytes. NG2-glia and perineuronal oligodendrocytes have a common lineage with myelinating oligodendrocytes, but they are each antigenically and functionally distinct.

*NG2-glia* are numerous throughout grey and white matter, and are considered a distinct fourth glial cell type (Butt *et al.*, 2005; Nishiyama *et al.*, 2009 – see Chapter 6 for the history of their discovery and discussion of their nomenclature). NG2-glia have an OPC antigenic phenotype (see Section 5.4.2) and are defined by their expression of the NG2 chondroitin sulphate proteoglycan (CSPG4) and the platelet-derived growth factor receptor alpha (PDGFRα), but they do not express markers for early OPCs, such as A2B5, or for myelinating oligodendrocytes, such as CNPase (Nishiyama *et al.*, 2009; Richardson *et al.*, 2011). Ultrastructurally, NG2-glia have elongate nuclei and a thin rim of pale organelle-poor cytoplasm (Peters, 2004). A highly specialised feature of NG2-glia is that they form functional synapses with neurones and respond to neurotransmitters released at synapses (Bergles *et al.*, 2000). The only defined function of NG2-glia is to serve as a pool of OPCs that generate oligodendrocytes in the adult brain (Richardson *et al.*, 2011), but it is not known whether this is their only function (see Chapter 6).

*Perineuronal oligodendrocytes* are restricted to grey matter areas, where they are directly apposed to neuronal cell bodies (Ludwin, 1979, 1984; Szuchet *et al.*, 2011; Takasaki *et al.*, 2010). In contrast to NG2-glia, perineuronal oligodendrocytes express A2B5 and CNPase, but do not express NG2 and have PDGFRαβ rather than PDGFRαα (Szuchet *et al.*, 2011; Takasaki *et al.*, 2010). Ultrastructurally, perineuronal oligodendrocytes are oval or polygonal cells that form a concave impression on the neurone to which they are tightly attached (Takasaki *et al.*, 2010). Perineuronal oligodendrocytes have a round nucleus, rich in dark heterochromatin (Takasaki *et al.*, 2010). Despite their direct apposition to neurones, perineuronal oligodendrocytes do not appear to receive synaptic input, unlike NG2-glia. The functions of perineuronal oligodendrocytes are unknown. They may fulfil a neurone metabolic support function and protect against neuronal apoptosis (Takasaki *et al.*, 2010; Taniike *et al.*, 2002). There is a deficit of perineuronal oligodendrocytes in schizophrenia, bipolar disorder and major depression, suggesting they may be involved in the pathophysiology of these neuropsychiatric disorders (Vostrikov *et al.*, 2007).

Myelination in the adult continues in cortical regions for up to 50 years in humans, and there is ongoing myelin breakdown that accelerates in the aging brain (Peters *et al.*, 2008). Hence, there is a requirement for a pool of cells capable of generating oligodendrocytes after the main developmental period. This is the only proven function of NG2-glia (adult OPCs) (Richardson *et al.*, 2011), and perineuronal oligodendrocytes may serve the same function (Ludwin, 1979). The need for enduring oligodendrogenesis to maintain higher cortical functions and to counteract the otherwise devastating effects of ongoing myelin loss may have been the evolutionary drive for preserving such a large surplus of NG2-glia, which otherwise appear to be functionally redundant. Deficiencies in NG2-glia are implicated in the decline in oligodendrocyte numbers that contributes to the cognitive deficits observed in the aging brain and in neuropsychiatric disorders (Fields, 2008b).

# 5.2   Myelin structure and function

## 5.2.1   Myelin and saltatory conduction

The myelin sheath imposes saltatory conduction on axons by dividing the axonal membrane into alternating conductive and non-conductive portions (Figure 5.3).

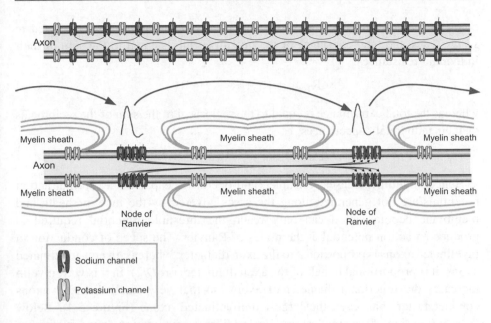

**Figure 5.3** Saltatory conduction.

The myelin sheath imposes saltatory conduction on axons by dividing the axonal membrane into alternating conductive portions localised to nodes of Ranvier, and non-conductive portions underneath the myelin sheath. Myelin increases the speed of conduction by dramatically increasing resistance and decreasing capacitance, so that action potentials are not generated along the areas covered by the myelin sheath, and membrane depolarisation can only reach the threshold potential required to produce an action potential at the nodes of Ranvier.

In addition to providing essential insulation that allows the action potential to be shunted from node to node through the low-resistance axoplasm, the myelin sheath is also critical for the specific clustering at nodes of sodium and potassium channels that generate the action potential (see Section 5.2.2). This method of propagation is extremely fast and safe, taking around 20 μseconds (or 0.00002 seconds) for an action potential to jump from node to node (internodal conduction time), with a safety factor >5 (defined as the ratio between current *available* and that *required* to stimulate a node of Ranvier).

Myelin increases *speed of conduction* by increasing *resistance* and decreasing *capacitance*. The speed of conduction is a function of the relationship between the low resistance of the axoplasm and the high resistance and capacitance of the axolemma; the phospholipid bilayer of the cell membrane has a high capacitance, because the hydrophobic centre is a good insulator and separates the good conductors of the extracellular and intracellular hydrophilic surfaces.

In non-myelinated axons, passive action potential propagation decays because the current leaks across the membrane, as a function of the membrane resistance, $R$, and the signal is reduced by the membrane capacitance, $C$. The myelin sheath is formed by multiple concentric layers of cell membrane wrapped around the axon many times, and each layer acts as another *resistor* and *capacitor* connected *in series*. Thus, the total resistance of the myelin sheath is equal to the sum of their individual resistances:

$$R_{Total} = R_1 + R_2 \ldots + R_n$$

whereas the total capacitance is equal to the reciprocal of the sum of the reciprocals of their individual capacitances:

$$1/C_{total} = 1/C_1 + 1/C_2 \ldots + 1/C_n.$$

Hence, myelin increases resistance and decreases capacitance, so that action potentials are not generated along the areas covered by the myelin sheath and membrane depolarisation can only reach the threshold potential required to produce an action potential at the nodes of Ranvier. The speed of conduction in myelinated axons is proportional to the axon diameter, whereas, in non-myelinated axons, it is proportional to half of the axon diameter ($v \propto D/2$). In this way, myelin increases the functional diameter of axons, so that very small diameter axons conduct faster than even the largest unmyelinated axons (Figure 5.4). Below 0.2 μm (the size of the smallest myelinated fibres), myelination does not increase the speed of conduction.

Periodicity of nodes of Ranvier and myelin thickness together determine the speed of conduction. Thick myelin sheaths provide proportionally much greater insulation than thin myelin sheaths, which allows for the action potential to be shunted between nodes separated by far greater internodal lengths (>500 μm) in

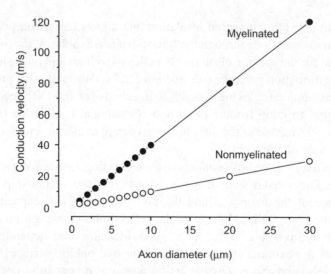

**Figure 5.4**  Relationship between conduction velocity and axon diameter.
Larger axons conduct faster than smaller axons, and the myelin sheath enables smaller diameter axons to conduct impulses much faster than the largest diameter unmyelinated axons. Myelin enables ultra-fast impulse generation, which is essential for the massive computing power of the brain.

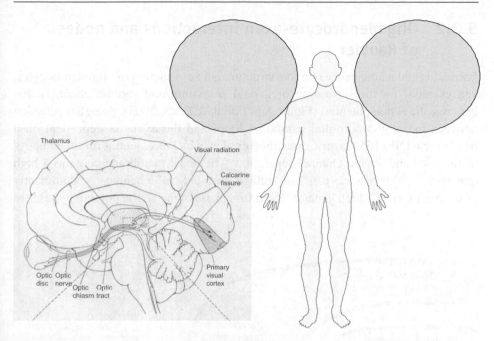

**Figure 5.5**   Myelin provides for the miniaturisation of the CNS.

To achieve the fastest conduction velocities observed in myelinated axons, unmyelinated axons would need to be as large as 500–1,000 μm (which is the case in invertebrates, such as the classic squid giant axon). In humans, this would mean that each optic nerve (cranial nerve II, which is CNS along its entire length) would need to be 0.75 m in diameter. The miniaturisation provided by myelin has allowed the development of highly complex nervous systems seen at their peak in the human cerebral cortex.

The drawing was kindly provided by Professor Helmut Kettenmann (MDC, Berlin).

large diameter fibres, compared to the smallest diameter axons, where nodal periodicity is $\leq 100$ μm. Hence, axons within type I/II units (0.2–2 μm diameter) have conduction velocities that are generally less than 20 m/s, whereas those in type III/IV oligodendrocyte-axon units (20–30 μm diameter) conduct the fastest, with conduction velocities of up to 80–120 m/s.

To achieve comparable speeds of action potential propagation, non-myelinated axons would need to be 500–1,000 μm diameter, such as that of the squid giant axon (Figure 5.4). Thus, oligodendrocytes and myelination provide for the miniaturisation and massive integrative computing power of the human brain (Figure 5.5). Consequently, the loss of oligodendrocytes and/or myelin has devastating effects on neural function; this can result from many causes, such as multiple sclerosis, as well as age-related degeneration of myelin sheaths (Peters, 2002). Remyelinated axons have much thinner myelin sheaths (reduced g-ratio) and shorter internodes than normal. This is sufficient to restore conduction, but conduction velocities are slower than in normal myelinated axons. This is believed to contribute to the cognitive deficits observed in normal aging and dementias.

## 5.2.2    Oligodendrocyte-axon interactions and nodes of Ranvier

Formation and maintenance of nodal structure is a key function of oligodendrocytes, and essential for the separation of axonal potassium and sodium channels that generate the action potential (Figure 5.6; Poliak & Peles, 2003). Axoglial adhesion between the oligodendroglial paranodal loops and the axons is dependent on a neurofascin (NF) 155-Caspr-Contactin complex, which is essential for the integrity of the node and for ion channel separation. The nodal membrane contains a high density ($>1,000$ channels/$\mu m^2$) of voltage-operated $Na^+$ channels predominantly of the $Na_v1.6$ type, which generate the initial phase of the action potential; these are

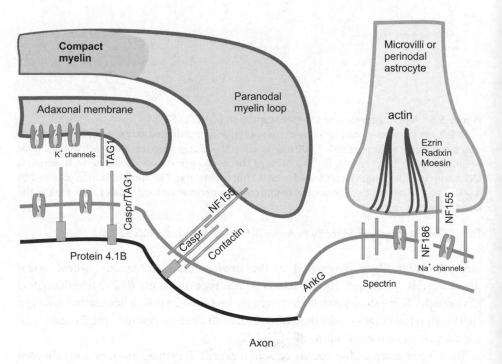

**Figure 5.6**  The node of Ranvier.
Axoglial junctions between the oligodendrocyte paranodal loops and the axolemma serve to separate sodium and potassium channels at nodes of Ranvier, which is essential for saltatory conduction. Paranodal axoglial adhesion is dependent on a NF155-Caspr-Contactin complex. Sodium channels that generate the rising phase of the action potential are concentrated in the nodal axolemma (predominantly $Na_v1.6$), whereas the potassium channels responsible for the repolarisation of the action potential are located in the juxtaparanodal region (mainly delayed rectifier $K^+$ channels $K_v1.1$ (KCNA1), $K_v1.2$ (KCNA2) and $K_v1.4$ (KCNA4)). The nodal membrane contains $K_v7.2$ (KCNQ2) and $K_v7.3$ (KCNQ3), which serve to stabilise the nodal membrane potential. Clustering of ion channels at nodes ($Na_v$ and KCNQ2/3) is dependent on neurofascin-186 (NF-186), ankyrinG (ankG), and $\beta IV$ spectrin. Accumulation of $K^+$ channels in the juxtaparanode depends on a *trans* interaction between axonal Caspr2-TAG1 heterodimer and TAG-1 expressed on the inner surface of the myelin sheath, and Caspr2 clustering requires protein 4.1B.

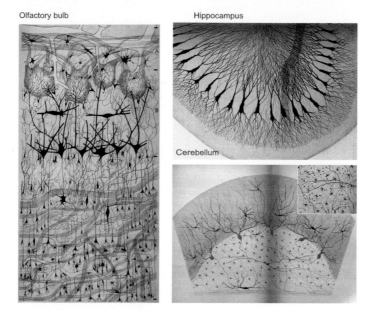

**Figure 1.6**

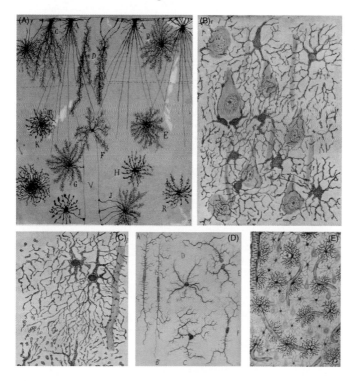

**Figure 1.18**

*See text for full figure legends.*

*Glial Physiology and Pathophysiology*, First Edition. Alexei Verkhratsky and Arthur Butt.
© 2013 by John Wiley & Sons, Ltd. Published 2013 by John Wiley & Sons, Ltd.

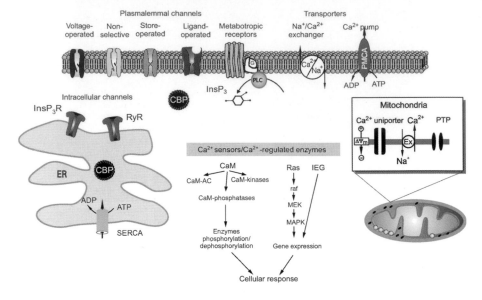

Figure 2.8

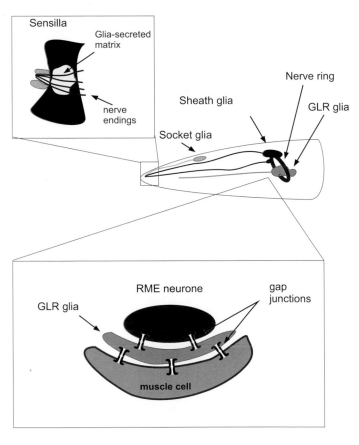

Figure 3.3

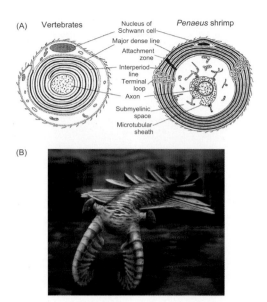

(A) Vertebrates

Penaeus shrimp

Nucleus of
Schwann cell
Major dense line
Attachment
zone
Interperiod
line
Terminal
loop
Axon
Submyelinic
space
Microtubular
sheath

(B)

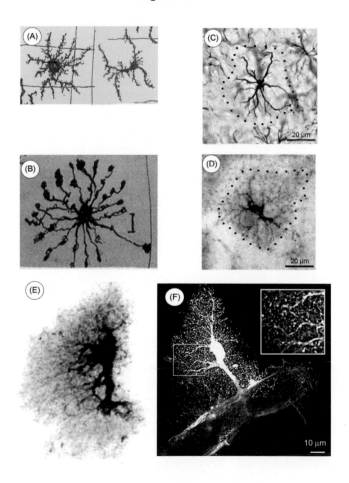

**Figure 3.6**

**Figure 4.3**

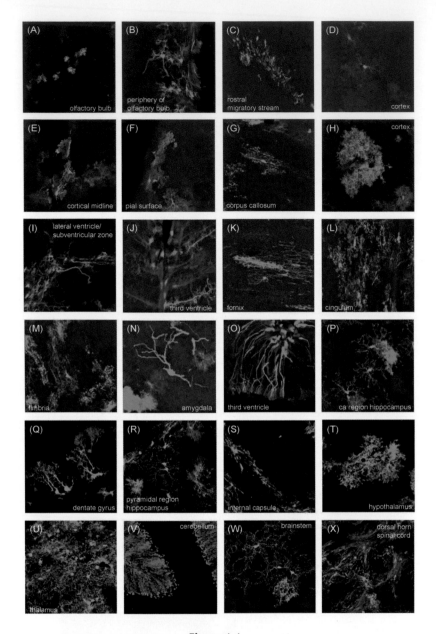

**Figure 4.4**

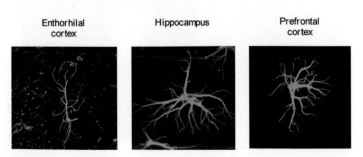

**Figure 4.5**

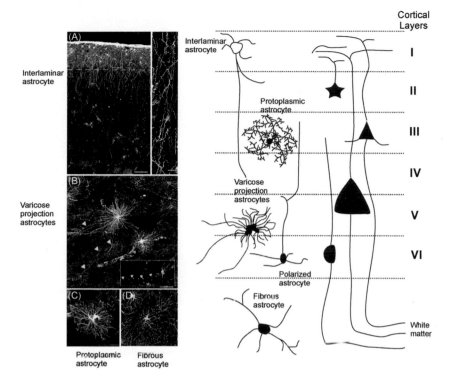

Figure 4.6

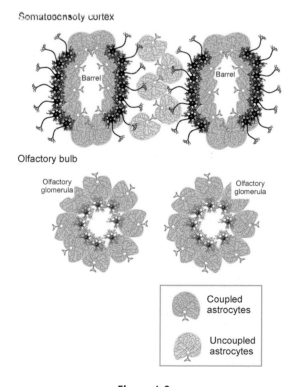

Figure 4.9

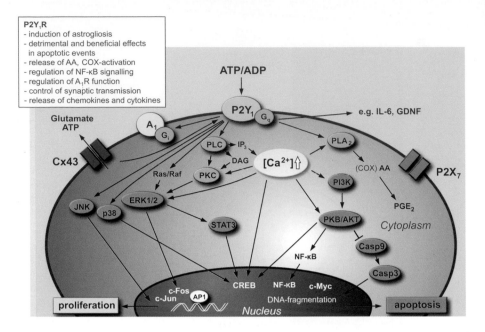

**Figure 4.15**

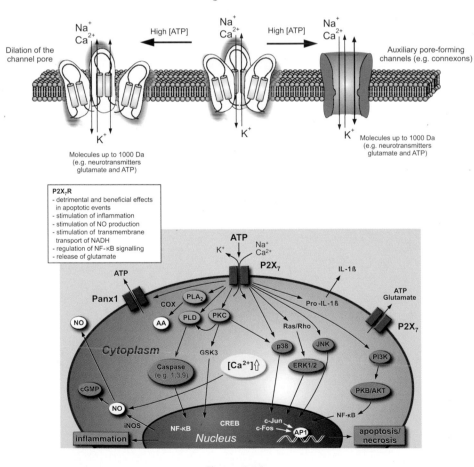

**Figure 4.16**

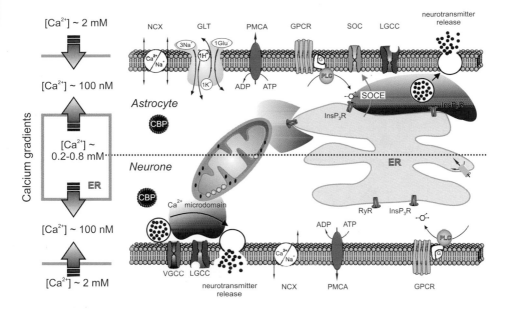

**Figure 4.20**

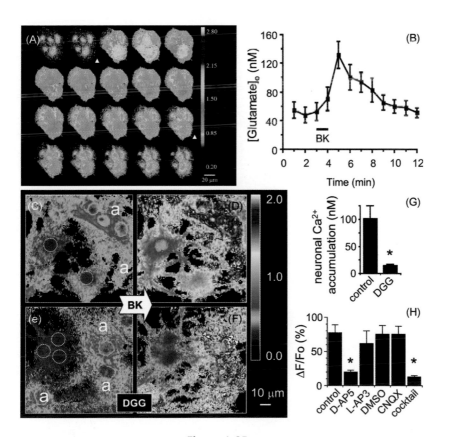

**Figure 4.25**

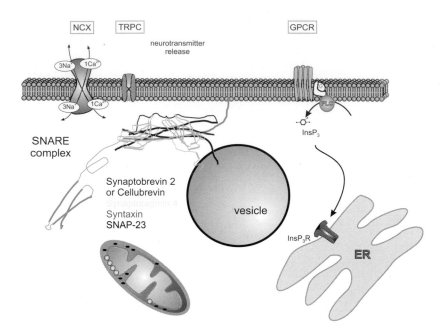

Figure 4.27

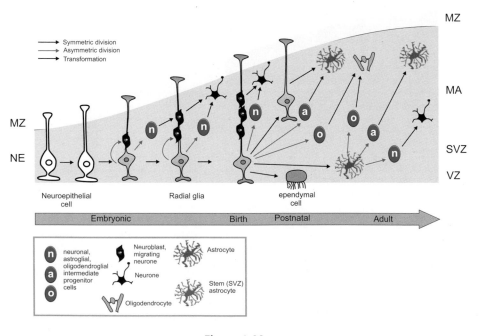

Figure 4.28

(A)

(B)

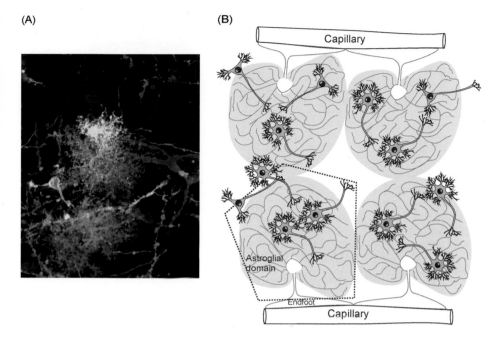

Capillary

Astroglial
domain

Endfoot

Capillary

Figure 4.33

(A)

(B)

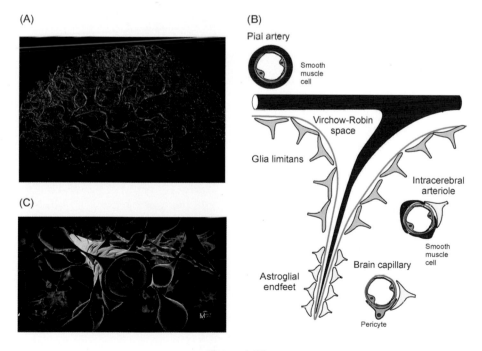

Pial artery

Smooth
muscle
cell

Virchow-Robin
space

Glia limitans

Intracerebral
arteriole

(C)

Smooth
muscle
cell

Astroglial
endfeet

Brain capillary

Pericyte

Figure 4.39

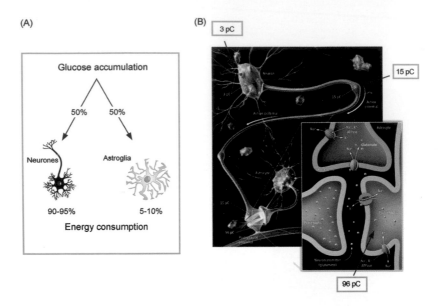

**Figure 4.41**

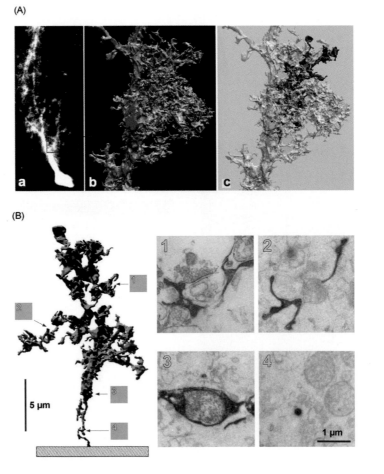

**Figure 4.50**

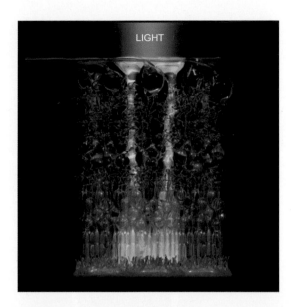

**Figure 4.58**

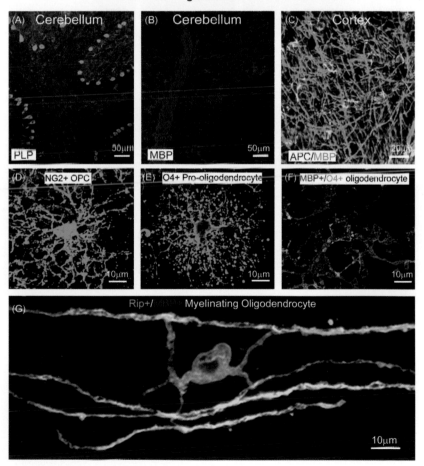

**Figure 5.7**

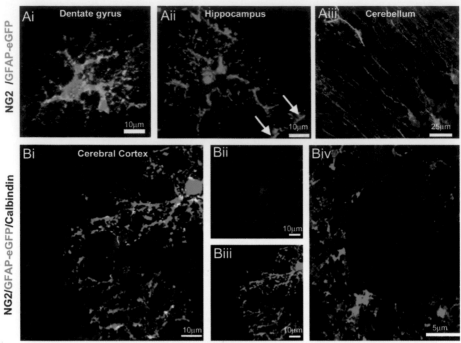

**Figure 6.4**

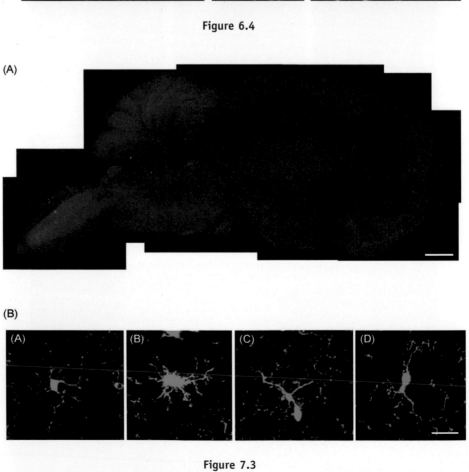

**Figure 7.3**

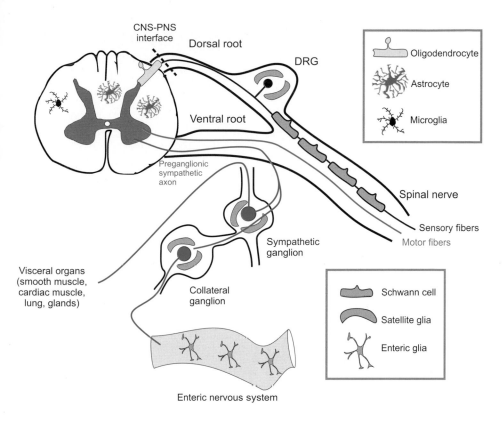

**Figure 8.1**

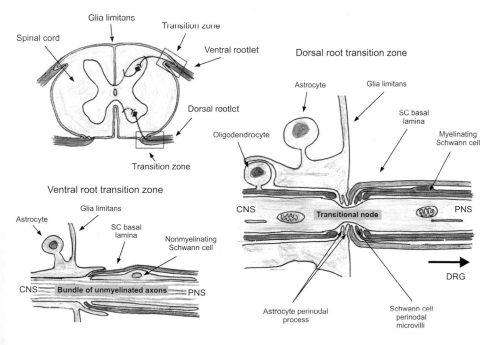

**Figure 8.4**

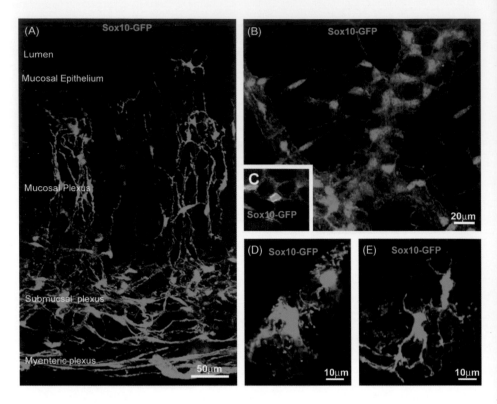

**Figure 8.16**

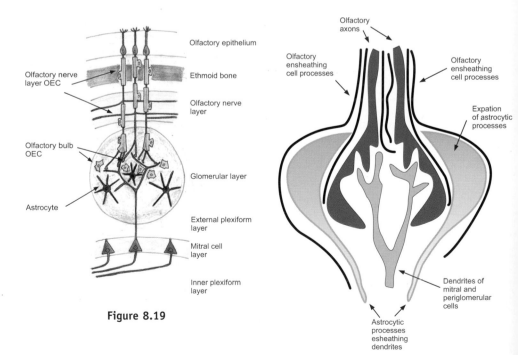

**Figure 8.19**

**Figure 8.20**

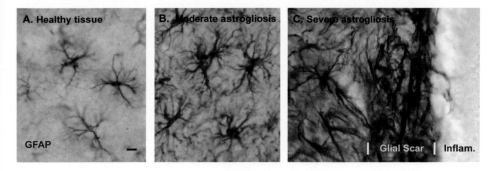

A. Healthy tissue

B. Moderate astrogliosis

C. Severe astrogliosis

GFAP

Glial Scar | Inflam.

Figure 9.4

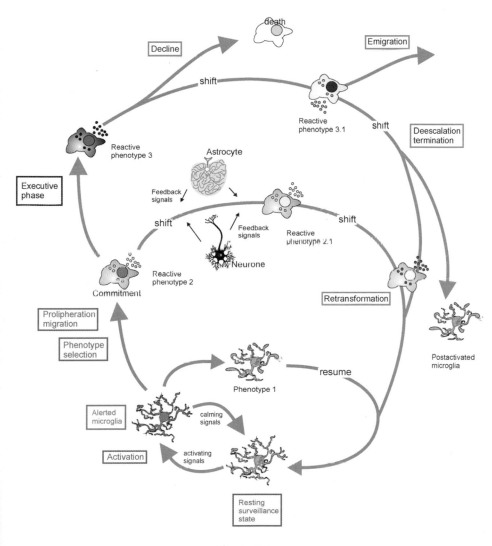

death

Decline

Emigration

shift

Reactive
phenotype 3.1

shift

Deescalation
termination

Reactive
phenotype 3

Astrocyte

Feedback
signals

Executive
phase

shift

Feedback
signals

shift

Reactive
phenotype 2.1

Neurone

Reactive
phenotype 2

Retransformation

Commitment

Proliperation
migration

Postactivated
microglia

Phenotype
selection

Phenotype 1

resume

Alerted
microglia

calming
signals

Activation

activating
signals

Resting
surveillance
state

Figure 9.9

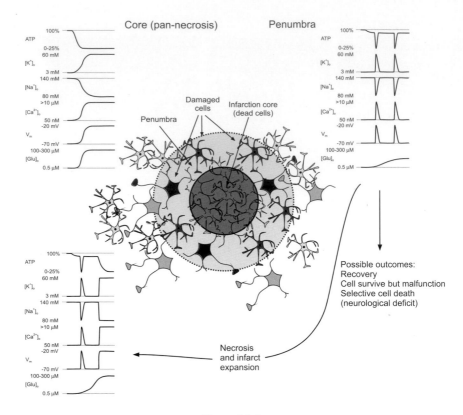

Figure 10.2

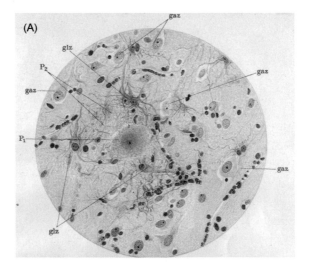

Figure 10.9

classical, very rapid, tetrodotoxin (TTX)-sensitive channels. Other sodium channel types ($Na_v1.2$ and TTX-resistant $Na_v1.8$) have also been detected within the nodal membranes. The density of $K^+$ channels responsible for repolarisation of the action potential is highest in the juxtaparanodal region under the myelin sheath, and they comprise mainly delayed rectifier $K^+$ channels $K_v1.1$ (KCNA1), $K_v1.2$ (KCNA2) and $K_v1.4$ (KCNA4), whereas the nodal membrane contains $K_v7.2$ (KCNQ2) and $K_v7.3$ (KCNQ3), which serve to stabilise the nodal membrane potential.

Clustering of ion channels at nodes ($Na_v$ and KCNQ2/3) is dependent on neurofascin-186 (NF-186), ankyrinG (ankG, ANK3), and βIV spectrin (Rasband, 2010; Thaxton et al., 2011). During development, soluble factors secreted by oligodendrocytes promote the clustering of $Na_v1.2$ α subunits at immature nodes of Ranvier, and myelin ensheathment induces the clustering of $Na_v1.6$ α subunits, which are characteristic of mature nodes (Boiko et al., 2001; Kaplan et al., 2001). Recruitment of ankG is required for the clustering of $Na^+$ channels, and the stability of these clusters is dependent on NF186 and βIV spectrin (Rasband & Trimmer, 2001). Genetic ablation of the neuron-specific isoform of NF186 in vivo results in nodal disorganization, including loss of $Na^+$ channel and AnkG enrichment at nodes.

As the myelin sheath becomes compacted, the lateral cytoplasmic ridges stack upon each other to form specialised axoglial contacts at paranodes, which depend on the presence of three cell adhesion molecules – NF 155 on the glial membrane and a complex of Caspr and contactin on the axon. Components of the paranodal cytoskeleton include ankyrinB (ANK2), αII spectrin and βII spectrin (Ogawa et al., 2006). Though not essential for the initial clustering of $Na^+$ channels, paranodal axoglial junctions are essential for the maintenance of the nodal complex, and mice lacking either Caspr or contactin have everted paranodal loops and absent transverse bands, resulting in displacement of $Na^+$ and $K^+$ channels. The juxtaparanodal accumulation of $K^+$ channels depends on a *trans* interaction between axonal Caspr2-TAG1 heterodimer and TAG-1 expressed on the inner surface of the myelin sheath (Poliak et al., 2003). In addition, Caspr2 clustering requires protein 4.1B, and loss of this protein also impairs assembly of the Kv1 channel-containing complexes at juxtaparanodes.

Disruption of paranodal junctions in demyelinating diseases results in the dispersal of ion channels from the nodes and exposes the $K^+$ channels under the internodal myelin, which very effectively dampens action potential propagation. Age-related changes in paranodal structure have also been noted, including $K_v1.2$ and Caspr, resulting in disruption of ion channel localisation at nodes and changes in axonal conduction (Hinman et al., 2006).

## 5.2.3 Myelin structure and metabolism

The dimensions of myelin sheaths are related to axon diameter (D) (Hildebrand et al., 1993). Axon diameter and the number of myelin lamellae is a strict 1 : 10 relationship, defined as the g-ratio, while axon diameter and internodal length have an approximate linear relationship, with a ratio of approximately 1 : 100 for the bulk of myelinated axons in white matter ($<4$ μm), which defines the nodal periodicity along the axon. There is an inverse, but not mathematically strict, relationship between axon diameter and the number of sheaths per unit (Butt *et al.*, 1998).

As noted above, remyelinated axons have much thinner myelin sheaths (reduced g-ratio) and shorter internodes. The volume of plasmalemma supported by individual oligodendrocytes is calculated as the internodal length (L), by the width ($\pi$.D), lamellar thickness (d) and the number of times the sheath is wrapped around the axon (number of lamellae, N), multiplied by the number of myelin sheaths within the oligodendrocyte unit (n). Thus, the volume of myelin supported by most oligodendrocytes in the grey and white matter, i.e. type II units, is approximately 500 $\mu m^3$, but is as great as 30,000–150,000 $\mu m^3$ in type III/IV oligodendrocytes (Butt *et al.*, 1998).

The energy cost of myelin synthesis has been calculated as $3.3 \times 10^{23}$ ATP molecules/g myelin, which is balanced by the reduced ATP cost of neuronal action potential propagation in myelinated axons (Harris & Attwell, 2012). Overall, the dramatic speeding-up action potential propagation provided by myelination is energy cost effective. Myelin biosynthesis in type II oligodendrocytes has been calculated to be $5–50 \times 103$ $\mu m^2$/cell/day (Baron & Hoekstra, 2010), and by extrapolation would be more than 100 times greater in type III/IV oligodendrocytes.

The morphology of type III/IV oligodendrocytes reflects the greater metabolic demand of supporting a much larger mass of myelin, with large cell bodies, thick connecting processes and prominent Schmidt-Lantermann incisures to expedite the distribution of substantial amounts of myelin components. In contrast, type I/II units have small somata and long, fine processes, reflecting the lower mass of myelin they support. Myelin comprises 50 per cent of the dry weight in human white matter, and supporting large volumes of cell membrane represents a major metabolic load on the brain as a whole, but this is balanced out by the benefits provided by myelination in terms of speed of neurotransmission, computing power and miniaturisation.

## 5.2.4    Myelin biochemistry

The main constituents of myelin are lipids (70 per cent of its dry weight) and proteins (30 per cent of the dry weight), many of which are specific to myelin. These proteins are used to identify oligodendrocytes by immunohistochemistry, or their genes are used to drive expression of fluorescent reporter proteins (Figures 5.7 and 5.8; Baumann & Pham-Dinh, 2001).

**(i)    Lipids**    Cholesterol is a major component of myelin (27 per cent), together with phospholipids and glycolipids, in ratios ranging from $4:3:2$ to $4:4:2$ (Jackman *et al.*, 2009). As a consequence, the concentration of unesterified cholesterol in the CNS is higher than in any other tissue (the CNS accounts for only 2.1 per cent of the body weight, but contains 23 per cent of the sterol), and its rate of synthesis is greatest during active myelination, increasing from 400 g in human newborn brain to 1,400 g in the adult (Dietschy & Turley, 2004). High levels

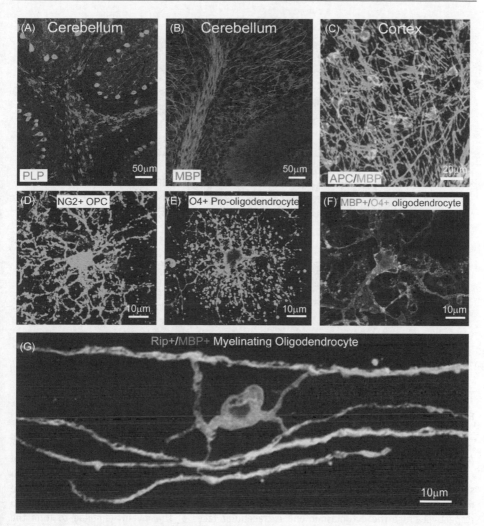

**Figure 5.7**  Immunolabelling of oligodendrocytes.
Oligodendrocytes are identified by their expression of specific myelin-related gene products.

A, B.   Oligodendrocytes in the cerebellum expressing the DsRed reporter driven by the gene for
PLP (A), and immunolabelled for MBP (red) (B).

C.   Double immunolabelling in the mouse cortex for APC (red) and MBP (green) identifies
oligodendroglial somata and myelin sheaths, respectively.

D–F.   Stages of oligodendrocyte differentiation identified *in vitro* by immunolabelling for NG2 in OPC
(D), O4 in pro-oligodendrocytes (E), and MBP (red) and O4 (green) in oligodendrocytes (F).

G.   Visualisation of three-dimensional morphology of mature oligodendrocyte *in vivo*, using
double immunolabelling with MBP (red) and the Rip antibody (green). Rip labels the entire
unit of the cell body, connecting processes and internodal myelin sheaths, whereas MBP is
found only in the compacted myelin sheaths of mature oligodendrocytes (co-localisation
appears yellow). (Full colour version in plate section.)

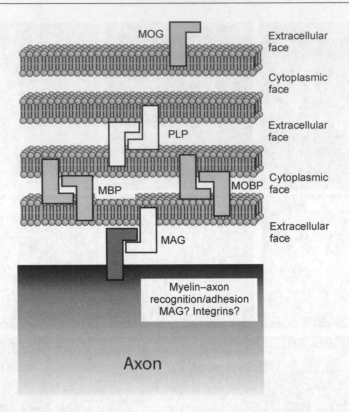

**Figure 5.8** Myelin composition.
The myelin sheath comprises multiple lamellae of expansions of the oligodendrocyte plasma-lemma. The main constituents are the phospholipids (70 per cent), together with myelin proteins (30 per cent), which serve mainly to bond the layers. The main component of myelin is cholesterol (27 per cent), together with the myelin glycosphingolipids, galactocerebroside (GalC), and their sulphated derivatives, sulphatides, recognised by the O4 antibody. The major myelin proteins are myelin basic protein (MBP) and proteolipid protein (PLP, and its isoform DM20), which respectively fuse the cytoplasmic and extracellular faces of the myelin lamellae to form the major dense line and intraperiod line. Other functionally important proteins include myelin associated glycoprotein (MAG), which is important in membrane-membrane interactions, myelin oligodendrocyte glycoprotein (MOG), which is specific to CNS myelin and is an autoantigen in experimental autoimmune encephalomyelitis (EAE), and myelin-associated/oligodendrocyte basic protein (MOBP), whose distribution and function appears to overlap with MBP.

of cholesterol are essential for myelination, and mice in which cholesterol synthesis was targeted in oligodendrocytes displayed severe perturbation of myelination, with ataxia and tremor (Saher *et al.*, 2005).

Myelin phospholipids are rich in glycosphingolipids, in particular galactocerebroside (GalC), and their sulphated derivatives, sulphatides, which are used immunohistochemically for identifying oligodendrocytes (Figure 5.7E, F) (see section 5.4.2). Studies in transgenic mice in which synthesis of GalC and/or sulphatides were disrupted (CGT-null mice, in which the enzyme UDP-galactose:

ceramide galactosyltransferase (CGT) is disrupted; and CST-null mice, in which cerebroside sulphotransferase (CST) is disrupted) showed that sulphatides negatively regulate oligodendrocyte differentiation, and that both GalC and sulphatides are essential for the formation of paranodal axoglial junctions, with a more severe phenotype in CGT-null mice (Jackman *et al.*, 2009). There are also several minor galactolipids, such as fatty esters of cerebroside, and a number of gangliosides, including GD3 (which can be used as an immunohistochemical marker of OPCs), as well as GM2 and GM3, which are implicated in myelination (Jackman *et al.*, 2009).

In co-cultures of neurones with OPCs from mice deficient in glycosyltransferases, deficiency of complex gangliosides resulted in the temporal disorganisation of ion channels at the nodes of Ranvier (Silajdzic *et al.*, 2009), while double-null mice unable to synthesise GM2 and GM3 developed severe CNS demyelination and axonal degeneration (Yamashita *et al.*, 2005).

**(ii)  Proteins**  Myelin proteins are mostly specific to myelin, and their expression is used to identify mature oligodendrocytes (Figure 5.7A–C). The major ones in the CNS are myelin basic protein (MBP) and proteolipid protein (PLP, and its isoform DM20), which constitute about 80 per cent of CNS protein. In addition, there are a number of proteins that make up a small but significant fraction of myelin, including $2',3'$-cyclic nucleotide-$3'$-phosphodiesterase (CNP, 4 per cent), myelin associated glycoprotein (MAG, <1 per cent), and myelin oligodendrocyte glycoprotein (MOG, <0.1 per cent) (see Figure 5.8). Other proteins include myelin/oligodendrocyte specific protein (MOSP), myelin-associated/oligodendrocyte basic protein (MOBP), oligodendrocyte-myelin glycoprotein (OMgp), Nogo, P2, transferrin, carbonic anhydrase, and members of the tetraspan-protein family, including oligodendrocyte specific protein (OSP/claudin-11), gap junction protein connexins (Cx32, Cx47), and tetraspan-2, together with a number of enzymes that are important for myelin formation and turnover.

*Myelin basic protein* (MBP) is a family of proteins with many isoforms, and constitutes as much as 30 per cent of myelin protein. There are four 'classic' MBP isoforms, the major ones (≈95 per cent of the MBPs) in the adult being 18.5- and 17.2-kDa isoforms in humans and 18.5 and 14 kDa in the mouse (Campagnoni & Skoff, 2001). These are encoded by the first seven exons of the MBP gene distributed over a 32-kb stretch in the mouse on chromosome 18. The entire MBP gene is substantially larger than this, at 105 kb in mice and 180 kb in humans, and encodes two families of proteins, the first comprising the myelin-associated MBPs and the second being the golli (gene expressed in the oligodendrocyte lineage)-MBP proteins. Golli and MBP families of transcripts are under independent developmental regulation and post-transcriptional modifications (Wegner, 2000).

A large deletion of the MBP gene in *shiverer* mutant mice results in the loss of the major dense line, providing direct evidence that the main function of MBP is in myelin compaction and adhesion of the cytoplasmic faces of the myelin sheath to form the major dense. MBP binds to negatively charged lipids on the cytosolic surface of oligodendrocytes and also acts as a scaffolding protein and binds actin filaments to the lipid bilayer (Boggs & Wang, 2004). An interesting aspect is that MBP is not translated within the cell body, but the mRNA is translocated to the myelin sheaths, where the protein is translated on site (see Section 5.2.5). Hence, MBP immunolabelling is only found within the compacted myelin sheaths in mature oligodendrocytes (Figure 5.7C, G); this compares to PLP, which is localised within the cell body and myelin (compare Figures 5.7A and 5.7B). Some isoforms of MBP are differentially expressed within oligodendrocyte somata and myelin, indicating they have multiple functions.

*Proteolipid protein* (PLP) constitutes up to 50 per cent of CNS myelin proteins, with the two isoforms PLP (25 kDa) and DM20 (20 kDa). There is a strong conservation of protein sequence between species, with 100 per cent identity between murine and human PLP proteins (Campagnoni & Skoff, 2001). PLP and DM20 are coded by the same gene, located on the X chromosome, as well as two additional variants – sr-PLP and sr-DM20 – derived from alternate splicing of the gene (Bongarzone *et al.*, 1999). The DM20 splice variant is expressed predominantly at early stages of oligodendrocyte differentiation, and it gradually declines as the myelin PLP splice variant becomes the major form in mature oligodendrocytes. There is considerable expression of DM20/PLP and the sr-DM20/PLP isoforms in non-myelinating cells, suggesting functions other than a myelin structural protein.

Myelin PLP comprises four hydrophobic α-helices spanning the whole thickness of the lipid bilayer, with two extracytoplasmic domains localised at the intraperiodic line of myelin and three cytoplasmic domains localised to the major dense line (Weimbs & Stoffel, 1992). Mutations involving the PLP gene (e.g. the jimpy (jp) mouse, myelin deficient (md) rats, the shaking pup and transgenic knockout mice) provide direct evidence that PLP is important for fusing the extracellular face of the myelin lamellae to form the intraperiod line (Griffiths *et al.*, 1998a). The absence of PLP/DM20 also results in axonal degeneration, particularly in small diameter axons (Griffiths *et al.*, 1998b). In addition, in jimpy mice, there are a number of developmental abnormalities, including premature oligodendrocyte cell death (Edgar *et al.*, 2004).

*CNP, 2′,3′-cyclic nucleotide-3′-phosphodiesterase* makes up four per cent of myelin and, in the CNS, it is specific to oligodendrocytes. Immunohistochemically, CNP is localised to the cell body and processes rather than compacted myelin (Lappe-Siefke *et al.*, 2003). There are two isoforms – CNP1 (46 kDa) and CNP2 (48 kDa) – and the two transcripts appear to be under the control of different promoters during oligodendrocyte differentiation. CNP2 is the only form expressed by OPCs, but both CNP1 and CNP2 are expressed by oligodendrocytes.

CNP is an enzyme that hydrolyses 2′,3′-cyclic nucleotides but, until recently, there were no known substrates for CNP in the brain, which led to the suggestion of alternative functions for CNP, such as interaction with the actin cytoskeleton and microtubules to regulate process outgrowth (Edgar & Nave, 2009). There is evidence that the 2′,3′-cAMP-adenosine pathway exists *in vivo* in both gray and white matter, and studies in CNPase knockout mice have indicated that CNPase is involved in the metabolism of endogenous $2',3'$-cAMP to $2'$-AMP and to adenosine (Verrier *et al.*, 2012).

Overexpression of CNP in transgenic mice has been shown to perturb myelin formation, and it creates aberrant oligodendrocyte membrane expansion (Gravel *et al.*, 1996). Studies in knockout mice indicate that CNP is critical for the formation of a normal inner tongue process in small diameter axons (Edgar *et al.*, 2009). A significant finding is that there is axonal degeneration in the absence of oligoden- droglial CNP, indicating an unresolved function in maintaining axoglial interactions (Edgar and Nave, 2009; Verrier *et al.*, 2012).

*Myelin associated glycoprotein* (MAG) is expressed in both CNS and PNS myelin (Schachner & Bartsch, 2000). It is only a minor component of myelin ($<1$ per cent in the CNS and 0.1 per cent in the PNS), but it is the major glycoprotein. MAG consists of two isoforms – S- (small, 67 kDa) and L- (large, 72 kDa) MAG – which are differentially expressed during development. L-MAG is the predominant form in early myelination, but it declines during development, while S-MAG is the predominant form in the adult. S-MAG is essential for normal myelination in the PNS, whereas L-MAG is the most important functionally in the CNS (Schachner and Bartsch, 2000).

In the CNS, MAG is confined to the periaxonal cytoplasmic ridges of the myelin sheath, contrasting with a broader distribution in the PNS. In knockout mice, the absence of MAG results in abnormal formation of the paranodal loops and periaxonal cytoplasmic ridge, indicating a role for MAG in axon-myelin inter- actions. MAG is a member of the immunoglobulin (Ig) gene superfamily, with significant homology to neural cell adhesion molecule (NCAM), and it is a member of the subgroup of sialic-acid-binding immunoglobulin-like lectins termed siglecs, which includes CD22 and CD33. The siglecs function in carbohydrate recognition and signalling important in cell-cell interactions, and also signalling functions in the haemopoietic, immune and nervous systems.

The extracellular domain of MAG possesses the L2/HNK-1 epitope and binds to specific gangliosides on the axon membrane, which participate in recognition and adhesion. The cytoplasmic domain of MAG has several phosphorylation sites, and it interacts with a number of transduction pathways, including Fyn, which is essential for myelination, and S100β protein, which regulates the cytoskeleton and signal transduction. Hence, MAG is likely to play a major role in signal transduction across the myelin membrane. MAG is also an inhibitor of axon growth, and it binds to the same receptor as Nogo and OMgp, with important implications for regeneration in the CNS.

*Myelin oligodendrocyte glycoprotein* (MOG) is specific to oligodendrocytes and is mostly located on the cell surface and outermost lamellae of compacted myelin in the CNS (Brunner *et al.*, 1989). MOG expression is developmentally regulated and it is one of the last myelin proteins to be expressed, making it a marker for mature oligodendrocytes. The function of MOG is unclear, but its topology indicates that there may be only one transmembrane domain member, like other members of the IgCAM superfamily, and it may have similar adhesive and intracellular functions to MAG and P0. CNS myelin does not have a basal lamina, so MOG may be important in adhesion and interactions between adjacent sheaths within axon fascicles. MOG is CNS-specific and is a key autoantigen for primary demyelination in multiple sclerosis (Clements *et al.*, 2003).

*Myelin-associated/oligodendrocyte basic proteins* (MOBPs) are expressed exclusively by oligodendrocytes in the CNS and are localised to the major dense line, like MBP. MOBPs comprise three isoforms (8.2, 9.7 and 11.7 kDa), which may have multiple functions, and they are derived by alternative splicing of a single gene. Expression of MOBPs occurs in the late stages of myelination, after MBPs, and they may overlap in function with MBP. Knockout mice did not display altered myelin compaction.

*Oligodendrocyte specific protein* (OSP/claudin-11) is an oligodendrocyte-specific protein and is the third most abundant protein in CNS myelin. Studies of OSP-deficient mice indicate that it is a tight junction protein important for the formation of the parallel arrays of tight junctions within myelin sheaths (Gow *et al.*, 1999). OSP/claudin-11 appears to modulate proliferation and migration of oligodendrocytes through interactions with $\beta 1$ integrin and $K_v 3.1$ (Tiwari-Woodruff *et al.*, 2006). Furthermore, there is evidence implicating OSP/claudin-11 as an autoantigen in the development of autoimmune demyelinating disease (Bronstein *et al.*, 2000).

*Connexins* in oligodendrocytes are predominantly Cx32 and Cx47, the latter being specific to oligodendrocytes in the CNS, as well as Cx29, which are crucial for CNS myelination (Kleopa *et al.*, 2010; Orthmann-Murphy *et al.*, 2008). Connexins most likely form gap junctions as a conduit for the movement of ions and water between cytoplasmic and compacted regions of the myelin sheath (see Section 5.3.7). Mutations in Cx47 can cause a devastating leukodystrophy called Pelizaeus-Merzbacher-like disease, whereas Cx32 mutations are found in the X-linked Charcot Marie Tooth disease (CMT1X), which causes progressive peripheral neuropathy and CNS myelin dysfunction (Kleopa *et al.*, 2010). Mice lacking either Cx47 or Cx32 are viable, but those lacking both connexins display marked abnormalities in CNS myelin, characterised by thin or absent myelin sheaths, vacuolation, enlarged periaxonal collars, oligodendrocyte cell death and axonal loss.

*Transferrin* (Tf) is an iron transport glycoprotein enriched in oligodendrocytes, and its developmental expression matches myelination. Oligodendrocytes contain the four proteins which are responsible for the regulation and management of iron: transferrin, transferrin receptor, ferritin and iron responsive protein. Iron is a cofactor for several enzymes, and it is a basic requirement for oxidative metabolism. Oligodendrocytes contain the highest levels of iron of any cell type in the brain, which may reflect the high metabolic load of myelin production. Iron is directly involved in myelin production, as a required co-factor for cholesterol and lipid biosynthesis, and indirectly because of its requirement for oxidative metabolism, which occurs in oligodendrocytes at a higher rate than other brain cells (Connor & Menzies, 1996). The susceptibility of oligodendrocytes to oxidative injury may be a result of their iron-rich cytoplasm, and differences in iron-mediated oxidative stress are most likely involved in susceptible oligodendrocyte populations (Todorich *et al.*, 2009).

*Carbonic anhydrases* (CA) are essential for intracellular pH regulation (see Section 5.3.6). They may play a role in ion and water movement in the myelin sheath, possibly in the extrusion of cytoplasm from compacted myelin, although no major abnormalities have been observed in the brains of CAII-deficient mice (Ghandour *et al.*, 1989).

## 5.2.5   Myelin transport

The formation of the myelin sheath is a highly complex process that involves a number of steps, from mRNA transcription to protein translation and assembly into the membranes. All of the myelin products have to be transported from the cell body and targeted to the 'workface' of the myelin sheath, over hundreds and potentially thousands of microns via the connecting branches in oligodendrocytes, and along the outer cytoplasmic ridge, down the paranodal loops, into the inner cytoplasmic ridge and Schmidt-Lanterman incisures.

PLP and the other main proteins are targeted to the myelin by multiple cellular pathways. In the 'direct' pathway, membrane proteins are translated within the cell body and sorted in the Golgi apparatus for transport to the distal myelin sheath by intracellular transport involving microtubules and other components of the cytoskeleton. In the 'indirect' pathway, proteins are first transported from the *trans* Golgi network and are then internalised by cholesterol-dependent and clathrin-independent endocytosis to a late endosome/lysmal compartment (Trajkovic *et al.*, 2006). This balance between endocytosis and exocytosis is believed to regulate myelin biogenesis (Simons & Trotter, 2007).

One of the most interesting aspects of protein targeting in myelinating cells is the phenomenon of MBP mRNA translocation from the cell body to the myelin sheaths. The MBPs are highly cationic polypeptides that interact with virtually any negatively charged molecule. Consequently, MBP is not translated in the cell body, where its interactions with other cellular components would impede its transport to the myelin sheath. Instead, the MBP mRNA is translocated in ribonucleoprotein granules along microtubules to the distal cytoplasmic ridges of the myelin sheath, where the protein is translated 'on site' (Figure 5.9).

Translocated MBP mRNA contains an A2RE element that binds the hnRNP A2 protein, and the mRNA granule-hnRNP A2 protein complex is transported along microtubules in the processes, dependent on the microtubule associated protein (MAP), TOG2 (Carson & Barbarese, 2005; Colman *et al.*, 1982; Kosturko *et al.*, 2006). Phosphorylation of hnRNPA2 and local translation of MBP is regulated by Fyn activation, which depends on the contact between the oligodendrocyte and axonal L1 (White *et al.*, 2008).

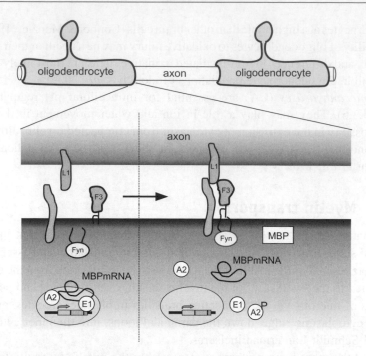

**Figure 5.9**   Local translation of MBP.

MBP is not translated in the cell body; instead, MBP mRNA is translocated in ribonucleoprotein granules along microtubules to the distal cytoplasmic ridges of the myelin sheath, where the protein is translated. MBP mRNA is translocated as part of an A2RE- hnRNP A2 protein complex, and activation of Fyn by axoglial signals (e.g. L1-F3 contactin) phosphorylates hnRNPA2, resulting in local translation of MBP.

Adapted from White *et al.*, 2008.

The two major MAPs in oligodendrocytes, MAP2 and tau, regulate microtubule assembly. Their importance is demonstrated in the taiep rat, where microtubular dysfunction results in the accumulation of MBP mRNA and myelin proteins in the cell bodies and dysmyelination (Song *et al.*, 2001). Also, oligodendrocytes are disrupted in familial multiple system tauopathy, and oligodendroglial degeneration is the histological hallmark of multiple system atrophy (MSA).

# 5.3   Physiology of oligodendrocytes

Oligodendrocytes express a wide range of ligand- and voltage-operated ion channels (Table 5.1), as well as G protein-coupled neurotransmitter receptors (Figure 5.10; Verkhratsky & Steinhauser, 2000); their properties are largely equivalent to those in astrocytes described in Chapter 4.

Oligodendroglial neurotransmitter receptors and ion channels are generally believed to be important for cell-cell communication with the neurones/axons

**Table 5.1** Ion channels in oligodendrocytes

| Ion channel | Molecular identity | Localisation | Main function |
|---|---|---|---|
| Voltage-independent $K^+$ channels | Two-pore domain $K^+$ channels: TREK1,2, TASK1,3 and TWIK1 | Uncertain; evidence that TASK1 localised to oligodendrocyte somata, whereas TREK2 localised to myelin. | Contribute to resting membrane potential during metabolic stress, e.g. acidosis. |
| Inward rectifier potassium channels | $K_{ir}4.1$ (predominant) $K_{ir}2.1$ $K_{ir}3.x?$ Kir5.1 $K_{ir}6.1, 6.2$ | $K_{ir}4.1$ in OPC and oligodendrocytes, expression may be heterogeneous. | Maintenance of resting membrane potential; $K^+$ and water transport in myelin; exit from cell cycle? $K^+$ buffering? |
| Delayed rectifier potassium channels $K_D$ | Mainly $K_V1.3$, $K_V1.5$ and $K_V2.6$ | Ubiquitous in OPCs; down-regulated in mature oligodendrocytes; $K_V1.5$ functionally predominant. | In OPCs, regulate proliferation, exit from cell cycle and differentiation. |
| Rapidly inactivating A-type potassium currents ($K_A$) | $K_V1.4$ | Predominant in OPCs and pro-oligodendrocytes, and re-expressed in EAE. | Suggested role in myelination. |
| $Ca^{2+}$-dependent $K^+$ channels | $K_{Ca}3.1$ | OPCs and oligodendrocytes, associated with OSP/claudin-11. | OPC proliferation and migration, and myelin sheath stabilisation. |
| M-type potassium currents (KCNQ) | $K_V7$ | OPCs but not oligodendrocytes. | Inhibiting migration? |
| Sodium channels | Principal CNS $Na_V$ | Fairly ubiquitous in OPCs and oligodendrocytes *in vitro* and in brain slices; Type I$\alpha$, II$\alpha$1, III$\alpha$ up-regulated in OPCs. | Unknown, but their loss in oligodendrocytes suggests a developmental function; controversy over 'spiking' OPCs. |

*(continued)*

**Table 5.1**  (*Continued*)

| Ion channel | Molecular identity | Localisation | Main function |
| --- | --- | --- | --- |
| Calcium channels | L- ($Ca_v1.2$, 1.3), N- ($Ca_v2.2$), P/Q- ($Ca_v2.1$), and T ($Ca_v3.1$, 3.2)<br><br>SOCC, CRAC | VOCCS in OPCs and oligodendrocytes *in vitro* and in brain slices<br><br>SOCC and CRAC indicated *in vitro*, but few details. | General down-regulation of VOCC with development and localisation to processes contacting axons indicates a role in myelination; functional interaction between VOCCs, SOCCs and the Golli-MBP proteins. |
| Transient receptor potential, TRP, channels | TRPC1, TRPC3 | Regional distribution is unknown. | Store-operated $Ca^{2+}$ entry; TRPC3 localised to oligodendrocytes; TRPC1 in OPCs associated with golli-MBP, with possible role in proliferation. |
| Chloride channels | CLC1, CLC2, CLC3<br>Volume-regulated anion channels of unknown identity | Ubiquitous? | Chloride transport; regulation of cell volume; possible role in ion and water transport from compacted myelin. |
| Acid-sensing ion channels (ASICs) | ASIC1a, 2a, 4 | Ubiquitous? | Likely metabolic role in the face of large pH shifts during axonal electrical activity; may be linked with expression of CAII. |

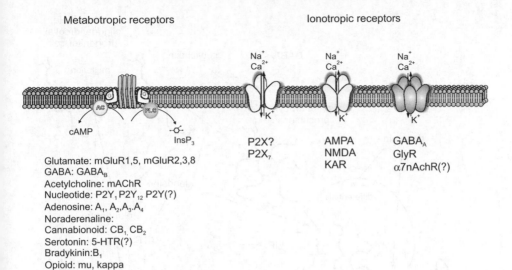

Figure 5.10   Neurotransmitter receptors in oligodendrocytes.

Oligodendrocytes have been reported to express most neurotransmitter receptors in various *in vitro* preparations, and some have been confirmed in brain slices from postnatal rodents or by immunohistochemistry/RT-PCR in cells of different ages and stages of development. This has made the picture confusing, since *in vitro* expression of GalC is generally taken as a sign of a mature oligodendrocyte and even, in some cases, O4 immunolabelling. However, GalC and O4 do not *per se* reflect a mature oligodendrocyte phenotype *in vivo*, which can be defined as a MBP+/PLP+/MAG+/MOG+ oligodendrocyte that supports compacted myelin sheaths. There have been very few electrophysiological studies on mature oligodendrocytes *in situ*, so we know little of the physiological significance of neurotransmitter receptors in these cells. In general, OPCs express most neurotransmitter receptors, although AMPA-type iGluR and GABA$_A$R predominate. Mature oligodendrocytes have been demonstrated to express AMPA-type iGluR on their somata and NMDA-R on their myelin sheaths, but neither appear to mediate functional currents activated by neuronal glutamate. P2YR and P2X$_7$R are present in OPCs and oligodendrocytes, and there is some evidence that they mediate raised intracellular calcium. By and large, however, the physiological function of all of these receptors are unproven, although they are presumed to mediate axoglial signalling and recognition (see Figure 5.11).

that they myelinate but, in most cases, their physiological significance in oligodendrocytes is unproven (Figure 5.11). Many regulate intracellular Ca$^{2+}$, which is known to be important during development and in pathology (Butt, 2006; Matute, 2011; Paez *et al.*, 2009b). A common theme appears to be that most voltage-operated ion channels and neurotransmitter receptors are highly active in OPCs, and that there is a developmental decline in their activity, suggesting specific roles during differentiation (Figure 5.11) (Frohlich *et al.*, 2011). However, it should be noted that most studies are either *in vitro*, where GalC+ oligodendrocytes are considered mature and studies on MBP+ myelin-forming oligodendrocytes are rare, or in brain slices from postnatal rodents younger than postnatal day 14. With a small number of exceptions, there are few studies on mature myelinating

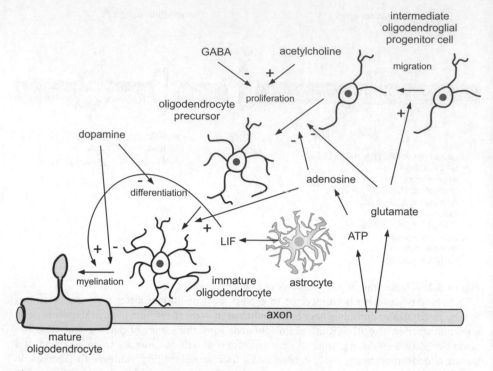

**Figure 5.11** Axon-oligodendrocyte signalling.

Oligodendrocytes express a number of neurotransmitter receptors that mediate axoglial interactions during differentiation and myelination. Glutamate and ATP, together with its breakdown product adenosine, stimulate OPC migration. Glutamate also inhibits OPC proliferation and differentiation, whereas adenosine inhibits proliferation and stimulates differentiation and myelination. ATP stimulates astrocytes to release leukemia inhibitory factor (LIF), which stimulates differentiation. OPC proliferation and differentiation are also altered by GABA and dopamine, which are inhibitory, and ACh, which is generally stimulatory.

oligodendrocytes *in vitro* or *in situ* (e.g. De Biase *et al.*, 2010; Gipson & Bordey, 2002; Kukley *et al.*, 2010). However, a key physiological feature of oligodendrocytes appears to be a general developmental decrease in excitability. This is associated with a developmental down-regulation of $K_v$ and up-regulation of $K_{ir}4.1$ potassium channels, and sustained expression of AMPA-type glutamate receptors and $P2X_7$ and $P2Y_1$ purinoceptors.

## 5.3.1  Voltage-operated ion channels

**(i)  Outwardly rectifying potassium channels** These channels are highly expressed in OPCs and are markedly down-regulated as they differentiate into oligodendrocytes, including the delayed rectifying $K^+$ channels (KD), rapidly-inactivating or transient A-type $K^+$ channels (KA), and calcium-activated $K^+$ channels (KCa; BK type, large conductance) (Verkhratsky & Steinhauser, 2000).

There are few studies on mature oligodendrocytes *in situ* but, overall, they appear to possess both large $K_{ir}$ currents and small voltage-activated $K_v$ currents (blocked by TEA and activated between $-40$ and $-50\,mV$), which together may facilitate clearance of $K^+$ released during axonal firing (Berger *et al.*, 1991; Gipson & Bordey, 2002; Sontheimer & Waxman, 1993).

Molecularly, OPC and oligodendrocytes have been shown to express $K_v1.2$, $K_v1.3$, $K_v1.4$, $K_v1.5$, and $K_v1.6$ (Attali *et al.*, 1997). $K_v1.3$, $K_v1.4$ and $K_v1.5$ stimulate OPC proliferation, whereas Kv1.6 inhibit OPC proliferation, and their expression is tightly regulated in different phases of the cell cycle, with selective up-regulation of $K_v1.3$ and $K_v1.5$ in the G1 phase of the cell cycle (Chittajallu *et al.*, 2002; Vautier *et al.*, 2004). Treatment of OPC with PDGF induces up-regulation of $K_v1.5$ and their blockade attenuates OPC proliferation, supporting the concept of a link between OPC proliferation and $K_v$ expression (Soliven *et al.*, 2003).

During development, $K_v1.4$ appear to be confined to OPCs and premyelinating oligodendrocytes, but not mature oligodendrocytes, although re-expression of $K_v1.4$ has been observed in experimental autoimmune encephalomyelitis (EAE), suggesting a role in myelination (Herrero-Herranz *et al.*, 2007). Pharmacological or AMPA receptor-mediated blockade of KD strongly inhibits OPC cell cycle progression and proliferation (Borges *et al.*, 1994; Chittajallu *et al.*, 2002; Gallo *et al.*, 1996; Tiwari-Woodruff *et al.*, 2006). In addition, $K_v7$/KCNQ channels (M-channels), which serve to stabilise the membrane potential in the presence of depolarising currents, are functional in OPCs, but not in differentiated oligodendrocytes, and their blockade promotes OPC migration *in vitro* (Wang *et al.*, 2011). $K_v3.1$, which are expressed mainly by fast-spiking neurones and are activated at very depolarised membrane potentials, are expressed both in OPCs and oligodendrocytes, associated with the oligodendrocyte-specific tight junction protein (OSP)/claudin-11, with functions in myelination as well as OPC proliferation and migration (Tiwari-Woodruff *et al.*, 2001).

**(ii) Inward rectifier potassium channels ($K_{ir}$)** The $K_{ir}$ channels are expressed in oligodendrocytes, where they are responsible for the high membrane permeability for $K^+$ ions and setting their strongly negative RMP (Bolton & Butt, 2006; Butt & Kalsi, 2006). The resting conductance in oligodendrocytes is mostly due to $K_{ir}4.1$, which are essential for the developmental negative shift in RMP and cell cycle exit and differentiation of oligodendrocytes (Knutson *et al.*, 1997; Neusch *et al.*, 2003). $K_{ir}4.1$ with Cx47 in oligodendroglial paranodal loops may be involved in buffering of $K^+$ ions released during propagation of action potentials (Menichella *et al.*, 2006).

Oligodendrocytes also express $K_{ir}5.1$ channels, which specifically associate with $K_{ir}4.1$ and $K_{ir}4.2$ to form highly pH-sensitive heterometric channels and may be most important in maintaining the RMP during metabolic stress (Butt and Kalsi, 2006). $K_{ir}2.1$ and $K_{ir}7.1$ are found in oligodendrocytes *in vivo* and *in vitro*, although their specific functions are unresolved (Butt and Kalsi, 2006).

ATP-dependent $K^+$ channels ($K_{ATP}$) $K_{ir}6.1$ and $K_{ir}6.2$ have also been demonstrated in cultured OPCs and oligodendrocytes, and their activation promotes cell proliferation and myelination (Fogal et al., 2011). $K_{ir}6.x$ channels are only active when ATP falls to very low levels, and their activation may help maintain oligodendrocytes and myelin during hypoxia. There is evidence that oligodendrocytes express two-pore domain $K^+$ channels ($K_{2P}$), which are responsible for the leak or background $K^+$ conductance and are implicated in oligodendrocyte damage during hypoxia (Butt and Kalsi, 2006).

**(iii)  Voltage-operated sodium channels ($Na_v$)**   The $Na_v$ channels have been found in OPCs in vitro and in brain slices, with functional properties similar to their neuronal counterparts, including rapid activation/inactivation kinetics and TTX sensitivity (Berger et al., 1992a; Chittajallu et al., 2004; De Biase et al., 2010; Karadottir et al., 2008; Paez et al., 2009a). A sub-population of OPCs that expresses high enough densities of $Na_v$ channels have been shown to generate action potentials upon depolarisation of their cell membrane (Karadottir et al., 2008). However, in general, the low density of $Na_v$, compared to the large $K^+$ conductances, prevents the initiation of regenerative spikes in OPCs (De Biase et al., 2010; Kukley et al., 2010).

The main CNS types of $Na_v$ (Type I$\alpha$, type II$\alpha$1, type III$\alpha$) are down-regulated as OPCs exit cell cycle and differentiate into mature myelinating oligodendrocytes (Berger et al., 1992a; De Biase et al., 2010), but transcripts for $Na_v$ continue to be detected in mature oligodendrocytes (De Biase et al., 2010). The function of $Na_v$ in OPCs is unknown, but their developmental decrease in mature oligodendrocytes suggests these channels have unresolved functions specifically in OPC development, as indicated for $K_v$. Sodium influx though $Na_v$ upon GABA-induced membrane depolarisation in OPCs triggers $Ca^{2+}$ influx via $Na^+/Ca^{2+}$ exchangers (NCXs) and is involved in OPC migration (Tong et al., 2009).

**(iv)  Voltage-operated calcium channels (VOCC, $Ca_v$)**   Calcium channels are expressed throughout the entire oligodendrocyte lineage (Paez et al., 2009a). VOCC identified in oligodendrocyte lineage cells are the low-voltage-activated channels (LVA, activation threshold of approximately $-60\,mV$), and the L-, N- and R-types of high-voltage-activated channels (HVA, activation threshold around $-30\,mV$). mRNA encoding the L-type channel isoforms $Ca_v1.2$ and $Ca_v1.3$ and the T-type channels $Ca_v3.1$ and $Ca_v3.2$ predominate in OPCs in situ, whereas transcripts for P/Q and N-type channels, $Ca_v2.1$ and $Ca_v2.2$, are less abundant, and mRNAs for $Ca_v1.4$, $Ca_v2.3$ and $Ca_v3.3$ have never been detected (Haberlandt et al., 2011).

It has become clear that the functions of $Ca_v$ and several of the earliest identified myelin protein genes regulate early developmental processes, including gene expression, cell proliferation, and cell migration (Fulton et al., 2010; Paez et al., 2009a). HVA channels are primarily located on cell bodies, whereas LVA channels are mostly on cell processes, suggesting differential activation of these channels in separate cellular domains as a signal for initiation of myelination (Kirischuk *et al.*, 1995b). There is a functional interaction between VOCC and myelin Golli proteins and store-operated calcium channels (SOCCs), suggesting they form myelin membrane sub-domains and modulate $Ca^{2+}$ entry along oligodendrocyte processes to regulate myelination (Paez *et al.*, 2009b, and see Section 5.4.1).

**(v) Chloride and acid-sensing ion channels (ASIC)** These types of channels have been identified in oligodendrocyte lineage cells (Feldman *et al.*, 2008; Williamson *et al.*, 1997). ASIC1a, 2a, and 4 mRNAs have been detected in OPC and decrease during differentiation (Feldman *et al.*, 2008). Chloride channels are important for ion and water transport, while ASICs may have a metabolic role in face of the large pH shifts during axonal activity in CNS white matter (Kettenmann *et al.*, 1990). Oligodendrocytes also express CAII (see Section 5.2.4), a key enzyme in cellular pH regulation which, together with $Na^+$-$H^+$ and $Na^+$-$HCO_3^-$ transporters, may act with ASICs to provide a mechanism for intracellular pH regulation in hypoxic stress (Ro & Carson, 2004). Transmembrane $Ca^{2+}$ influx through ASICs may contribute to the vulnerability of oligodendrocyte lineage cells to CNS ischaemia (Feldman *et al.*, 2008).

## 5.3.2 Glutamate receptors

Glutamate is the main excitatory neurotransmitter in the brain, and oligodendrocytes, like neurones, express a wide variety of ionotropic and metabotropic glutamate receptors (Frohlich *et al.*, 2011; Gallo & Ghiani, 2000; for further details, see Section 4.3.3(i) and Figure 4.13).

**(i) Ionotropic glutamate receptors (iGluRs)** The ionotropic glutamate receptors of the AMPA, kainate and NMDA types are abundantly expressed throughout the oligodendrocyte lineage. All iGluRs are ligand-gated non-selective cation channels which allow the flow of $K^+$, $Na^+$ and $Ca^{2+}$ in response to glutamate binding. The receptors are tetramers, and heterogeneity within each class arises from the homo-oligomeric or hetero-oligomeric assembly of distinct subunits, which determines their properties and ion permeability. The classification of these subunits has recently been re-addressed by NC-IUPHAR (Collingridge *et al.*, 2009), which recommends a revised nomenclature for ionotropic glutamate receptor subunits. The original classification of the subunits is indicated in parentheses, but their continued use is not recommended.

*AMPA receptors* (AMPAR) assemble as homomers or heteromers from four subunits – GluA1 (GluR1), GluA2 (GluR2), GluA3 (GluR3) or GluA4 (GluR4). GluA1–4 can exist as two variants generated by alternative splicing (termed 'flip' and 'flop'). AMPAR subunits GluA2, GluA3, and GluA4 have been detected by RT-PCR and western blot in oligodendrocytes (De Biase *et al.*, 2010; Itoh *et al.*,

2002). RNA encoding the GluA2 subunit undergoes extensive RNA editing of the Q/R site, and AMPA receptors lacking RNA-edited GluA2 subunits are permeable to $Ca^{2+}$, which is a feature of AMPAR in OPCs (Bergles *et al.*, 2000; Haberlandt *et al.*, 2011; Hamilton *et al.*, 2010). However, it is not clear whether this is due to non-edited GluA2 subunits or to the complete absence of GluA2 subunits (Li & Stys, 2000), although immmunoprecipitation experiments have indicated that protein complexes in oligodendrocytes form exclusively of GluA3 and GluA4 (Itoh *et al.*, 2002).

AMPAR function, subunit expression and $Ca^{2+}$ permeability appear to be strongly down-regulated during oligodendrocyte development (De Biase *et al.*, 2010; Itoh *et al.*, 2002; Kukley *et al.*, 2010). It is suggested that AMPAR activation in oligodendrocyte lineage cells mediates signalling from axons and, in particular, regulates OPC differentiation and myelination (Figure 5.11) (Wake *et al.*, 2011).

*Kainate receptors* can be expressed as homomers of GluK1 (GluR5), GluK2 (GluR6) or GluK3 (GluR7) subunits, and GluK1–3 subunits are also capable of assembling into heterotetramers. Two additional kainate receptor subunits – GluK4 (KA1) and GluK5 (KA2) – can form heteromers when co-expressed with GluK1–3 subunits, but they lack function when expressed individually. Kainate receptors in oligodendrocyte lineage cells have properties consistent with ones lacking the GluK1 subunit (Kukley & Dietrich, 2009). Kainate receptors may be less important in OPCs than oligodendrocytes, which express GluK2, GluK3, GluK4, and GluK5 (De Biase *et al.*, 2010; Sanchez-Gomez & Matute, 1999).

*NMDA receptors* (NMDAR) assemble as heteromers of GluN1 (NR1), GluN2A (NR2A), GluN2B (NR2B), GluN2C (NR2C), GluN2D (NR2D), GluN3A (NR3A) and GluN3B (NR3B) subunits. The minimal requirement for efficient functional expression of NMDA receptors is a di-heteromeric assembly of GluN1 and at least one GluN2 subunit variant, although they can assemble as complex tri-heteromeric assemblies incorporating GluN1 with multiple subtypes of GluN2 or GluN3 subunits. All NMDAR subunits have been detected in the optic nerve, including novel splice variants of GluN3B that modulate the $Mg^{2+}$ sensitivity (Burzomato *et al.*, 2011; Domingues *et al.*, 2011; Salter & Fern, 2005).

Functional NMDARs in oligodendrocytes appear to be tri-heteromers of GluN1, GluN2C, and GluN3A/B subunits (Burzomato *et al.*, 2011; Salter and Fern, 2005), a combination associated with decreased $Mg^{2+}$ block (Cavara & Hollmann, 2008), which is compatible with the properties of oligodendrocyte NMDA-evoked currents (Karadottir *et al.*, 2005). Immunohistochemical labelling has showed that NMDAR are clustered in oligodendrocyte cell processes, in contrast to AMPAR, which appear to be localised to the somata (Salter and Fern, 2005).

NMDARs in both OPCs and mature oligodendrocytes induce intracellular $Ca^{2+}$ transients when activated, suggesting that they do not contain GluN3B subunits, which have reduced permeability to $Ca^{2+}$ (Micu *et al.*, 2006). However, specific

GluN1 knockout in oligodendrocyte lineage cells had no effect on developmental functional properties or their response to demyelination in EAE (De Biase *et al.*, 2011; Guo *et al.*, 2012). The physiological importance of oligodendroglial NMDAR is unresolved, and they are apparently not activated significantly by the synaptic release of glutamate from neurones (De Biase *et al.*, 2010). Co-expression of GluN1, GluN3A and GluN3B form glycine-activated receptors in mammalian cells (Smothers & Woodward, 2007), so oligodendroglial NMDAR, with this composition (Domingues *et al.*, 2011), may be activated by glycine and D-serine, which has been shown in optic nerve myelin (Pina-Crespo *et al.*, 2010).

**(ii)  Metabotropic glutamate receptors (mGluRs)**   These receptors belong to one of three groups, which have all been demonstrated in oligodendrocytes (Bagayogo & Dreyfus, 2009; Luyt *et al.*, 2003, 2006). Group I receptors (mGluR1 and mGlur5) are positively coupled to phospholipase C (PLC), and their activation increases intracellular inositol 1,4,5-triphosphate (InsP$_3$), which subsequently triggers Ca$^{2+}$ release of from intracellular ER stores. Group II (mGluR2 and mGluR3) and Group III (mGluR4, mGluR6–8) are coupled to adenylate cyclase and regulate cAMP production.

Group I mGluRs mediate [Ca$^{2+}$]$_i$ elevations in OPCs, although these receptors have not been shown to be activated by synaptic release of glutamate (Haberlandt *et al.*, 2011). They also regulate expression of Ca$^{2+}$-permeable AMPARs in OPCs via elevation of Ca$^{2+}$ and release of InsP$_3$ (Zonouzi *et al.*, 2011). Expression levels of mGluRs are developmentally down-regulated as OPC differentiate into mature oligodendrocytes, and their activation attenuates excitotoxicity, by a mechanism distinct from regulating expression of AMPARs (Deng *et al.*, 2004).

## 5.3.3  Purinergic receptors

Purine receptors are broadly divided into adenosine (P1) and ATP (P2) receptors, and there is evidence for expression of both groups in oligodendrocyte lineage cells, where they are important in development and myelin maintenance (Figure 5.11; Butt, 2011; Matute & Cavaliere, 2011). ATP is released as a neurotransmitter and gliotransmitter fairly ubiquitously throughout the CNS, and it is rapidly broken down by ectonucleotidases into ADP and adenosine (see Section 4.4.3(ii) and Figure 4.14).

**(i)  P1 purinergic receptors**   There are four subtypes of adenosine receptors: A$_1$ and A$_3$ receptors inhibit cAMP via G$_{i/o}$, whereas A$_{2A}$ and A$_{2B}$ receptors stimulate cAMP via G$_s$. Messenger RNA for all four subtypes has been detected by RT-PCR in cultures of OPC (Stevens *et al.*, 2002), but *in vivo* evidence of adenosine receptors in mature myelinating oligodendrocytes is lacking. Adenosine receptors regulate OPC migration, proliferation, and differentiation (Othman *et al.*, 2003; Stevens *et al.*, 2002).

**(ii)   P2X receptors**   There are seven mammalian P2X subunits ($P2X_{1-7}$), which assemble as trimers to form homomeric and heteromeric receptors with a diverse range of properties. P2X receptors are cationic ligand-gated channels permeable to $Na^+$, $K^+$ and $Ca^{2+}$; most are activated at low concentrations of ATP, with $EC_{50s}$ of $1–10\,\mu M$, and they can be distinguished by their relative ion permeabilities, gating kinetics and sensitivity to ATP and a range of agonists and antagonists. $P2X_7$ receptors are only activated at high concentrations of ATP, in the millimolar range, and are capable of pore formation, resulting in sustained influx of $Ca^{2+}$. Oligodendrocytes and OPCs exhibit robust expression of $P2X_7$ receptors (Agresti *et al.*, 2005a, 2005b; Matute *et al.*, 2007).

Furthermore, ATP released by astrocytes can evoke a rapid and transient rise in intracellular $Ca^{2+}$ in OPCs involving $P2X_7$ receptors (Hamilton *et al.*, 2010). These data suggest an unresolved physiological function of $P2X_7$ receptors in oligodendrocytes, possibly related to myelin maintenance, by providing a mechanism by which oligodendrocytes sense their environment. As well as raised $[Ca^{2+}]_i$, activation of $P2X_7$ receptors is linked to multiple intracellular pathways, including MAPK, PKC, and PI3K (see Figure 4.16), all of which are known to regulate oligodendrocyte proliferation, survival, differentiation and myelination (see Section 5.4.6 and Figure 5.16). In addition, $P2X_7$ receptors are implicated in the loss of oligodendrocytes and myelin in ischaemia and demyelination (Domercq *et al.*, 2010).

**(iii)   P2Y receptors**   Eight subtypes of the P2Y receptor have been cloned in mammals, and they exhibit differential sensitivity to the adenine nucleotides ATP/ADP ($P2Y_{1,11,12,13}$), the uracil nucleotides UTP/UDP ($P2Y_{4,6}$), both adenine and uracil nucleotides ($P2Y_2$), or UDP-glucose ($P2Y_{14}$). All P2Y receptors are G-protein-coupled and, broadly speaking, activate phospholipase C/inositol triphosphate ($InsP_3$) and $Ca^{2+}$-release from the smooth endoplasmic reticulum via $G\alpha_{q/11}$ ($P2Y_1$, $P2Y_2$, $P2Y_4$, $P2Y_6$, and $P2Y_{11}$), or inhibit adenylyl cyclase via $G\alpha_s$ and $G\alpha_{i/o}$ ($P2Y_{12}$, $P2Y_{13}$, and $P2Y_{14}$) (see Figure 4.15).

The specific subtypes expressed in oligodendrocytes are less clearly defined (Butt, 2011), but a key feature is the prominent expression of $P2Y_1$ receptors and their prominant role in mediating ATP-evoked $Ca^{2+}$ signals coupled to $InsP_3$ (Agresti *et al.*, 2005a; Agresti *et al.*, 2005b). $P2Y_1$ $Ca^{2+}$ responses may be developmentally regulated, since only late OPC and mature oligodendrocytes appear to exhibit significant ATP-induced $Ca^{2+}$ elevations, although in OPCs $P2Y_1R$ activation stimulates cell migration, inhibits mitogenic response to PDGF, and promotes differentiation (Agresti *et al.*, 2005a; Agresti *et al.*, 2005b). $P2Y_1$ receptors are linked to MAPK, JNK, PKC, and PI3K pathways (see Figure 4.15), which regulate OPC proliferation and survival, as well as differentiation and myelination (see Section 5.4.6 and Figure 5.16). In addition, $P2Y_{12}$ receptors are enriched in oligodendrocytes and are implicated in MS (Amadio *et al.*, 2010).

*GPR17* is a P2Y-like receptor that responds to both uracil nucleotides (e.g. UDP-glucose) and cysteinyl-leukotrienes (e.g. LTD4 and LTC4). GPR17 is highly expressed on OPCs during development and NG2-glia in the adult, and it is implicated in the timing of differentiation and injury (Boda *et al.*, 2011; Ceruti *et al.*, 2009; Fumagalli *et al.*, 2011). GPR17 expression sensitises OPCs to adenine nucleotide-induced cytotoxicity, whereas activation with uracil nucleotides promotes differentiation (Ceruti *et al.*, 2011).

## 5.3.4 GABA receptors

*Ionotropic GABA$_A$R* are Cl$^-$ channels that have been demonstrated to be functional in OPCs and oligodendrocytes in culture and in brain slices (Berger *et al.*, 1992b; Kirchhoff & Kettenmann, 1992; Lin & Bergles, 2004; Velez-Fort *et al.*, 2010; Von Blankenfeld *et al.*, 1991). The exact composition of GABA$_A$Rs in oligodendrocytes remains to be determined: GABA$_A$Rs are pentamers usually made of two $\alpha$ subunits, two $\beta$ subunits, and one $\gamma$ subunit, and their diversity is greatly increased by the existence of six different $\alpha$ subunits ($\alpha1$–$\alpha6$), three different $\beta$ subunits ($\beta1$–$\beta3$) and three different $\gamma$ subunits ($\gamma1$–$\gamma3$). GABAergic synapses from neurones are known to contact OPCs (Lin and Bergles, 2004), and there is evidence that GABA$_A$Rs expressed by OPCs switch from a synaptic to an extra-synaptic localisation during development (Velez-Fort *et al.*, 2010).

In oligodendrocytes, as in astrocytes, because intracellular [Cl$^-$] is maintained higher than in neurones, activation of GABA$_A$R receptors leads to Cl$^-$ efflux and cell depolarisation (see Section 4.4.3(iii) for further details). This can result in GABA$_A$R-mediated activation of VOCC and intracellular Ca$^{2+}$ increases in OPC and oligodendrocytes (Kirchhoff and Kettenmann, 1992; Velez-Fort *et al.*, 2010). Another possible mechanism for Ca$^{2+}$ entry is reversal of the Na$^+$/Ca$^{2+}$ exchanger (NCX1) due to raised intracellular Na$^+$ (Tong *et al.*, 2009).

The physiological function of GABA$_A$R in the early oligodendroglial lineage is to inhibit their proliferation, although this may not be a major control mechanism for cell cycle progression (Yuan *et al.*, 1998). The localisation and function of GABA$_A$R in mature oligodendrocytes is unknown, and the endogenous source of GABA to activate these receptors is unresolved, although extra-synaptic oligodendroglial GABA$_A$R could be activated by spillover release of GABA from neurones or astrocytes (Figure 5.11) (Velez-Fort *et al.*, 2010). Similar to other neurotransmitter receptors, GABA$_A$R expression appears to be strongly down-regulated in mature oligodendrocytes (Von Blankenfeld *et al.*, 1991).

*Metabotropic GABA$_B$R* are expressed by OPCs and stimulate proliferation and migration (Luyt *et al.*, 2007), and are down-regulated in myelinating oligodendrocytes (Charles *et al.*, 2003). They can be composed of two major types of subunits – B1$_{a/b}$ and B2, which have been identified in OPCs and oligodendrocytes *in vitro* (Luyt *et al.*, 2007).

## 5.3.5   Other neurotransmitter receptors

*Glycine receptors (GlyRs)* have been described in OPCs (Belachew *et al.*, 1998a; Belachew *et al.*, 1998b; Kirchhoff *et al.*, 1996). The composition of oligodendroglial glycine receptors is uncertain. Transcripts of the $\alpha 1$ subunit, but not of $\alpha 2$ or $\alpha 3$ subunits, have been reported in spinal cord cells (Kirchhoff *et al.*, 1996), whereas cultured OPCs of newborn rat cortex expresses $\alpha 2$ and $\beta$ subunits (Belachew *et al.*, 1998b). As for most other ligand-gated ion channels, GlyR expression seems to peak at the OPC stage and decrease thereafter (Belachew *et al.*, 1998a).

*Acetylcholine receptors (AChRs)*, both ionotropic nicotinic and metabotropic muscarinic (nAChRs and mAChRs) have been identified in oligodendrocytes. RT-PCR analysis and immunocytochemistry in OPCs cultured from rat corpus callosum have detected expression of nAChR subunits $\alpha 3$, $\alpha 4$, $\alpha 5$, $\alpha 7$, $\beta 2$, and $\beta 4$ (Rogers *et al.*, 2001). The presence of $Ca^{2+}$-permeable $\alpha 7$-containing nAChRs has been demonstrated in OPCs recorded from mouse hippocampus slices (Velez-Fort *et al.*, 2009) and, in cultured OPCs, nAChR can induce increased intracellular $Ca^{2+}$ involving VOCC (Rogers *et al.*, 2001). It is not clear whether nAChRs persist in myelinating oligodendrocytes.

OPCs and oligodendrocytes express functional mAChRs *in vitro*, and their activation triggers intracellular signals such as MAPK, $InsP_3$, and $Ca^{2+}$ mobilisation (Cui *et al.*, 2006; Kastritsis & McCarthy, 1993; Ragheb *et al.*, 2001). At the RNA level, expression of all mAChR subtypes has been reported in both OPCs and oligodendrocytes, but expression is decreased during maturation (De Angelis *et al.*, 2011, Ragheb *et al.*, 2001). The predominant mAChR subtype expressed in oligodendrocytes is M3, followed by M4, M2, M1, and M5 (Ragheb *et al.*, 2001). In OPCs, mAChR activation significantly increases proliferation and inhibits their differentiation into myelinating oligodendrocytes, and receptors may be developmentally down-regulated (Figure 5.11) (De Angelis *et al.*, 2011; Ragheb *et al.*, 2001).

*Dopamine receptors* comprising $D_2$ and $D_3$ subtypes have been reported in oligodendrocyte lineage cells (Bongarzone *et al.*, 1998; Niu *et al.*, 2010; Rosin *et al.*, 2005). $D_3R$ expression occurs in OPCs and immature oligodendrocytes in the corpus callosum and *in vitro* (Bongarzone *et al.*, 1998). The reports of $D_3R$ function in OPCs are conflicting, with blockade being shown both to stimulate and to inhibit OPC differentiation *in vitro* (Figure 5.11; Bongarzone *et al.*, 1998; Niu *et al.*, 2010), which may be related to changes in relative expression of $D_2R$ and $D_3R$ during differentiation. Both $D_2R$ and $D_3R$ mRNA have been shown in differentiated rat cortical oligodendrocytes and protects them against glutamate-mediated excitoxicity (Rosin *et al.*, 2005).

A variety of receptors to *neuromodulators* are reported to be expressed by OPCs and/or oligodendrocytes, such as bradykinin receptors (Stephens *et al.*, 1993), opioid $\mu$ and $\kappa$ receptors (Knapp *et al.*, 2009), and cannabinoid $CB_1$ and $CB_2$

receptors (Gomez *et al.*, 2011; Molina-Holgado *et al.*, 2002), and adrenaline α1 receptors (Cohen & Almazan, 1993), which have also been detected in NG2-glia *in vivo*, but not in mature oligodendrocytes (Papay *et al.*, 2006).

## 5.3.6 Transporters and exchangers

Oligodendrocytes express all the major cation and anion transporters seen in astrocytes, including Na-K-ATPase, Ca-ATPase, Na-Ca exchanger, and a variety of anion transport proteins (see Section 4.4.4 and Figures 4.19, 4.20 and 4.23 for further details). The $Na^+/K^+$-ATPase catalyses the active transport of $Na^+$ and $K^+$, and has two principal subunits (α and β); the β3 isoform predominates in oligodendrocytes and co-localises with CAII (Martin-Vasallo *et al.*, 2000). CAII is critical for $H^+$ buffering and exists in oligodendrocytes as a freely diffusing protein throughout the cell, as well as in microdomains associated with $Na^+$-$H^+$ exchangers in the somata and Na-$HCO_3$-cotransporter in the processes. Also, together with the Na-independent $Cl^-$-$HCO_3^-$ exchanger, CAII regulates intracellular pH in oligodendrocytes (Boussouf & Gaillard, 2000; Ro & Carson, 2004). $Na^+/K^+/Cl^-$ (NKCC1) and $K^+/Cl^-$ co-transporters are also expressed in oligodendrocytes and myelin (Chen & Sun, 2005; Malek *et al.*, 2003). $Na^+/K^+/Cl^-$ co-transport can promote pathological $Na^+$ entry into oligodendrocytes, which then triggers reversal of the $Na^+$-$Ca^{2+}$ exchanger, resulting in $Ca^{2+}$ entry and additional $Ca^{2+}$-dependent injury (Chen *et al.*, 2007). Oligodendrocytes express $Na^+$-$Ca^{2+}$ exchangers NCX1, NCX2, and NCX3 (Boscia *et al.*, 2012).

*Glutamate transporters* are developmentally expressed by oligodendrocyte lineage cells, with EAAT1/GLAST being localised to myelinating oligodendrocytes and EAAT3/EAAC1 being localised to OPC (Domercq *et al.*, 1999). In addition, oligodendrocytes express glutamine synthetase, a key enzyme in glutamate metabolism. Basal release of glutamate is substantial, even in white matter, and impairment of uptake causes severe damage to oligodendrocytes in particular.

## 5.3.7 Gap junctions

Oligodendrocytes predominantly express Cx32 and Cx47, as well as Cx29 (Figure 5.12; Kleopa *et al.*, 2010; Orthmann-Murphy *et al.*, 2008; and see Section 4.3.1 and Figure 4.5 for further details on gap junctions). Cx47 is expressed by all types of oligodendrocytes both in the white and grey matter and forms gap junctions (GJs) on cell bodies and proximal processes, as well as most of the GJs with astrocytes. Cx32 is expressed mostly by white matter oligodendrocytes and forms GJs in Schmidt-Lanterman incisures and between paranodal loops, and is associated with Caspr at paranodes (Kamasawa *et al.*, 2005). Cx29 appears to be restricted to oligodendrocytes that myelinate small calibre fibres and most likely form hemichannels (Altevogt *et al.*, 2002).

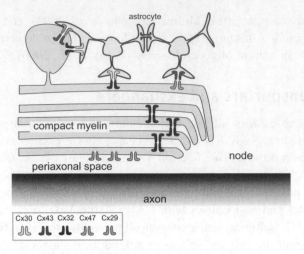

**Figure 5.12** Connexins in oligodendrocytes

Oligodendrocytes predominantly express Cx32 and Cx47, as well as Cx29. Autologous Cx32 gap junctions are localised to the paranodal loops, whereas Cx29 form hemi-channels along the inner face of myelin. Cx47 and Cx32 form gap junctions with astrocytes to act as conduits for long-distance intracellular and intercellular movement of ions and water.

Thus, Cx47-Cx32 containing GJs act as conduits for long-distance intracellular and intercellular movement of ions and associated osmotic water, and place oligodendrocytes within astroglial segregated networks (see Figures 4.9 and 4.33). The autologous Cx32 GJs may regulate paranodal electrical properties during saltatory conduction. Mice lacking either Cx47 or Cx32 are viable, but those lacking both connexins display marked abnormalities in CNS myelin, characterised by thin or absent myelin sheaths, vacuolation, enlarged periaxonal collars, oligodendrocyte cell death and axonal loss.

## 5.3.8   Intracellular calcium

A wide range of agents evoke an increase in $[Ca^{2+}]_i$ in oligodendrocytes, including growth factors and neurotransmitters, and have been shown to regulate their development and pathology (Butt, 2006). As in astrocytes, raised $[Ca^{2+}]_i$ in oligodendrocytes occurs by triggering $Ca^{2+}$ influx through plasmalemmal $Ca^{2+}$ channels or release from intracellular stores (see Section 4.4.5 and Figure 4.20 for further details). The maintenance of $[Ca^{2+}]_i$ is brought about by sequestration of $Ca^{2+}$ into the sarcoplasmic/endoplasmic reticulum via $Ca^{2+}$-ATPases (SERCA pumps), into mitochondria, and by extrusion of $Ca^{2+}$ into the extracellular milieu via plasma membrane ATP-dependent $Ca^{2+}$-pumps (PCMAs) and $Na^+$-$Ca^{2+}$ exchangers (NCX) (Alberdi *et al.*, 2005; Verkhratsky *et al.*, 1998).

*Calcium influx* across the oligodendroglial plasmalemma can occur through a number of routes:

1. ligand-operated channels, such as P2X purinoceptors and AMPA/kainate iGluR;

2. voltage-operated $Ca^{2+}$ channels (VOCC), activated in response to receptor-mediated cell membrane depolarisation – this occurs, for example, in response to raised extracellular $[K^+]$ during neuronal activity, or $Na^+$ influx during activation of AMPA/kainate iGluR or amino acid transporters, or $Cl^-$ efflux during activation of $GABA_AR$ and GlyR;

3. store-operated $Ca^{2+}$ channels (SOCC) or capacitive $Ca^{2+}$ entry (CRAC) in response to depletion of intracellular stores (see Section 5.4).

The localized expression of VOCC indicates $Ca^{2+}$ influx would be restricted to the tips of oligodendrocyte processes, providing a mechanism for regulating directional process growth and axon ensheathment in response to axonal action potentials.

*Intracellular calcium release* is via $InsP_3$ receptor-mediated efflux from ER intracellular stores in response to G protein coupled receptor activation of phospholipase C (PLC) and the formation of diaglycerol (DAG) (Butt, 2006). OPCs and oligodendrocytes express $InsP_3$ receptors (Simpson *et al.*, 1998) and ryanodine receptors (RyR), and their activation mediates calcium-induced calcium release (CICR) (Simpson *et al.*, 1997, 1998; see Figure 4.21).

Calcium events triggered by $InsP_3$-R and RyR are respectively termed 'puffs' and 'sparks', and both have been shown to occur along the processes of cultured OPCs, but only puffs are able to trigger $Ca^{2+}$ waves (Haak *et al.*, 2001). Depletion of ER stores results in the opening of SOCC and capacitive $Ca^{2+}$ entry across the plasmalemma, which replenishes ER stores and prolongs the cytoplasmic $Ca^{2+}$ signal after the original agonist-evoked signal has ended (Simpson & Russell, 1997).

In addition, mitochondria can also release $Ca^{2+}$ into the cytosol and contribute to the propagation of $Ca^{2+}$ signals in oligodendrocytes (Haak *et al.*, 2000, 2002; Simpson *et al.*, 1997, 1998). One mechanism for mitochondrial $Ca^{2+}$ efflux is via the mitochondria permeability transition pore (PTP), which is constitutively active in OPCs and accompanies agonist evoked $Ca^{2+}$ signals (Smaili & Russell, 1999).

*Intracellular calcium signal amplification microdomains*, containing high densities of $InsP_3R$ co-localised with SERCA pumps, RyR and mitochondria, serve to propagate $InsP_3$-mediated $Ca^{2+}$ signals along oligodendrocyte processes (Haak *et al.*, 2000, 2001, 2002; Simpson *et al.*, 1997). The concentration of both cell membrane VOCC and intracellular wave-amplification sites on oligodendrocyte processes which contact axons suggests that they serve to mediate highly localised events during axon-to-oligodendrocyte signalling and regulate process growth during myelination.

*Multiple calcium-dependent intracellular signalling pathways* are regulated by extracellular and axon-dependent factors, including MAP kinases and CREB, which regulate oligodendrocyte cell proliferation, survival, growth and differentiation (Soliven, 2001). Many neurotransmitters evoke raised $[Ca^{2+}]_i$ signals in OPCs and influence OPC development, most notably ATP, which is a potent mediator of $Ca^{2+}$ signalling in OPCs and regulates their migration, proliferation and differentiation, primarily via metabotropic P2Y receptors (Agresti *et al.*, 2005b).

Activation of muscarinic cholinergic receptors (mAChR) in OPCs increases $[Ca^{2+}]_i$ and activates $Ca^{2+}$-dependent gene transcription, activation of MAP kinases and proliferation (Cohen *et al.*, 1996; Pende *et al.*, 1997; Ragheb *et al.*, 2001; Sato-Bigbee *et al.*, 1999). Calcium signalling via AChR, glutamate, and purinoceptors depends on neuronal contact and/or electrical signalling, supporting a role for these neurotransmitters in regulating OPC differentiation and myelination (He *et al.*, 1996; Wake *et al.*, 2011).

*Glutamate affects early oligodendrocyte development* via activation of plasma-lemmal GluR (Gallo & Ghiani, 2000). AMPA receptors in OPCs allow $Ca^{2+}$ entry to stimulate OPC migration (Gudz *et al.*, 2006), and inhibit OPC proliferation and lineage progression (Gallo *et al.*, 1996; Yuan *et al.*, 1998). Physiological action potential propagation in the optic nerve activates AMPA receptors on NG2-glia (OPCs) but does not normally induce somatic $[Ca^{2+}]_i$ elevations, suggesting that $[Ca^{2+}]_i$ signals in NG2-glia may be restricted to their processes, where VOCC are clustered (Haberlandt *et al.*, 2011; Hamilton *et al.*, 2010). Glutamate released from electrically active axons stimulates Fyn activation, which promotes process growth and myelination (Wake *et al.*, 2011). Although OPCs also express NMDA receptors, and their blockade inhibits OPC migration *in vitro* (Wang *et al.*, 1996), specific NR1 knockout in the oligodendrocyte lineage has been shown to have no effect on OPC development (De Biase *et al.*, 2011), and specific knockout of NR1 or NR3A does not affect their response to demyelination in EAE (Guo *et al.*, 2012).

*ATP and adenosine mediate axonal control of myelination* via raised $[Ca^{2+}]_i$ in OPCs and immature oligodendrocytes (Ishibashi *et al.*, 2006; Stevens *et al.*, 2002). In the optic nerve, adenosine and ATP released from electrically active axons and from astrocytes triggers $Ca^{2+}$ transients in OPCs (Hamilton *et al.*, 2010; Stevens *et al.*, 2002). Adenosine acts directly to inhibit OPC proliferation and promote their differentiation and myelination (Stevens *et al.*, 2002), whereas ATP acts on astrocytes to trigger the release of LIF, which in turn acts on oligodendrocytes to promote myelination (Figure 5.11; Ishibashi *et al.*, 2006). Adenosine, acting via A1 receptors, and ATP, acting via $P2Y_1$ receptors, also regulate the migration of OPCs (Agresti *et al.*, 2005a; Othman *et al.*, 2003).

*Mature oligodendrocytes express receptors for neurotransmitters,* but to date their physiological role is undefined (Butt, 2006). Oligodendrocytes express $P2Y_1$ receptors and $P2X_7$ receptors and there is evidence they mediate raised $[Ca^{2+}]_i$ (James & Butt, 2001; Kirischuk *et al.*, 1995a; Matute *et al.*, 2007; Moran-Jimenez & Matute, 2000). Similarly, oligodendrocytes express AMPA receptors on their cell somata and NMDA receptors in myelin, but evidence is lacking that they mediate $Ca^{2+}$ influx under physiological conditions (Micu *et al.*, 2006). In contrast, there is a clear function for glutamate and ATP in oligodendrocyte pathology (Matute, 2011).

## 5.4  Oligodendrocyte development

Oligodendrocytes are generated from OPCs that arise from multipotent neural stem cells (NSCs) in the subventricular zone (SVZ) (Figure 5.13; see also Section 4.5.1 and Figures 4.28–4.30; Richardson *et al.*, 2006). From these focal sources, OPCs migrate to populate the entire CNS, where they undergo local proliferation and differentiate into oligodendrocytes. In addition, a significant population of OPCs do not differentiate, and persist as adult OPCs or NG2-glia, which reside throughout the brain parenchyma and generate oligodendrocytes into adulthood and following demyelination (see Chapters 6 and 9).

The specification, migration, proliferation and differentiation of oligodendrocytes are regulated by the highly complex interplay between intrinsic and extrinsic factors, which both negatively and positively influence oligodendrocyte generation and myelination. These include sonic hedgehog (Shh), Notch signalling, and key

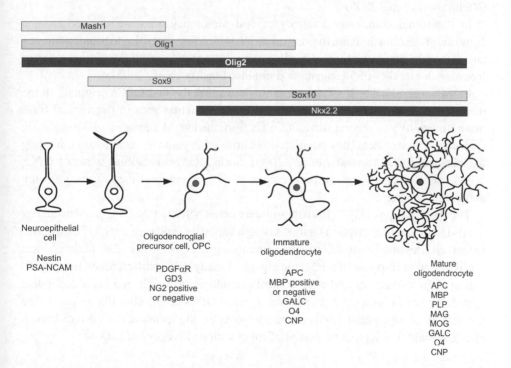

**Figure 5.13**  Stages of oligodendrocyte differentiation.
Oligodendrocytes are generated from OPCs that arise from neuroepithelial cells, which pass through several distinct differentiation stages that can be identified by specific markers and are under the regulation of a series of transcription factors.

growth factors such as platelet-derived growth factor (PDGF) and fibroblast growth factor (FGF) (see Figure 4.30).

Transcription factors are part of the gene regulatory machinery and some, such as Sox10, are cornerstones of myelination. Crosstalk between transcription factors and epigenetic modulators of gene expression also play key roles in regulating oligodendrocyte differentiation, including histone modifications and microRNAs (miRNAs). Many of these factors are also involved in oligodendrocyte pathologies and regulate regeneration and remyelination in diseases such as multiple sclerosis.

## 5.4.1   Developmental origins of oligodendrocytes

The embryonic origins of oligodendrocytes are well defined in the rodent spinal cord and forebrain (Richardson *et al.*, 2006). Oligodendrocyte origins in the diencephalon, midbrain and hind brain remain unclear; in the cerebellum, oligodendrocytes migrate in from the midbrain, but they may also be derived from endogenous sources within the cerebellum. In the embryonic forebrain and spinal cord, the majority of oligodendrocytes arise first from restricted ventral zones around embryonic day (E) 12.5, but after E15 there is a second wave of generation from dorsal regions (Richardson *et al.*, 2006).

In the spinal cord, oligodendrocytes and motor neurones are derived from a common progenitor domain, the ventral pMN, which first gives rise to motor neurones and then to the majority of spinal cord oligodendrocytes. Later, oligodendrocytes arise from the dorsal dP3-dP5 progenitor domains (Fogarty *et al.*, 2005).

In the forebrain, Cre-lox fate mapping shows that the first OPCs originate in the medial ganglionic eminence and anterior entopeduncular area in the ventral forebrain, followed by a second wave of OPCs from the lateral and/or caudal ganglionic eminences, from where they populate the entire embryonic telencephalon including the cerebral cortex (Kessaris *et al.*, 2006). Soon after birth, a third wave of OPCs arises from the dorsal subventricular zone (SVZ) to colonise the corpus callosum and cerebral cortex.

The specification of OPCs from neural stem cells (NSCs) in the SVZ is controlled by local signals and transcription factors. Using a variety of guidance cues, OPCs migrate from their sites of origin to their final destinations in the CNS, where they undergo local proliferation in response to mitogenic signals. Finally, OPCs differentiate into myelinating oligodendrocytes under the control of multiple diffusible and axon-dependent signals, or persist as a large population of adult OPCs (NG2-glia) that populate the entire white and grey matter and continue to generate oligodendrocytes into adulthood, after the main developmental period of myelination (Rivers *et al.*, 2008).

## 5.4.2   Stages of oligodendrocyte differentiation

A range of stage-specific markers and transcription factors have enabled discrete phases of oligodendrocyte differentiation to be identified and studied, from early

OPCs to late OPCs and pro-oligodendrocytes, through premyelinating oligodendrocytes, and finally into mature myelinating oligodendrocytes (Figure 5.13). Most often, these markers have been used to identify oligodendrocyte lineage cells immunohistochemically, and to isolate and purify cells for *in vitro* studies and, more recently, genomic and proteomic analyses. Increasingly, many markers are used to drive the cell- and stage-specific expression of reporter genes and using Cre/loxP technology for fate mapping studies. Expression studies, the use of global knock-outs and targeted gene deletion have identified functions for most of the key markers for oligodendrocyte differentiation and myelination.

*OPCs* can be defined by their expression of PDGFRα and the NG2 chondroitin sulphate proteoglycan (cspg4) (Nishiyama *et al.*, 2009; Richardson *et al.*, 2011). PDGFRα mediate the potent mitogenic actions of PDGF on OPC, but the functions of the NG2 CSPG in OPCs are unknown (see Chapter 6). Early OPCs can also be identified by the A2B5 antibody, but A2B5 is not specific to OPCs and it is also expressed by neuroblasts and glial-restricted precursor cells (GRPs) (Noble *et al.*, 2003). In addition, the NSC marker CD133 (Prominin-1/PROM1) is highly expressed by foetal and adult human OPCs, although it appears to be a marker for NSCs in rodents (Uchida *et al.*, 2000).

Most OPCs appear to differentiate directly from NSCs and sequentially express the basic helix-loop-helix (bHLH) transcription factors Olig1/Olig2 (oligodendrocyte lineage transcription factor 1 and 2), Sox10 (SRY (Sex determining region Y)-box 10), and the homeodomain transcription factor Nkx2.2. These transcription factors are essential for OPC specification and their differentiation into oligodendrocytes, although Olig1/Olig2 expressing cells also generate motor neurones and astrocytes (see Section 5.4.3). Mash1 is also broadly expressed by SVZ and migratory OPCs, as well as neural progenitors, and it cooperates with Olig2 in OPC specification from the postnatal SVZ (Parras *et al.*, 2004; Wang *et al.*, 2001).

*Late OPC/ pro-oligodendrocytes* gain expression of the antigens recognised by the O4 antibody, without losing PDGFRα/NG2 and prior to gaining expression of GalC (Bansal, 2002). O4 first labels oligodendrocyte lineage cells at the migratory stage, and the antigens recognised by O4 include sulphatide, seminolipid, sulphated and non-sulphated cholesterol, together with an unidentified pro-oligodendroblast antigen (POA) (Bansal *et al.*, 1992).

*Premyelinating oligodendrocytes* lose expression of PDGFRα and NG2 (but not O4) and gain expression of GalC and CNPase which, in the CNS, are specifically expressed by oligodendrocytes and myelin (see Section 5.2.4). These are useful early markers of terminal differentiation, since they are expressed by multiple process-bearing, non-proliferative and non-migratory premyelinating oligodendrocytes, prior to most other myelin-related proteins.

*Mature myelin-forming oligodendrocytes* can be identified by their expression of myelin-related proteins, mainly PLP and MBP (see Section 5.2.4). However, PLP and MBP, along with MAG, are first expressed at the late premyelinating stage and onwards. PLP/DM20 may also be expressed by OPCs early in development, and embryonically PLP/DM20 cells have been shown to differentiate into neurones (Delaunay *et al.*, 2008). MOG is one of the last myelin proteins to be expressed, and is useful for identifying the final stages of oligodendrocyte differentiation.

### 5.4.3   Trophic factors and oligodendrocyte differentiation

*Growth factors and hormones* that have been shown to regulate oligodendrocyte generation and differentiation *in vitro* are numerous (Taveggia *et al.*, 2010). Notable amongst these are PDGF, FGF2 and IGF1, which have been shown to be key regulators of oligodendrocyte differentiation *in vitro*, and studies in transgenic mice are beginning to unravel how they act in concert to achieve the exquisitely fine regulation of the complex process of oligodendrocyte development and myelination.

*Platelet derived growth factor* (PDGF) is produced by both astrocytes and neurones, and *in vitro* is a survival factor, motogen and potent mitogen for OPCs. PDGF is only effective in OPCs, because PDGFRα are lost at the O4+ stage of oligodendrocyte maturation. Studies in transgenic mice have demonstrated profound reductions in the numbers of OPCs and oligodendrocytes in PDGF-A deficient mice, and increased OPCs in transgenic mice overexpressing PDGF-A (Calver *et al.*, 1998; Fruttiger *et al.*, 1999).

*FGF2* (also called basic FGF, bFGF) has multiple actions at different stages of oligodendrocyte differentiation (Bansal, 2002). FGF2 is a potent mitogen and motogen for OPCs *in vitro*. FGF2 inhibits OPC differentiation *in vitro*, in part by maintaining the expression of PDGFRα to increase the developmental period during which OPCs respond to PDGF. FGF2 is highly expressed in the developing CNS and its effects on oligodendrocytes are mediated by FGF receptors-1, -2 and -3 (FGFR1-3), which mediate diverse stage-specific effects *in vitro* and *in vivo* (Bansal, 2002; Fortin *et al.*, 2005).

*In vitro*, FGFR1 mediates OPC proliferation, while FGFR3 inhibits terminal OPC differentiation and FGFR2 mediate process growth and myelination in oligodendrocytes. Knockout studies confirm that FGFR3 positively regulates the timing of oligodendrocyte differentiation and myelination (Oh *et al.*, 2003), but inactivation of FGFR2 in oligodendrocyte lineage cells does not affect oligodendrocyte numbers or myelination (Kaga *et al.*, 2006). Furthermore, there were no effects reported in the studies on OPC proliferation and differentiation in mice lacking both FGFR1 and FGFR2 in oligodendrocyte-lineage cells, although myelin thickness was reduced, indicating a role for FGF receptor signalling in regulation of myelin growth (Furusho *et al.*, 2012).

*Insulin-like growth factor I (IGF-I)* stimulates proliferation of OPCs and O4+ preoligodendrocytes, and it is a survival factor throughout the lineage *in vitro* (McMorris & McKinnon, 1996). Oligodendrocytes express type 1 IGF receptor

(IGFR1) at all stages, and IGF1 increases oligodendrocyte number, stimulates their differentiation and increases the amount of myelin they produce. IGF1 over-expression in transgenic mice results in hypermyelination, whereas IGF1 ablation results in impaired myelination (Carson *et al.*, 1993; Ye *et al.*, 1995; Zeger *et al.*, 2007). However, there are also reduced neurones in the IGF-I null mouse with associated hypomyelination (Cheng *et al.*, 1998).

*Other growth factors* that regulate oligodendrocyte differentiation include *neurotrophin-3* (NT-3), *brain-derived neurotrophic factor* (BDNF), and *nerve growth factor* (NGF) (Taveggia *et al.*, 2010). NGF, acting via TrkA receptors on axons and p75$^{NTR}$ on oligodendrocytes, exerts an inhibitory effect on oligoden-drocyte maturation and myelination (Lee *et al.*, 2007; Mi *et al.*, 2004). BDNF, acting through TrkB receptors, up-regulates the expression of myelin proteins in oligodendrocytes (Du *et al.*, 2006). NT-3, acting through the TrkC receptor, is a mitogen and survival factor for OPCs in combination with other factors (Barres *et al.*, 1993). In addition, the hormones progesterone and thyroid hormone positively regulate oligodendrocyte differentiation and myelination (Calza *et al.*, 2010; Schumacher *et al.*, 2012).

*Cytokines and chemokines* act on oligodendrocytes and OPCs through a wide range of receptors (Schmitz & Chew, 2008). TNF-$\alpha$ and IFN-$\gamma$ are inhibitory for OPC differentiation in culture (Agresti *et al.*, 1996; Chew *et al.*, 2005). Many of the interleukins (ILs) regulate OPC proliferation and differentiation, including IL-6 (Pizzi *et al.*, 2004) and astrocyte-derived IL-11 (Zhang *et al.*, 2006). In addition, there is evidence that IL-1$\beta$ inhibits OPC proliferation (Vela *et al.*, 2002), while IL-2 induces proliferation and differentiation, or induces cell death, in oligodendro-cytes (Otero & Merrill, 1997).

LIF (leukemia inhibitory factor) is released by astrocytes in response to ATP released by electrically active axons, and it is required for correct myelination during a precise developmental time window (Ishibashi *et al.*, 2006, 2009). Several molecules can act through the LIF receptor, or gp130 signalling chain, to have similar effects on oligodendrocytes, including CNTF (ciliary neurotrophic factor), which can act as a comitogen with PDGF in OPCs and promotes oligodendrocyte survival (Butzkueven *et al.*, 2006). TGF-$\beta$ inhibits OPC proliferation and promotes oligodendrocyte development (McKinnon *et al.*, 1993).

Chemokines are often triggered by inflammatory mediators, but some are constitutively expressed, such as CXCL1 and CXCL12 in neurones and astrocytes, respectively. CXCL1 signalling through CXCR2 directs migration of OPCs in the spinal cord (Tsai *et al.*, 2002). In addition, CXCL1 and CXCL12 both stimulate OPC proliferation and promote MBP synthesis (Kadi *et al.*, 2006). CXCL1 has been shown to directly increase OPC numbers in the dysmyelinating mutant jimpy mouse (Wu *et al.*, 2000). Astrocytes have been shown to be a source of CXCL1 that enhances the proliferative response of OPCs to PDGF (Robinson *et al.*, 1998).

The importance of signalling through CXCR2 was demonstrated in CXCR2 KO mice, in which spinal cord myelination was severely disrupted (Padovani-Claudio *et al.*, 2006). Taken together, there is good evidence that cytokines and chemokines play important roles in normal oligodendrocyte development, but increased production by activated astrocytes, microglia and blood-borne cells, indicates their impact on oligodendrocyte pathology may be more important.

### 5.4.4    Regulation of oligodendrocyte differentiation

Oligodendrocyte specification, migration, proliferation and differentiation are controlled by a series of intrinsic and extrinsic factors (Wegner, 2008).

*Specification* of oligodendrocyte lineage cells in the ventral spinal cord and telencephalon is strongly and positively dependent on Shh, whereas later emergence of OPCs from dorsal origins is Shh-independent and strongly FGF2 dependent (Kessaris *et al.*, 2004). In addition to the induction signals of Shh and FGF2 in the ventral spinal cord, specification of oligodendrocytes is inhibited by Wnts and bone morphogenetic proteins (BMPs), secreted from the dorsal spinal cord.

Two classes of transcription families, the bHLH proteins Olig1 and Olig2, and homeodomain protein Nkx2.2, are highly Shh concentration-dependent and act in concert to control neurone versus glial fate (Fu *et al.*, 2002; Lu *et al.*, 2000, 2002; Zhou & Anderson, 2002; Zhou *et al.*, 2001). Olig2 is required for production of both motor neurones and OPCs, but OPC specification requires both Olig1 and Olig2. At early stages, the bHLH transcription factors Neurogenin-1 and Neurogenin-2 promote Olig2-dependent motor neurone production and prevent OPC production. At later stages, Neurogenin-1 and Neurogenin-2 are down-regulated and gliogenic factors, including Sox9 and Notch, regulate Olig2 function to produce glia instead of neurones (Finzsch *et al.*, 2008; Li *et al.*, 2011; Stolt *et al.*, 2006; Zhou *et al.*, 2001). Also, the involvement of histone methylation in the transition from NSC to OPC is suggested by experimental evidence on the role of PcG proteins in repressing neurogenin, especially Ezh2, and components from both PRC2 and PRC1 complexes also appear to be critical (Liu & Casaccia, 2010).

OPC specification is marked by the induction of the high mobility group (HMG) domain protein Sox10, which is a direct target of Olig2 in OPC (Kuspert *et al.*, 2011), and Olig2 and Sox10 are retained throughout the lineage (Lu *et al.*, 2000; Stolt *et al.*, 2006; Zhou and Anderson, 2002). Sox10, together with Sox9, promote oligodendrocyte specification and are required to maintain PDGFRα in OPC (Finzsch *et al.*, 2008). In addition, OPC express group D Sox transcription factors Sox5 and Sox6, which have the opposite effect to group E Sox proteins and repress OPC terminal differentiation (Stolt *et al.*, 2006). The transcription factor Nkx2.2 is also developmentally up-regulated and is essential for expansion of OPC, but it is not essential for their specification (Qi *et al.*, 2001; Zhou *et al.*, 2001).

*Migration* of OPCs from the ventricular zone is regulated by a wide range of chemo-attractants and repellents, among them contact-mediated mechanisms (adhesion molecules) and long-range cues (chemotropic molecules) (de Castro & Bribian, 2005). Newly specified OPCs are highly migratory and disperse widely in response to PDGF acting on PDGFRα. The stimulatory effects of PDGF may be counterbalanced by the chemokines CXCL1 and CXCL12, which inhibit OPC migration via receptors CXCR2 and CXCR4 and, thereby, help to fine tune the dispersal of OPC (Dziembowska *et al.*, 2005; Tsai *et al.*, 2002).

This theme of counterbalance is replicated by a wide range of chemo-attractants and repellents. For example, FGF2, acting via FGFR1, is a potent motogen for OPCs, and its effects in OPCs are counteracted by Anosmin-1 (Bribian *et al.*, 2006). In NPs, FGF2 and Anosmin-1 co-operate as chemotropic agents in the embryonic brain (Garcia-Gonzalez *et al.*, 2011). Similarly, the chemo-repellents Sema3a and netrin1, and the astrocyte-derived chemo-attractant endothelin-1 (ET-1), co-function to promote OPC migration from ventral sources (Gadea *et al.*, 2009). Neuregulin-1/ErbB4 signalling controls the migration of OPCs selectively during early stages of CNS development (Ortega *et al.*, 2012a).

In addition to OPC specification and proliferation, Shh also regulates migration of OPCs through the multiligand receptor megalin (or LRP-2) (Ortega *et al.*, 2012b). Similarly, by maintaining PDGFRα in OPC, Sox10 and Sox9 promote OPC migration (Finzsch *et al.*, 2008). OPC migration is also dependent on multiple components of the extracellular matrix (ECM), including tenascin-C, which inhibits migration, while fibronectin and the laminin family member merosin promote migration.

OPC migration depends on the rearrangement of the actin cytoskeleton, and modulators of actin polymerisation in oligodendrocytes include the Src family receptor tyrosine kinase Fyn, a key regulator of oligodendrocyte differentiation and myelination (see Section 5.4.5). PDGF stimulates OPC migration through activation of Fyn kinase (Miyamoto *et al.*, 2008), whereas Slit2 inhibits OPC migration by decreasing the association between Robo1 and Fyn (Lin *et al.*, 2012). OPC also express a range of neurotransmitter receptors and ion channels that regulate their migration, which includes a role for Golli MBP through modulation of voltage-operated calcium channels (Paez *et al.*, 2009c), as well as glutamate, GABA, muscarinic receptors, and ATP and its breakdown product adenosine (Butt, 2006; see Section 5.3).

*Proliferation* of OPCs is strongly dependent on PDGF-A, as demonstrated in transgenic mice lacking or overexpressing PDGF-A (Calver *et al.*, 1998; Fruttiger *et al.*, 1999), and a key mitogenic role has also been identified for FGF-2 (Bansal, 2002). PDGF and FGF2 are critical for the expansion of OPC from sub-ventricular zone sources and are also potent motogens (see above). In addition, local proliferation of OPC following migration is essential to generate sufficient oligodendrocytes for myelination and is dependent on growth factors and axon-derived signals (Miller, 2002).

A number of other factors have been identified that stimulate OPC proliferation and survival, but in general their functions *in vivo* are unclear (see Section 5.4.3). The proliferative actions of PDGF, FGF2 and IGF-I act are mediated at least in part by PI3K/Akt, which in turn inhibit GSK3β, a key negative regulator of OPC proliferation (Azim and Butt, 2011; Bansal, 2002; Cui & Almazan, 2007). Cell cycle progression in OPCs is controlled by cyclin-dependent kinases (Cdks) and their inhibitors. Proliferating OPCs display higher activities of both cyclin D1-cdk4/6 and cyclin E-cdk2, and permanent withdrawal from the cycle is associated with a decrease in the formation of these complexes (Ghiani & Gallo, 2001). The recruitment of OPCs into cell cycle by FGF-2 involves induction of cyclin D1-cdk4/6 complexes and disinhibition of cyclin E-cdk2 by decreasing levels of the cdk inhibitor p27(Kip1); IGF-I acts synergistically to enhance the effects of FGF-2 (Frederick & Wood, 2004). miRNAs regulate crucial developmental genes in oligodendrocytes, and the miR-17-92 cluster is highly enriched in OPCs and promotes their proliferation via the down-regulation of PTEN translation and disinhibition of Akt signalling (Budde et al., 2010).

ECM components also regulate OPC proliferation. For example, the glycoprotein tenascin-C is expressed by OPCs and is required for their responsiveness to PDGF (Garwood et al., 2004), and NG2 may also interact with ECM components to promote OPC proliferation (Kucharova & Stallcup, 2010). Local proliferation of OPCs is also dependent on electrical activity of axons (Barres & Raff, 1993), and is regulated through neurotransmitter receptors and ion channels (Butt, 2006; see Section 5.3).

*Cell cycle exit* is essential for the initiation of OPC terminal differentiation. The transcription factors Yin Yang 1 (YY1) and Sox17 regulate the transition of OPCs from cell cycle to differentiation. YY1 acts as a lineage-specific repressor of transcriptional inhibitors of myelin gene expression (TCF4 and ID4), by recruiting HDAC1 to their promoters during oligodendrocyte differentiation (He et al., 2007). Sox17 appears in the interphase between OPCs and pro-oligodendrocytes (Sohn et al., 2006), and acts by inhibiting PDGF-induced cyclin D1 activity and by counteracting β-catenin, the downstream effector of Wnt signalling, which inhibits OPC differentiation (Chew et al., 2011). Several different receptor-ligand pairs that regulate OPC differentiation are induced or reduced by axonal electrical activity (see below), and electrical activity also results in the release of adenosine, which inhibits OPC proliferation and stimulates differentiation (Stevens et al., 2002).

*Inhibition of premature differentiation in OPCs* determines the developmental timing of myelination and possibly helps maintain adult OPCs in their non-myelinating state (Figure 5.14; Taveggia et al., 2010). Key negative regulators of oligodendrocyte differentiation include BMP, Wnt and Notch signalling. OPCs express high levels of ID2 and ID4, which are downstream effectors of BMP signalling and inhibit myelin gene expression, at least in part by heterodimerising Olig1/2 proteins (Kondo & Raff, 2000; Wang et al., 2001).

Canonical Wnt-β-catenin signalling inhibits OPC differentiation and myelination by suppressing Olig2 via a complex transcriptional and epigenetic modulation of gene expression (Fancy et al., 2009; Feigenson et al., 2009; Tawk et al., 2011; Ye et al., 2009). The endogenous source of Wnt is unknown, but by binding to its receptor frizzled it inhibits GSK-3β to enable translocation of β-catenin to the

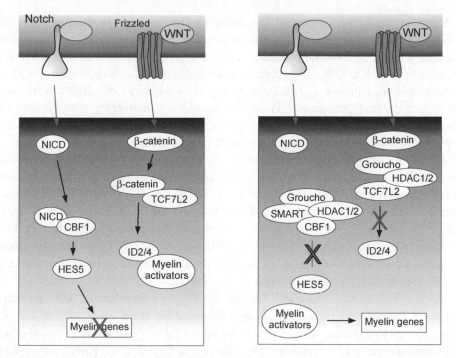

**Figure 5.14**   Interplay of extracellular signals and epigenetic factors in controlling oligodendrocyte differentiation.

A.  Negative regulators of oligodendrocyte differentiation such as Wnt, BMP or Notch signalling,
    acting through β-catenin, Smads or NICD induce the transcription of differentiation inhibitors
    such as ID2, ID4 and Hes1/5. ID2/4 sequestrate Olig1/2 away from myelin gene promoters,
    whereas Hes1/5 bind to regulatory elements of genes required for oligodendrocyte maturation.

B.  HDAC1/2, with co-repressors such as Groucho, compete with or displace Wnt, BMP and Notch
    signalling components to cause disinhibition, thereby activating the transcription of myelin
    genes.

Adapted from Yu *et al.*, 2010.

nucleus, where it forms a complex with the transcription factor TCF4 (T-cell
factor/lymphoid enhancing factor or TCF/LEF) to activate or repress target genes.
Inhibition of GSK-3β is sufficient to profoundly increase oligodendrocyte differentiation and myelination *in vivo* (Azim & Butt, 2011). The complex formation of
TCF4 with β-catenin is prevented by HDAC1/2, which thereby antagonise Wnt
signalling to stimulate oligodendrocyte differentiation (Ye *et al.*, 2009). The
developmental down-regulation of TCF4 (TCF7L2) prevents efficient Wnt signalling and allows myelin gene transcription (Rosenberg & Chan, 2009). OPC terminal
differentiation is also inhibited by activation of their Notch1 receptors by axonal
Jagged1 (Wang *et al.*, 1998), while interactions between OPC Notch/Deltex1 and
axonal F3/contactin promote differentiation (Hu *et al.*, 2003).

Selective inhibition of Notch1 signalling in OPCs using the Cre/loxP system established the widespread function for Notch1 in the correct spatial and temporal regulation of OL differentiation in the CNS (Genoud *et al.*, 2002). One of the genes induced by Notch in OPCs is the bHLH factor Hes5, which interacts with Sox10 to prevent it from stimulating myelin gene expression (Liu *et al.*, 2006). Sox5 and Sox6 also prevent premature OPC differentiation by interfering with binding of Sox10 to regulatory regions of myelin genes, as well as recruiting HDACs, which repress transcription of myelin genes (Stolt *et al.*, 2006).

*Promotion of OPC differentiation into oligodendrocytes* is stimulated by multiple extracellular and axon-derived factors. Among these are the transcription factors Nkx2.2 and Mash1, which combine with Sox10 and Olig proteins to initiate terminal differentiation and myelination (Qi *et al.*, 2001; Sugimori *et al.*, 2008). There are complex reciprocal interactions between these transcription factors. For example, Olig2 activates Sox10 directly (Kuspert *et al.*, 2011), and Sox10 alone is sufficient to induce oligodendrocyte differentiation, but Sox10 also modulates expression of Olig2 and Nkx2.2 (Liu *et al.*, 2007).

Histone modifications and miRNAs further regulate interactions between transcription factors and oligodendrocyte differentiation (Lau *et al.*, 2008; Liu & Casaccia, 2010). Histone acetylation is regulated by the balance between histone acetyltransferase (HATs) and histone deacetylases (HDACs). Knockout studies have confirmed that HDAC1 and HDAC2 are required for oligodendrocyte differentiation *in vivo*, by competing with β-catenin, which negatively regulates oligodendrocyte differentiation via the canonical Wnt pathway (Ye *et al.*, 2009).

Conditional ablation of the zinc finger protein YY1 has shown that it is essential for OPC differentiation by recruiting HDAC1 to repress transcriptional inhibitors of myelin gene expression TCF7L2 and ID4 (He *et al.*, 2007). In addition, YY1 has been reported to enhance transcription of PLP, possibly by direct action on the Plp1 gene (Berndt *et al.*, 2001). However, another study indicated that YY1 appears to function as a repressor of the Plp1 gene in immature oligodendrocytes (Zolova & Wight, 2011).

Similarly, processing of miRNAs depends on Dicer1, and conditional deletion of this enzyme in oligodendrocytes has provided proof that miRNAs are required for terminal oligodendrocyte differentiation and myelination, with key roles being indicated for miR-219 and miR-338 (Budde *et al.*, 2010; Dugas *et al.*, 2010; Zhao *et al.*, 2010). miR-219 and miR-338 are up-regulated during the transition from late OPC to pro-oligodendrocyte, and their targets include Sox6 and Hes5. This strongly suggests that miR-219 and miR-338 directly stimulate oligodendrocyte differentiation by promoting the degradation of transcripts for these myelination inhibitors (Liu and Casaccia, 2010).

*Terminal oligodendrocyte differentiation* is characterised by myelin gene expression and active myelination of axons. This is related to a progressive decrease of transcriptional inhibitors and up-regulation of myelin gene activators. The two-tier regulatory system, combining direct transcriptional activation of myelin genes with epigenetic repression of transcriptional inhibitors, provides a precise mechanism for genetic control of the myelination program (Li *et al.*, 2009).

Myelin gene regulatory factor (MRF) is a transcriptional regulator that is required for CNS myelination, and it appears in pro-oligodendrocytes shortly before the onset of myelination (Emery *et al.*, 2009). In the absence of MRF, there is no myelin gene expression, analogous to Krox20 in Schwann cells. MRF, Sox10 and Olig proteins cooperate to activate expression of myelin genes and maintain the myelination program. Olig1 knockout results in severe myelination defects, whereas oligodendrocyte specification is minimally affected, indicating that Olig1, unlike Olig 2, is more functional for terminal differentiation and myelination (Rowitch *et al.*, 2002).

The transit of oligodendrocytes from an active state of myelination into steady state myelin maintenance requires a further change in the gene regulatory network. The P2Y-like G protein-coupled receptor GPR17 is restricted to oligodendrocyte lineage cells during the peak in myelination, and it negatively regulates the transition between immature and myelinating oligodendrocytes (Chen *et al.*, 2009). Overexpression of GPR17 inhibits oligodendrocyte differentiation and maturation both *in vivo* and *in vitro*, while Gpr17 knockout mice show early onset of oligodendrocyte myelination. GPR17 functions at least in part to increase nuclear translocation of the potent oligodendrocyte differentiation inhibitors ID2/4 and oppose the action of Olig1. In mature oligodendrocytes, Olig1 is removed from the nucleus (Arnett *et al.*, 2004) and Nkx2.2 and Nkx6.2 become re-expressed (Cai *et al.*, 2010). The function of Nkx2.2 in mature oligodendrocytes is unclear, but Nkx6.2 is essential for the maintenance of axoglial interactions, and its genetic deletion results in myelin abnormalities and alteration of paranodal proteins (Southwood *et al.*, 2004).

## 5.4.5 Axoglial interactions regulating oligodendrocyte differentiation and myelination

The developmental onset of myelination involves a number of axoglial recognition and adhesion events that regulate the production of myelin-related gene products and radial axon growth (Figure 5.15). Myelination within units then occurs in a series of distinct axoglial interdependent phases (Butt & Berry, 2000):

1. Axonal contact and recognition by OPCs.

2. Induction phase, in which OPCs extend initiator processes along receptive axons to form short ensheathing segments, triggering the differentiation of OPCs into premyelinating oligodendrocytes and the initiation of axonal ion channel clustering.

3. Remodelling phase, in which non-myelinating processes within the unit are lost, and radial and longitudinal growth of myelinating processes forms incipient internodal segments, inducing axon radial growth and establishing nodes of Ranvier.

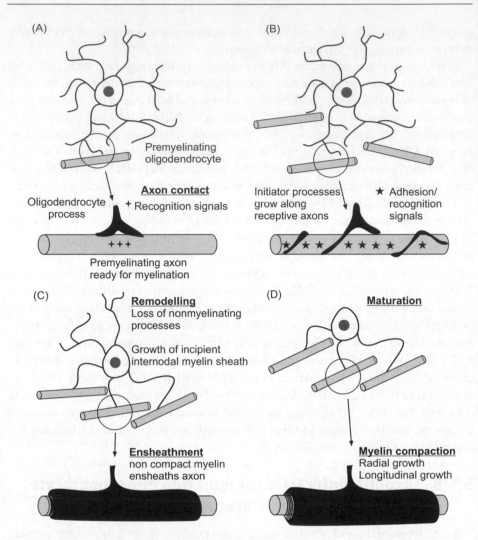

**Figure 5.15**  Axoglial interactions regulate myelination.

A number of axoglial recognition and adhesion events regulate the developmental onset of myelination. Laminin-integrin interactions can be considered an axonal signal that promotes oligodendrocyte differentiation upon axon contact, with a key role for Fyn activation. Differentiation and myelination are regulated by axonal signals, including down-regulation of axonal Jagged, an increase in electrical activity and receptor-ligand interactions between NRG1-ErbB2/3 and laminin-integrinβ1.

4. Maturation phase, in which axons and myelin sheaths within units undergo interdependent growth to establish adult dimensions of axon diameter, myelin sheath g-ratios and internodal lengths.

5. Late developing oligodendrocytes fill unmyelinated gaps along axons as part of normal growth into adulthood, as well as in response to remodelling and demyelination/remyelination.

The factors controlling the different stages are complex and largely unresolved, but axonal electrical activity provides an obvious potential signal by which oligodendrocytes recognise axons and myelination is regulated (Fields, 2008a).

A number of receptor-ligand pairs that are known to be important for oligoden-drocyte differentiation have been shown to be induced or reduced by axonal electrical activity, including neuregulin (NRG1)-ErbB2/3, NGF-TrkA, and Notch-Jagged or -F3/contactin interactions (see above). For example, NGF acting via TrkA receptors modulates the expression of Lingo1 (Lee *et al.*, 2007), which is expressed on axons and oligodendrocytes and is thought to exert an inhibitory effect on oligodendrocyte maturation and myelination via *cis* interactions with Nogo receptor 1 (NgR1) and p75$^{NTR}$ (Mi *et al.*, 2004). Axonal regulation of myelination will be discussed further below.

*Axon-oligodendrocyte recognition* is the first event between OPC processes and an axonal segment that is receptive for myelination (Piaton *et al.*, 2010). The axonal adhesion molecules L1 and NCAM are candidates for negative and positive recognition signals (Camara *et al.*, 2009). Disappearance of NCAM from the axonal surface is coincident with the onset of myelination, whereas L1 is expressed by premyelinated axons and is down-regulated during myelination. Suppression of NCAM stimulates myelination, whereas L1 has an inductive role for myelination. Thus, myelinating cells may distinguish axons that are, and are not, ready for myelination by their differential expression of NCAM and L1.

In addition, laminin expressed by the axon can be considered an axonal signal that promotes oligodendrocyte differentiation upon axon contact (Colognato *et al.*, 2002). Laminin2 (LN2)- α6β1 integrin signalling is a positive regulator of myelina-tion; the loss of LN2-integrin signalling leads to defective myelination and delay in myelination of small-diameter axons (Camara *et al.*, 2009; Chun *et al.*, 2003). N-cadherin may be important for the initial contact between myelinating oligoden-drocytes and axons, and process extension is regulated by neurofascin specifically expressed by oligodendrocytes at myelination onset (Collinson *et al.*, 1998). Interactions between axonal Caspr and oligodendroglial NF155 are also indicated in early myelination, with axonal Caspr distributing as a helical coil that winds around the axon to interact with NF155 on the overlying myelinating process (Pedraza *et al.*, 2009). Neurofascin is also a ligand for the axonal L1 CAM family, which are likely to play a later role in myelination.

*Myelin initiation* is stimulated following contact with axons. The growth factor NRG1, expressed on the surface of axons, is a major trigger for myelination, acting through oligodendroglial ErbB2 and ErbB3 receptors (Lemke, 2006). The switch of axonal NRG1 from a proliferation signal to a differentiation signal is related to axonal activity and depends on axonal laminin, which interacts with oligodendro-glial integrin β1 to mediate a switch from PI3K to MAPK signalling pathways (Lemke, 2006). Down-regulation of axonal Jagged is required for the onset of myelination, and interactions between axonal contactin and oligodendroglial Notch receptors play an instructive role by promoting OPC differentiation and up-regulation of myelin proteins. In addition, activation of Fyn when oligodendrocytes contact axonal laminins regulates integrin-driven myelin formation and reverses the capacity of NRG1 to inhibit OPC differentiation (Colognato *et al.*, 2002).

Laminins regulate myelination through interactions with both integrin receptors and dystroglycan receptors (Colognato *et al.*, 2007), to modulate Fyn regulatory molecules (Relucio *et al.*, 2009). The dystroglycan receptor for laminin also induces the pro-differentiation effects of IGF-1 (Galvin *et al.*, 2010). Fyn regulates process growth and oligodendrocyte morphology through the Rho-family GTPases RhoA, Cdc42 and Rac1 (Liang *et al.*, 2004), and by recruiting microtubules to stablise the cytoskelton (via its SH2 and SH3 protein binding domains and the microtubule associated protein Tau) (Klein *et al.*, 2002). Fyn also mediates Netrin1-dependent growth of oligodendrocyte processes and myelin-like membrane sheet formation; by forming a complex binding with the Dcc (Deleted in Colorectal Cancer) intracellular domain that includes FAK and N-WASP, resulting in the inhibition of RhoA and inducing process remodelling (Rajasekharan *et al.*, 2010). N-WASP regulates process extension, involving F-actin, WAVE1, contactin, Cdc42 and Rac proteins present at tips, cell body and processes (Bacon *et al.*, 2007). WAVE1 is essential for subsequent oligodendrocyte morphogenesis and myelination (Suetsugu & Takenawa, 2003). These essential steps in oligodendroglial maturation facilitate the detection of target axons, a key step towards myelination.

*Remodelling and maturation* from the premyelinating to mature myelinating oligodendrocyte involves the loss of non-myelinating processes and the radial and longitudinal growth of myelinating processes. Remodelling occurs in response to contact-mediated recognition signals derived from axons within the unit. This is followed by inter-dependent growth of the axon and the myelin sheath (Buckley *et al.*, 2010; Colello *et al.*, 1994), involving interactions between oligodendroglial ligands integrin α6β1 and/or dystroglycan, and their respective axonal receptors L1 and laminin-2 (Baron & Hoekstra, 2010; Camara *et al.*, 2009; Laursen *et al.*, 2009).

Myelin growth depends on laminin2-α6β1 integrin and neuregulin1-ErbB signalling (Chun *et al.*, 2003; Roy *et al.*, 2007). Axonal L1 binding to oligodendrocytes, and interactions between oligodendroglial integrin and axonal contactin, regulate myelin formation by controlling Fyn activity (Laursen *et al.*, 2009; White *et al.*, 2008). Neurones stimulate the transport of PLP to the plasma membrane (Trajkovic *et al.*, 2006), and axonal electrical activity stimulates localised synthesis of MBP through Fyn kinase-dependent signalling (Wake *et al.*, 2011). Neurones also regulate PLP trafficking in oligodendrocytes, whereby PLP is internalised and stored in late endosomes/lysosomes (LEs/Ls), and a cAMP-dependent neuronal signal triggers the transport of PLP from LEs/Ls to the plasma membrane (Trajkovic *et al.*, 2006). Likewise, myelin proteins are essential for axon radial growth. For example, when both OSP/claudin-11 and PLP genes are knocked out, mice exhibit markedly smaller axon diameters (Chow *et al.*, 2005).

In addition to controlling axon growth, oligodendrocytes are also essential for axon integrity (Edgar & Nave, 2009). Mice have been shown to develop widespread axon degeneration in the absence of PLP-DM20 (Griffiths *et al.*, 1998b) or CNP1 (Lappe-Siefke *et al.*, 2003), and mice deficient in both CNP and PLP display more severe axonal degeneration (Edgar *et al.*, 2009). A study in sulphatide-null mice indicated an interesting function for this myelin lipid, which played a limited role in myelin development, but was essential for myelin maintenance and axonal integrity in aged animals. In the absence of sulphatide, axons displayed degenerating myelin sheaths, deteriorating nodal/paranodal structure and decreased axonal calibre (Marcus *et al.*, 2006). Thus, the growth of the myelin sheath and axons and establishment of mature oligodendrocyte-axon units are interdependent.

## 5.4.6 Downstream signalling cascades that regulate oligodendrocyte differentiation and myelination

*Fyn kinase* and α6β1-integrin, as noted above, mediate many of the axoglial signals that control CNS myelination, including Dcc, Lingo-1 and F3/contactin (Kramer-Albers & White, 2011; Sperber *et al.*, 2001). It has been further proposed that axonal electrical activity and the release of glutamate stimulates Fyn (Wake *et al.*, 2011). Fyn acts through three major downstream signalling pathways to:

1.  regulate oligodendrocyte morphology through the Rho-family GTPases RhoA, Cdc42 and Rac1 (Liang *et al.*, 2004);

2.  interact with the microtubule associated protein Tau to recruit microtubules, which is essential for the transport of myelin-cargo to the axoglial contact site (Klein *et al.*, 2002); and

3.  activate MBP translation by stimulating the phosphorylation of hnRNPA2 (White *et al.*, 2008).

*PI3K-Akt signalling* is critical for CNS myelination and is activated through various receptors, including the receptor tyrosine kinases (RTKs), such as IGF-1 (Figure 5.16) (Flores *et al.*, 2008). PI3K (phosphatidylinositol 3-kinase) phosphorylates the membrane lipid PIP2 (phosphatidylinositol (4,5)-biphosphate), which produces the key second messenger PIP3 (phosphatidylinositol (3,4,5)-triphosphate), and PIP3 in turn activates Akt (Ser-473 phosphorylation). PIP2 is an essential determinant for stable membrane binding of MBP (Nawaz *et al.*, 2009).

The major Akt target regulating myelination is mTOR (mammalian target of rapamycin) and its downstream substrates p70S6 kinase and S6 ribosomal protein (Flores *et al.*, 2008; Narayanan *et al.*, 2009). mTOR is required for myelination, by forming complexes with mTORC1 and mTORC2, defined by the presence of the adaptor proteins raptor and rictor, respectively. mTORC2 regulates myelin gene expression at the mRNA level, whereas mTORC1 influences MBP by an alternative mechanism (Tyler *et al.*, 2009). The actions of PI3K are regulated by PTEN (phosphatase and tensin homolog), which dephosphorylates PIP3 back to PIP2.

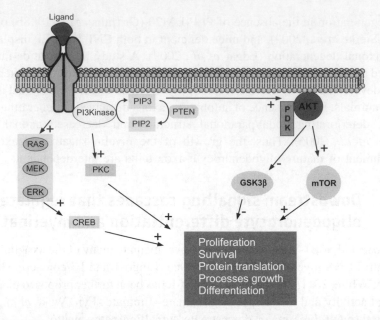

**Figure 5.16**  Intracellular signalling cascades regulating oligodendrocyte differentiation.
Many ligands, including growth factors and neurotransmitters, mediate their effects on oligodendrocytes by activation of PI3 kinase and/or the MAPK pathways. PI3K (phosphatidylinositol 3-kinase) phosphorylates the membrane lipid PIP2 (phosphatidylinositol (4,5)-biphosphate), which produces the key second messenger PIP3 (phosphatidylinositol (3,4,5)-triphosphate), and PIP3, in turn, activates Akt (Ser-473 phosphorylation). The major Akt target regulating myelination is mTOR (mammalian target of rapamycin). The actions of PI3K are regulated by PTEN (phosphatase and tensin homolog), which dephosphorylates PIP3 back to PIP2. The MAPK (mitogen-activated protein kinase) and CREB (cAMP response element binding protein) pathways mediate many of the effects of growth factors and neurotransmitters.

Targeted disruption of PTEN in oligodendrocytes results in increased PIP3 and mTOR and its downstream kinases, enhancing myelin gene expression and widespread hypermyelination (Goebbels *et al.*, 2010; Harrington *et al.*, 2010). Laminin 2 (LN-2) signals oligodendrocyte myelin formation through a PI3K-dependent mechanism and integrin-linked kinase.

*MAPK and CREB* pathways mediate the mitogenic effects of PDGF, FGF2 and NT3 in OPCs, and activation of protein kinase C (PKC) has been found to be necessary for their mitogenic activity, whereas cAMP-dependent kinase A (PKA) inhibits the mitogenic effects of FGF2 (Baron *et al.*, 2000; Kumar *et al.*, 1998; Pende *et al.*, 1997). Neurotransmitters activate the MAPK (mitogen-activated protein kinase) pathway in OPCs, which mediates CREB (cAMP response element binding protein) phosphorylation in response to $Ca^{2+}$ influx, PKC activation and growth factors (Pende *et al.*, 1997; Sato-Bigbee *et al.*, 1999). BDNF mediates its effects in oligodendrocytes via the MAPK pathway (Du *et al.*, 2006).

*JAK/STAT* pathways are active in OPC and play a role during injury and demyelination (Dell'Albani *et al.*, 1998). Cytokines and chemokines, including PDGF and CNTF, activate JAK1, JAK2, STAT1$\alpha$/$\beta$ and STAT3 in OPCs (see Figure 4.18).

## 5.5 Concluding remarks

Oligodendrocytes are defined by their myelinating function in the CNS. Myelination provides rapid nervous transmission and miniaturisation, without which the brain could not achieve its massive computing power. Oligodendrocytes and the axons they myelinate are completely interdependent functional units – neither element functions correctly without the other. Oligodendrocyte and/or myelin dysfunction results in axon degeneration and neuronal death, whereas oligodendrocytes are redundant without axons. This level of interdependence was present evolutionarily in the first vertebrates and independently in higher invertebrates, such as cephalopods. It requires a phenomenal degree of axoglial signalling and interactions, which we barely understand.

A great deal of oligodendroglial research is driven by the search for an understanding of the demyelinating disease multiple sclerosis. Compared to astrocytes, for example, we know a great deal about the factors regulating oligodendrocyte generation from their progenitors in the developing CNS and the adult. In contrast, while physiological functions of astrocytes are an area of intense research, we know little about the physiological attributes of oligodendrocytes, with regards to their complement of ion channels and neurotransmitter receptors.

There is evidence of pathological roles for neurotransmitter receptors in oligodendrocyte cell death and demyelination, but fundamental questions remain about their physiological roles. Moreover, it is clear that myelin disruption occurs in the normal ageing brain and in dementias, as well as in neuropsychological diseases, such as bipolar disorder and schizophrenia. The underlying causes of oligodendrocyte dysfunction are unknown, but it is becoming evident that they are an important element of cognitive decline in these conditions. To answer these questions, in the future we will need to move from current studies on cultures of embryonic cells and brain slices from postnatal rodents, and focus our attention to the normal physiological functions of oligodendrocytes and their interactions with neurones in the ageing brain.

## References

Agresti C, D'Urso D, Levi G. (1996). Reversible inhibitory effects of interferon-gamma and tumour necrosis factor-alpha on oligodendroglial lineage cell proliferation and differentiation *in vitro*. *European Journal of Neuroscience* **8**(6), 1106–16.

Agresti C, Meomartini ME, Amadio S, Ambrosini E, Serafini B, Franchini L, Volonte C, Aloisi F, Visentin S. (2005a). Metabotropic P2 receptor activation regulates oligodendrocyte progenitor migration and development. *Glia* **50**(2), 132–44.

Agresti C, Meomartini ME, Amadio S, Ambrosini E, Volonte C, Aloisi F, Visentin S. (2005b). ATP regulates oligodendrocyte progenitor migration, proliferation, and differentiation: involvement of metabotropic P2 receptors. *Brain Research Brain Research Reviews* **48**(2), 157–65.

Alberdi E, Sanchez-Gomez MV, Matute C. (2005). Calcium and glial cell death. *Cell Calcium* **38**(3–4), 417–25.

Almeida RG, Czopka T, Ffrench-Constant C, Lyons DA. (2011). Individual axons regulate the myelinating potential of single oligodendrocytes *in vivo*. *Development* **138**(20), 4443–50.

Altevogt BM, Kleopa KA, Postma FR, Scherer SS, Paul DL. (2002). Connexin29 is uniquely distributed within myelinating glial cells of the central and peripheral nervous systems. *Journal of Neuroscience* **22**(15), 6458–70.

Amadio S, Montilli C, Magliozzi R, Bernardi G, Reynolds R, Volonte C. (2010). P2Y12 receptor protein in cortical gray matter lesions in multiple sclerosis. *Cerebral Cortex* **20**(6), 1263–73.

Arnett HA, Fancy SP, Alberta JA, Zhao C, Plant SR, Kaing S, Raine CS, Rowitch DH, Franklin RJ, Stiles CD. (2004). bHLH transcription factor Olig1 is required to repair demyelinated lesions in the CNS. *Science* **306**(5704), 2111–5.

Azim K, Butt AM. (2011). GSK3beta negatively regulates oligodendrocyte differentiation and myelination *in vivo*. *Glia* **59**(4), 540–53.

Bacon C, Lakics V, Machesky L, Rumsby M. (2007). N-WASP regulates extension of filopodia and processes by oligodendrocyte progenitors, oligodendrocytes, and Schwann cells-implications for axon ensheathment at myelination. *Glia* **55**(8), 844–58.

Bagayogo IP, Dreyfus CF. (2009). Regulated release of BDNF by cortical oligodendrocytes is mediated through metabotropic glutamate receptors and the PLC pathway. *ASN Neuro* **1**(1).

Bansal R. (2002). Fibroblast growth factors and their receptors in oligodendrocyte development: implications for demyelination and remyelination. *Developmental Neuroscience* **24**(1), 35–46.

Bansal R, Stefansson K, Pfeiffer SE. (1992). Proligodendroblast antigen (POA), a developmental antigen expressed by A007/O4-positive oligodendrocyte progenitors prior to the appearance of sulfatide and galactocerebroside. *Journal of Neurochemistry* **58**(6), 2221–9.

Baron W, Hoekstra D. (2010). On the biogenesis of myelin membranes: Sorting, trafficking and cell polarity. *FEBS Letters* **584**(9), 1760–1770.

Baron W, Metz B, Bansal R, Hoekstra D, de Vries H. (2000). PDGF and FGF-2 signaling in oligodendrocyte progenitor cells: regulation of proliferation and differentiation by multiple intracellular signaling pathways. *Molecular and Cellular Neurosciences* **15**(3), 314–29.

Barres BA, Raff MC. (1993). Proliferation of oligodendrocyte precursor cells depends on electrical activity in axons. *Nature* **361**(6409), 258–60.

Barres BA, Schmid R, Sendnter M, Raff MC. (1993). Multiple extracellular signals are required for long-term oligodendrocyte survival. *Development* **118**(1), 283–95.

Baumann N, Pham-Dinh D. (2001). Biology of oligodendrocyte and myelin in the mammalian central nervous system. *Physiological Reviews* **81**(2), 871–927.

Belachew S, Malgrange B, Rigo JM, Rogister B, Coucke P, Mazy-Servais C, Moonen G. (1998a). Developmental regulation of neuroligand-induced responses in cultured oligodendroglia. *Neuroreport* **9**(6), 973–80.

Belachew S, Rogister B, Rigo JM, Malgrange B, Mazy-Servais C, Xhauflaire G, Coucke P, Moonen G. (1998b). Cultured oligodendrocyte progenitors derived from cerebral cortex express a glycine receptor which is pharmacologically distinct from the neuronal isoform. *European Journal of Neuroscience* **10**(11), 3556–64.

Berger T, Schnitzer J, Kettenmann H. (1991). Developmental changes in the membrane current pattern, K+ buffer capacity, and morphology of glial cells in the corpus callosum slice. *Journal of Neuroscience* **11**(10), 3008–24.

Berger T, Schnitzer J, Orkand PM, Kettenmann H. (1992a). Sodium and calcium currents in glial cells of the mouse corpus callosum Slice. *European Journal of Neuroscience* **4**(12), 1271–1284.

Berger T, Walz W, Schnitzer J, Kettenmann H. (1992b). GABA- and glutamate-activated currents in glial cells of the mouse corpus callosum slice. *Journal of Neuroscience Research* **31**(1), 21–7.

Bergles DE, Roberts JD, Somogyi P, Jahr CE. (2000). Glutamatergic synapses on oligodendrocyte precursor cells in the hippocampus. *Nature* **405**(6783), 187–91.

Berndt JA, Kim JG, Tosic M, Kim C, Hudson LD. (2001). The transcriptional regulator Yin Yang 1 activates the myelin PLP gene. *Journal of Neurochemistry* **77**(3), 935–42.

Berry M, Ibrahim M, Carlile J, Ruge F, Duncan A, Butt AM. (1995). Axon-glial relationships in the anterior medullary velum of the adult rat. *Journal of Neurocytology* **24**(12), 965–83.

Bjartmar C, Hildebrand C, Loinder K. (1994). Morphological heterogeneity of rat oligodendrocytes: electron microscopic studies on serial sections. *Glia* **11**(3), 235–44.

Boda E, Vigano F, Rosa P, Fumagalli M, Labat-Gest V, Tempia F, Abbracchio MP, Dimou L, Buffo A. (2011). The GPR17 receptor in NG2 expressing cells: Focus on *in vivo* cell maturation and participation in acute trauma and chronic damage. *Glia* **59**(12), 1958–73.

Boggs JM, Wang H. (2004). Co-clustering of galactosylceramide and membrane proteins in oligodendrocyte membranes on interaction with polyvalent carbohydrate and prevention by an intact cytoskeleton. *Journal of Neuroscience Research* **76**(3), 342–55.

Boiko T, Rasband MN, Levinson SR, Caldwell JH, Mandel G, Trimmer JS, Matthews G. (2001). Compact myelin dictates the differential targeting of two sodium channel isoforms in the same axon. *Neuron* **30**(1), 91–104.

Bolton S, Butt AM. (2006). Cyclic AMP-mediated regulation of the resting membrane potential in myelin-forming oligodendrocytes in the isolated intact rat optic nerve. *Experimental Neurology* **202**(1), 36–43.

Bongarzone ER, Howard SG, Schonmann V, Campagnoni AT. (1998). Identification of the dopamine D3 receptor in oligodendrocyte precursors: potential role in regulating differentiation and myelin formation. *Journal of Neuroscience* **18**(14), 5344–53.

Bongarzone ER, Campagnoni CW, Kampf K, Jacobs EC, Handley VW, Schonmann V, Campagnoni AT. (1999). Identification of a new exon in the myelin proteolipid protein gene encoding novel protein isoforms that are restricted to the somata of oligodendrocytes and neurons. *Journal of Neuroscience* **19**(19), 8349–57.

Borges K, Ohlemeyer C, Trotter J, Kettenmann H. (1994). AMPA/kainate receptor activation in murine oligodendrocyte precursor cells leads to activation of a cation conductance, calcium influx and blockade of delayed rectifying $K^+$ channels. *Neuroscience* **63**(1), 135–49.

Boscia F, D'Avanzo C, Pannaccione A, Secondo A, Casamassa A, Formisano L, Guida N, Annunziato L. (2012). Silencing or knocking out the $Na^+/Ca^{2+}$ exchanger-3 (NCX3) impairs oligodendrocyte differentiation. *Cell Death & Differentiation* **19**(4), 562–72.

Boussouf A, Gaillard S. (2000). Intracellular pH changes during oligodendrocyte differentiation in primary culture. *Journal of Neuroscience Research* **59**(6), 731–9.

Bribian A, Barallobre MJ, Soussi-Yanicostas N, de Castro F. (2006). Anosmin-1 modulates the FGF-2-dependent migration of oligodendrocyte precursors in the developing optic nerve. *Molecular and Cellular Neurosciences* **33**(1), 2–14.

Bronstein JM, Tiwari-Woodruff S, Buznikov AG, Stevens DB. (2000). Involvement of OSP/-claudin-11 in oligodendrocyte membrane interactions: role in biology and disease. *Journal of Neuroscience Research* **59**(6), 706–11.

Brunner C, Lassmann H, Waehneldt TV, Matthieu JM, Linington C. (1989). Differential ultrastructural localization of myelin basic protein, myelin/oligodendroglial glycoprotein, and 2′,3′-

cyclic nucleotide 3′-phosphodiesterase in the CNS of adult rats. *Journal of Neurochemistry* **52**(1), 296–304.

Buckley CE, Marguerie A, Alderton WK, Franklin RJ. (2010). Temporal dynamics of myelination in the zebrafish spinal cord. *Glia* **58**(7), 802–12.

Budde H, Schmitt S, Fitzner D, Opitz L, Salinas-Riester G, Simons M. (2010). Control of oligodendroglial cell number by the miR-17-92 cluster. *Development* **137**(13), 2127–32.

Bunge RP. (1968). Glial cells and the central myelin sheath. *Physiological Reviews* **48**(1), 197–251.

Burzomato V, Frugier G, Perez-Otano I, Kittler JT, Attwell D. (2011). The receptor subunits generating NMDA receptor mediated currents in oligodendrocytes. *Journal of Physiology* **588**(Pt 18), 3403–14.

Butt AM. (2006). Neurotransmitter-mediated calcium signalling in oligodendrocyte physiology and pathology. *Glia* **54**(7), 666–75.

Butt AM. (2011). ATP: a ubiquitous gliotransmitter integrating neuron-glial networks. *Seminars in Cell and Developmental Biology* **22**(2), 205–13.

Butt AM, Ransom BR. (1989). Visualization of oligodendrocytes and astrocytes in the intact rat optic nerve by intracellular injection of lucifer yellow and horseradish peroxidase. *Glia* **2**(6), 470–5.

Butt AM, Berry M. (2000). Oligodendrocytes and the control of myelination *in vivo*: new insights from the rat anterior medullary velum. *Journal of Neuroscience Research* **59**(4), 477–88.

Butt AM, Kalsi A. (2006). Inwardly rectifying potassium channels (Kir) in central nervous system glia: a special role for Kir4.1 in glial functions. *Journal of Cellular and Molecular Medicine* **10**(1), 33–44.

Butt AM, Colquhoun K, Tutton M, Berry M. (1994). Three-dimensional morphology of astrocytes and oligodendrocytes in the intact mouse optic nerve. *Journal of Neurocytology* **23**(8), 469–85.

Butt AM, Ibrahim M, Berry M. (1997). The relationship between developing oligodendrocyte units and maturing axons during myelinogenesis in the anterior medullary velum of neonatal rats. *Journal of Neurocytology* **26**(5), 327–38.

Butt AM, Ibrahim M, Berry M. (1998). Axon-myelin sheath relations of oligodendrocyte unit phenotypes in the adult rat anterior medullary velum. *Journal of Neurocytology* **27**(4), 259–69.

Butt AM, Duncan A, Hornby MF, Kirvell SL, Hunter A, Levine JM, Berry M. (1999). Cells expressing the NG2 antigen contact nodes of Ranvier in adult CNS white matter. *Glia* **26**(1), 84–91.

Butt AM, Hamilton N, Hubbard P, Pugh M, Ibrahim M. (2005). Synantocytes: the fifth element. *Journal of Anatomy* **207**(6), 695–706.

Butzkueven H, Emery B, Cipriani T, Marriott MP, Kilpatrick TJ. (2006). Endogenous leukemia inhibitory factor production limits autoimmune demyelination and oligodendrocyte loss. *Glia* **53**(7), 696–703.

Cai J, Zhu Q, Zheng K, Li H, Qi Y, Cao Q, Qiu M. (2010). Co-localization of Nkx6.2 and Nkx2.2 homeodomain proteins in differentiated myelinating oligodendrocytes. *Glia* **58**(4), 458–68.

Calver AR, Hall AC, Yu WP, Walsh FS, Heath JK, Betsholtz C, Richardson WD. (1998). Oligodendrocyte population dynamics and the role of PDGF *in vivo*. *Neuron* **20**(5), 869–82.

Calza L, Fernandez M, Giardino L. (2010). Cellular approaches to central nervous system remyelination stimulation: thyroid hormone to promote myelin repair via endogenous stem and precursor cells. *Journal of Molecular Endocrinology* **44**(1), 13–23.

Camara J, Wang Z, Nunes-Fonseca C, Friedman HC, Grove M, Sherman DL, Komiyama NH, Grant SG, Brophy PJ, Peterson A *et al.* (2009). Integrin-mediated axoglial interactions initiate myelination in the central nervous system. *Journal of Cell Biology* **185**(4), 699–712.

Campagnoni AT, Skoff RP. (2001). The pathobiology of myelin mutants reveal novel biological functions of the MBP and PLP genes. *Brain Pathology* **11**(1), 74–91.

Carson JH, Barbarese E. (2005). Systems analysis of RNA trafficking in neural cells. *Biology of The Cell* **97**(1), 51–62.

Carson MJ, Behringer RR, Brinster RL, McMorris FA. (1993). Insulin-like growth factor I increases brain growth and central nervous system myelination in transgenic mice. *Neuron* **10**(4), 729–40.

Cavara NA, Hollmann M. (2008). Shuffling the deck anew: how NR3 tweaks NMDA receptor function. *Molecular Neurobiology* **38**(1), 16–26.

Ceruti S, Villa G, Genovese T, Mazzon E, Longhi R, Rosa P, Bramanti P, Cuzzocrea S, Abbracchio MP. (2009). The P2Y-like receptor GPR17 as a sensor of damage and a new potential target in spinal cord injury. *Brain* **132**(Pt 8), 2206–18.

Ceruti S, Vigano F, Boda E, Ferrario S, Magni G, Boccazzi M, Rosa P, Buffo A, Abbracchio MP. (2011). Expression of the new P2Y-like receptor GPR17 during oligodendrocyte precursor cell maturation regulates sensitivity to ATP-induced death. *Glia* **59**(3), 363–78.

Charles KJ, Deuchars J, Davies CH, Pangalos MN. (2003). GABA B receptor subunit expression in glia. *Molecular and Cellular Neurosciences* **24**(1), 214–23.

Chen H, Kintner DB, Jones M, Matsuda T, Baba A, Kiedrowski L, Sun D. (2007). AMPA-mediated excitotoxicity in oligodendrocytes: role for Na(+)-K(+)-Cl(−) co-transport and reversal of Na(+)/Ca$^{2+}$ exchanger. *Journal of Neurochemistry* **102**(6), 1783–95.

Chen H, Sun D. (2005). The role of Na-K-Cl co-transporter in cerebral ischemia. *Neurological Research* **27**(3), 280–6.

Chen Y, Wu H, Wang S, Koito H, Li J, Ye F, Hoang J, Escobar SS, Gow A, Arnett HA *et al.* (2009). The oligodendrocyte-specific G protein-coupled receptor GPR17 is a cell-intrinsic timer of myelination. *Nature Neuroscience* **12**(11), 1398–406.

Cheng CM, Joncas G, Reinhardt RR, Farrer R, Quarles R, Janssen J, McDonald MP, Crawley JN, Powell-Braxton L, Bondy CA. (1998). Biochemical and morphometric analyses show that myelination in the insulin-like growth factor 1 null brain is proportionate to its neuronal composition. *Journal of Neuroscience* **18**(15), 5673–81.

Chew LJ, King WC, Kennedy A, Gallo V. (2005). Interferon-gamma inhibits cell cycle exit in differentiating oligodendrocyte progenitor cells. *Glia* **52**(2), 127–43.

Chew LJ, Shen W, Ming X, Senatorov VV, Jr., Chen HL, Cheng Y, Hong E, Knoblach S, Gallo V. (2011). SRY-box containing gene 17 regulates the Wnt/beta-catenin signaling pathway in oligodendrocyte progenitor cells. *Journal of Neuroscience* **31**(39), 13921–35.

Chittajallu R, Chen Y, Wang H, Yuan X, Ghiani CA, Heckman T, McBain CJ, Gallo V. (2002). Regulation of Kv1 subunit expression in oligodendrocyte progenitor cells and their role in G1/S phase progression of the cell cycle. *Proceedings of The National Academy Of Sciences Of The United States Of America* **99**(4), 2350–5.

Chittajallu R, Aguirre A, Gallo V. (2004). NG2-positive cells in the mouse white and grey matter display distinct physiological properties. *Journal of Physiology* **561**(Pt 1), 109–22.

Chow E, Mottahedeh J, Prins M, Ridder W, Nusinowitz S, Bronstein JM. (2005). Disrupted compaction of CNS myelin in an OSP/Claudin-11 and PLP/DM20 double knockout mouse. *Molecular and Cellular Neurosciences* **29**(3), 405–13.

Chun SJ, Rasband MN, Sidman RL, Habib AA, Vartanian T. (2003). Integrin-linked kinase is required for laminin-2-induced oligodendrocyte cell spreading and CNS myelination. *Journal of Cell Biology* **163**(2), 397–408.

Clements CS, Reid HH, Beddoe T, Tynan FE, Perugini MA, Johns TG, Bernard CC, Rossjohn J. (2003). The crystal structure of myelin oligodendrocyte glycoprotein, a key autoantigen in multiple sclerosis. *Proceedings of The National Academy Of Sciences Of The United States Of America* **100**(19), 11059–64.

Cohen RI, Almazan G. (1993). Norepinephrine-stimulated PI hydrolysis in oligodendrocytes is mediated by alpha 1A-adrenoceptors. *Neuroreport* **4**(9), 1115–8.

Cohen RI, Molina-Holgado E, Almazan G. (1996). Carbachol stimulates c-fos expression and proliferation in oligodendrocyte progenitors. *Brain Research. Molecular Brain Research* **43**(1–2), 193–201.

Colello RJ, Pott U, Schwab ME. (1994). The role of oligodendrocytes and myelin on axon maturation in the developing rat retinofugal pathway. *Journal of Neuroscience* **14**(5 Pt 1), 2594–605.

Collingridge GL, Olsen RW, Peters J, Spedding M. (2009). A nomenclature for ligand-gated ion channels. *Neuropharmacology* **56**(1), 2–5.

Collinson JM, Marshall D, Gillespie CS, Brophy PJ. (1998). Transient expression of neurofascin by oligodendrocytes at the onset of myelinogenesis: implications for mechanisms of axon-glial interaction. *Glia* **23**(1), 11–23.

Colman DR, Kreibich G, Frey AB, Sabatini DD. (1982). Synthesis and incorporation of myelin polypeptides into CNS myelin. *Journal of Cell Biology* **95**(2 Pt 1), 598–608.

Colognato H, Baron W, Avellana-Adalid V, Relvas JB, Baron-Van Evercooren A, Georges-Labouesse E, ffrench-Constant C. (2002). CNS integrins switch growth factor signalling to promote target-dependent survival. *Nature Cell Biology* **4**(11), 833–41.

Colognato H, Galvin J, Wang Z, Relucio J, Nguyen T, Harrison D, Yurchenco PD, Ffrench-Constant C. (2007). Identification of dystroglycan as a second laminin receptor in oligodendrocytes, with a role in myelination. *Development* **134**(9), 1723–36.

Connor JR, Menzies SL. (1996). Relationship of iron to oligodendrocytes and myelination. *Glia* **17**(2), 83–93.

Cui QL, Almazan G. (2007). IGF-I-induced oligodendrocyte progenitor proliferation requires PI3K/Akt, MEK/ERK, and Src-like tyrosine kinases. *Journal of Neurochemistry* **100**(6), 1480–93.

Cui QL, Fogle E, Almazan G. (2006). Muscarinic acetylcholine receptors mediate oligodendrocyte progenitor survival through Src-like tyrosine kinases and PI3K/Akt pathways. *Neurochemistry International* **48**(5), 383–93.

De Angelis F, Bernardo A, Magnaghi V, Minghetti L, Tata AM. (2011). Muscarinic receptor subtypes as potential targets to modulate oligodendrocyte progenitor survival, proliferation and differentiation. *Developmental Neurobiology*.

De Biase LM, Nishiyama A, Bergles DE. (2010). Excitability and synaptic communication within the oligodendrocyte lineage. *Journal of Neuroscience* **30**(10), 3600–11.

De Biase LM, Kang SH, Baxi EG, Fukaya M, Pucak ML, Mishina M, Calabresi PA, Bergles DE. (2011). NMDA receptor signaling in oligodendrocyte progenitors is not required for oligodendrogenesis and myelination. *Journal of Neuroscience* **31**(35), 12650–62.

de Castro F, Bribian A. (2005). The molecular orchestra of the migration of oligodendrocyte precursors during development. *Brain Research Brain Research Reviews* **49**(2), 227–41.

Delaunay D, Heydon K, Cumano A, Schwab MH, Thomas JL, Suter U, Nave KA, Zalc B, Spassky N. (2008). Early neuronal and glial fate restriction of embryonic neural stem cells. *Journal of Neuroscience* **28**(10), 2551–62.

Dell'Albani P, Kahn MA, Cole R, Condorelli DF, Giuffrida-Stella AM, de Vellis J. (1998). Oligodendroglial survival factors, PDGF-AA and CNTF, activate similar JAK/STAT signaling pathways. *Journal of Neuroscience Research* **54**(2), 191–205.

Deng W, Wang H, Rosenberg PA, Volpe JJ, Jensen FE. (2004). Role of metabotropic glutamate receptors in oligodendrocyte excitotoxicity and oxidative stress. *Proceedings of The National Academy Of Sciences Of The United States Of America* **101**(20), 7751–6.

Dietschy JM, Turley SD. (2004). Thematic review series: brain Lipids. Cholesterol metabolism in the central nervous system during early development and in the mature animal. *Journal of Lipid Research* **45**(8), 1375–97.

Domercq M, Sanchez-Gomez MV, Areso P, Matute C. (1999). Expression of glutamate transporters in rat optic nerve oligodendrocytes. *European Journal of Neuroscience* **11**(7), 2226–36.

Domercq M, Perez-Samartin A, Aparicio D, Alberdi E, Pampliega O, Matute C. (2010). P2X7 receptors mediate ischemic damage to oligodendrocytes. *Glia* **58**(6), 730–40.

Domingues AM, Neugebauer KM, Fern R. (2011). Identification of four functional NR3B isoforms in developing white matter reveals unexpected diversity among glutamate receptors. *Journal of Neurochemistry* **117**(3), 449–60.

Du Y, Lercher LD, Zhou R, Dreyfus CF. (2006). Mitogen-activated protein kinase pathway mediates effects of brain-derived neurotrophic factor on differentiation of basal forebrain oligodendrocytes. *Journal of Neuroscience Research* **84**(8), 1692–702.

Dugas JC, Cuellar TL, Scholze A, Ason B, Ibrahim A, Emery B, Zamanian JL, Foo LC, McManus MT, Barres BA. (2010). Dicer1 and miR-219 Are required for normal oligodendrocyte differentiation and myelination. *Neuron* **65**(5), 597–611.

Dziembowska M, Tham TN, Lau P, Vitry S, Lazarini F, Dubois-Dalcq M. (2005). A role for CXCR4 signaling in survival and migration of neural and oligodendrocyte precursors. *Glia* **50**(3), 258–69.

Edgar JM, Nave KA. (2009). The role of CNS glia in preserving axon function. *Current Opinion In Neurobiology* **19**(5), 498–504.

Edgar JM, McLaughlin M, Barrie JA, McCulloch MC, Garbern J, Griffiths IR. (2004). Age-related axonal and myelin changes in the rumpshaker mutation of the Plp gene. *Acta Neuropathologica* **107**(4), 331–5.

Edgar JM, McLaughlin M, Werner HB, McCulloch MC, Barrie JA, Brown A, Faichney AB, Snaidero N, Nave KA, Griffiths IR. (2009). Early ultrastructural defects of axons and axon-glia junctions in mice lacking expression of Cnp1. *Glia* **57**(16), 1815–24.

Emery B, Agalliu D, Cahoy JD, Watkins TA, Dugas JC, Mulinyawe SB, Ibrahim A, Ligon KL, Rowitch DH, Barres BA. (2009). Myelin gene regulatory factor is a critical transcriptional regulator required for CNS myelination. *Cell* **138**(1), 172–85.

Fanarraga ML, Griffiths IR, Zhao M, Duncan ID. (1998). Oligodendrocytes are not inherently programmed to myelinate a specific size of axon. *Journal of Comparative Neurology* **399**(1), 94–100.

Fancy SP, Baranzini SE, Zhao C, Yuk DI, Irvine KA, Kaing S, Sanai N, Franklin RJ, Rowitch DH. (2009). Dysregulation of the Wnt pathway inhibits timely myelination and remyelination in the mammalian CNS. *Genes and Development* **23**(13), 1571–85.

Feigenson K, Reid M, See J, Crenshaw EB, 3rd, Grinspan JB. (2009). Wnt signaling is sufficient to perturb oligodendrocyte maturation. *Molecular and Cellular Neurosciences* **42**(3), 255–65.

Feldman DH, Horiuchi M, Keachie K, McCauley E, Bannerman P, Itoh A, Itoh T, Pleasure D. (2008). Characterization of acid-sensing ion channel expression in oligodendrocyte-lineage cells. *Glia* **56**(11), 1238–49.

Fields RD. (2008a). Oligodendrocytes changing the rules: action potentials in glia and oligodendrocytes controlling action potentials. *Neuroscientist* **14**(6), 540–3.

Fields RD. (2008b). White matter in learning, cognition and psychiatric disorders. *Trends In Neurosciences* **31**(7), 361–70.

Finzsch M, Stolt CC, Lommes P, Wegner M. (2008). Sox9 and Sox10 influence survival and migration of oligodendrocyte precursors in the spinal cord by regulating PDGF receptor alpha expression. *Development* **135**(4), 637–46.

Flores AI, Narayanan SP, Morse EN, Shick HE, Yin X, Kidd G, Avila RL, Kirschner DA, Macklin WB. (2008). Constitutively active Akt induces enhanced myelination in the CNS. *Journal of Neuroscience* **28**(28), 7174–83.

Fogal B, McClaskey C, Yan S, Yan H, Rivkees SA. (2011). Diazoxide promotes oligodendrocyte precursor cell proliferation and myelination. *PLoS One* **5**(5), e10906.

Fogarty M, Richardson WD, Kessaris N. (2005). A subset of oligodendrocytes generated from radial glia in the dorsal spinal cord. *Development* **132**(8), 1951–9.

Fortin D, Rom E, Sun H, Yayon A, Bansal R. (2005). Distinct fibroblast growth factor (FGF)/FGF receptor signaling pairs initiate diverse cellular responses in the oligodendrocyte lineage. *Journal of Neuroscience* **25**(32), 7470–9.

Frederick TJ, Wood TL. (2004). IGF-I and FGF-2 coordinately enhance cyclin D1 and cyclin E-cdk2 association and activity to promote G1 progression in oligodendrocyte progenitor cells. *Molecular and Cellular Neurosciences* **25**(3), 480–92.

Frohlich N, Nagy B, Hovhannisyan A, Kukley M. (2011). Fate of neuron-glia synapses during proliferation and differentiation of NG2 cells. *Journal of Anatomy* **219**(1), 18–32.

Fruttiger M, Karlsson L, Hall AC, Abramsson A, Calver AR, Bostrom H, Willetts K, Bertold CH, Heath JK, Betsholtz C *et al.* (1999). Defective oligodendrocyte development and severe hypomyelination in PDGF-A knockout mice. *Development* **126**(3), 457–67.

Fu H, Qi Y, Tan M, Cai J, Takebayashi H, Nakafuku M, Richardson W, Qiu M. (2002). Dual origin of spinal oligodendrocyte progenitors and evidence for the cooperative role of Olig2 and Nkx2.2 in the control of oligodendrocyte differentiation. *Development* **129**(3), 681–93.

Fulton D, Paez PM, Campagnoni AT. (2010). The multiple roles of myelin protein genes during the development of the oligodendrocyte. *ASN Neuro* **2**(1), e00027.

Fumagalli M, Daniele S, Lecca D, Lee PR, Parravicini C, Fields RD, Rosa P, Antonucci F, Verderio C, Trincavelli ML *et al.* (2011). Phenotypic changes, signaling pathway, and functional correlates of GPR17-expressing neural precursor cells during oligodendrocyte differentiation. *Journal of Biological Chemistry* **286**(12), 10593–604.

Furusho M, Dupree JL, Nave KA, Bansal R. (2012). Fibroblast growth factor receptor signaling in oligodendrocytes regulates myelin sheath thickness. *Journal of Neuroscience* **32**(19), 6631–41.

Gadea A, Aguirre A, Haydar TF, Gallo V. (2009). Endothelin-1 regulates oligodendrocyte development. *Journal of Neuroscience* **29**(32), 10047–62.

Gallo V, Ghiani CA. (2000). Glutamate receptors in glia: new cells, new inputs and new functions. *Trends In Pharmacological Sciences* **21**(7), 252–8.

Gallo V, Zhou JM, McBain CJ, Wright P, Knutson PL, Armstrong RC. (1996). Oligodendrocyte progenitor cell proliferation and lineage progression are regulated by glutamate receptor-mediated K+ channel block. *Journal of Neuroscience* **16**(8), 2659–70.

Galvin J, Eyermann C, Colognato H. (2010). Dystroglycan modulates the ability of insulin-like growth factor-1 to promote oligodendrocyte differentiation. *Journal of Neuroscience Research* **88**(15), 3295–307.

Garcia-Gonzalez D, Clemente D, Coelho M, Esteban PF, Soussi-Yanicostas N, de Castro F. (2011). Dynamic roles of FGF-2 and Anosmin-1 in the migration of neuronal precursors from the subventricular zone during pre- and postnatal development. *Experimental Neurology* **222**(2), 285–95.

Garwood J, Garcion E, Dobbertin A, Heck N, Calco V, ffrench-Constant C, Faissner A. (2004). The extracellular matrix glycoprotein Tenascin-C is expressed by oligodendrocyte precursor cells and required for the regulation of maturation rate, survival and responsiveness to platelet-derived growth factor. *European Journal of Neuroscience* **20**(10), 2524–40.

Genoud S, Lappe-Siefke C, Goebbels S, Radtke F, Aguet M, Scherer SS, Suter U, Nave KA, Mantei N. (2002). Notch1 control of oligodendrocyte differentiation in the spinal cord. *Journal of Cell Biology* **158**(4), 709–18.

Ghandour MS, Skoff RP, Venta PJ, Tashian RE. (1989). Oligodendrocytes express a normal phenotype in carbonic anhydrase II-deficient mice. *Journal of Neuroscience Research* **23**(2), 180–90.

Ghiani C, Gallo V. (2001). Inhibition of cyclin E-cyclin-dependent kinase 2 complex formation and activity is associated with cell cycle arrest and withdrawal in oligodendrocyte progenitor cells. *Journal of Neuroscience* **21**(4), 1274–82.

Gipson K, Bordey A. (2002). Analysis of the K+ current profile of mature rat oligodendrocytes *in situ*. *Journal of Membrane Biology* **189**(3), 201–12.

Goebbels S, Oltrogge JH, Kemper R, Heilmann I, Bormuth I, Wolfer S, Wichert SP, Mobius W, Liu X, Lappe-Siefke C *et al.* (2010). Elevated phosphatidylinositol 3,4,5-trisphosphate in glia triggers cell-autonomous membrane wrapping and myelination. *Journal of Neuroscience* **30**(26), 8953–64.

Gomez O, Sanchez-Rodriguez A, Le M, Sanchez-Caro C, Molina-Holgado F, Molina-Holgado E. (2011). Cannabinoid receptor agonists modulate oligodendrocyte differentiation by activating PI3K/Akt and the mammalian target of rapamycin (mTOR) pathways. *British Journal of Pharmacology* **163**(7), 1520–32.

Gow A, Southwood CM, Li JS, Pariali M, Riordan GP, Brodie SE, Danias J, Bronstein JM, Kachar B, Lazzarini RA. (1999). CNS myelin and sertoli cell tight junction strands are absent in Osp/claudin-11 null mice. *Cell* **99**(6), 649–59.

Gravel M, Peterson J, Yong VW, Kottis V, Trapp B, Braun PE. (1996). Overexpression of 2′,3′-cyclic nucleotide 3′-phosphodiesterase in transgenic mice alters oligodendrocyte development and produces aberrant myelination. *Molecular and Cellular Neurosciences* **7**(6), 453–66.

Griffiths I, Klugmann M, Anderson T, Thomson C, Vouyiouklis D, Nave KA. (1998a). Current concepts of PLP and its role in the nervous system. *Microscopy Research and Technique* **41**(5), 344–58.

Griffiths I, Klugmann M, Anderson T, Yool D, Thomson C, Schwab MH, Schneider A, Zimmermann F, McCulloch M, Nadon N *et al.* (1998b). Axonal swellings and degeneration in mice lacking the major proteolipid of myelin. *Science* **280**(5369), 1610–3.

Gudz TI, Komuro H, Macklin WB. (2006). Glutamate stimulates oligodendrocyte progenitor migration mediated via an alphav integrin/myelin proteolipid protein complex. *Journal of Neuroscience* **26**(9), 2458–66.

Guo F, Maeda Y, Ko EM, Delgado M, Horiuchi M, Soulika A, Miers L, Burns T, Itoh T, Shen H *et al.* (2012). Disruption of NMDA receptors in oligodendroglial lineage cells does not alter their susceptibility to experimental autoimmune encephalomyelitis or their normal development. *Journal of Neuroscience* **32**(2), 639–45.

Haak LL, Grimaldi M, Russell JT. (2000). Mitochondria in myelinating cells: calcium signaling in oligodendrocyte precursor cells. *Cell Calcium* **28**(5–6), 297–306.

Haak LL, Song LS, Molinski TF, Pessah IN, Cheng H, Russell JT. (2001). Sparks and puffs in oligodendrocyte progenitors: cross talk between ryanodine receptors and inositol trisphosphate receptors. *Journal of Neuroscience* **21**(11), 3860–70.

Haak LL, Grimaldi M, Smaili SS, Russell JT. (2002). Mitochondria regulate $Ca^{2+}$ wave initiation and inositol trisphosphate signal transduction in oligodendrocyte progenitors. *Journal of Neurochemistry* **80**(3), 405–15.

Haberlandt C, Derouiche A, Wyczynski A, Haseleu J, Pohle J, Karram K, Trotter J, Seifert G, Frotscher M, Steinhauser C *et al.* (2011). Gray matter NG2 cells display multiple $Ca^{2+}$-signaling pathways and highly motile processes. *PLoS One* **6**(3), e17575.

Hamilton N, Vayro S, Wigley R, Butt AM. (2010). Axons and astrocytes release ATP and glutamate to evoke calcium signals in NG2-glia. *Glia* **58**(1), 66–79.

Harrington EP, Zhao C, Fancy SP, Kaing S, Franklin RJ, Rowitch DH. (2010). Oligodendrocyte PTEN is required for myelin and axonal integrity, not remyelination. *Annals of Neurology* **68**(5), 703–16.

Harris JJ, Attwell D. (2012). The energetics of CNS white matter. *Journal of Neuroscience* **32**(1), 356–71.

He M, Howe DG, McCarthy KD. (1996). Oligodendroglial signal transduction systems are regulated by neuronal contact. *Journal of Neurochemistry* **67**(4), 1491–9.

He Y, Dupree J, Wang J, Sandoval J, Li J, Liu H, Shi Y, Nave KA, Casaccia-Bonnefil P. (2007). The transcription factor Yin Yang 1 is essential for oligodendrocyte progenitor differentiation. *Neuron* **55**(2), 217–30.

Herrero-Herranz E, Pardo LA, Bunt G, Gold R, Stuhmer W, Linker RA. (2007). Re-expression of a developmentally restricted potassium channel in autoimmune demyelination: Kv1.4 is implicated in oligodendroglial proliferation. *American Journal of Pathology* **171**(2), 589–98.

Hildebrand C, Remahl S, Persson H, Bjartmar C. (1993). Myelinated nerve fibres in the CNS. *Progress In Neurobiology* **40**(3), 319–84.

Hinman JD, Peters A, Cabral H, Rosene DL, Hollander W, Rasband MN, Abraham CR. (2006). Age-related molecular reorganization at the node of Ranvier. *Journal of Comparative Neurology* **495**(4), 351–62.

Hirano A. (1968). A confirmation of the oligodendroglial origin of myelin in the adult rat. *Journal of Cell Biology* **38**(3), 637–40.

Hu QD, Ang BT, Karsak M, Hu WP, Cui XY, Duka T, Takeda Y, Chia W, Sankar N, Ng YK *et al.* (2003). F3/contactin acts as a functional ligand for Notch during oligodendrocyte maturation. *Cell* **115**(2), 163–75.

Ishibashi T, Dakin KA, Stevens B, Lee PR, Kozlov SV, Stewart CL, Fields RD. (2006). Astrocytes promote myelination in response to electrical impulses. *Neuron* **49**(6), 823–32.

Ishibashi T, Lee PR, Baba H, Fields RD. (2009). Leukemia inhibitory factor regulates the timing of oligodendrocyte development and myelination in the postnatal optic nerve. *Journal of Neuroscience Research* **87**(15), 3343–55.

Itoh T, Beesley J, Itoh A, Cohen AS, Kavanaugh B, Coulter DA, Grinspan JB, Pleasure D (2002). AMPA glutamate receptor-mediated calcium signaling is transiently enhanced during development of oligodendrocytes. *Journal of Neurochemistry* **81**(2), 390–402.

Jackman N, Ishii A, Bansal R. (2009). Oligodendrocyte development and myelin biogenesis: parsing out the roles of glycosphingolipids. *Physiology (Bethesda)* **24**, 290–7.

James G, Butt AM. (2001). P2X and P2Y purinoreceptors mediate ATP-evoked calcium signalling in optic nerve glia *in situ*. *Cell Calcium* **30**(4), 251–9.

Kadi L, Selvaraju R, de Lys P, Proudfoot AE, Wells TN, Boschert U. (2006). Differential effects of chemokines on oligodendrocyte precursor proliferation and myelin formation in vitro. *Journal of Neuroimmunology* **174**(1–2), 133–46.

Kaga Y, Shoemaker WJ, Furusho M, Bryant M, Rosenbluth J, Pfeiffer SE, Oh L, Rasband M, Lappe-Siefke C, Yu K *et al.* (2006). Mice with conditional inactivation of fibroblast growth factor receptor-2 signaling in oligodendrocytes have normal myelin but display dramatic hyperactivity when combined with Cnp1 inactivation. *Journal of Neuroscience* **26**(47), 12339–50.

Kamasawa N, Sik A, Morita M, Yasumura T, Davidson KG, Nagy JI, Rash JE. (2005). Connexin-47 and connexin-32 in gap junctions of oligodendrocyte somata, myelin sheaths, paranodal loops and Schmidt-Lanterman incisures: implications for ionic homeostasis and potassium siphoning. *Neuroscience* **136**(1), 65–86.

Kaplan MR, Cho MH, Ullian EM, Isom LL, Levinson SR, Barres BA. (2001). Differential control of clustering of the sodium channels Na(v)1.2 and Na(v)1.6 at developing CNS nodes of Ranvier. *Neuron* **30**(1), 105–19.

Karadottir R, Cavelier P, Bergersen LH, Attwell D. (2005). NMDA receptors are expressed in oligodendrocytes and activated in ischaemia. *Nature* **438**(7071), 1162–6.

Karadottir R, Hamilton NB, Bakiri Y, Attwell D (2008). Spiking and nonspiking classes of oligodendrocyte precursor glia in CNS white matter. *Nature Neuroscience* **11**(4), 450–6.

Kastritsis CH, McCarthy KD. (1993). Oligodendroglial lineage cells express neuroligand receptors. *Glia* **8**(2), 106–13.

Kessaris N, Jamen F, Rubin LL, Richardson WD. (2004). Cooperation between sonic hedgehog and fibroblast growth factor/MAPK signalling pathways in neocortical precursors. *Development* **131**(6), 1289–98.

Kessaris N, Fogarty M, Iannarelli P, Grist M, Wegner M, Richardson WD. (2006). Competing waves of oligodendrocytes in the forebrain and postnatal elimination of an embryonic lineage. *Nature Neuroscience* **9**(2), 173–9.

Kettenmann H, Ransom BR, Schlue WR. (1990). Intracellular pH shifts capable of uncoupling cultured oligodendrocytes are seen only in low HCO3– solution. *Glia* **3**(2), 110–7.

Kirchhoff F, Kettenmann H. (1992). GABA Triggers a [$Ca^{2+}$]$_i$ Increase in Murine Precursor Cells of the Oligodendrocyte Lineage. *European Journal of Neuroscience* **4**(11), 1049–1058.

Kirchhoff F, Mulhardt C, Pastor A, Becker CM, Kettenmann H. (1996). Expression of glycine receptor subunits in glial cells of the rat spinal cord. *Journal of Neurochemistry* **66**(4), 1383–90.

Kirischuk S, Scherer J, Kettenmann H, Verkhratsky A. (1995a). Activation of P2-purinoreceptors triggered $Ca^{2+}$ release from InsP3-sensitive internal stores in mammalian oligodendrocytes. *Journal of Physiology* **483**(Pt 1), 41–57.

Kirischuk S, Scherer J, Moller T, Verkhratsky A, Kettenmann H. (1995b). Subcellular heterogeneity of voltage-operated $Ca^{2+}$ channels in cells of the oligodendrocyte lineage. *Glia* **13**(1), 1–12.

Klein C, Kramer EM, Cardine AM, Schraven B, Brandt R, Trotter J. (2002). Process outgrowth of oligodendrocytes is promoted by interaction of fyn kinase with the cytoskeletal protein tau. *Journal of Neuroscience* **22**(3), 698–707.

Kleopa KA, Orthmann-Murphy J, Sargiannidou I. (2010). Gap junction disorders of myelinating cells. *Reviews in the Neurosciences* **21**(5), 397–419.

Knapp PE, Adjan VV, Hauser KF. (2009). Cell-specific loss of kappa-opioid receptors in oligodendrocytes of the dysmyelinating jimpy mouse. *Neuroscience Letters* **451**(2), 114–8.

Knutson P, Ghiani CA, Zhou JM, Gallo V, McBain CJ. (1997). K+ channel expression and cell proliferation are regulated by intracellular sodium and membrane depolarization in oligodendrocyte progenitor cells. *Journal of Neuroscience* **17**(8), 2669–82.

Kondo T, Raff M. (2000). Basic helix-loop-helix proteins and the timing of oligodendrocyte differentiation. *Development* **127**(14), 2989–98.

Kosturko LD, Maggipinto MJ, Korza G, Lee JW, Carson JH, Barbarese E. (2006). Heterogeneous nuclear ribonucleoprotein (hnRNP) E1 binds to hnRNP A2 and inhibits translation of A2 response element mRNAs. *Molecular Biology of The Cell* **17**(8), 3521–33.

Kramer-Albers EM, White R. (2011). From axon-glial signalling to myelination: the integrating role of oligodendroglial Fyn kinase. *Cellular and Molecular Life Sciences* **68**(12), 2003–12.

Kucharova K, Stallcup WB. (2010). The NG2 proteoglycan promotes oligodendrocyte progenitor proliferation and developmental myelination. *Neuroscience* **166**(1), 185–94.

Kukley M, Dietrich D. (2009). Kainate receptors and signal integration by NG2 glial cells. *Neuron Glia Biology* **5**(1–2), 13–20.

Kukley M, Nishiyama A, Dietrich D. (2010). The fate of synaptic input to NG2 glial cells: neurons specifically downregulate transmitter release onto differentiating oligodendroglial cells. *Journal of Neuroscience* **30**(24), 8320–31.

Kumar S, Kahn MA, Dinh L, de Vellis J. (1998). NT-3-mediated TrkC receptor activation promotes proliferation and cell survival of rodent progenitor oligodendrocyte cells *in vitro* and *in vivo*. *Journal of Neuroscience Research* **54**(6), 754–65.

Kuspert M, Hammer A, Bosl MR, Wegner M. (2011). Olig2 regulates Sox10 expression in oligodendrocyte precursors through an evolutionary conserved distal enhancer. *Nucleic Acids Research* **39**(4), 1280–93.

Lappe-Siefke C, Goebbels S, Gravel M, Nicksch E, Lee J, Braun PE, Griffiths IR, Nave KA. (2003). Disruption of Cnp1 uncouples oligodendroglial functions in axonal support and myelination. *Nature Genetics* **33**(3), 366–74.

Lau P, Verrier JD, Nielsen JA, Johnson KR, Notterpek L, Hudson LD. (2008). Identification of dynamically regulated microRNA and mRNA networks in developing oligodendrocytes. *Journal of Neuroscience* **28**(45), 11720–30.

Laursen LS, Chan CW, ffrench-Constant C. (2009). An integrin-contactin complex regulates CNS myelination by differential Fyn phosphorylation. *Journal of Neuroscience* **29**(29), 9174–85.

Lee X, Yang Z, Shao Z, Rosenberg SS, Levesque M, Pepinsky RB, Qiu M, Miller RH, Chan JR, Mi S. (2007). NGF regulates the expression of axonal LINGO-1 to inhibit oligodendrocyte differentiation and myelination. *Journal of Neuroscience* **27**(1), 220–5.

Lemke G. (2006). Neuregulin-1 and myelination. *Science's STKE: Signal Transduction Knowledge Environment* 2006 (325), pe11.

Li H, He Y, Richardson WD, Casaccia P. (2009). Two-tier transcriptional control of oligodendrocyte differentiation. *Current Opinion In Neurobiology* **19**(5), 479–85.

Li H, de Faria JP, Andrew P, Nitarska J, Richardson WD. (2011). Phosphorylation regulates OLIG2 cofactor choice and the motor neuron-oligodendrocyte fate switch. *Neuron* **69**(5), 918–29.

Li S, Stys PK. (2000). Mechanisms of ionotropic glutamate receptor-mediated excitotoxicity in isolated spinal cord white matter. *Journal of Neuroscience* **20**(3), 1190–8.

Liang X, Draghi NA, Resh MD. (2004). Signaling from integrins to Fyn to Rho family GTPases regulates morphologic differentiation of oligodendrocytes. *Journal of Neuroscience* **24**(32), 7140–9.

Lin SC, Bergles DE. (2004). Synaptic signaling between GABAergic interneurons and oligodendrocyte precursor cells in the hippocampus. *Nature Neuroscience* **7**(1), 24–32.

Liu A, Li J, Marin-Husstege M, Kageyama R, Fan Y, Gelinas C, Casaccia-Bonnefil P. (2006). A molecular insight of Hes5-dependent inhibition of myelin gene expression: old partners and new players. *EMBO Journal* **25**(20), 4833–42.

Liu J, Casaccia P. (2010). Epigenetic regulation of oligodendrocyte identity. *Trends In Neurosciences* **33**(4), 193–201.

Liu X, Lu Y, Zhang Y, Li Y, Zhou J, Yuan Y, Gao X, Su Z, He C. (2012). Slit2 Regulates the Dispersal of Oligodendrocyte Precursor Cells via Fyn/RhoA Signaling. *Journal of Biological Chemistry*.

Liu Z, Hu X, Cai J, Liu B, Peng X, Wegner M, Qiu M. (2007). Induction of oligodendrocyte differentiation by Olig2 and Sox10: evidence for reciprocal interactions and dosage-dependent mechanisms. *Developmental Biology* **302**(2), 683–93.

Lu QR, Yuk D, Alberta JA, Zhu Z, Pawlitzky I, Chan J, McMahon AP, Stiles CD, Rowitch DH. (2000). Sonic hedgehog-regulated oligodendrocyte lineage genes encoding bHLH proteins in the mammalian central nervous system. *Neuron* **25**(2), 317–29.

Lu QR, Sun T, Zhu Z, Ma N, Garcia M, Stiles CD, Rowitch DH. (2002). Common developmental requirement for Olig function indicates a motor neuron/oligodendrocyte connection. *Cell* **109**(1), 75–86.

Ludwin SK. (1979). The perineuronal satellite oligodendrocyte. A role in remyelination. *Acta Neuropathologica* **47**(1), 49–53.

Ludwin SK. (1984). The function of perineuronal satellite oligodendrocytes: an immuno-histochemical study. *Neuropathology and Applied Neurobiology* **10**(2), 143–9.

Luyt K, Varadi A, Molnar E. (2003). Functional metabotropic glutamate receptors are expressed in oligodendrocyte progenitor cells. *Journal of Neurochemistry* **84**(6), 1452–64.

Luyt K, Varadi A, Durant CF, Molnar E. (2006). Oligodendroglial metabotropic glutamate receptors are developmentally regulated and involved in the prevention of apoptosis. *Journal of Neurochemistry* **99**(2), 641–56.

Luyt K, Slade TP, Dorward JJ, Durant CF, Wu Y, Shigemoto R, Mundell SJ, Varadi A, Molnar E. (2007). Developing oligodendrocytes express functional GABA(B) receptors that stimulate cell proliferation and migration. *Journal of Neurochemistry* **100**(3), 822–40.

Malek SA, Coderre E, Stys PK. (2003). Aberrant chloride transport contributes to anoxic/ischemic white matter injury. *Journal of Neuroscience* **23**(9), 3826–36.

Marcus J, Honigbaum S, Shroff S, Honke K, Rosenbluth J, Dupree JL. (2006). Sulfatide is essential for the maintenance of CNS myelin and axon structure. *Glia* **53**(4), 372–81.

Martin-Vasallo P, Wetzel RK, Garcia-Segura LM, Molina-Holgado E, Arystarkhova E, Sweadner KJ. (2000). Oligodendrocytes in brain and optic nerve express the beta3 subunit isoform of Na, K-ATPase. *Glia* **31**(3), 206–18.

Matute C. (2011). Glutamate and ATP signalling in white matter pathology. *Journal of Anatomy* **219**(1), 53–64.

Matute C, Cavaliere F. (2011). Neuroglial interactions mediated by purinergic signalling in the pathophysiology of CNS disorders. *Seminars in Cell and Developmental Biology* **22**(2), 252–9.

Matute C, Torre I, Perez-Cerda F, Perez-Samartin A, Alberdi E, Etxebarria E, Arranz AM, Ravid R, Rodriguez-Antiguedad A, Sanchez-Gomez M *et al.* (2007). P2X(7) receptor blockade prevents ATP excitotoxicity in oligodendrocytes and ameliorates experimental autoimmune encephalomyelitis. *Journal of Neuroscience* **27**(35), 9525–33.

McKinnon RD, Piras G, Ida JA, Jr., Dubois-Dalcq M. (1993). A role for TGF-beta in oligodendrocyte differentiation. *Journal of Cell Biology* **121**(6), 1397–407.

McMorris FA, McKinnon RD. (1996). Regulation of oligodendrocyte development and CNS myelination by growth factors: prospects for therapy of demyelinating disease. *Brain Pathology* **6**(3), 313–29.

Menichella DM, Majdan M, Awatramani R, Goodenough DA, Sirkowski E, Scherer SS, Paul DL. (2006). Genetic and physiological evidence that oligodendrocyte gap junctions contribute to spatial buffering of potassium released during neuronal activity. *Journal of Neuroscience* **26**(43), 10984–91.

Mi S, Lee X, Shao Z, Thill G, Ji B, Relton J, Levesque M, Allaire N, Perrin S, Sands B *et al.* (2004). LINGO-1 is a component of the Nogo-66 receptor/p75 signaling complex. *Nature Neuroscience* **7**(3), 221–8.

Micu I, Jiang Q, Coderre E, Ridsdale A, Zhang L, Woulfe J, Yin X, Trapp BD, McRory JE, Rehak R *et al.* (2006). NMDA receptors mediate calcium accumulation in myelin during chemical ischaemia. *Nature* **439**(7079), 988–92.

Miller RH. (2002). Regulation of oligodendrocyte development in the vertebrate CNS. *Progress In Neurobiology* **67**(6), 451–67.

Miyamoto Y, Yamauchi J, Tanoue A. (2008). Cdk5 phosphorylation of WAVE2 regulates oligodendrocyte precursor cell migration through nonreceptor tyrosine kinase Fyn. *Journal of Neuroscience* **28**(33), 8326–37.

Molina-Holgado E, Vela JM, Arevalo-Martin A, Almazan G, Molina-Holgado F, Borrell J, Guaza C. (2002). Cannabinoids promote oligodendrocyte progenitor survival: involvement of cannabinoid receptors and phosphatidylinositol-3 kinase/Akt signaling. *Journal of Neuroscience* **22**(22), 9742–53.

Moran-Jimenez MJ, Matute C. (2000). Immunohistochemical localization of the P2Y(1) purinergic receptor in neurons and glial cells of the central nervous system. *Brain Research. Molecular Brain Research* **78**(1–2), 50–8.

Murtie JC, Macklin WB, Corfas G. (2007). Morphometric analysis of oligodendrocytes in the adult mouse frontal cortex. *Journal of Neuroscience Research* **85**(10), 2080–6.

Narayanan SP, Flores AI, Wang F, Macklin WB. (2009). Akt signals through the mammalian target of rapamycin pathway to regulate CNS myelination. *Journal of Neuroscience* **29**(21), 6860–70.

Nawaz S, Kippert A, Saab AS, Werner HB, Lang T, Nave KA, Simons M. (2009). Phosphatidylinositol 4,5-bisphosphate-dependent interaction of myelin basic protein with the plasma membrane in oligodendroglial cells and its rapid perturbation by elevated calcium. *Journal of Neuroscience* **29**(15), 4794–807.

Neusch C, Weishaupt JH, Bahr M. (2003). Kir channels in the CNS: emerging new roles and implications for neurological diseases. *Cell and Tissue Research* **311**(2), 131–8.

Nishiyama A, Komitova M, Suzuki R, Zhu X. (2009). Polydendrocytes (NG2 cells): multifunctional cells with lineage plasticity. *Nature Reviews Neuroscience* **10**(1), 9–22.

Niu J, Mei F, Li N, Wang H, Li X, Kong J, Xiao L. (2010). Haloperidol promotes proliferation but inhibits differentiation in rat oligodendrocyte progenitor cell cultures. *Biochemistry and Cell Biology* **88**(4), 611–20.

Noble M, Arhin A, Gass D, Mayer-Proschel M. (2003). The cortical ancestry of oligodendrocytes: common principles and novel features. *Developmental Neuroscience* **25**(2–4), 217–33.

Ogawa Y, Schafer DP, Horresh I, Bar V, Hales K, Yang Y, Susuki K, Peles E, Stankewich MC, Rasband MN. (2006). Spectrins and ankyrinB constitute a specialized paranodal cytoskeleton. *Journal of Neuroscience* **26**(19), 5230–9.

Oh LY, Denninger A, Colvin JS, Vyas A, Tole S, Ornitz DM, Bansal R. (2003). Fibroblast growth factor receptor 3 signaling regulates the onset of oligodendrocyte terminal differentiation. *Journal of Neuroscience* **23**(3), 883–94.

Ortega MC, Bribian A, Peregrin S, Gil MT, Marin O, de Castro F. (2012a). Neuregulin-1/ErbB4 signaling controls the migration of oligodendrocyte precursor cells during development. *Experimental Neurology* **235**(2), 610–20.

Ortega MC, Cases O, Merchan P, Kozyraki R, Clemente D, de Castro F. (2012b). Megalin mediates the influence of sonic hedgehog on oligodendrocyte precursor cell migration and proliferation during development. *Glia* **60**(6), 851–66.

Orthmann-Murphy JL, Abrams CK, Scherer SS. (2008). Gap junctions couple astrocytes and oligodendrocytes. *Journal of Molecular Neuroscience* **35**(1), 101–16.

Otero GC, Merrill JE. (1997). Response of human oligodendrocytes to interleukin-2. *Brain, Behavior, and Immunity* **11**(1), 24–38.

Othman T, Yan H, Rivkees SA. (2003). Oligodendrocytes express functional A1 adenosine receptors that stimulate cellular migration. *Glia* **44**(2), 166–72.

Padovani-Claudio DA, Liu L, Ransohoff RM, Miller RH. (2006). Alterations in the oligodendrocyte lineage, myelin, and white matter in adult mice lacking the chemokine receptor CXCR2. *Glia* **54**(5), 471–83.

Paez PM, Fulton D, Colwell CS, Campagnoni AT. (2009a). Voltage-operated $Ca^{2+}$ and $Na^{+}$ channels in the oligodendrocyte lineage. *Journal of Neuroscience Research* **87**(15), 3259–66.

Paez PM, Fulton DJ, Spreuer V, Handley V, Campagnoni CW, Campagnoni AT. (2009b). Regulation of store-operated and voltage-operated $Ca^{2+}$ channels in the proliferation and death of oligodendrocyte precursor cells by golli proteins. *ASN Neuro* **1**(1).

Paez PM, Fulton DJ, Spreuer V, Handley V, Campagnoni CW, Macklin WB, Colwell C, Campagnoni AT. (2009c). Golli myelin basic proteins regulate oligodendroglial progenitor cell migration through voltage-operated $Ca^{2+}$ influx. *Journal of Neuroscience* **29**(20), 6663–76.

Papay R, Gaivin R, Jha A, McCune DF, McGrath JC, Rodrigo MC, Simpson PC, Doze VA, Perez DM. (2006). Localization of the mouse alpha1A-adrenergic receptor (AR) in the brain: alpha1AAR is expressed in neurons, GABAergic interneurons, and NG2 oligodendrocyte progenitors. *Journal of Comparative Neurology* **497**(2), 209–22.

Parras CM, Galli R, Britz O, Soares S, Galichet C, Battiste J, Johnson JE, Nakafuku M, Vescovi A, Guillemot F. (2004). Mash1 specifies neurons and oligodendrocytes in the postnatal brain. *EMBO Journal* **23**(22), 4495–505.

Pedraza L, Huang JK, Colman D. (2009). Disposition of axonal caspr with respect to glial cell membranes: Implications for the process of myelination. *Journal of Neuroscience Research* **87**(15), 3480–91.

Pende M, Fisher TL, Simpson PB, Russell JT, Blenis J, Gallo V. (1997). Neurotransmitter- and growth factor-induced cAMP response element binding protein phosphorylation in glial cell progenitors: role of calcium ions, protein kinase C, and mitogen-activated protein kinase/ribosomal S6 kinase pathway. *Journal of Neuroscience* **17**(4), 1291–301.

Penfield W. (1932). *Cytology & cellular pathology of the nervous system*. New York: P.B. Hoeber, Inc.

Peters A. (1964). Observations on the Connexions between Myelin Sheaths and Glial Cells in the Optic Nerves of Young Rats. *Journal of Anatomy* **98**, 125–34.

Peters A. (2002). The effects of normal aging on myelin and nerve fibers: a review. *Journal of Neurocytology* **31**(8–9), 581–93.

Peters A. (2004). A fourth type of neuroglial cell in the adult central nervous system. *Journal of Neurocytology* **33**(3), 345–57.

Peters A, Sethares C. (2004). Oligodendrocytes, their progenitors and other neuroglial cells in the aging primate cerebral cortex. *Cerebral Cortex* **14**(9), 995–1007.

Peters A, Verderosa A, Sethares C. (2008). The neuroglial population in the primary visual cortex of the aging rhesus monkey. *Glia* **56**(11), 1151–61.

Piaton G, Gould RM, Lubetzki C. (2010). Axon-oligodendrocyte interactions during developmental myelination, demyelination and repair. *Journal of Neurochemistry* **114**(5), 1243–60.

Pina-Crespo JC, Talantova M, Micu I, States B, Chen HS, Tu S, Nakanishi N, Tong G, Zhang D, Heinemann SF *et al.* (2010). Excitatory glycine responses of CNS myelin mediated by NR1/NR3 "NMDA" receptor subunits. *Journal of Neuroscience* **30**(34), 11501–5.

Pizzi M, Sarnico I, Boroni F, Benarese M, Dreano M, Garotta G, Valerio A, Spano P. (2004). Prevention of neuron and oligodendrocyte degeneration by interleukin-6 (IL-6) and IL-6 receptor/IL-6 fusion protein in organotypic hippocampal slices. *Molecular and Cellular Neurosciences* **25**(2), 301–11.

Poliak S, Peles E. (2003). The local differentiation of myelinated axons at nodes of Ranvier. *Nature Reviews Neuroscience* **4**(12), 968–80.

Poliak S, Salomon D, Elhanany H, Sabanay H, Kiernan B, Pevny L, Stewart CL, Xu X, Chiu SY, Shrager P *et al.* (2003). Juxtaparanodal clustering of Shaker-like $K^+$ channels in myelinated axons depends on Caspr2 and TAG-1. *Journal of Cell Biology* **162**(6), 1149–60.

Qi Y, Cai J, Wu Y, Wu R, Lee J, Fu H, Rao M, Sussel L, Rubenstein J, Qiu M. (2001). Control of oligodendrocyte differentiation by the Nkx2.2 homeodomain transcription factor. *Development* **128**(14), 2723–33.

Ragheb F, Molina-Holgado E, Cui QL, Khorchid A, Liu HN, Larocca JN, Almazan G. (2001). Pharmacological and functional characterization of muscarinic receptor subtypes in developing oligodendrocytes. *Journal of Neurochemistry* **77**(5), 1396–406.

Rajasekharan S, Bin JM, Antel JP, Kennedy TE. (2010). A central role for RhoA during oligodendroglial maturation in the switch from netrin-1-mediated chemorepulsion to process elaboration. *Journal of Neurochemistry* **113**(6), 1589–97.

Ransom BR, Butt AM, Black JA. (1991). Ultrastructural identification of HRP-injected oligodendrocytes in the intact rat optic nerve. *Glia* **4**(1), 37–45.

Rasband MN. (2010). Clustered K+ channel complexes in axons. *Neuroscience Letters* **486**(2), 101–6.

Rasband MN, Trimmer JS. (2001). Developmental clustering of ion channels at and near the node of Ranvier. *Developmental Biology* **236**(1), 5–16.

Relucio J, Tzvetanova ID, Ao W, Lindquist S, Colognato H. (2009). Laminin alters fyn regulatory mechanisms and promotes oligodendrocyte development. *Journal of Neuroscience* **29**(38), 11794–806.

Remahl S, Hildebrand C. (1990). Relation between axons and oligodendroglial cells during initial myelination. I. The glial unit. *Journal of Neurocytology* **19**(3), 313–28.

Richardson WD, Kessaris N, Pringle N. (2006). Oligodendrocyte wars. *Nature Reviews Neuroscience* **7**(1), 11–8.

Richardson WD, Young KM, Tripathi RB, McKenzie I. (2011). NG2-glia as multipotent neural stem cells: fact or fantasy? *Neuron* **70**(4), 661–73.

Rivers LE, Young KM, Rizzi M, Jamen F, Psachoulia K, Wade A, Kessaris N, Richardson WD. (2008). PDGFRA/NG2 glia generate myelinating oligodendrocytes and piriform projection neurons in adult mice. *Nature Neuroscience* **11**(12), 1392–401.

Ro HA, Carson JH. (2004). pH microdomains in oligodendrocytes. *Journal of Biological Chemistry* **279**(35), 37115–23.

Robinson S, Tani M, Strieter RM, Ransohoff RM, Miller RH. (1998). The chemokine growth-regulated oncogene-alpha promotes spinal cord oligodendrocyte precursor proliferation. *Journal of Neuroscience* **18**(24), 10457–63.

Rogers SW, Gregori NZ, Carlson N, Gahring LC, Noble M. (2001). neuronal nicotinic acetylcholine receptor expression by O2A/oligodendrocyte progenitor cells. *Glia* **33**(4), 306–13.

Rosenberg SS, Chan JR. (2009). Modulating myelination: knowing when to say Wnt. *Genes and Development* **23**(13), 1487–93.

Rosin C, Colombo S, Calver AA, Bates TE, Skaper SD. (2005). Dopamine D2 and D3 receptor agonists limit oligodendrocyte injury caused by glutamate oxidative stress and oxygen/glucose deprivation. *Glia* **52**(4), 336–43.

Rowitch DH, Lu QR, Kessaris N, Richardson WD. (2002). An 'oligarchy' rules neural development. *Trends In Neurosciences* **25**(8), 417–22.

Roy K, Murtie JC, El-Khodor BF, Edgar N, Sardi SP, Hooks BM, Benoit-Marand M, Chen C, Moore H, O'Donnell P *et al.* (2007). Loss of erbB signaling in oligodendrocytes alters myelin and dopaminergic function, a potential mechanism for neuropsychiatric disorders. *Proceedings of The National Academy Of Sciences Of The United States Of America* **104**(19), 8131–6.

Saher G, Brugger B, Lappe-Siefke C, Mobius W, Tozawa R, Wehr MC, Wieland F, Ishibashi S, Nave KA. (2005). High cholesterol level is essential for myelin membrane growth. *Nature Neuroscience* **8**(4), 468–75.

Salter MG, Fern R. (2005). NMDA receptors are expressed in developing oligodendrocyte processes and mediate injury. *Nature* **438**(7071), 1167–71.

Sanchez-Gomez MV, Matute C. (1999). AMPA and kainate receptors each mediate excitotoxicity in oligodendroglial cultures. *Neurobiology of Disease* **6**(6), 475–85.

Sandell JH, Peters A. (2003). Disrupted myelin and axon loss in the anterior commissure of the aged rhesus monkey. *Journal of Comparative Neurology* **466**(1), 14–30.

Sato-Bigbee C, Pal S, Chu AK. (1999). Different neuroligands and signal transduction pathways stimulate CREB phosphorylation at specific developmental stages along oligodendrocyte differentiation. *Journal of Neurochemistry* **72**(1), 139–47.

Schachner M, Bartsch U. (2000). Multiple functions of the myelin-associated glycoprotein MAG (siglec-4a) in formation and maintenance of myelin. *Glia* **29**(2), 154–65.

Schmitz T, Chew LJ. (2008). Cytokines and myelination in the central nervous system. *ScientificWorldJournal* **8**, 1119–47.

Schumacher M, Hussain R, Gago N, Oudinet JP, Mattern C, Ghoumari AM. (2012). Progesterone synthesis in the nervous system: implications for myelination and myelin repair. *Frontiers in Neuroscience* **6**, 10.

Silajdzic E, Willison HJ, Furukawa K, Barnett SC. (2009). *In vitro* analysis of glial cell function in ganglioside-deficient mice. *Journal of Neuroscience Research* **87**(11), 2467–83.

Simons M, Trotter J. (2007). Wrapping it up: the cell biology of myelination. *Current Opinion In Neurobiology* **17**(5), 533–40.

Simpson PB, Holtzclaw LA, Langley DB, Russell JT. (1998). Characterization of ryanodine receptors in oligodendrocytes, type 2 astrocytes, and O-2A progenitors. *Journal of Neuroscience Research* **52**(4), 468–82.

Simpson PB, Russell JT. (1997). Role of sarcoplasmic/endoplasmic-reticulum $Ca^{2+}$-ATPases in mediating $Ca^{2+}$ waves and local $Ca^{2+}$-release microdomains in cultured glia. *Biochemical Journal* **325**(Pt 1), 239–47.

Simpson PB, Mehotra S, Lange GD, Russell JT. (1997). High density distribution of endoplasmic reticulum proteins and mitochondria at specialized $Ca^{2+}$ release sites in oligodendrocyte processes. *Journal of Biological Chemistry* **272**(36), 22654–61.

Smaili SS, Russell JT. (1999). Permeability transition pore regulates both mitochondrial membrane potential and agonist-evoked $Ca^{2+}$ signals in oligodendrocyte progenitors. *Cell Calcium* **26**(3–4), 121–30.

Smothers CT, Woodward JJ. (2007). Pharmacological characterization of glycine-activated currents in HEK 293 cells expressing N-methyl-D-aspartate NR1 and NR3 subunits. *Journal of Pharmacology and Experimental Therapeutics* **322**(2), 739–48.

Sohn J, Natale J, Chew LJ, Belachew S, Cheng Y, Aguirre A, Lytle J, Nait-Oumesmar B, Kerninon C, Kanai-Azuma M et al. (2006). Identification of Sox17 as a transcription factor that regulates oligodendrocyte development. *Journal of Neuroscience* **26**(38), 9722–35.

Soliven B. (2001). Calcium signalling in cells of oligodendroglial lineage. *Microscopy Research and Technique* **52**(6), 672–9.

Soliven B, Ma L, Bae H, Attali B, Sobko A, Iwase T. (2003). PDGF upregulates delayed rectifier via Src family kinases and sphingosine kinase in oligodendroglial progenitors. *American Journal of Physiology. Cell Physiology* **284**(1), C85–93.

Song J, Goetz BD, Kirvell SL, Butt AM, Duncan ID. (2001). Selective myelin defects in the anterior medullary velum of the taiep mutant rat. *Glia* **33**(1), 1–11.

Sontheimer H, Waxman SG. (1993). Expression of voltage-activated ion channels by astrocytes and oligodendrocytes in the hippocampal slice. *Journal of Neurophysiology* **70** (5), 1863–73.

Southwood C, He C, Garbern J, Kamholz J, Arroyo E, Gow A. (2004). CNS myelin paranodes require Nkx6-2 homeoprotein transcriptional activity for normal structure. *Journal of Neuroscience* **24**(50), 11215–25.

Sperber BR, Boyle-Walsh EA, Engleka MJ, Gadue P, Peterson AC, Stein PL, Scherer SS, McMorris FA. (2001). A unique role for Fyn in CNS myelination. *Journal of Neuroscience* **21**(6), 2039–47.

Stensaas LJ, Stensaas SS. (1968). Astrocytic neuroglial cells, oligodendrocytes and microgliacytes in the spinal cord of the toad. I. Light microscopy. *Zeitschrift Fur Zellforschung und Mikroskopische Anatomie* **84**(4), 473–89.

Stephens GJ, Marriott DR, Djamgoz MB, Wilkin GP. (1993). Electrophysiological and biochemical evidence for bradykinin receptors on cultured rat cortical oligodendrocytes. *Neuroscience Letters* **153**(2), 223–6.

Stevens B, Porta S, Haak LL, Gallo V, Fields RD. (2002). Adenosine: a neuron-glial transmitter promoting myelination in the CNS in response to action potentials. *Neuron* **36**(5), 855–68.

Stolt CC, Schlierf A, Lommes P, Hillgartner S, Werner T, Kosian T, Sock E, Kessaris N, Richardson WD, Lefebvre V and others. (2006). SoxD proteins influence multiple stages of oligodendrocyte development and modulate SoxE protein function. *Developmental Cell* **11**(5), 697–709.

Suetsugu S, Takenawa T. (2003). Translocation of N-WASP by nuclear localization and export signals into the nucleus modulates expression of HSP90. *Journal of Biological Chemistry* **278**(43), 42515–23.

Sugimori M, Nagao M, Parras CM, Nakatani H, Lebel M, Guillemot F, Nakafuku M. (2008). Ascl1 is required for oligodendrocyte development in the spinal cord. *Development* **135**(7), 1271–81.

Szuchet S, Nielsen JA, Lovas G, Domowicz MS, de Velasco JM, Maric D, Hudson LD. (2011). The genetic signature of perineuronal oligodendrocytes reveals their unique phenotype. *European Journal of Neuroscience* **34**(12), 1906–22.

Takasaki C, Yamasaki M, Uchigashima M, Konno K, Yanagawa Y, Watanabe M. (2010). Cytochemical and cytological properties of perineuronal oligodendrocytes in the mouse cortex. *European Journal of Neuroscience* **32**(8), 1326–36.

Taniike M, Mohri I, Eguchi N, Beuckmann CT, Suzuki K, Urade Y. (2002). Perineuronal oligodendrocytes protect against neuronal apoptosis through the production of lipocalin-type prostaglandin D synthase in a genetic demyelinating model. *Journal of Neuroscience* **22**(12), 4885–96.

Taveggia C, Feltri ML, Wrabetz L. (2010). Signals to promote myelin formation and repair. *Nature Reviews Neurology* **6**(5), 276–87.

Tawk M, Makoukji J, Belle M, Fonte C, Trousson A, Hawkins T, Li H, Ghandour S, Schumacher M, Massaad C. (2011). Wnt/beta-catenin signaling is an essential and direct driver of myelin gene expression and myelinogenesis. *Journal of Neuroscience* **31**(10), 3729–42.

Thaxton C, Pillai AP, Pribisko AL, Dupree JL, Bhat MA. (2011). Nodes of Ranvier act as barriers to restrict invasion of flanking paranodal domains in myelinated axons. *Neuron* **69**(2), 244–257.

Tiwari-Woodruff S, Beltran-Parrazal L, Charles A, Keck T, Vu T, Bronstein J. (2006). K+ channel KV3.1 associates with OSP/claudin-11 and regulates oligodendrocyte development. *American Journal of Physiology. Cell Physiology* **291**(4), C687–98.

Tiwari-Woodruff SK, Buznikov AG, Vu TQ, Micevych PE, Chen K, Kornblum HI, Bronstein JM. (2001). OSP/claudin-11 forms a complex with a novel member of the tetraspanin super family and beta1 integrin and regulates proliferation and migration of oligodendrocytes. *Journal of Cell Biology* **153**(2), 295–305.

Todorich B, Pasquini JM, Garcia CI, Paez PM, ConnorJR. (2009). Oligodendrocytes and myelination: the role of iron. *Glia* **57**(5), 467–78.

Tong XP, Li XY, Zhou B, Shen W, Zhang ZJ, Xu TL, Duan S. (2009). Ca$(^{2+})$ signaling evoked by activation of Na(+) channels and Na(+)/Ca$(^{2+})$ exchangers is required for GABA-induced NG2 cell migration. *Journal of Cell Biology* **186**(1), 113–28.

Trajkovic K, Dhaunchak AS, Goncalves JT, Wenzel D, Schneider A, Bunt G, Nave K-A, Simons M. (2006). Neuron to glia signaling triggers myelin membrane exocytosis from endosomal storage sites. *Journal of Cell Biology* **172**(6), 937–948.

Tripathi RB, Clarke LE, Burzomato V, Kessaris N, Anderson PN, Attwell D, Richardson WD. (2011). Dorsally and ventrally derived oligodendrocytes have similar electrical properties but myelinate preferred tracts. *Journal of Neuroscience* **31**(18), 6809–19.

Tsai HH, Frost E, To V, Robinson S, Ffrench-Constant C, Geertman R, Ransohoff RM, Miller RH. (2002). The chemokine receptor CXCR2 controls positioning of oligodendrocyte precursors in developing spinal cord by arresting their migration. *Cell* **110**(3), 373–83.

Tyler WA, Gangoli N, Gokina P, Kim HA, Covey M, Levison SW, Wood TL. (2009). Activation of the mammalian target of rapamycin (mTOR) is essential for oligodendrocyte differentiation. *Journal of Neuroscience* **29**(19), 6367–78.

Uchida N, Buck DW, He D, Reitsma MJ, Masek M, Phan TV, Tsukamoto AS, Gage FH, Weissman IL. (2000). Direct isolation of human central nervous system stem cells. *Proceedings of The National Academy Of Sciences Of The United States Of America* **97**(26), 14720–5.

Vautier F, Belachew S, Chittajallu R, Gallo V. (2004). Shaker-type potassium channel subunits differentially control oligodendrocyte progenitor proliferation. *Glia* **48**(4), 337–45.

Vela JM, Molina-Holgado E, Arevalo-Martin A, Almazan G, Guaza C. (2002). Interleukin-1 regulates proliferation and differentiation of oligodendrocyte progenitor cells. *Molecular and Cellular Neurosciences* **20**(3), 489–502.

Velez-Fort M, Audinat E, Angulo MC. (2009). Functional alpha 7-containing nicotinic receptors of NG2-expressing cells in the hippocampus. *Glia* **57**(10), 1104–14.

Velez-Fort M, Maldonado PP, Butt AM, Audinat E, Angulo MC. (2010). Postnatal switch from synaptic to extrasynaptic transmission between interneurons and NG2 cells. *Journal of Neuroscience* **30**(20), 6921–9.

Velumian AA, Samoilova M, Fehlings MG. (2011). Visualization of cytoplasmic diffusion within living myelin sheaths of CNS white matter axons using microinjection of the fluorescent dye Lucifer Yellow. *Neuroimage* **56**(1), 27–34.

Verkhratsky A, Steinhauser C. (2000). Ion channels in glial cells. *Brain Research Brain Research Reviews* **32**(2–3), 380–412.

Verkhratsky A, Orkand RK, Kettenmann H. (1998). Glial calcium: homeostasis and signaling function. *Physiological Reviews* **78**(1), 99–141.

Verrier JD, Jackson TC, Bansal R, Kochanek PM, Puccio AM, Okonkwo DO, Jackson EK. (2012). The brain *in vivo* expresses the 2′,3′-cAMP-adenosine pathway. *Journal of Neurochemistry*.

Von Blankenfeld G, Trotter J, Kettenmann H. (1991). Expression and Developmental Regulation of a GABAA Receptor in Cultured Murine Cells of the Oligodendrocyte Lineage. *European Journal of Neuroscience* **3**(4), 310–316.

Vostrikov VM, Uranova NA, Orlovskaya DD. (2007). Deficit of perineuronal oligodendrocytes in the prefrontal cortex in schizophrenia and mood disorders. *Schizophrenia Research* **94**(1–3), 273–80.

Wake H, Lee PR, Fields RD. (2011). Control of local protein synthesis and initial events in myelination by action potentials. *Science* **333**(6049), 1647–51.

Wang C, Pralong WF, Schulz MF, Rougon G, Aubry JM, Pagliusi S, Robert A, Kiss JZ. (1996). Functional N-methyl-D-aspartate receptors in O-2A glial precursor cells: a critical role in regulating polysialic acid-neural cell adhesion molecule expression and cell migration. *Journal of Cell Biology* **135**(6 Pt 1), 1565–81.

Wang S, Sdrulla AD, diSibio G, Bush G, Nofziger D, Hicks C, Weinmaster G, Barres BA. (1998). Notch receptor activation inhibits oligodendrocyte differentiation. *Neuron* **21**(1), 63–75.

Wang S, Sdrulla A, Johnson JE, Yokota Y, Barres BA. (2001). A role for the helix-loop-helix protein Id2 in the control of oligodendrocyte development. *Neuron* **29**(3), 603–14.

Wang W, Gao XF, Xiao L, Xiang ZH, He C. (2011). K(V)7/KCNQ channels are functionally expressed in oligodendrocyte progenitor cells. *PLoS One* **6**(7), e21792.

Wegner M. (2000). Transcriptional control in myelinating glia: flavors and spices. *Glia* **31**(1), 1–14.

Wegner M. (2008). A matter of identity: transcriptional control in oligodendrocytes. *Journal of Molecular Neuroscience* **35**(1), 3–12.

Weimbs T, Stoffel W. (1992). Proteolipid protein (PLP) of CNS myelin: positions of free, disulfide-bonded, and fatty acid thioester-linked cysteine residues and implications for the membrane topology of PLP. *Biochemistry* **31**(49), 12289–96.

Weruaga-Prieto E, Eggli P, Celio MR. (1996). Topographic variations in rat brain oligodendrocyte morphology elucidated by injection of Lucifer Yellow in fixed tissue slices. *Journal of Neurocytology* **25**(1), 19–31.

White R, Gonsior C, Krämer-Albers EM, Stöhr N, Hüttelmaier S, Trotter J. (2008). Activation of oligodendroglial Fyn kinase enhances translation of mRNAs transported in hnRNP A2-dependent RNA granules. *Journal of Cell Biology* **181**(4), 579–586.

Williamson AV, Compston DA, Randall AD. (1997). Analysis of the ion channel complement of the rat oligodendrocyte progenitor in a commonly studied *in vitro* preparation. *European Journal of Neuroscience* **9**(4), 706–20.

Wu Q, Miller RH, Ransohoff RM, Robinson S, Bu J, Nishiyama A. (2000). Elevated levels of the chemokine GRO-1 correlate with elevated oligodendrocyte progenitor proliferation in the jimpy mutant. *Journal of Neuroscience* **20**(7), 2609–17.

Yamashita T, Wu YP, Sandhoff R, Werth N, Mizukami H, Ellis JM, Dupree JL, Geyer R, Sandhoff K, Proia RL. (2005). Interruption of ganglioside synthesis produces central nervous system degeneration and altered axon-glial interactions. *Proceedings of The National Academy Of Sciences Of The United States Of America* **102**(8), 2725–30.

Ye F, Chen Y, Hoang T, Montgomery RL, Zhao XH, Bu H, Hu T, Taketo MM, van Es JH, Clevers H. *et al.* (2009). HDAC1 and HDAC2 regulate oligodendrocyte differentiation by disrupting the beta-catenin-TCF interaction. *Nature Neuroscience* **12**(7), 829–38.

Ye P, Carson J, D'Ercole AJ. (1995). *In vivo* actions of insulin-like growth factor-I (IGF-I) on brain myelination: studies of IGF-I and IGF binding protein-1 (IGFBP-1) transgenic mice. *Journal of Neuroscience* **15**(11), 7344–56.

Yu Y, Casaccia P, Lu QR. (2010). Shaping the oligodendrocyte identity by epigenetic control. *Epigenetics* **5**(2), 124–8.

Yuan X, Eisen AM, McBain CJ, Gallo V. (1998). A role for glutamate and its receptors in the regulation of oligodendrocyte development in cerebellar tissue slices. *Development* **125**(15), 2901–14.

Zeger M, Popken G, Zhang J, Xuan S, Lu QR, Schwab MH, Nave KA, Rowitch D, D'Ercole AJ, Ye P. (2007). Insulin-like growth factor type 1 receptor signaling in the cells of oligodendrocyte lineage is required for normal *in vivo* oligodendrocyte development and myelination. *Glia* **55**(4), 400–11.

Zhang Y, Taveggia C, Melendez-Vasquez C, Einheber S, Raine CS, Salzer JL, Brosnan CF, John GR. (2006). Interleukin-11 potentiates oligodendrocyte survival and maturation, and myelin formation. *Journal of Neuroscience* **26**(47), 12174–85.

Zhao X, He X, Han X, Yu Y, Ye F, Chen Y, Hoang T, Xu X, Mi QS, Xin M. *et al.* (2010). MicroRNA-mediated control of oligodendrocyte differentiation. *Neuron* **65**(5), 612–26.

Zhou Q, Anderson DJ. (2002). The bHLH transcription factors OLIG2 and OLIG1 couple neuronal and glial subtype specification. *Cell* **109**(1), 61–73.

Zhou Q, Choi G, Anderson DJ. (2001). The bHLH transcription factor Olig2 promotes oligodendrocyte differentiation in collaboration with Nkx2.2. *Neuron* **31**(5), 791–807.

Zolova OE, Wight PA. (2011). YY1 negatively regulates mouse myelin proteolipid protein (Plp1) gene expression in oligodendroglial cells. *ASN Neuro* **3**(4).

Zonouzi M, Renzi M, Farrant M, Cull-Candy SG. (2011). Bidirectional plasticity of calcium-permeable AMPA receptors in oligodendrocyte lineage cells. *Nature Neuroscience* **14**(11), 1430–8.

# 6
# NG2-glial Cells

## 6.1   Definition of NG2-glia

Since their discovery in the 1980s, NG2-glial cells have been a point of controversy (for review see Richardson *et al.*, 2011). The identification of NG2-glia was made possible by the development of antibodies to the chondroitin sulphate proteoglycan NG2 (cspg4)

*Glial Physiology and Pathophysiology*, First Edition. Alexei Verkhratsky and Arthur Butt.
© 2013 by John Wiley & Sons, Ltd. Published 2013 by John Wiley & Sons, Ltd.

by Stallcup and colleagues (Levine & Card, 1987; Stallcup, 1981; Stallcup & Beasley, 1987). NG2-glia are equivalent to O-2A cells identified by Raff and colleagues (Ffrench-Constant & Raff, 1986; Raff *et al.*, 1984; Stallcup and Beasley, 1987; see Chapter 2).

Most researchers consider NG2-glia to be oligodendrocyte progenitor cells (OPCs), since they express PDGFRα, and NG2+/PDGFRα+ cells generate oligo-dendrocytes in the developing and adult CNS (Kang *et al.*, 2010; Rivers *et al.*, 2008; Zhu *et al.*, 2011; see Chapter 5). There can be no reasonable doubt that most, although possibly not all, NG2-glia have an oligodendrocyte lineage. Similarly, in the developing brain, most NG2+ cells are OPCs that migrate from their sources to populate the entire CNS and generate oligodendrocytes.

So what is the controversy? Why are NG2-glia not simply called OPCs and be done with it? It is because very few NG2-glia appear to generate oligodendrocytes in the adult CNS, and it is far from clear this is their *raison d'être* (Butt *et al.*, 2002). NG2-glia are a ubiquitous population throughout the adult CNS, and many located in grey matter do not appear to generate oligodendrocytes (Dimou *et al.*, 2008; Figure 6.1). Furthermore, NG2-glia have unique features among glia in that they form synapses with neurones and display spontaneous and evoked synaptic currents (see review by Bergles *et al.*, 2010). As a result, NG2-glia have been considered a fourth distinct glial cell type, after astrocytes, oligodendrocytes and microglia.

Alternative names for NG2-glia, besides OPCs, are synantocytes (Butt *et al.*, 2002) and polydendrocytes (Nishiyama *et al.*, 2009). Here, we will use the term NG2-glia to define cells with the following features in the adult CNS:

1.  First and foremost, they are defined by their co-expression of NG2 *and* PDGFRα, but not GFAP, myelin genes (e.g. MBP, PLP etc) or markers for microglia.

2.  NG2-glia have a stellate morphology, with highly branched processes that extend for 50-100 μm from a centrally located cell body, which is irregularly shaped, with thin cytoplasm, and is organelle poor.

3.  They are slowly proliferating cells that undergo asymmetric cell division and increase proliferation in response to CNS insults.

4.  They generate oligodendrocytes in the adult CNS *in vivo*.

5.  They receive synaptic input from neurones, at dendrites and axons (Bergles *et al.*, 2010).

However, even these definitions are not clear cut. For example, there is not 100 per cent overlap of the NG2+ and PDGFRα+ populations in the adult CNS, and there is heterogeneous expression of other OPC/oligodendrocyte lineage markers in NG2-glia (e.g. Olig2 and Nkx2.2). Expression of NG2 *per se* is not definitive for NG2-glia, since pericytes also express NG2. However, pericytes and NG2-glia can be distin-guished by their expression of PDGFRβ and PDGFRα, respectively. Even so, it is not certain how complete this segregation is. In transgenic reporter mice, some NG2-glia

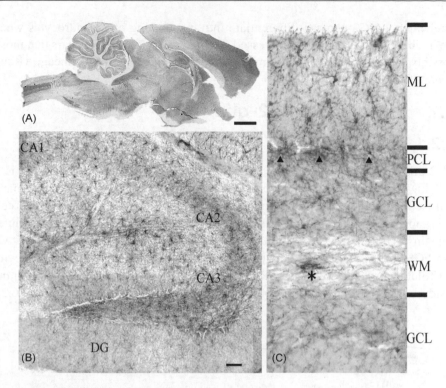

**Figure 6.1** Distribution of NG2-glia in the adult brain.
Saggital section of adult rat brain immunolabelled with anti-NG2 antibody. (A) Low magnification illustrates that NG2 immunostaining highlights the architecture of the brain and distinguishes the neuronal layers. This is illustrated further in the hippocampus (B) and the cerebellum (C). NG2-glia are abundant in grey and white matter and form a 'mosaic' covering the entire brain (B). NG2-glia densely populate regions where myelination is not evident in the adult, such as the molecular layer of the cerebellum (C).
From Butt *et al.*, 2005, with permission.

express reporters for astrocytes (e.g. GFAP) and oligodendrocytes (e.g. PLP1) and, following injury, microglia may express NG2 (Gao *et al.*, 2010). In addition, NG2-glia have been reported to express the 'astrocyte markers' S100β and glutamine synthetase. Moreover, at most only 50 per cent of NG2-glia appear to be in cell cycle (Kukley *et al.*, 2008; Psachoulia *et al.*, 2009), and a similar proportion do not appear to be involved in generating oligodendrocytes in the adult CNS *in vivo* (Dimou *et al.*, 2008; Ehninger *et al.*, 2011). This provokes questions of whether all NG2-glia have an OPC function. Even direct synaptic input may be a feature of the postnatal brain, and there appears to be a developmental shift to a rather non-specific diffuse volume (spillover) extrasynaptic mode of transmission (Maldonado *et al.*, 2011).

It is likely that NG2-glia display heterogeneous properties, and this reflects the diversity of a single cell type, depending on its location within the CNS and its proliferation/differentiation status at a particular point of time. For example, in regions where myelin is not normally found – such as in the molecular layer of the cerebellum – NG2-glia can differentiate into myelinating oligodendrocytes when the inhibitory environment is suppressed (Givogri *et al.*, 2002). It appears that most, possibly all, NG2-glia remain committed to the oligodendrocyte lineage (Kang *et al.*, 2010).

# 6.2    Structure of NG2-glia

## 6.2.1    Identification

NG2-glia are identified by their expression of NG2 and PDGFRα. NG2 is a 300 kDa membrane-spanning core glycoprotein with binding sites for many extracellular and intracellular proteins implicated in the regulation of cell migration and proliferation (Stallcup & Huang, 2008). The NG2 extracellular domain has binding sites for α1 integrins and growth factors, including PDGF-AA and FGF2. The cytoplasmic domain has a PDZ-binding motif that interacts with scaffolding proteins MUPP1, GRIP1 and syntenin-1, together with threonine residues that are sites of phosphorylation by PKCα and ERK (Figure 6.2).

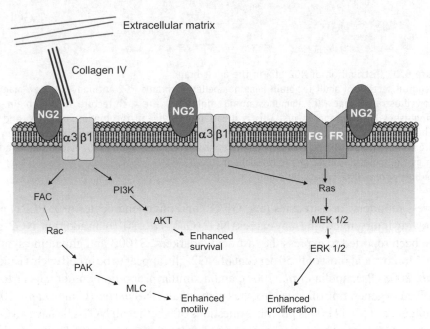

**Figure 6.2**   Functional interactions of the NG2 CSPG.

NG2 provides a linkage between the cell surface and the extracellular matrix via its interaction with type VI collagen, and it activates α3β1 integrin signalling on the cell surface to promote enhanced motility through the FAC/Rac pathway. NG2-α3β1 integrin signalling also promotes survival (via the PI3/AKT pathway) and proliferation (via MAPK). NG2 also potentiates growth factor receptor signalling to promote cell proliferation, here illustrated by the FGFR dimer.

Drawn from (Stallcup & Huang, 2008).

PDGFRα mediates the survival, proliferation and migration effects of PDGF-AA on OPCs (see Chapter 5), although its effects on adult NG2-glia have not been studied in detail.

Transgenic mouse lines that express reporter proteins driven by OPC genes identify NG2-glia, e.g. Pdgfra- and Olig2-EGFP mice. Similarly, mouse lines that express reporters driven by NG2 express PDGFRα and other OPC markers, e.g. NG2-YFP knock-in mice (Karram *et al.*, 2008) and NG2-DsRed BAC mice (Zhu *et al.*, 2008). In NG2-YFP knock-in mice, NG2-glia displayed heterogeneity with regard to expression of astroglial markers S100β and glutamine synthetase, and in their electrophysiological properties. Notably, there is no discernible developmental or behavioural phenotype in heterozygous NG2-YFP mice that lack one allele of the Cspg-4 gene as a consequence of the YFP knock-in. Similarly, NG2 null mice display only a subtle phenotype, with a decrease in OPC proliferation and delayed myelination (Kucharova & Stallcup, 2010). This contrasts dramatically with PDGFRα in OPCs, which are essential for the generation of OPCs and oligodendrocytes (see Chapter 5). In short, the functions of the NG2 CSPG in NG2-glia are unresolved.

## 6.2.2   Morphology and distribution

NG2-glia have a multi-processed morphology, with their process domains or territories overlapping slightly at their edges (Leoni *et al.*, 2009).This is most evident in grey matter, where NG2-glia are distributed as a 'mosaic' (Figure 6.3).

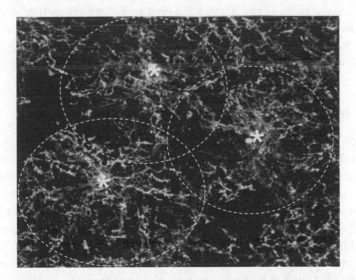

**Figure 6.3**   NG2-glial cell domains. Confocal microscopic images of coronal sections of the pons from adult mice immunolabelled for NG2. NG2-glia have a multi-processed morphology, with their process domains or territories overlapping slightly at their edges (circles).

In white matter, NG2-glia have an elongated appearance, extending processes along the axonal axis and, in the compacted white matter, individual cellular domains are difficult to distinguish (Butt *et al.*, 1999). Ultrastructurally, NG2-glia have a quiescent appearance, with elongate nuclei, with little chromatin and a thin rim of pale organelle-poor cytoplasm containing some short, rough endoplasmic reticulum, small mitochondria and few free polyribosomes (Peters, 2004). NG2-glia constitute 8–9 per cent of total cells in the white matter and 2–3 per cent of total cells in the gray matter, with an estimated density of 10–140 per mm$^2$ in the adult CNS (Nishiyama *et al.*, 2009). The ratio of NG2-glia to oligodendrocytes ranges from 1: 1 in the rat hippocampus to 1: 10 in the cat spinal cord. In grey matter, the cell bodies of NG2-glia are often applied directly to neuronal somata.

## 6.2.3   Relationship of NG2-glia with neuroglial domains

NG2-glia and astrocytes have overlapping domains (Figure 6.4). Indeed, the somata of NG2-glia and astrocytes are often adjacent and there is extensive inter-digitation of their overlapping process fields (Wigley & Butt, 2009). NG2-glia and astrocytes serve the same neurones, but whereas astroglia interact with hundreds of thousands of synapses (see Chapter 4), NG2-glia on average may form electrophysiologically active contacts with less than 20 synapses (Bergles *et al.*, 2010).

However, extrasynaptic transmission may be more important in adult NG2-glia (Velez-Fort *et al.*, 2010). The overlapping domain organization of NG2-glia and astrocytes may also be important for glia-glia signalling (Hamilton *et al.*, 2010). The domain organisation of astrocytes is considered to be important for integrated activity at the synapses in their domain (see Chapter 4), but the significance of NG2-glial cell domains is uncertain.

## 6.2.4   NG2-glia and synapses

EM studies show that NG2-glia contact synapses in grey matter and electro-physiological studies show they display both GABAergic and glutamatergic inputs (Figure 6.5; Bergles *et al.*, 2010). In white matter, NG2-glia respond to glutamate via processes that contact nodes of Ranvier in myelinated axons, and synaptic sites in unmyelinated axons (Butt *et al.*, 1999; Hamilton *et al.*, 2010; Kukley *et al.*, 2007). Dividing NG2-glia retain their synaptic inputs (Ge *et al.*, 2009; Kukley *et al.*, 2008) and synaptic input disappears as NG2-glia differentiate into oligodendrocytes (De Biase *et al.*, 2010; Kukley *et al.*, 2010). In NG2-glia that do not differentiate into oligodendrocytes, there is a postnatal switch from synaptic to extrasynaptic transmission (Figure 6.6; Velez-Fort *et al.*, 2010).

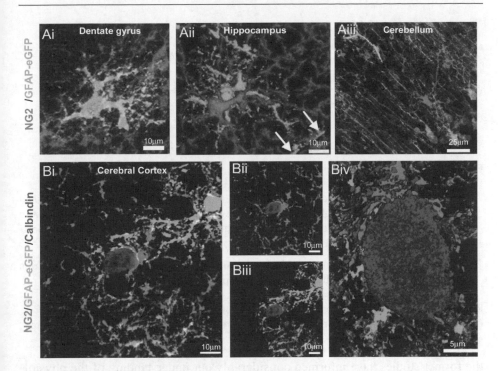

**Figure 6.4**  Domain structure of NG2-glia and astroglia.

Confocal microscopic images of sagittal sections from brain of adult GFAP-eGFP mice, to identify astrocytes (green), and immunolabelled for NG2 (red) and calbindin (blue) to identify NG2-glia and neurones, respectively.

A.  NG2-glia and astroglia are arranged in overlapping radial domains throughout grey matter, as illustrated in the dentate gyrus (Ai). NG2-glial cell and astrocyte somata are often directly apposed and have completely overlapping domains, with processes that interdigitate extensively, often extending to end on blood vessels (Aii, arrows). In the cerebellum, NG2-glia traverse the different layers to associate with multiple Bergmann glia and velate astrocytes (Aiii). The process of NG2-glia and primary process of Bergmann glia are extensively apposed along their length.

B.  NG2-glia and astrocytes serve the same neurones, as illustrated here in the cortex. NG2-glia and astrocytes are associated with ten or more neurones within their overlapping domains, and their processes almost circumnavigate the same neuronal somata. (Full colour version in plate section.)

# 6.3  Physiology of NG2-glia

The terms OPCs and NG2-glia are often used interchangeably. Indeed, there have been considerable electrophysiological studies on cultured OPCs since the 1980s, which are mostly derived from embryonic or postnatal brains. It is not easy to extrapolate directly from studies on cultured OPCs to NG2-glia *in situ*, although

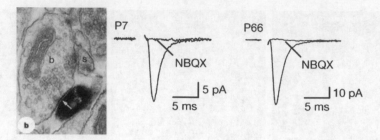

**Figure 6.5**   Synaptic relationships of NG2-glia.

A.   Electronmicrograph of a process (black, peroxidase reaction) from a physiologically identified, biocytin-labelled NG2-glial cell receiving a synapse (arrow) from a bouton (b) that also
gives a synapse to a dendritic spine(s). The NG2-glial cell process approaches the spine post-
synaptic density to within 110 nm.

B.   Excitatory post-synaptic currents (EPSCs) from NG2-glia in hippocampal slices prepared from
different age animals were blocked by NBQX (5 μM).

Reproduced, with permission, from Bergles, D. E., Roberts, D. B., Somogyl, P. and Jahr, C. E.
(2000) Glutamatergic synapses on oligodendrocyte precursor cells in the hippocampus. Nature
405: 6783. © Nature Publishing Group.

the former studies have informed considerably our understanding of the physiology of NG2-glia in the developing brain.

In more recent times, there have been far more studies on NG2-glia *in situ*.
However, these are most often in the postnatal brain, where NG2-glia either
generate oligodendrocytes (i.e. behave as OPCs) or are destined to persist as adult
NG2-glia. Hence, considerable care must be taken in interpreting the available
literature with respect to the physiological properties of adult NG2-glia. The
following account refers to NG2-glia *in situ*, and where they are known, differences
between postnatal and adult NG2-glia are noted.

## 6.3.1   Membrane properties

Whole-cell recordings from NG2-glia in brain slices isolated from young adult mice
indicate that they have a total cell capacitance of approximately 20 pF, consistent with
their modest size. NG2-glia in postnatal brain slices are reported to have a highly
negative resting membrane potential of approximately −90 mV and a membrane
resistance of 300 MΩ, suggesting a primary role for $K^+$ channels that are open at rest.

## 6.3.2   Gap junctional coupling

NG2-glia do not display dye coupling or electrical coupling (Lin and Bergles,
2002). Analysis of transgenic mice expressing beta-Gal under regulatory elements
of the Cx43 promoter revealed the absence of Cx43 in cells with the

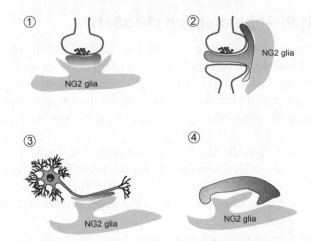

**Figure 6.6** Different modes of transmission between neurones and NG2-glia.

1. Synaptic transmission. Vesicle-containing pre-synaptic compartments directly contact an NG2-glial cell process, forming specialised synaptic junctions similar to those described in neurones. Released neurotransmitters diffuse across a narrow cleft to rapidly activate high densities of post-synaptic receptors.

2. Local spillover transmission. NG2-glial cell processes passing very close to neuronal synapses sense locally neurotransmitters spilling out of the synaptic cleft. No miniature events would be detectable in this case.

3. Ectopic transmission. Neurotransmitters are released at non-synaptic sites from small 'synaptic-like' vesicles located at varicosities along axons to activate extrasynaptic receptors expressed at these sites in NG2-glia.

4. Diffuse volume transmission. Diffuse transmission may occur at non-synaptic sites and, compared to other types of transmission modes, released neurotransmitters would have to cross large distances (typically $> 1\,\mu m$) before reaching a targeted cell.
   Notably, modes (2) and (4) would include neurotransmitters release from astrocytes, which are closely apposed to NG2-glia (see Figure 6.4), although direct synaptic communication akin to those illustrated in (1) and (3) have not been identified between NG2-glia and astrocytes.

Redrawn based on (Kukley *et al.*, 2010).

electrophysiological features of NG2-glia (Wallraff *et al.*, 2004). Connexin32 gap junction protein has been localised to a subset of NG2+/PDGFRα + early OPCs in the dentate gyrus of adult mice and, in Cx32-deficient mice, there was an increase in the total number of proliferating nestin+/NG2+ progenitors in the sub-granular zone and a defect in oligodendrogenesis in this subpopulation (Melanson-Drapeau *et al.*, 2003). However, it seems that most NG2-glia in the brain parenchyma do not express gap junctions.

## 6.3.3   Voltage-operated ion channels

*Potassium channels*: There is evidence for both A-type and delayed-rectifier $K^+$ channels in NG2-glia, and molecularly they are likely to comprise $K_v1.3$ and $K_v1.5$ channels (Chittajallu *et al.*, 2004). In addition, NG2-glia express $K_{ir}$ currents, and studies in $K_{ir}4.1$ knockout mice indicate they are the dominant resting conductance in NG2-glia and play a dominant role in controlling the resting potential (Djukic *et al.*, 2007).

*Sodium channels*: NG2-glia express TTX-sensitive $Na_v$. In most NG2-glia in the mature CNS, injection of depolarizing current does not elicit a regenerative, $Na^+$-dependent action potential (De Biase *et al.*, 2010). However, one or more $Na^+$ spikes can be elicited in some NG2-glia upon depolarisation (Chittajallu *et al.*, 2004; Karadottir *et al.*, 2008).

*Calcium channels*: Whole-cell recordings from NG2-glia have revealed the presence of L-type ($Ca_v1.2$, 1.3) and T-type ($Ca_v3.1$, 3.2) $Ca^{2+}$ channels (Haberlandt *et al.*, 2011). These currents are rather small, indicating that the overall density is low. There is also evidence of $Ca^{2+}$-induced $Ca^{2+}$ release (CICR), $Na^+$-dependent $Ca^{2+}$ exchange and plasma membrane store operated channels such as TRPC1 (Haberlandt *et al.*, 2011; Paez *et al.*, 2011; Tong *et al.*, 2009). At rest, the membrane potential of NG2-glia is more negative than $-30$mV, activation threshold of $Ca_v$s, suggesting that NG2-glia would require substantive depolarization for $Ca^{2+}$ influx through these channels. This may occur within microdomains at process terminals contacting axons and synapses.

## 6.3.4   Neurotransmitter receptors

*Glutamate Receptors*: A key feature of most NG2-glia studied is their prominent expression of AMPA-type glutamate receptors. Activation of AMPA receptors in NG2-glia in brain slices triggers inward currents (Figure 6.5; Bergles *et al.*, 2000). Analysis of mRNA expression by single cell analysis in OPCs suggested a predominance of GluA4 (Seifert *et al.*, 1997). A small number of kainate receptors also appear to be expressed by NG2-glia (Kukley & Dietrich, 2009). NG2-glia express NMDA receptors with reduced sensitivity to block by external $Mg^{2+}$, suggesting that they could contribute to significant $Ca^{2+}$ influx at resting membrane potential (De Biase *et al.*, 2010; Karadottir *et al.*, 2005; Ziskin *et al.*, 2007). Not all NG2-glia express NMDA receptors.

*GABA receptors*: NG2-glia that are associated with GABAergic neurones express functional $GABA_A$ receptors (Lin & Bergles, 2004; Velez-Fort *et al.*, 2010). $GABA_A$ currents in NG2-glia reverse at $-43$ mV, about 30 mV more positive than the $GABA_A$ reversal potential in neurones at this age, indicating that NG2-glia maintain a high intracellular $Cl^-$ concentration. The expression of $GABA_A$ receptors by NG2-glia appears to reflect the level of neuronal GABAergic fibres in the region.

*Other Neurotransmitter Receptors*: NG2-glia have been reported to express nAChR, mGluR, $\alpha_1$ adrenergic receptors and P2 purinergic receptors (Haberlandt *et al.*, 2011; Hamilton *et al.*, 2010; Papay *et al.*, 2004; Velez-Fort *et al.*, 2009). Indeed, gene expression studies in OPCs (Cahoy *et al.*, 2008) suggest that NG2-glia may have the capacity to express most, if not all, neurotransmitter receptors, most likely reflecting the neurones they are associated with. However, a systematic assessment of the expression and function of different neurotransmitters by NG2-glia in different brain regions is lacking.

## 6.3.5 Neurone-NG2-glial cell signalling at synapses

*Excitatory post-synaptic currents (EPSCs)* mediated by AMPA receptors are evident in NG2-glia in brain slices from all brain regions where these cells has been studied (Figure 6.5), suggesting that this mode of communication is a conserved property of these glial cells (Bergles *et al.*, 2010). EPSCs have the same stochastic, spontaneous vesicle fusion events that occur at synapses between neurones. EM studies have demonstrated pre-synaptic boutons containing small vesicles $\approx 30$ nm in diameter in direct apposition to the processes of NG2-glia (Figure 6.5; Bergles *et al.*, 2000; Haberlandt *et al.*, 2011; Kukley *et al.*, 2007). In contrast to most neuronal glutamatergic synapses, NMDARs contribute little to spontaneous or evoked EPSCs (De Biase *et al.*, 2010), suggesting that NMDAR in NG2 glia are either predominantly extrasynaptic, or that there are only a small number of receptors present at each synapse.

*Spontaneous, miniature and evoked GABA$_A$ receptor-mediated currents* have been observed in recordings from NG2-glia in the hippocampus, cortex and cerebellum (Maldonado *et al.*, 2011). In the cortex, there is an age-dependent shift from direct activation of these receptors at synapses to indirect activation through spillover (Figure 6.6; Velez-Fort *et al.*, 2010). Thus, direct GABAergic synapses are restricted to the first postnatal month in cortical NG2-glia, whereas glutamatergic inputs appear to remain prominent into adulthood.

*The function of NG2-glial cell synapses is unresolved.* There is a dramatic loss of synapses when NG2-glia differentiate into oligodendrocytes, suggesting they may have a role in regulating proliferation and differentiation of NG2-glia (De Biase *et al.*, 2010; Kukley *et al.*, 2010). Evaluation of the function of neurotransmitter signalling in NG2-glia *in situ* is complicated by indirect actions on neurones and astrocytes. For example, pharmacological studies indicate functional NMDA receptors in NG2-glia, but selective deletion of GluN1 in NG2-glia demonstrated that NMDA receptor signalling is redundant in these cells (De Biase *et al.*, 2011).

It is assumed that synaptic signalling onto NG2-glia controls their behaviour and, in particular, their function of oligodendrocyte generation. However, the response of NG2-glia to glutamatergic and GABAergic synaptic inputs is minimal and is insufficient to activate voltage-operated ion channels. The permeability of

AMPA and NMDA receptors to $Ca^{2+}$ provides a potential mechanism by which they could regulate NG2-glial cell behaviour (Haberlandt et al., 2011). However, it is unclear whether activation of AMPA or NMDA receptors mediates physiological $Ca^{2+}$ signals in NG2-glia in situ and, if they do, it is likely to be within microdomains (Hamilton et al., 2010). It is possible that rapid neuronal synaptic communication onto NG2-glia controls aspects of their physiology that we have not yet discovered, and which is unrelated to their potential to develop into oligodendrocytes.

## 6.4    Proliferation of NG2-glia and generation of oligodendrocytes

### 6.4.1    Normal adult brain

Developmentally, there is no distinction between NG2-glia and OPCs, and they refer to the same cell. In the postnatal brain, OPCs can be defined as constantly dividing cells that give rise to myelinating oligodendrocytes and adult NG2-glia, as demonstrated unequivocally in fate-mapping studies (Dimou et al., 2008; Kang et al., 2010; Rivers et al., 2008; Zhu et al., 2011). In the adult CNS, only 50 per cent of NG2-glia are in cell cycle, and the cell cycle time is >70 days, compared to 2–3 days in the early postnatal brain (Kukley et al., 2008; Psachoulia et al., 2009).

Despite their abundance, little is known about the fate of constantly proliferating NG2-glia in the adult CNS. In the adult, it has been estimated that 17 to 30 per cent of oligodendrocytes are generated de novo from NG2-glia within a period of 2–3 months in young adult mice (Rivers et al., 2008; Zhu et al., 2011). This contributes to the gradual rise in the total number of oligodendrocytes in the adult brain, as well as the replacement of existing or degenerating oligodendrocytes (Peters & Sethares, 2004).

Fate mapping in Olig2-Cre mice demonstrated that NG2-glia are involved in the continuous generation of myelinating oligodendrocytes in white matter, but those in grey matter generated mostly post-mitotic NG2-glia and not oligodendrocytes (Dimou et al., 2008). This implies there is either a constant turnover of NG2-glia or a gradual rise in their number with age. Hence, it is unclear whether heterogeneity in the proliferation status of NG2-glia, and their contribution to the generation of oligodendrocytes, represents distinct functional subtypes of NG2-glia. In this respect, the G protein-coupled membrane receptor GPR17 and the tetraspanin protein CD9 may be useful for distinguishing between NG2-glia that are, and are not, actively involved in generating oligodendrocytes in the adult mammalian brain. GPR17 specifically identifies slowly proliferating NG2-glia that form pre-oligodendrocytes (Fumagalli et al., 2011), whereas CD9 is expressed when NG2-glia differentiate into premyelinating oligodendrocytes and not by adult NG2-glia (Terada *et al.*, 2002).

### 6.4.2   Are NG2-glia multipotent stem cells?

Fate mapping studies have also indicated that during development, NG2-glia generate more than 40 per cent of protoplasmic astrocytes in the ventral forebrain, but not those in the white matter or dorsal forebrain (Zhu *et al.*, 2008). In contrast, there is little evidence that NG2-glia in the adult brain generate astrocytes. A small population of NG2-glia in the adult also generate neurones in the piriform cortex (Guo *et al.*, 2010; Rivers *et al.*, 2008). However, most fate mapping studies conclude that NG2-glia generate only oligodendrocytes at all ages (Kang *et al.*, 2010; Zhu *et al.*, 2011). The current consensus is that NG2-glia do not contribute significantly to the generation of new astrocytes or neurones in the normal adult brain (Richardson *et al.*, 2011).

### 6.4.3   Response of NG2-glia to injury and demyelination

NG2-glia respond to a variety of insults to the CNS by increased proliferation and dramatically altering their morphology, often seen as shortening and thickening of their processes and a strong up-regulation of NG2 expression (Figure 6.7). Genetic fate mapping studies using Pdgfra-creER mice have provided direct evidence that NG2-glia in the spinal cord generate new oligodendrocytes that remyelinate demyelinated lesions (Tripathi *et al.*, 2010; Zawadzka *et al.*, 2010). NG2-glial cell senescence may contribute to reduced remyelination efficiency in the ageing brain (see Chapter 5). In addition, NG2 is an important component of the glial scar follow injury, although it is not clear that NG2-glia are the predominant source of NG2 at the lesion site.

## 6.5   Relationship between NG2-glia and CNS pericytes

### 6.5.1   Identification of pericytes

In addition to NG2-glia in the CNS, pericytes strongly express the NG2 CSPG and are abundantly distributed perivascularly throughout the CNS (Figure 6.8; for review, see (Krueger & Bechmann, 2010). Notably, CNS pericytes are derived from neural crest cells in common with PNS glia (see Chapter 8, Section 8.1.2), and the transcription factor Sox10 plays a key role in their development, as it does in NG2-glia and other oligodendroglial cells (see Chapter 5, Section 5.4.2; Simon

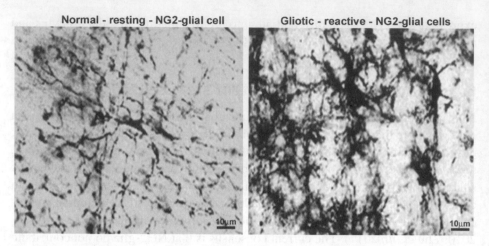

**Figure 6.7**   NG2-glia are highly reactive cells.

NG2 immunolabelling in the anterior medullary velum of the rat. Normal NG2-glia, in their resting or quiescent state, have a typical stellate morphology with a small irregular cell body, from which emanate delicate processes that extend radially and branch occasionally. Following most, if not all, insults to the CNS, NG2-glia undergo a reactive response akin to astrocytes and microglia, characterised by increased proliferation and a dramatic change in their morphology. Reactive NG2-glia display a strong up-regulation of NG2, with enlarged cell bodies and shortened and thickened processes that have a fibrous appearance. There is an overall increase in the density of NG2-glia within damaged areas.

*et al.*, 2012). Pericytes are defined by their location on the outer face of vascular endothelial cells, with which they share a common basal lamina, and they can be identified by their expression of NG2, PDGFR$\beta$ and $\alpha$-smooth muscle actin ($\alpha$SMA) (Stallcup, 2002; Winkler *et al.*, 2010).

Pericytes are prominent in transgenic mice in which reporter proteins are driven by NG2 (Figure 6.8), and they can be distinguished from NG2-glia by their respective and exclusive expression of PDGFR$\beta$ and PDGFR$\alpha$ in the adult mouse brain. The name pericyte literally means 'around the cell', after their intimate and defining association with endothelial cells, with one pericyte wrapping around multiple endothelial cells which line the lumen of the blood vessel. The basal lamina of the cerebral micro-vasculature surrounds the endothelial cells and pericytes and is in direct contact with astrocyte perivascular end-feet, which together form the elements of the blood-brain barrier. The precise functions of pericytes are not fully resolved, but they are known to play important roles during angiogenesis and maintenance of the vasculature.

## 6.5.2   Developmental origin of pericytes

The generation of an inducible Sox10-iCreERT2 BAC transgenic mouse line demonstrated that pericytes are derived embryonically from Sox10+ neural crest cells (NCC) (Simon *et al.*, 2012). Fate-mapping in the Sox10-iCreERT2 mouse line

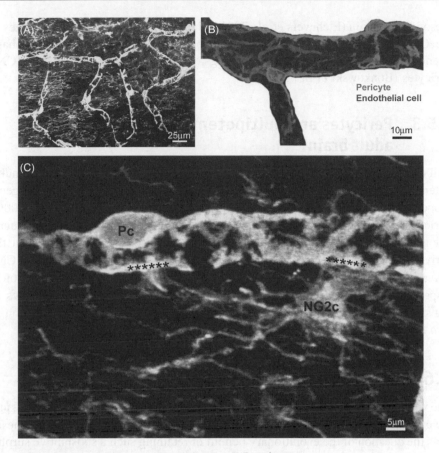

**Figure 6.8**  Relationship between NG2-glia and CNS pericytes.
NG2 immunolabelling in sections of optic nerve from adult mice.

A.  Pericytes strongly express NG2 and are abundantly distributed on blood vessels; parenchymal stellate NG2-glia are distributed between the blood vessels.

B.  The name pericyte literally means 'around the cell', after their intimate and defining association with blood vessels, with one pericyte wrapping around multiple endothelial cells which line the lumen of the blood vessel.

C.  Periocytes (Pc) and NG2-glia (NG2c) form expanded sites of contact (asterisks) which, at the confocal microscopic level, are often too close to separate.

showed that, following induction in the embryo, the progeny of Sox10+ cells in the cerebral grey matter were oligodendrocytes, NG2-glia and pericytes. This study provided direct evidence in support of earlier studies in chick embryos showing that pericytes are derived from cranial NCC, but not endothelial cells, which are exclusively mesoderm-derived (Etchevers *et al.*, 2001; Korn *et al.*, 2002). Studies in the chick indicated that NCC-derived pericytes specifically supply the capillaries of the forebrain, while the rest of the CNS capillaries are populated by pericytes of mesodermal origin (Etchevers *et al.*, 2001). Hence, the origin of all the pericytes in the CNS remains an open question. CNS pericytes can take on a macrophage phenotype in culture, evidence supporting a mesenchymal origin of some CNS pericytes (Bonkowski *et al.*, 2011).

### 6.5.3 Pericytes are multipotent stem cells in the adult brain

Cell culture experiments have provided evidence that CNS pericytes exhibit multi-potential stem cell characteristics and differentiate into cells displaying the antigenic properties of astrocytes, neurones and oligodendrocytes (Dore-Duffy *et al.*, 2006). Pericytes are nestin+/NG2+ and, in response to FGF2, they differentiate into neural lineage cells. It remains to be seen whether this is also possible *in vivo*, but the perivascular niche has emerged as a key element of neurogenesis in the adult CNS (Tavazoie *et al.*, 2008). In addition, pericytes migrate from their vascular location in response to stress injury (Dore-Duffy *et al.*, 2000). The ability of pericytes to transform into NG2+ OPCs *in vitro* and migrate from their vascular location *in vivo* raises questions about their relationship with parenchymal NG2-glia.

## 6.6 Evolution of NG2-glia

The very limited production of oligodendrocytes in the adult mammalian CNS, and the evidence that not all NG2-glia are actively involved in oligodendrogliogenesis, begs the question of the evolutionary benefit of retaining such a substantive surplus of cells. In contrast to mammals, the brain of adult non-mammalian vertebrates exhibits a higher proliferative and neurogenic activity. As is the case in mammals, proliferation and neurogenesis in lower vertebrates occurs around the telencephalic ventricular zones, although proliferative activity has been observed in the brain parenchyma of some species of adult fish and frogs (Marz *et al.*, 2010; Simmons *et al.*, 2008). However, the main proliferating and neurogenic cells in fish and frogs are radial glia, not parenchymal NG2-glia, which are a largely non-proliferative population (Almli & Wilczynski, 2007; Marz *et al.*, 2010).

It is not certain that NG2-glia (adult OPCs) regenerate oligodendrocytes or are responsible for remyelination in fish or frogs. In adult fish, for example, following CNS axon transection, there is efficient regeneration and remyelination, although the latter appears to be performed mainly by Schwann cells (Nona *et al.*, 1992, 2000). Interestingly, slowly proliferating Olig2-expressing cells with the appearance of NG2-glia have been identified within the parenchyma of the telencephalon of the adult zebra fish, and these cells did not display a profound increase in proliferation in response to injury (Marz *et al.*, 2011).

In conclusion, the phylogeny of NG2-glia is unclear, and it is possible that NG2-glia as defined above (Section 6.1) are a mammalian evolutionary development.

In mammals, there is continued generation of oligodendrocytes in the adult brain and, in its absence, there would be devastating effects on cognitive function. This would be a strong evolutionary drive for maintaining a substantial population of NG2-glia long after the main period of myelination.

## 6.7 Concluding remarks

It has now become widely accepted that NG2-glia represent a fourth resident glial cell population in the normal adult CNS. In the postnatal CNS, NG2-glia equate with OPCs, although a substantial population do not generate oligodendrocytes at any stage of development or in the adult. It seems likely that all adult NG2-glia are OPCs, but it remains to be resolved whether this is their sole function. Myelination is essential for the miniaturization and massive computing power of the mammalian brain, and it proceeds long into adulthood. Hence, there is a clear need for a population of NG2-glia to generate oligodendrocytes throughout life. This ability of NG2-glia is related to their synaptic connectivity, but the precise functions of synaptic signalling in NG2-glia is unresolved.

Physiological and comprehensive ultrastructural studies *in vivo* in the adult brain are essential to address these questions and to provide insight into the roles of NG2-glia in CNS circuits. In addition, conditional ablation of NG2-glia in the adult brain is likely to be the only way to address their importance in normal CNS function and pathology of the young and ageing brain.

## References

Almli LM, Wilczynski W. (2007). Regional distribution and migration of proliferating cell populations in the adult brain of Hyla cinerea (Anura, Amphibia). *Brain Research* **1159**, 112–8.

Bergles DE, Roberts JD, Somogyi P, Jahr CE. (2000). Glutamatergic synapses on oligodendrocyte precursor cells in the hippocampus. *Nature* **405**(6783), 187–91.

Bergles DE, Jabs R, Steinhauser C. (2010). Neuron-glia synapses in the brain. *Brain Research Reviews* **63**(1–2), 130–7.

Bonkowski D, Katyshev V, Balabanov RD, Borisov A, Dore-Duffy P. (2011). The CNS microvascular pericyte: pericyte-astrocyte crosstalk in the regulation of tissue survival. *Fluids and Barriers of the CNS* CNS **8**(1), 8.

Butt AM, Duncan A, Hornby MF, Kirvell SL, Hunter A, Levine JM, Berry M. (1999). Cells expressing the NG2 antigen contact nodes of Ranvier in adult CNS white matter. *Glia* **26**(1), 84–91.

Butt AM, Kiff J, Hubbard P, Berry M. (2002). Synantocytes: new functions for novel NG2 expressing glia. *Journal of Neurocytology* **31**(6–7), 551–65.

Butt AM, Hamilton N, Hubbard P, Pugh M, Ibrahim M. (2005). Synantocytes: the fifth element. *Journal of Anatomy* **207**(6), 695–706.

Cahoy JD, Emery B, Kaushal A, Foo LC, Zamanian JL, Christopherson KS, Xing Y, Lubischer JL, Krieg PA, Krupenko S.A. *et al.* (2008). A transcriptome database for astrocytes, neurons, and oligodendrocytes: a new resource for understanding brain development and function. *Journal of Neuroscience* **28**(1), 264–78.

Chittajallu R, Aguirre A, Gallo V. (2004). NG2-positive cells in the mouse white and grey matter display distinct physiological properties. *Journal of Physiology* **561**(Pt 1), 109–22.

De Biase LM, Nishiyama A, Bergles DE. (2010). Excitability and synaptic communication within the oligodendrocyte lineage. *Journal of Neuroscience* **30**(10), 3600–11.

De Biase LM, Kang SH, Baxi EG, Fukaya M, Pucak ML, Mishina M, Calabresi PA, Bergles DE. (2011). NMDA receptor signaling in oligodendrocyte progenitors is not required for oligodendrogenesis and myelination. *Journal of Neuroscience* **31**(35), 12650–62.

Dimou L, Simon C, Kirchhoff F, Takebayashi H, Gotz M. (2008). Progeny of Olig2-expressing progenitors in the gray and white matter of the adult mouse cerebral cortex. *Journal of Neuroscience* **28**(41), 10434–42.

Djukic B, Casper KB, Philpot BD, Chin LS, McCarthy KD. (2007). Conditional knock-out of Kir4.1 leads to glial membrane depolarization, inhibition of potassium and glutamate uptake, and enhanced short-term synaptic potentiation. *Journal of Neuroscience* **27**(42), 11354–65.

Dore-Duffy P, Owen C, Balabanov R, Murphy S, Beaumont T, Rafols JA. (2000). Pericyte migration from the vascular wall in response to traumatic brain injury. *Microvascular Research* **60**(1), 55–69.

Dore-Duffy P, Katychev A, Wang X, Van Buren E. (2006). CNS microvascular pericytes exhibit multipotential stem cell activity. *Journal of Cerebral Blood Flow and Metabolism* **26**(5), 613–24.

Ehninger D, Wang LP, Klempin F, Romer B, Kettenmann H, Kempermann G. (2011). Enriched environment and physical activity reduce microglia and influence the fate of NG2 cells in the amygdala of adult mice. *Cell and Tissue Research* **345**(1), 69–86.

Etchevers HC, Vincent C, Le Douarin NM, Couly GF. (2001). The cephalic neural crest provides pericytes and smooth muscle cells to all blood vessels of the face and forebrain. *Development* **128**(7), 1059–68.

Ffrench-Constant C, Raff MC. (1986). Proliferating bipotential glial progenitor cells in adult rat optic nerve. *Nature* **319**(6053), 499–502.

Fumagalli M, Daniele S, Lecca D, Lee PR, Parravicini C, Fields RD, Rosa P, Antonucci F, Verderio C, Trincavelli M.L. *et al.* (2011). Phenotypic changes, signaling pathway, and functional correlates of GPR17-expressing neural precursor cells during oligodendrocyte differentiation. *Journal of Biological Chemistry* **286**(12), 10593–604.

Gao Q, Lu J, Huo Y, Baby N, Ling EA, Dheen ST. (2010). NG2, a member of chondroitin sulfate proteoglycans family mediates the inflammatory response of activated microglia. *Neuroscience* **165**(2), 386–94.

Ge WP, Zhou W, Luo Q, Jan LY, Jan YN. (2009). Dividing glial cells maintain differentiated properties including complex morphology and functional synapses. *Proceedings of The National Academy Of Sciences Of The United States Of America* **106**(1), 328–33.

Givogri MI, Costa RM, Schonmann V, Silva AJ, Campagnoni AT, Bongarzone ER. (2002). Central nervous system myelination in mice with deficient expression of Notch1 receptor. *Journal of Neuroscience Research* **67**(3), 309–20.

Guo F, Maeda Y, Ma J, Xu J, Horiuchi M, Miers L, Vaccarino F, Pleasure D. (2010). Pyramidal neurons are generated from oligodendroglial progenitor cells in adult piriform cortex. *Journal of Neuroscience* **30**(36), 12036–49.

Haberlandt C, Derouiche A, Wyczynski A, Haseleu J, Pohle J, Karram K, Trotter J, Seifert G, Frotscher M, Steinhauser C and others. (2011). Gray matter NG2 cells display multiple $Ca^{2+}$-signaling pathways and highly motile processes. *PLoS One* **6**(3), e17575.

Hamilton N, Vayro S, Wigley R, Butt AM. (2010). Axons and astrocytes release ATP and glutamate to evoke calcium signals in NG2-glia. *Glia* **58**(1), 66–79.

Kang SH, Fukaya M, Yang JK, Rothstein JD, Bergles DE. (2010). NG$^{2+}$ CNS glial progenitors remain committed to the oligodendrocyte lineage in postnatal life and following neuro-degeneration. *Neuron* **68**(4), 668–81.

Karadottir R, Cavelier P, Bergersen LH, Attwell D. (2005). NMDA receptors are expressed in oligodendrocytes and activated in ischaemia. *Nature* **438**(7071), 1162–6.

Karadottir R, Hamilton NB, Bakiri Y, Attwell D. (2008). Spiking and nonspiking classes of oligodendrocyte precursor glia in CNS white matter. *Nature Neuroscience* **11**(4), 450–6.

Karram K, Goebbels S, Schwab M, Jennissen K, Seifert G, Steinhauser C, Nave KA, Trotter J. (2008). NG2-expressing cells in the nervous system revealed by the NG2-EYFP-knockin mouse. *Genesis* **46**(12), 743–57.

Korn J, Christ B, Kurz H. (2002). Neuroectodermal origin of brain pericytes and vascular smooth muscle cells. *Journal of Comparative Neurology* **442**(1), 78–88.

Krueger M, Bechmann I. (2010). CNS pericytes: concepts, misconceptions, and a way out. *Glia* **58**(1), 1–10.

Kucharova K, Stallcup WB. (2010). The NG2 proteoglycan promotes oligodendrocyte progenitor proliferation and developmental myelination. *Neuroscience* **166**(1), 185–94.

Kukley M, Capetillo-Zarate E, Dietrich D. (2007). Vesicular glutamate release from axons in white matter. *Nature Neuroscience* **10**(3), 311–20.

Kukley M, Kiladze M, Tognatta R, Hans M, Swandulla D, Schramm J, Dietrich D. (2008). Glial cells are born with synapses. *The FASEB Journal* **22**(8), 2957–69.

Kukley M, Dietrich D. (2009). Kainate receptors and signal integration by NG2 glial cells. *Neuron Glia Biology* **5**(1–2), 13–20.

Kukley M, Nishiyama A, Dietrich D. (2010). The fate of synaptic input to NG2 glial cells: neurons specifically downregulate transmitter release onto differentiating oligodendroglial cells. *Journal of Neuroscience* **30**(24), 8320–31.

Leoni G, Rattray M, Butt AM. (2009). NG2 cells differentiate into astrocytes in cerebellar slices. *Molecular and Cellular Neurosciences* **42**(3), 208–18.

Levine JM, Card JP. (1987). Light and electron microscopic localization of a cell surface antigen (NG2) in the rat cerebellum: association with smooth protoplasmic astrocytes. *Journal of Neuroscience* **7**(9), 2711–20.

Lin SC, Bergles DE. (2002). Physiological characteristics of NG2-expressing glial cells. *Journal of Neurocytology* **31**(6–7), 537–49.

Lin SC, Bergles DE. (2004). Synaptic signaling between GABAergic interneurons and oligo-dendrocyte precursor cells in the hippocampus. *Nature Neuroscience* **7**(1), 24–32.

Maldonado PP, Velez-Fort M, Angulo MC. (2011). Is neuronal communication with NG2 cells synaptic or extrasynaptic? *Journal of Anatomy* **219**(1), 8–17.

Marz M, Schmidt R, Rastegar S, Strahle U. (2010). Expression of the transcription factor Olig2 in proliferating cells in the adult zebrafish telencephalon. *Developmental Dynamics* **239**(12), 3336–49.

Marz M, Schmidt R, Rastegar S, Strahle U. (2011). Regenerative response following stab injury in the adult zebrafish telencephalon. *Developmental Dynamics* **240**(9), 2221–31.

Melanson-Drapeau L, Beyko S, Dave S, Hebb AL, Franks DJ, Sellitto C, Paul DL, Bennett SA. (2003). Oligodendrocyte progenitor enrichment in the connexin32 null-mutant mouse. *Journal of Neuroscience* **23**(5), 1759–68.

Nishiyama A, Komitova M, Suzuki R, Zhu X. (2009). Polydendrocytes (NG2 cells): multi-functional cells with lineage plasticity. *Nature Reviews Neuroscience* **10**(1), 9–22.

Nona SN, Duncan A, Stafford CA, Maggs A, Jeserich G, Cronly-Dillon JR. (1992). Myelination of regenerated axons in goldfish optic nerve by Schwann cells. *Journal of Neurocytology* **21**(6), 391–401.

Nona SN, Thomlinson AM, Bartlett CA, Scholes J. (2000). Schwann cells in the regenerating fish optic nerve: evidence that CNS axons, not the glia, determine when myelin formation begins. *Journal of Neurocytology* **29**(4), 285–300.

Paez PM, Fulton D, Spreuer V, Handley V, Campagnoni AT. (2011). Modulation of canonical transient receptor potential channel 1 in the proliferation of oligodendrocyte precursor cells by the golli products of the myelin basic protein gene. *Journal of Neuroscience* **31**(10), 3625–37.

Papay R, Gaivin R, McCune DF, Rorabaugh BR, Macklin WB, McGrath JC, Perez DM. (2004). Mouse alpha1B-adrenergic receptor is expressed in neurons and NG2 oligodendrocytes. *Journal of Comparative Neurology* **478**(1), 1–10.

Peters A. (2004). A fourth type of neuroglial cell in the adult central nervous system. *Journal of Neurocytology* **33**(3), 345–57.

Peters A, Sethares C. (2004). Oligodendrocytes, their progenitors and other neuroglial cells in the aging primate cerebral cortex. *Cerebral Cortex* **14**(9), 995–1007.

Psachoulia K, Jamen F, Young KM, Richardson WD. (2009). Cell cycle dynamics of NG2 cells in the postnatal and ageing brain. *Neuron Glia Biology* **5**(3–4), 57–67.

Raff MC, Williams BP, Miller RH. (1984). The *in vitro* differentiation of a bipotential glial progenitor cell. *EMBO Journal* **3**(8), 1857–64.

Richardson WD, Young KM, Tripathi RB, McKenzie I. (2011). NG2-glia as multipotent neural stem cells: fact or fantasy? *Neuron* **70**(4), 661–73.

Rivers LE, Young KM, Rizzi M, Jamen F, Psachoulia K, Wade A, Kessaris N, Richardson WD. (2008). PDGFRA/NG2 glia generate myelinating oligodendrocytes and piriform projection neurons in adult mice. *Nature Neuroscience* **11**(12), 1392–401.

Seifert G, Rehn L, Weber M, Steinhauser C. (1997). AMPA receptor subunits expressed by single astrocytes in the juvenile mouse hippocampus. *Brain Research. Molecular Brain Research* **47** (1–2), 286–94.

Simmons AM, Horowitz SS, Brown RA. (2008). Cell proliferation in the forebrain and midbrain of the adult bullfrog, Rana catesbeiana. *Brain, Behavior and Evolution* **71**(1), 41–53.

Simon C, Lickert H, Gotz M, Dimou L. (2012). Sox10-iCreER(T2): A mouse line to inducibly trace the neural crest and oligodendrocyte lineage. *Genesis*.

Stallcup WB. (1981). The NG2 antigen, a putative lineage marker: immunofluorescent localization in primary cultures of rat brain. *Developmental Biology* **83**(1), 154–65.

Stallcup WB. (2002). The NG2 proteoglycan: past insights and future prospects. *Journal of Neurocytology* **31**(6–7), 423–35.

Stallcup WB, Beasley L. (1987). Bipotential glial precursor cells of the optic nerve express the NG2 proteoglycan. *Journal of Neuroscience* **7**(9), 2737–44.

Stallcup WB, Huang FJ. (2008). A role for the NG2 proteoglycan in glioma progression. *Cell Adhesion & Migration* **2**(3), 192–201.

Tavazoie M, Van der Veken L, Silva-Vargas V, Louissaint M, Colonna L, Zaidi B, Garcia-Verdugo JM, Doetsch F. (2008). A specialized vascular niche for adult neural stem cells. *Cell Stem Cell* **3**(3), 279–88.

Terada N, Baracskay K, Kinter M, Melrose S, Brophy PJ, Boucheix C, Bjartmar C, Kidd G, Trapp BD. (2002). The tetraspanin protein, CD9, is expressed by progenitor cells committed to oligodendrogenesis and is linked to beta1 integrin, CD81, and Tspan-2. *Glia* **40**(3), 350–9.

Tong XP, Li XY, Zhou B, Shen W, Zhang ZJ, Xu TL, Duan S. (2009). Ca$^{2+}$ signaling evoked by activation of Na(+) channels and Na(+)/Ca$^{2+}$ exchangers is required for GABA-induced NG2 cell migration. *Journal of Cell Biology* **186**(1), 113–28.

Tripathi RB, Rivers LE, Young KM, Jamen F, Richardson WD. (2010). NG2 glia generate new oligodendrocytes but few astrocytes in a murine experimental autoimmune encephalomyelitis model of demyelinating disease. *Journal of Neuroscience* **30**(48), 16383–90.

Velez-Fort M, Audinat E, Angulo MC. (2009). Functional alpha 7-containing nicotinic receptors of NG2-expressing cells in the hippocampus. *Glia* **57**(10), 1104–14.

Velez-Fort M, Maldonado PP, Butt AM, Audinat E, Angulo MC. (2010). Postnatal switch from synaptic to extrasynaptic transmission between interneurons and NG2 cells. *Journal of Neuroscience* **30**(20), 6921–9.

Wallraff A, Odermatt B, Willecke K, Steinhauser C. (2004). Distinct types of astroglial cells in the hippocampus differ in gap junction coupling. *Glia* **48**(1), 36–43.

Wigley R, Butt AM. (2009). Integration of NG2-glia (synantocytes) into the neuroglial network. *Neuron Glia Biology* **5**(1–2), 21–8.

Winkler EA, Bell RD, Zlokovic BV. (2010). Pericyte-specific expression of PDGF beta receptor in mouse models with normal and deficient PDGF beta receptor signaling. *Molecular Neurodegeneration* **5**, 32.

Zawadzka M, Rivers LE, Fancy SP, Zhao C, Tripathi R, Jamen F, Young K, Goncharevich A, Pohl H, Rizzi M. *et al.* (2010). CNS-resident glial progenitor/stem cells produce Schwann cells as well as oligodendrocytes during repair of CNS demyelination. *Cell Stem Cell* **6**(6), 578–90.

Zhu X, Hill RA, Nishiyama A. (2008). NG2 cells generate oligodendrocytes and gray matter astrocytes in the spinal cord. *Neuron Glia Biology* **4**(1), 19–26.

Zhu X, Hill RA, Dietrich D, Komitova M, Suzuki R, Nishiyama A. (2011). Age-dependent fate and lineage restriction of single NG2 cells. *Development* **138**(4), 745–53.

Ziskin JL, Nishiyama A, Rubio M, Fukaya M, Bergles DE. (2007). Vesicular release of glutamate from unmyelinated axons in white matter. *Nature Neuroscience* **10**(3), 321–30.

# 7
# Microglia

*Glial Physiology and Pathophysiology*, First Edition. Alexei Verkhratsky and Arthur Butt.
© 2013 by John Wiley & Sons, Ltd. Published 2013 by John Wiley & Sons, Ltd.

# 7.1    Definition of microglia

Microglial cells are CNS tissue macrophages which determine the organ's innate immunity. These cells are also known under colourful names, e.g. a 'CNS alarm system' or 'sensor of pathology'. Several reviews which provide an exhaustive characterisation of microglia have been published in recent years (Biber *et al.*, 2007; Graeber, 2010; Graeber *et al.*, 2011; Hanisch & Kettenmann, 2007; Kettenmann *et al.*, 2011; Prinz & Mildner, 2011; Ransohoff & Perry, 2009; Tremblay *et al.*, 2011); the reader is referred to these papers for extended reference lists and many fine details that are beyond the scope of this book. The main properties of microglia were defined by Pio del Rio-Hortega in his chapter on 'Microglia' (Del Rio-Hortega, 1932), which was written for the landmark publication *Cytology and Cellular Pathology of the Nervous System*, edited by Wilder Penfield in 1932.

1.    Microglia enter the brain during early development.

2.    These invading cells have amoeboid morphology and are of mesodermal origin.

3.    They use vessels and white matter tracts as guiding structures for migration and enter all brain regions.

4.    They transform into a branched, ramified morphological phenotype in the more mature brain – known today as the resting microglia.

5.    In the mature brain, they are found almost evenly dispersed throughout the central nervous system and display little variation.

6.    Each cell seems to occupy a defined territory.

7.    After a pathological event, these cells undergo a transformation.

8.    Transformed cells acquire amoeboid morphology similar to the one observed early in development.

9.    Amoeboid microglia cells have the capacity to migrate, proliferate and phagocytose.

In the years since, del Rio-Hortega's observations have been confirmed and further elaborated. Three major microglial phenotypes are defined. Embryonic microglia have an *amoeboid* phenotype and are phagocytic and immune competent cells. At developmental maturity, amoeboid microglia transform into the *resting* or *ramified* phenotype, which down-regulates its phagocytic activity and immune markers. In response to CNS insults, microglia become *activated* and *in extremis* regain their amoeboid phagocytic and immune competent phenotype.

These terms are inadequate. The term 'resting' microglia is a *non sequitur*, since in this state microglia are probably the most active cells in the brain, constantly extending and contracting their process to survey their environment. Hence, microglia are never inactive, and the term 'activated' is another *non sequitur*. Moreover, the 'activated' phenotype does not describe a single state, but a diverse range of multiple activation stages between resting microglia and the fully activated amoeboid phenotype. Thus, it is important to avoid oversimplifications and misconceptions when describing the state of microglia. Nonetheless, microglial phenotypes all have in common that they serve to support and protect the structural and functional integrity of the CNS.

## 7.2 Microglial origin and development

Microglial cells are of mesodermal/mesenchymal origin; microglia derive from progenitors that migrated into the CNS from the periphery. The microglial precursors are not simply blood macrophages, but rather derive from primitive myeloid progenitors that originate from the extraembryonic yolk sac (Ginhoux *et al.*, 2010). These progenitors enter the brain tissue in several batches during embryonic development (between embryonic days 10 and 19 in rodents) and in the perinatal period (up to postnatal day 10 in rodents), before the closure of blood-brain barrier. There is evidence that the early embryonic invaders are not macrophages, but rather are myeloid progenitors.

Monocytes enter the brain in several immigration spots (most notably around the choroid plexuses), which have been defined by Kershman (1939) as 'microglia fountains' (Figure 7.1). The invading monocytes have an amoeboid morphology and thus can be easily recognised by light microscopy in acute slices (for example of the corpus callosum) based on their shape and motility (Brockhaus *et al.*, 1993; Haas *et al.*, 1996).

At this stage, amoeboid microglia can be relatively easily approached by patch electrodes that readily form giga-seals, and the cells can be afterwards lifted from the surface of the slice for further electrophysiological studies (Figure 7.2). After the sealing of the blood-brain barrier, the monocyte exchange between blood and neural tissue terminates, and essentially the number of microglial cells remains stable throughout life.

## 7.3 Morphology of microglia

### 7.3.1 Morphology in the healthy tissue: resting or survelliant phenotype

After invading the central nervous system, microglial precursors disseminate throughout the brain parenchyma and rapidly transform into the *ramified* phenotype. This

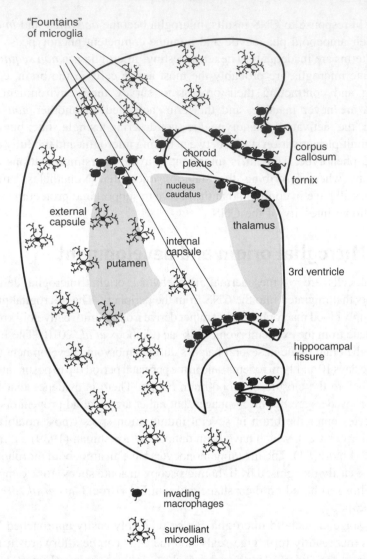

**Figure 7.1**  Microglial immigration into the brain and fountains of microglia.

Drawn based on Kershman, 1939.

metamorphosis is a striking example of epigenetic regulation, since the appearance of ramified microglia is far from the morphology of macrophages. Microglial cells are homogeneously distributed throughout the CNS, with more or less similar densities in different regions (Figure 7.3). The microglial cells in the healthy CNS have small cell bodies ($\approx 5\ \mu$m) from which several main processes are extending. Microglial primary processes are rather thin and produce even thinner distal arborisations.

The morphology of microglia is not absolutely uniform, with several general subtypes being observed (Figure 7.3); nonetheless, the morphological diversity is

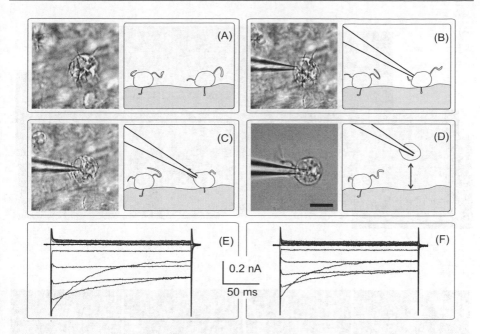

**Figure 7.2** Method of isolation of single amoeboid microglial cells from the surface of corpus callosum slice and inward rectifier K$^+$ currents recorded from these cells.

A–D.  Combinations of images taken by means of infrared video microscopy (left panels) and schematic drawings showing the method of cell isolation.

A.  Initial position of amoeboid microglial cells situated on the surface of a corpus callosum slice.

B.  A single microglial cell was approached with a micropipette and a whole-cell patch clamp configuration was established.

C.  After 2–3 min the cell partially spread over the pipette, intensifying the cell-to-pipette contact.

D.  Finally, the cell was lifted for 200 µm over the slice surface. Scale bar in (D) = 10 µm.

E,F.  Voltage-activated whole cell currents recorded from a single cell at stages indicated in (B) and (D) respectively. Currents were activated by depolarisation and hyperpolarisation voltage steps (duration 200 ms, increment 10 mV) from the holding potential −70 mV. The lifting of the cell did not affect the ionic current pattern.

Reproduced with permission from Haas, S. et al. (1996) ATP-induced membrane currents in ameboid microglia acutely isolated from mouse brain slices. Neuroscience 75:1, pp. 257-262 © Elsevier

far less pronounced than, for example, astrocytes. What is similar to astrocytes, however, is the domain organisation; every microglial cell has its own territory, about 30–50 µm diameter, and there is very little (if any) overlap of microglial cell distal processes (Figure 7.4).

(A)

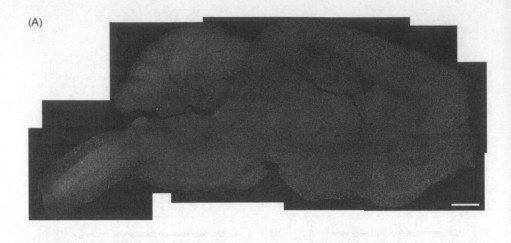

(B)

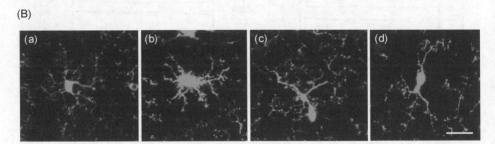

**Figure 7.3**   Distribution and morphological heterogeneity of microglial cells in the brain.

A.   Montage of a brain sagittal section showing the distribution of microglia in mice, in which microglial cells specifically expressed green fluorescent protein (GFP) under control of the fractalkine (or CX3C) receptor promoter.

B.   Different types of brain microglial cell morphology. Brain microglial cells were classified as ramified (a), hypertrophied (b), monopolarised (c) and bipolarised (d). Hypertrophied microglia were defined as having large soma and short, thick and radially projecting processes. Ramified microglial cells were defined as possessing thin, slender, radially projecting processes with well-developed ramifications. Monopolarised microglial cells were defined as having one thick process with well developed ramifications extending toward one direction. Bipolarized microglial cells were defined as having two thick processes emanating from the opposing poles of the cell and projecting in the opposite directions. Bar = 1 μm in A, 20 μm in B.

Reproduced with permission from Zhang *et al.*, 2008. (Full colour version in plate section.)

The microglial phenotype described above is generally referred to as *ramified* or *resting*. However, defining this phenotype as 'resting' is deceptive, and these cells in the unperturbed brain are far from being quiescent. The processes of ramified microglial cells are constantly moving through their territory; this is a relatively

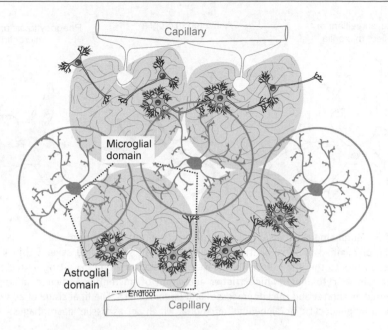

**Figure 7.4**  Domain organisation of microglia in the CNS.

rapid movement, with a speed of about 1.2–1.5 μm/min. At the same time, microglial processes also constantly send out and retract small protrusions, which can grow and shrink by 2–3 μm/min.

At first glance, the movement of microglial processes does not appear to have any evident pattern, and they seem to be randomly scanning their domains. Considering the velocity of this movement, the brain parenchyma can be completely scanned by microglial processes every few hours. The motility of the processes is not affected by neuronal firing, but it is sensitive to pharmacological modulation of various neurotransmitter receptors, most notably of purinoceptors. Some microglial processes seem to have a purposeful motility as they stop near synapses, presumably identifying their functional state (see Section 7.6). This continuous scanning of brain tissue allows microglial cells to integrate and interpret various environmental cues that control microglial behaviour. Hence, the ramified phenotype represents the *survelliant* state in which 'resting' microglial cells are ready to rapidly initiate various activation programmes in response to threats to the CNS.

## 7.3.2  Morphology in pathological tissue: activated phenotype

Insulting the brain tissue triggers *microglial activation*, which is accompanied by marked morphological changes (microglial activation will be discussed in detail in

Resting, surveillant or          Activated microglia          Phagocytic or "amoeboid"
"ramified" microglia                                          microglia

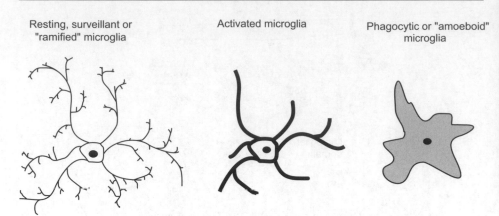

**Figure 7.5** Morphological transformation of microglia during activation.
   Resting, or ramified or survelliant, microglia have small somata and several thin and long
processes. Insults to the brain result in release of vascular, neuronal or astroglial factors (e.g.
ATP, thrombin or cytokines), which trigger activation of microglia. Activated microglia are
characterised by shorter and thicker processes and larger somata. The final stage of activation is
represented by phagocytic or 'amoeboid' microglia, which act as tissue macrophages.

Chapter 9). In general, during activation, microglial cells retract the branches of
their processes so that they are reabsorbed into the cell body. There are several
intermediate stages, characterised by processes withdrawal, transition or hyper-
ramification, and subsequent formation of new protrusions along with increased
motility (Figure 7.5).

## 7.3.3   Morphology in the dish

Most of our knowledge about microglial physiology has been acquired using *in vitro*
microglial cultures as experimental preparations. It is important to consider that
microglia, being the primary defensive cells of the CNS, are extremely sensitive to
environmental changes, and therefore cell isolation from the tissue inevitably
triggers microglial activation. As a result, the activation state of these cells should
always be considered when experimenting with microglial cell cultures.
   As a rule, microglial cells *in vitro* usually do not have the ramified structure
typical of the healthy CNS. Primary cultured microglial cells show heterogeneous
morphology, ranging from spindle and rod-shaped, or amoeboid varieties, displaying short thick processes, expanded lamellipodia, or even rounded cells. Further
morphological remodelling can be induced by exposure to activating signals such as
components of bacterial walls (*lypopolysaccharide* or *LPS* being the most commonly used activation agent). This *in vitro* activation favours acquisition of the
phagocytic phenotype and promotes secretion of inflammatory factors. The activated cells tend to acquire multiple shapes, with bushy, or bi- and tripolar, spindle-
or rod-shaped morphologies. At the same time, changes to the ramified morphology

can also be induced in cell cultures by exposing them to astroglial conditioning medium or to increased levels of ATP/adenosine.

Morphological transformations of cultured microglial cells are prominent and rapid. These changes are often accompanied with increased motility of microglial cells that requires filopodia protrusion and dynamic rebuilding of the cellular cytoskeleton. Cultured cells may also demonstrate phagocytic activity, which is also accompanied by rapid morphological metamorphosis.

### 7.3.4   Identification of microglial cells in neural tissues

Identification of microglia in the brain has been facilitated by the development of numerous staining techniques and transgenic animals expressing various markers under control of microglial promoters. An important issue for all microglia-specific probes is their selectivity and ability to distinguish resident microglia from peripheral macrophages, which may infiltrate CNS in various (usually pathological) conditions.

In addition to classical staining techniques, several immunological techniques have been developed, usually targeting molecules localised at the plasma membrane. Tomato lectin staining (in which tomato lectin is fused with fluorescent markers, e.g. Texas Red) targets oligosaccharides with N-acetylglucosamine oligomers and is successfully used for localising microglial cells in brain slices for electrophysiological experiments. In fixed preparations, microglial cells can be labelled with numerous antibodies, the most popular being those raised against ionised calcium-binding adaptor molecule 1 (Iba-1), antibodies against $\alpha_M\beta_2$ integrin (CD11b/18), antibodies against leukocyte common antigen (CD45), the F4/80 antigen (which belongs to the family of epidermal growth factor heptahelical receptors), etc. (see Kettenmann et al., 2011) for detailed review). Good results have also been obtained with immunolabelling for glucose transporter 5 (GLUT5), which seems to be selectively expressed in human microglia.

Recently, several transgenic animals expressing fluorescent proteins in microglial cells under control of fractalkin ($CX_3CR1$) receptor gene or Iba1 gene have been developed. These models greatly facilitate identification of microglia in situ and in vivo.

## 7.4   General physiology of microglia

### 7.4.1   Membrane potential and ion distribution

Ion gradients in microglia are similar to those in other neuroglia. Measurements mostly performed on cultured microglia show that their cytoplasm contains a high concentration of $K^+$ (120–140 mM), cytosolic free $Ca^{2+}$ is $\approx100$ nM, and $Na^+$ concentration has been estimated at $\approx10$ mM. Membrane potentials of microglial cells have been measured in vitro and in situ in acutely isolated brain slices. In primary cultures, the $V_m$ of microglial cells is $\approx-50$ mV (Kettenmann et al., 1990; Norenberg et al., 1994), whereas in situ microglial membrane polarisation is lower, being in the range of $-20\,mV$ in the cortex, striatum and facial nucleus from young adult (8–12 weeks old) rats and in adult humans (Bordey & Spencer, 2003; Boucsein *et al.*, 2000). In young mice, the $V_m$ of ramified microglial cells was determined at $\approx -40\,mV$. Amoeboid microglial cells studied in corpus callosum slices from neonatal mice (these cells are migrating monocytes which had just entered the brain) had a resting membrane potential ranging between $-10$ and $-70\,mV$ (Brockhaus *et al.*, 1993).

Low levels of membrane polarisation in microglial cells *in situ* coincides with low resting membrane conductances. Ramified microglial cells in acute brain slices have high input resistance and very small voltage-operated membrane currents (Figure 7.6). Stimulation of microglial activation in cultures (by exposure to LPS) or *in vivo* (by lesioning facial nerve) resulted in up-regulation of expression of voltage-operated channels (primarily $K^+$ channels) and an increase in membrane polarisation.

## 7.4.2   Ion channels in microglia

Microglial cells express a wide variety of ion channels (see Table 7.1), expression of which can be substantially modified by their functional state. Essentially, expression of ion channels increases in activated microglia and may even be activation stage-specific.

**(i)   Sodium channels**   Sodium currents activated by membrane depolarisation have been observed only in cultured microglia from rat and human brain. These currents were similar to typical $Na^+$ currents in excitable cells in their fast kinetics and sensitivity to tetrodotoxin (TTX). The proportion of microglial cells expressing $Na^+$ currents was highest in microglia obtained from brain tissues of patients with brain tumours, which may indicate a specific reaction. There are some indications that expression of microglial $Na^+$ channels can increase in other CNS pathologies, such as experimental autoimmune encephalomyelitis, an animal model for multiple sclerosis.

At the molecular level, three types of $Na^+$ channels were identified immunologically in rat microglial cultures – $Na_v1.1$, $Na_v1.6$ (TTX-sensitive) and $Na_v1.5$ (TTX-insensitive). All in all, however, there is little evidence for functional activity of voltage-operated $Na^+$ channels in microglial cells *in vivo* in the healthy CNS.

**(ii)   Calcium-permeable channels**   There is no evidence for functional expression of classical voltage-operated $Ca^{2+}$ channels in microglia in the CNS tissues *in vivo* or *in situ*. Two main classes of $Ca^{2+}$ permeable channels in microglia are represented by store-operated channels and channels of the TRP family. Microglial cells, similar to other non-excitable cells, are in possession of store-operated $Ca^{2+}$ entry, which is mediated by $Ca^{2+}$-release activated channels and, possibly, by TRP channels.

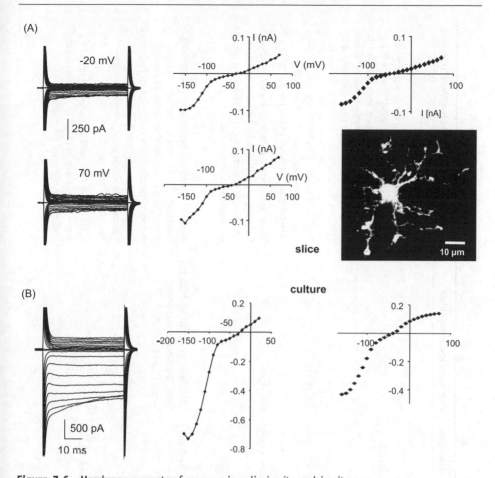

**Figure 7.6** Membrane currents of mouse microglia *in situ* and *in vitro*.

A. Membrane currents from cells in the acute slice were recorded during de- and hyperpolarising voltage steps from a holding potential of −20 mV (upper graph) or −70 mV
   (lower graph). The current traces are displayed on the left and the resulting current-
   voltage curve (I–V curve) in the middle. On the right, the average currents (mean ± SEM)
   from 89 cells are shown. The confocal photomicrograph, shows a microglial cell after
   recording and filling with Lucifer yellow. It displays the typical morphology of a resting
   microglial cell.

B. Membrane current recordings were also obtained from cultured microglial cells. The
   holding potential was −70 mV. The average current-voltage curve on the right
   indicates that the membrane conductance of the cultured cells is on average approximately four times larger compared with cells in the slice (note the difference in current
   scale)

**Table 7.1** Ion channels in microglia (modified from Kettenmann *et al.*, 2011)

| Channel type/subunit | Experimental preparation/technique | Pharmacology: antagonists | Biophysical properties and functional relevance |
|---|---|---|---|
| *Sodium channels* | | | |
| TTX-sensitive $I_{Na}$ | Rat, human/cultured primary microglia/whole-cell voltage clamp | TTX | In rat cultured microglia $I_{Na}$ was detected in $\approx20$ per cent of cells; in human cells this was $\approx95$ per cent; human cultures, however, were prepared from patients with brain tumours. Co-culturing rat cells with astrocytes increased proportion of cells with $I_{Na}$. |
| $Na_v1.1$, $Na_v1.5$ (TTX-sensitive), $Na_v1.6$ (TTX-resistant) | Rat/cultured primary microglia/specific antibodies | TTX, phenytoin | Treatment of LPS-activated microglia with TTX or phenytoin reduced IL-$\alpha1$, IL-1$\beta$ and TNF-$\alpha$ secretion and decreased motility responses to ATP. |
| $Na_v1.6$ | EAE mice/post-mortem MS human spinal cord/immunocytochemistry/ *in situ* hybridization | Phenytoin | The protein and mRNA for $Na_v1.6$ were detected in EAE mice spinal cord and optic nerve, as well as in MS-affected human spinal cord. Phenytoin reduced microglial activation in EAE. |
| *Calcium-permeable channels* | | | |
| ORAI1/CRAC | Rat/cultured primary microglia/whole-cell voltage clamp/RT-PCR | $Gd^{3+}$, SKF-96365, diethylstilbestrol (DES), 2-aminoethoxydiphenyl borate (2_APB; 50 $\mu$M). | High-$Ca^{2+}$ selective channel activated following depletion of ER $Ca^{2+}$ stores. Activation of $I_{CRAC}$ participates in formation of sustained phase of metabotropically induced $Ca^{2+}$ signals. Profound ER store depletion may cause persisting (tens of minutes) activation of $I_{CRAC}$-mediated store-operated $Ca^{2+}$ entry. |
| TRPM7; TRPC6; TRPM2, TRPV1; TRPM4 and to a lesser extend other TRPs | Rat, mouse, microglial cell lines/whole-cell voltage clamp/RT-PCR | | Activation of TRPs participates in microglial $Ca^{2+}$ signalling and may be linked to IL-6 release and initiation of microglial cell death. |

### Potassium channels

| Channel | Species/preparation/method | Blockers | Comments |
|---|---|---|---|
| Inward rectifier potassium channels $IK_{IR}$, Kir2.1 | Rat, mouse, human/culture, amoeboid microglia from acute juvenile corpus callosum slices/whole-cell voltage clamp | $Ba^{2+}$, $Cs^+$, TEA, quinine | Generally expressed in activated microglia; very low densities in resting microglia. |
| $IK_{DR}$; $K_v1.1$; $K_v1.2$; $K_v1.3$; $K_v1.5$ | Rat, mouse/cultured primary microglia; slices/whole-cell voltage clamp/RT-PCR/immunocytochemistry | $Cd^{2+}$, $Zn^{2+}$, $Ba^{2+}$, TEA, 4-AP, CTX, KTX, NTX, MTX | $IK_{DR}$ is up-regulated following microglial activation in both *in vitro* and *in situ* preparations. $K_v1.3$ and $K_v1.5$ channels are required for $IK_{DR}$ in adult activated microglia. $K_v1.1$ and $K_v1.2$.channels are expressed in amoeboid postnatal microglia; hypoxic insults increase $K_v1.2$ expression in adult microglial cells. Both $K_v1.3$ and $K_v1.5$ channels are linked to various functional responses of activated microglia, from regulation of motility ($K_v1.3$) to release of NO ($K_v1.5$) |
| $Ca^{2+}$-dependent potassium ($K_{Ca}$) channels IK(Ca): BK/ $K_{Ca}1.1$; KCNN1/SK1 KCNN3/SK2 KCNN3/SK3 KCNN4/SK4; | Calf, rat, mouse, human, adult and newborn rat/ primary cultures; slices/ sections of striatum/whole-cell voltage clamp/ RT-PCR/ immunohistochemistry | Apamin (KCNN2), clotrimazole (KCNN4), Apamin (100 nM-KCNN3), Tapamin (5 nM-KCNN3) | BK channels were identified based on their single channel conductance (140–240 pS). SK channels are linked to NO release, MAPK signalling and respiratory burst. KCNN3/SK3 channels were predominantly expressed in both cultures and healthy striatum tissue; LPS treatment or ischaemic insult increased the level of expression. Inhibition of KCNN3/SK3 affected microglial activation and reduced microglial neurotoxicity. |
| G-protein activated $K^+$ channels | Mouse/Primary cultures/ whole-cell voltage clamp | 4-AP, PTX | Currents were activated following stimulation of G-protein coupled metabotropic receptors. |

### Anion channels

| Channel | Species/preparation/method | Blockers | Comments |
|---|---|---|---|
| Volume-regulated $Cl^-$ channels, Best family of channels | Mouse; microglial cell lines/Primary cultures/ whole-cell voltage clamp/qRT-PCR | flufenamic acid; DIDS, SITS, DIOA, NPPB, IAA-94 | Single channel conductances 1–3.5 pS. Volume activate channels are involved in setting the resting |

(continued)

**Table 7.1**  (*Continued*)

| Channel type/subunit | Experimental preparation/technique | Pharmacology: antagonists | Biophysical properties and functional relevance |
|---|---|---|---|
| CLIC-1 chloride channels | Rat; microglial cell lines/ primary cultures/whole-cell voltage clamp | IAA-94 | Vm, regulation of microglia proliferation, phagocytosis and morphological phenotype. Single channel conductance 6.5–8 pS. CLIC-1 channels are involved in microglia proliferation and ROS-generation. |
| *Other channels* | | | |
| Proton channels<br>$H_v1$ voltage-activated $H^+$ channels | Mouse, rat, human, microglial cell lines/primary cultures/ whole-cell voltage clamp | TEA, bi- and trivalent cations | Single channel conductance $\approx$ fS range. Highly sensitive to extracellular pH; probably are associated with generation of respiratory burst. Disruption of cytoskeleton leads to a $\approx$50 per cent reduction in $H^+$ current amplitude, whereas cell swelling potentiates $H^+$ currents. |
| Aquaporins<br>AQP4 | Rat/RT-PCR/Western blotting | ? | Expression of AQP4 was observed in activated microglial cells following LPS injection into substantia nigra. |
| Connexins<br>Cx43, Cx36, Cx32, Cx45 | Rat, human, mouse/RT-PCR, immunocytochemistry, imaging, whole-cell voltage clamp | ? | No indications for connexins in resting microglia *in situ*. Traumatic brain lesion resulted in an appearance of Cx43 immunoreactivity. Cx32, Cx6, Cx43, and Cx45 were identified in cultured microglia. |

$Ca^{2+}$ *release activated* $Ca^{2+}$ *currents* ($I_{CRAC}$) have been identified in cultured rodent microglia; the amplitude of these currents was decreased after activation of microglia with LPS. At the molecular level, $I_{CRAC}$ occurs after activation of the complex of *ORAI/STIM* proteins; in this complex, ORAI[1] acts as a pore-forming protein, whereas STIM proteins serve as $Ca^{2+}$ sensors in the ER lumen (Feske *et al.*, 2006). Microglial cells express all 3 types of ORAI proteins with maximal expression of ORAI3 (Ohana *et al.*, 2009). Microglial cells also express several types of *TRPM*, *TRPV* and *TRPC* channels, which have substantial $Ca^{2+}$ permeability. Activation of these channels in cultured microglia produced intracellular $Ca^{2+}$ signals and may regulate release of cytokines.

**(iii)   Potassium channels**   The *inward rectifier* $K^+$ *currents* are generally present in activated microglia. These currents are always recorded from microglial cells in cultures. Similarly, inward rectifier $K^+$ currents are the main component of membrane permeability of amoeboid invading microglia in early perinatal tissues. However, these currents are either very small or are undetectable in ramified microglia in brain slices. Activation of microglia by pathological insults, such as ischaemic attack or surgical lesion of facial nerve, induces a several-fold increase in the amplitudes of inward rectifier $K^+$ channels (Boucsein *et al.*, 2000; Eder, 1998).

Activation of microglia in cultures with LPS or interferon-γ also induces significant up-regulation of *delayed (outward) rectifier* $K^+$ *channels* (Norenberg *et al.*, 1992). Likewise, an increase in delayed rectifier channel densities was observed in microglial cells *in situ* following activation by axotomy (Boucsein *et al.*, 2000). Increased delayed rectifier $K^+$ currents also accompanies microglial activation caused by other pathogenic stimuli, such as exposure to β-amyloid or HIV-1 regulatory protein Tat.

The main types of delayed rectifier $K^+$ channels in microglia are represented by $K_v1.2$, $K_v1.3$ and $K_v1.5$; early migrating amoeboid microglial cells also express $K_v1.1$ and $K_v1.2$ channels, which disappear in the postnatal period. Up-regulation of $K_v1.3$ and $K_v1.5$ channels seems to be responsible for increased delayed rectifier currents in activated microglia. Increased expression of delayed rectifier channels is linked to various functional responses of activated microglia – including, for example, proliferation and release of nitric oxide.

Cultured microglial cells also express $Ca^{2+}$-*dependent potassium* ($K_{Ca}$) *channels*, including high-conductance (BK) and small conductance (KCNN4/$K_{Ca}3.1$/ SK4/$I_K1$) types. These channels (and especially channels of the SK4 type) are involved in regulation of microglial activation, production of NO and controlling the respiratory burst. Expression of SK3 $Ca^{2+}$-dependent $K^+$ channels is increased in ischaemic conditions (Schlichter *et al.*, 2010).

---

[1] So-named after the Greek goddesses Orai (Harmony, Justice and Peace), who were the keepers of Heaven's gate (Feske *et al.*, 2006).

**(iv)  Anion channels**  Cultured microglial cells express *volume-regulated Cl⁻ channels* that are responsible for regulatory volume decrease, can be involved in regulation of proliferation and phagocytic activity, may contribute to setting microglial resting potential, and are somehow involved in controlling ramified morphology of resting microglia (Eder, 1998; Schlichter *et al.*, 1996). These channels are activated by hypo-osmotic shock. Microglial cells in culture also express the chloride intracellular channel-1 (CLIC-1). Expression of CLIC-1 channels is strongly potentiated by exposure to β-amyloid; this treatment also promotes translocation of Cl⁻ channels to the plasmalemma. These channels are potentially important for release of pro-inflammatory factors from microglia in the presence of β-amyloid (Milton *et al.*, 2008).

**(v)  Proton channels**  Cultured microglial cells express voltage-operated proton channels, which have low single-channel conductance ($\approx$ several fA) and very high selectivity to $H^+$; their voltage-dependence is strongly regulated by extracellular pH (Eder & DeCoursey, 2001). Activation of microglia in the dish decreases $H^+$ current amplitude.

The functional role of $H^+$ channels can be connected to regulation of the so-called respiratory burst which accompanies phagocytosis. The respiratory burst stems from activation of NADPH oxidase, which produces superoxide anions and protons; the $H^+$ channels can provide an efflux pathway for these extra protons, thus protecting the cytosol against acidification.

## 7.4.3  Calcium signalling in microglia

Calcium signalling plays an important role in microglial function, being readily activated in response to numerous physiological and pathological environmental factors. The main pathway in triggering microglial $Ca^{2+}$ signals is associated with $Ca^{2+}$ release from the endoplasmic reticulum store (Figure 7.7). The main route for the generation of microglial $Ca^{2+}$ signals is associated with InsP₃ receptors (Kettenmann *et al.*, 2011), which are activated by a wide variety of metabotropic receptors expressed in microglia (see Section 7.4.5).

Microglial cells also express ryanodine receptors, which can be activated by cyclic ADP ribose and by 4-chloro-*m*-cresol in millimolar concentrations. The state of the ER $Ca^{2+}$ store can be regulated by microglial activation and various pathological contexts. For example, InsP₃-mediated $Ca^{2+}$ release (following the stimulation of purinoceptors or PAF receptors) was reduced by more than 50 per cent in microglial cells obtained from the brains of Alzheimer's disease patients, possibly indicating chronic depletion of the ER store (McLarnon *et al.*, 2005).

Depletion of ER stores in the presence of metabotropic agonists triggers *store-operated Ca²⁺ entry* or *SOCE* (see also Section 7.4.2), which plays an important role in shaping $Ca^{2+}$ signalling in microglia. SOCE is mainly responsible for producing and maintaining the plateau phase of microglial $[Ca^{2+}]_i$ transients triggered by

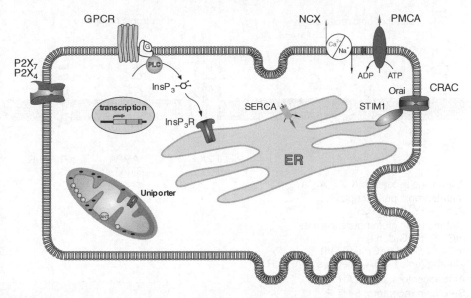

**Figure 7.7**   Calcium signalling in microglia. The main calcium signalling cascades in microglial cells are represented by:

(i)   $InsP_3$-induced $Ca^{2+}$ release from the ER. $InsP_3$ is generated by PLC, coupled with multiple G-protein coupled receptors (GPCR). Depletion of the ER $Ca^{2+}$ store activates store-operated channels (CRAC), which are likely to be formed through interactions between STIM1/Orai proteins.

(ii)  $Ca^{2+}$ influx through P2X$_7$ and/or P2X$_4$ receptors constitutively expressed in microglia. The extrusion of $Ca^{2+}$ from the cytosol is accomplished by (i) $Ca^{2+}$ uptake into the ER via SERCA; (ii) $Ca^{2+}$ accumulation into mitochondria through $Ca^{2+}$-selective uniporters; (iii) $Ca^{2+}$ extrusion to the extracellular space by plasmalemmal $Ca^{2+}$ ATPase (PMCA) and $Na^+/Ca^{2+}$ exchangers (NCX).

metabotropic agonists. SOCE is activated following stimulation of metabotropic purinoceptors, PAF receptors, lysophosphatidic acid receptors, complement fragment receptors, endothelin and bradykinin receptors, etc.

SOCE is particularly prominent in human microglial cells, in which metabotropically induced $Ca^{2+}$ signals strongly depend on $Ca^{2+}$ influx. Strong stimulation of microglia (e.g. with prolonged exposure to relatively high concentrations of ATP or UTP) results in the chronic activation of SOCE (Toescu *et al.*, 1998), which remains operative for tens of minutes after removal of the agonists, and essentially produces steady-state $Ca^{2+}$ influx, thus increasing resting $[Ca^{2+}]_i$. Similarly, the resting $[Ca^{2+}]_i$ is increased after treating microglial cells with activating stimuli, such as LPS, interferon-$\gamma$ or $\beta$-amyloid. Long-lasting increases in $[Ca^{2+}]_i$ are believed to be critically important for regulating various responses of activated microglia that include the release of nitric oxide, cytokines and chemokines (Hoffmann *et al.*, 2003). These long-lasting $[Ca^{2+}]_i$ increases involve SOCE and may also be regulated by mitochondrial $Ca^{2+}$ uptake.

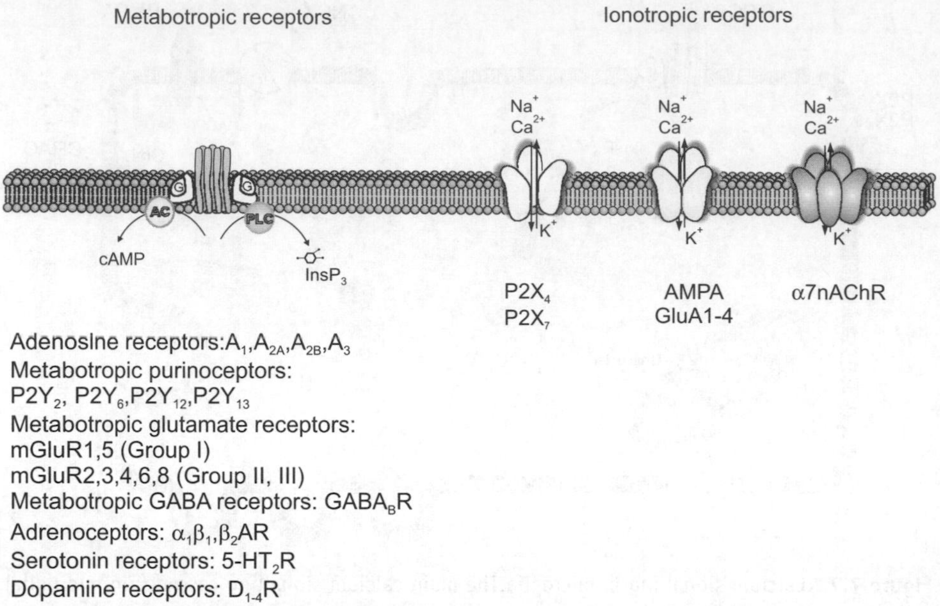

Metabotropic receptors                              Ionotropic receptors

cAMP                              InsP$_3$

                                         P2X$_4$        AMPA        α7nAChR
                                         P2X$_7$        GluA1-4

Adenosine receptors:A$_1$,A$_{2A}$,A$_{2B}$,A$_3$
Metabotropic purinoceptors:
P2Y$_2$, P2Y$_6$,P2Y$_{12}$,P2Y$_{13}$
Metabotropic glutamate receptors:
mGluR1,5 (Group I)
mGluR2,3,4,6,8 (Group II, III)
Metabotropic GABA receptors: GABA$_B$R
Adrenoceptors: α$_1$β$_1$,β$_2$AR
Serotonin receptors: 5-HT$_2$R
Dopamine receptors: D$_{1-4}$R

**Figure 7.8**  Neurotransmitter receptors in microglia.

Plasmalemmal transport of $Ca^{2+}$ ions in microglia is controlled by plasmalemmal $Ca^{2+}$ ATP-ases and by sodium-calcium exchangers, NCX. All three isoforms of NCX (NCX1–3) are expressed in microglial cells, with NCX1 being the predominant type. NCXs in microglia most likely operate in reverse mode because of the low membrane potential, and thus act as an additional pathway for $Ca^{2+}$ influx. NCX-mediated $Ca^{2+}$ influx is important for regulation of microglial motility (Ifuku *et al.*, 2007).

## 7.4.4  Neurotransmitter receptors

Acquisition of neurotransmitter receptors arguably represents the most profound departure of microglia from their monocyte ancestors (summarised in Figure 7.8). By acquiring these receptors, microglia have adapted to the CNS environment and have attained the ability to sense chemical signals employed in communication between neural cells. These chemical signals, in turn, regulate microglial physiology and control activation programmes, either by inducing microglial activation ('On' signals) or by promoting maintenance of the resting, surveillance state ('Off' signals, see also Chapter 9).

**(i)  Purinoceptors**  Microglial cells express several types of purinoceptors activated by ATP, adenosine and related nucleotides. These receptors regulate a variety of microglial functions and are involved in the control of microglial activation, reflecting the fact that ATP is an ancient 'danger' signal, because massive ATP release invariably accompanies cell death (Burnstock & Verkhratsky, 2009). Sudden increases in ATP concentration in the CNS tissue often reflect lesion, and this initiates rapid microglial responses, represented by converging movement of processes towards the lesion site (Davalos *et al.*, 2005; Nimmerjahn *et al.*, 2005).

Purinoceptors also regulate microglial motility, growth of processes and the release of various pro-inflammatory factors (Farber & Kettenmann, 2006; Ferrari *et al.*, 1997). Exposure of cultured microglia to millimolar ATP concentrations induces rapid activation. At the same time, lower concentrations of ATP and, especially, adenosine, may promote acquisition of the resting state. Purinoceptors control microglial $Ca^{2+}$ signalling through both ER $Ca^{2+}$ release (metabotropic receptors) and $Ca^{2+}$ entry (ionotropic receptors). In addition, microglial cells express the full complement of ecto-nucleotidases (nucleoside triphosphate diphosphohydrolases or NTDPases and, especially, NTDPase2 or CD39, nucleoside diphosphatase (NDPase), ecto-5'-nucleotidase and purine nucleoside phosphorylase (PNPase)), that degrade ATP to related nucleotides and to adenosine.

Expression of purinoceptors in microglia varies depending on the environment and activation status. It is not yet known (although possible) that microglial cells in different regions of the brain express different complements of purinoceptors. *In vitro*, even within the confines of the same culture dish, the pharmacological profile of purinergic responses differs between individual microglia. This might reflect their state of activation, which affects purinoceptor expression and the pharmacology of purinoceptor-mediated responses (Moller *et al.*, 2000). Microglial activation state also affects expression of ecto-nucleotidases.

Activation of microglial cells remodels purinoceptor expression both *in vitro* and *in vivo* in different pathological models. Exposure of microglial cultures to LPS increases expression of metabotropic P2Y receptors and down-regulates ionotropic P2X receptors. In the kainate-induced status epilepticus model, up-regulation of both P2X and P2Y receptors was observed and resulted in an increase in ATP-mediated $Ca^{2+}$ signalling and microglial motility. In the transgenic mouse model for amyotrophic lateral sclerosis (expressing mutant superoxide dismutase 1), microglial cells expressed higher levels of $P2X_4$, $P2X_7$ and $P2Y_6$ receptors. Similarly, various changes in expression of purinoceptors were found in acute trauma, during oxygen and glucose deprivation, and in various models of neuropathic pain (see Verkhratsky *et al.*, 2009 for detailed review).

The *adenosine (P1) receptors*, of which all four types ($A_1$, $A_{2A}$, $A_{2B}$ and $A_3$) are detected in microglia, regulate a wide variety of metabotropic and trophic responses. Adenosine receptors are neuroprotective and generally reduce activation of microglia. Stimulation of adenosine receptors in cultured microglia regulates $K^+$ channels, stimulates expression and release of nerve growth factor and prostaglandin E2, in addition to regulating proliferation.

Microglial cells express two types of *ionotropic P2X purinoceptors*, represented by homomeric $P2X_4$ and $P2X_7$ receptors. These are both cation ($Na^+/K^+/Ca^{2+}$) channels, with relatively large $Ca^{2+}$ permeability; the $P_{Ca}/P_{monovalent}$ ratio for $P2X_4$ receptors is $\approx 4-6$, whereas the $Ca^{2+}$ permeability of $P2X_7$ receptors varies depending on the pore status. $P2X_4$ receptors are activated by micromolar ATP concentrations ($EC_{50} \approx 2-7\,\mu M$), and are involved in various aspects of microglial activation, in particular in the context of neuropathic pain (see Chapter 9).

$P2X_7$ receptors are abundantly and constitutively expressed by microglia. In this respect, microglial cells are similar to other immune cells, which ubiquitously express $P2X_7$ receptors, and activation of these receptors participates in many immune responses. Functional $P2X_7$ receptors have been characterised in microglial cells in primary cultures and in amoeboid microglia from early postnatal corpus callosum slices (Ferrari *et al.*, 1996; Haas *et al.*, 1996). $P2X_7$ receptors require high ATP concentrations ($>1$ mM) for activation, which makes them ideal sensors of cell damage in the CNS. The $P2X_7$ receptors do not have specific agonists; $2',3'$-(benzoyl-4-benzoyl)-ATP (BzATP), which is often used as such, activates most other P2X receptors with high potency. Inhibitors of $P2X_7$ receptors generally used in experimental practice include Brilliant Blue G (BBG), which is effective blocking concentrations $\approx 100-200$ nM, and oxidised ATP (oxATP), which is effective in $100-300\,\mu M$ concentrations. Recently, many specific and potent $P2X_7$ receptor antagonists have been synthesised (see Syed & Kennedy, 2012 for details).

In the healthy CNS, microglial cells expressing $P2X_7$ receptors are diffusely scattered throughout virtually all areas (Yu *et al.*, 2008). Practically every sort of damage to nervous tissue results in prominent up-regulation of microglial expression of $P2X_7$ receptors (Collo *et al.*, 1997), e.g. middle cerebellar artery occlusion (model for stroke), experimental autoimmune encephalomyelitis (model for multiple sclerosis), injection of β-amyloid (model for Alzheimer's disease), etc. Increased levels of $P2X_7$ receptors in microglia are also found in human tissues affected by different neurological diseases, including stroke, multiple sclerosis, Alzheimer's disease, amyotrophic lateral sclerosis, encephalitis and meningitis.

Activation of microglial $P2X_7$ has many effects, both cytotoxic and trophic. First and foremost, $P2X_7$ receptors control microglial activation. Overexpression of $P2X_7$ receptors induces microglial activation even without additional stimulation, and this activation can be blocked by the $P2X_7$ receptor antagonist oxATP (Monif *et al.*, 2009). Microglial activation in response to intra-hippocampal injection of β-amyloid was critically dependent on $P2X_7$ receptors, and this activation was completely absent in $P2X_7$ receptor deficient animals (Sanz *et al.*, 2009). $P2X_7$ receptors are also obligatory for activation of the inflammasome and for stimulating release of interleukins and pro-inflammatory factors from activated microglia.

Furthermore, $P2X_7$ receptors are classical mediators of cell death. Overstimulation of $P2X_7$ receptors kills cultured microglia, mainly through apoptosis; this cell death was absent in animals with genetic deletion of $P2X_7$ receptor (Brough *et al.*, 2002). Similarly, $P2X_7$ receptors mediated death of activated microglia in organotypic hippocampal rat slices. In addition, $P2X_7$ receptors regulate microglial autophagy through release of autolysosomes (Takenouchi *et al.*, 2009). Stimulation of $P2X_7$ receptors also promotes microglial neurotoxicity through release of superoxide or nitric oxide, this neurotoxicity being inhibited by $P2X_7$ antagonists.

In addition, $P2X_7$ receptors mediate numerous trophic effects through activation of intracellular transcription factors such as cAMP response element-binding factor (CREB). In certain conditions, activation of microglial $P2X_7$ receptors can even induce neuroprotection, for example in conditions of acute ischaemia.

The main types of *metabotropic P2Y purinoceptors* in microglia are represented by $P2Y_2$, $P2Y_6$, $P2Y_{12}$, and $P2Y_{13}$ receptors (Inoue, 2008). Activation of these receptors activates $K^+$ channels and triggers microglial $Ca^{2+}$ signalling and $[Ca^{2+}]_i$ oscillations (which both heavily involve activation of store-operated $Ca^{2+}$ entry). The P2Y receptors also control secretion of interleukins and other pro-inflammatory factors. The UDP-preferring $P2X_6$ receptors are responsible for activation of microglia mediated through initiation of $Ca^{2+}$ signals and $P2Y_6$ receptors also regulate microglial phagocytosis (Inoue *et al.*, 2009). The ADP-preferring $P2Y_{12}$ receptors act as key mediators of rapid microglial responses to injury in the CNS.

$P2Y_{12}$ receptors in the brain and in the spinal cord are predominantly expressed in microglia and are localised in microglial processes. These receptors are primarily responsible for microglial activation and chemotaxis in response to local injury (Haynes *et al.*, 2006). In the brain, $P2X_{12}$ receptors are down-regulated in activated microglia, whereas in the spinal cord $P2X_{12}$ receptors are up-regulated and are involved in neuropathic pain (see Chapter 9). Activated microglial cells also express the P2Y-like receptor GRP17, which is activated by UDP, UDP-glucose, UDP-galactose and by cysteinyl-leukotrienes LTD4 and LTC4 (Lecca *et al.*, 2008).

**(ii)    Glutamate receptors**    Microglial cells in primary cultures express all four subtypes of *AMPA receptors* (GluA1–4), which, upon activation produce membrane currents, regulate release of TNF-$\alpha$ and are involved in regulation of microglial chemotaxis (Noda *et al.*, 2000). Activation of AMPA receptors also induces remodelling of the cytoskeleton, manifested by condensation of cytoplasmic actin filaments, their rapid de- and re-polymerisation, and cytoplasmic redistribution of condensed actin bundles. These changes play a role in the regulation of motility and phagocytosis of activated microglial cells (Christensen *et al.*, 2006). Recently functional NMDA receptors, linked to calcium signalling and possibly to activation, were found in cortical murine microglia (Kaindl et al., 2012).

Microglial cells express metabotropic glutamate receptors of all three groups. The mGluR5 (which belong to group I) triggers $Ca^{2+}$ release from the ER through the InsP$_3$ signalling cascade. Stimulation of the group II receptors (of which mGluR2 and mGluR3 receptors were detected in microglia) triggers microglial activation and release of TNF-$\alpha$, the latter mediating neurotoxicity. In contrast, stimulation of group III receptors (mGluR4, mGluR6 and mGluR8) is neuroprotective.

**(iii)    GABA receptors**    The main CNS inhibitory neurotransmitter, GABA, has a well-documented neuroprotective effect which is, at least in part, mediated through its action on microglia. Microglial cells express *metabotropic GABA$_B$ receptors*, which are linked to $K^+$ channels and $Ca^{2+}$ signalling. Stimulation of GABA$_B$ receptors attenuates microglial activation and reduces their release of interleukins (Kuhn *et al.*, 2004).

**(iv)   Acetylcholine receptors**   Cholinergic systems in the CNS are known to exert general anti-inflammatory effects, representing the endogenous 'cholinergic anti-inflammatory pathway' (Shytle *et al.*, 2004). Weakening of cholinergic transmission in certain neurodegenerative diseases (e.g. Alzheimer's disease or Parkinson's disease) may contribute to progression of neuroinflammation. Cholinergic input into microglia is mediated mainly through $\alpha 7$ (neuronal type) nicotinic receptors, activation of which inhibits immune responses of microglial cells. Nicotinic cholinoreceptors also mediate microglial $Ca^{2+}$ signalling, through both $Ca^{2+}$ influx and stimulation of ER $Ca^{2+}$ release (by yet unknown mechanisms).

**(v)   Adrenergic receptors**   Microglial adrenergic receptors are mainly represented by $\alpha_1$, $\beta_1$ and $\beta_2$ adrenoceptors, stimulation of which increase synthesis of cyclic AMP, and attenuate expression and release of interleukins (IL-1, IL6), NO and TNF-$\alpha$ (Farber *et al.*, 2005; Prinz *et al.*, 2001). Adrenoceptors are also involved in regulation of microglial motility and phagocytosis.

**(vi)   Dopamine receptors**   Four dopamine receptors (D$_{1-4}$) have been identified in microglia in cultures and *in situ* (Farber *et al.*, 2005). Activation of these receptors by exogenous ligands activated $K^+$ channels, whereas chronic exposure to dopamine receptors agonists enhanced microglial motility and chemotaxis. There are some indications that expression of dopamine receptors in activated microglia can contribute to pathogenesis of Parkinson's disease (Mastroeni *et al.*, 2008); it is also worth noting that the density of microglia in the substantia nigra is the highest in the brain. Dopamine receptors may also be involved in enhancing microglial activation in the spinal cord in amyotrophic lateral sclerosis.

**(vii)   Serotonin receptors**   Microglial cells express *5-HT$_2$ serotonin receptors* which modulate $K^+$ currents and trigger $Ca^{2+}$ signals. Activation of these receptors also enhances motility of microglial processes in response to local injury and attenuates phagocytic activity (Krabbe *et al.*, 2012).

## 7.4.5   Receptors for neurohormones and neuromodulators

Microglial cells express an impressive variety of receptors to various neurohormones and neuromediators that may mediate both physiological and pathological reactions (see Table 7.2). Expression of many of these receptors is modulated by the activation status of microglia. Microglia in the healthy brain

**Table 7.2** Microglial receptors for neurohormones and neuromodulators (modified from Kettenmann *et al.*, 2011)

| Receptor type | Properties and functional role |
| --- | --- |
| PAF receptors | In the brain, PAF receptors are predominantly expressed in microglia. Stimulation of PAF receptors triggers $[Ca^{2+}]_i$ elevation, resulting from ER $Ca^{2+}$ release and long-lasting activation of $Ca^{2+}$ entry. $Ca^{2+}$ entry increases IL-6 expression in cultured microglia. |
| Bradykinin receptors, $B_1$, $B_2$ | Resting microglia express only $B_2$ receptors; activation by LPS up-regulates $B_1$ expression. Stimulation of $B_2$ receptors triggers $IK_{Ca}$ following $[Ca^{2+}]_i$ increase. $B_1$ receptors induce chemotaxis and activate NCX. |
| Histamine receptors | Histamine triggers $Ca^{2+}$ release from the ER. |
| Endothelin receptors, $ET_B$ | Stimulation of microglia with ET-1 and ET-3 triggers $Ca^{2+}$ release and SOCE in 13 per cent of mouse and in 80 per cent of human cells. $Ca^{2+}$ responses are inhibited by $ET_B$ antagonist BQ788, and are mimicked by $ET_B$ agonist BQ3020 |
| Cannabinoid receptors $CB_1$, $CB_2$ | Resting microglia express $CB_1$ receptors; activation causes up-regulation of $CB_2$ receptors. High expression of $CB_2$ receptors is found in mice with experimental autoimmune encephalomyelitis. Stimulation of CB receptors stimulates proliferation and reduces neurotoxicity. |
| Angiotensin II receptors, $AT_1$, $AT_2$ | Unstimulated microglia express $AT_2$ receptors; LPS triggers up-regulation of $AT_1$ receptor. Inhibition of $AT_1$ receptors by losartan suppresses microglial activation and reduces production of NO and IL-1$\beta$. |
| Somatostatin receptors, sst2, sst3, sst4 | Activation of sst receptors induces protein phosphorylation and inhibits microglial proliferation |
| Glucocorticoid and mineralocorticoid receptors | Microglia expresses both glucocorticoid and mineralocorticoid receptors; stimulation of glucocorticoid receptors inhibits proliferation of cultured microglia and enhances lysosomal formation. |
| Opioid receptors KOR, MOR | Stimulation of MOR inhibits chemotaxis towards C5a, increases migration and up-regulates $P2X_4$ expression in rat. |
| Neurokinin (Substance P) receptors, NK-1 | Stimulation of NK-1 receptors triggers activation of NF-$\kappa$B. |
| VIP receptors $VPAC_1$ | Stimulation of $VPAC_1$ receptors inhibits LPS-induced activation and secretion of pro-inflammatory factors TNF-$\alpha$, IL-1$\beta$ and NO. |
| Neurotrophin receptors, Trk-B1 | BDNF triggers sustained $[Ca^{2+}]_i$ elevation resulting from $PLC/InsP_3$-medaietd $Ca^{2+}$ release followed by a long-lasting activation of SOCE. The Trk-B1 receptors are identified by RT-PCR. |

express *bradykinin receptors* of the $B_2$ *subtype*, which mediate $Ca^{2+}$ signalling. Activation of microglial cells induces a substantial increase in expression of $B_2$ receptors and additionally evokes expression of $B_1$ receptors. These receptors are activated by bradykinin released into the nerve tissue in pathology and regulate microglial chemotaxis; they also provide for neuroprotection by attenuating microglial release of pro-inflammatory factors (Noda *et al.*, 2007). Some cultured microglia also express *histamine receptors* linked to $Ca^{2+}$ release from the ER. Similarly, microglial $Ca^{2+}$ signalling is induced through activation of *endothelin receptors,* predominantly of $ET_B$ *type*; expression of these receptors is increased in ischaemic nervous tissue.

Another very potent activator of microglial $Ca^{2+}$ signalling is *platelet-activating factor* (PAF), acting through specific *PAF receptors*, which are highly expressed in microglial cells. These PAF receptors are G-protein coupled receptors linked to $InsP_3$ production and ER $Ca^{2+}$ release; they also stimulate mitogen-activated protein kinase (MAPK). Stimulation of PAF receptors triggers massive $Ca^{2+}$ release, with subsequent long-lasting store-operated $Ca^{2+}$ entry. This $Ca^{2+}$ entry regulates expression of interleukin 6 and microglial response factor-1 (Sattayaprasert *et al.*, 2005).

Microglial activation and neurotoxicity are negatively controlled by *cannabinoid receptors*, of which $CB_1$ and $CB_2$ receptors are expressed in microglial cells (see Stella, 2010 for comprehensive overview). The expression of both receptors in healthy microglia is very low; the exception are perivascular microglial cells in white matter of human cerebellum that express $CB_2$ receptors. Activation of microglia results in rapid and very substantial up-regulation of expression of $CB_1$ and $CB_2$ receptors; the up-regulation of $CB_2$ receptors is particularly high in EAE (model for MS). Similarly, $CB_2$ receptor levels increase in patients with Alzheimer's disease, amyotrophic lateral sclerosis and HIV-associated dementia. Expression of microglial $CB_2$ receptors can also be induced by acute treatment with 3,4-Methylenedioxymethamphetamine, popularly known as 'ecstasy' (Torres *et al.*, 2010).

Cultured microglia have been reported to express *angiotensin II receptors type 1 and 2* ($AT_1/AT_2$), which may stimulate microglial activation. Microglial activation is also stimulated by opiate alkaloid-selective mu3 receptors; this activation can be blocked by the specific inhibitor naloxone. Receptors to *Substance P,* also known as *neurokinin-1 (NK-1) receptors,* enhance activation and inflammatory responses of microglial cells exposed to bacteria. In contrast, *somatostatin receptors* (of sst2, sst3 and sst4 types) decrease microglial activation.

Similarly, microglial activation and inflammatory responses can be down-regulated by *vasoactive intestinal peptide (VIP),* acting through specific *VIP/pituitary adenylate cyclase-activating peptide receptors 1 and 2 (VPAC$_1$/VPAC$_2$).* The neurotrophins (nerve growth factor, NGF, brain-derived growth factor, BDNF and neurotrophins 3, 4, NT-3/4 act on microglia through the so-called *Trk receptors*; activation of these receptors by BDNF results in sustained $[Ca^{2+}]_i$ elevation and decreases release of nitric oxide from activated microglia.

## 7.4.6   Cytokines and chemokines receptors

Receptors to cytokines and chemokines generally modulate microglial motility and chemotaxis, and may regulate release of various pro-inflammatory factors. The *chemokines* are a specific class of chemoattractive cytokines; they are small proteins of 8–12 kDa, classified into four subgroups – the C, CC, CXC and $CX_3C$ chemokines (Laing & Secombes, 2004). The chemokines are expressed by neurones and neuroglia.

Cellular effects of chemokines are mediated through 7-TM G-protein coupled receptors, classified into CCR, CXCR or $CX_3CR$ subtypes. These receptors are coupled to intercellular signalling cascades which include adenylate cyclase, phospholipases, GTPases and some kinases, such as mitogen-activated protein kinase (MAPK) or phosphatidyl inositol-3 kinase (PI3-K) (Biber *et al.*, 2008; Gebicke-Haerter *et al.*, 2001).

Chemokine receptors have a degree of promiscuity and can be activated by several cytokines, albeit at different concentrations. In microglia, activation of chemokine receptors (in particular $CX_3CR1$, the receptor for $CX_3CL1$ or fractalkine) triggers $Ca^{2+}$ signalling through $InsP_3$-mediated $Ca^{2+}$ release from the ER and store-operated $Ca^{2+}$ entry (Boddeke *et al.*, 1999). One of the consequences of $Ca^{2+}$ release is the activation of $Ca^{2+}$-dependent $K^+$ channels. CXCR3 receptors have also been reported to activate volume-regulated $Cl^-$ channels linked to microglial migration. These chemokine receptors also generally suppress microglial secretion of pro-inflammatory factors. As a rule, activated microglia up-regulate expression of chemokine receptors and chemokines. Release of chemokines from neurones can guide chemotaxis and provide for fine tuning of microglial activation.

Chemokine signalling is altered in various types of neuropathology, for example in multiple sclerosis, in Alzheimer's disease and in neuropathic pain. These pathologies are often accompanied with increased expression of CCR3 and CCR5 chemokine receptors (Gebicke-Haerter *et al.*, 2001).

Microglial effects of *cytokines* are mediated through receptors to *tumour necrosis factor* α (TNF-α) and receptors to various interleukins. TNF-α acts through *TNF-α receptor 1* (*TNRF1*), which have been identified in microglia. Activation of these receptors facilitates microglial activation and enhances phagocytosis. TNF-α receptors are also positively linked to microglial release of TNF-α, providing positive autocrine feedback that further increases microglial activation (Kuno *et al.*, 2005).

Interleukins are an extended family of cytokines (of which at least 35 types, IL-1 to IL-35, are identified) that mediate various trophic and immune effects. mRNA transcripts of many interleukin receptors have been detected in cultured microglia (IL-1RI, IL-1RII, IL-5R, IL-6R, IL-8R, IL-9R, IL-10R, IL-12R, IL-13R, and

**Table 7.3**  Cytokines and chemokines receptors in microglia (modified from Kettenmann *et al.*, 2011)

| Receptor type | Properties and functional relevance |
| --- | --- |
| *Chemokine receptors* | |
| CCR1, CCR2, CCR5 | Stimulation of CCR2 and CCR5 triggered $[Ca^{2+}]_i$ transients; activation of microglia by LPS increased these $Ca^{2+}$ responses. |
| CXCR1, CXCR3 and CCR3 | Receptor expression was increased following treatments with TNF-$\alpha$ and IFN-$\gamma$. |
| CCR5 | Hypoxia/ischaemia increased CCR5 mRNA expression. |
| CCR5 | Stimulation with MIP-1$\alpha$ increased the amplitude of $K^+$ currents. |
| CXCR3 | Activation of CXCR3 receptors activated volume-regulated $Cl^-$ channels. |
| *TNF-$\alpha$ receptors* | |
| TNFR1 and TNFR2 | Reduced microglial activation along with increased neuronal damage in receptor-deficient mice challenged by ischaemia and seizures, up-regulation of TLR2. |
| *Interferon (IFN) receptors* | |
| IFN$\gamma$R | Regulation and massive reorganization of induced cytokine and chemokine production, up-regulation of MHC II, induction of immunoproteasome, induction of neuronal markers and a neuroprotective phenotype, instruction of a M1-like reactive phenotype. |
| IFNAR, type I IFN receptor | Suppression of glutamate and superoxide production, regulation of gene expression, involvement in the control of microglial functions *in vivo* and *ex vivo*. |
| *Interleukin receptors* | |
| IL-1R1/IL-1R2 and related molecules | Induction of inflammatory mediators, like PGE2 and IL-6, activation of NF-$\kappa$B, p38, JNK and ERK1/2. |
| IL-2R$\alpha$/$\beta$/$\gamma$ ($\gamma_c$) | Augmented NO production, increased growth and viability, indirect evidence for recruitment of MHC II$^+$ and CD11b$^+$ microglia to lesions. |
| IL-4R | Induction of cytokines and chemokines with M2-like profile, enhanced $\beta$-amyloid clearance, regulation of scavenger receptor expression, oligodendrocyte markers and dendritic cell (DC) marker, CD11c, down-regulation of pro-inflammatory cytokines, induction of a M2-alternatively activated phenotype. |
| IL-10R | Induction of a M2-deactivated phenotype. |
| IL-13R | Induction of cytokines and chemokines with M2-like profile. |
| IL-15R$\alpha$ (sharing IL-2R$\beta$ and $\gamma$ for signalling) | Induction of intracellular signalling via JAK1 recruitment, support of microglial survival, reduction of NO production, indirect evidence for recruitment of MHC II$^+$ microglia to lesions. |
| IL-18R (IL-1-related) | Inducible signalling by IRAK and TRAF6 recruitment, regulation (attenuation) of induced IL-12 production. |

IL-15R) (Lee *et al.*, 2002). Expression of these receptors is usually higher in activated microglia.

## 7.4.7 Pattern-recognition receptors

An important group of microglial receptors is represented by the pattern recognition receptors (defined also as *pathogen-associated molecular patterns* or *PAMPs*), whose primary function is to detect invading exogenous pathogens associated mostly with bacteria and viruses. These receptors regulate microglial activation through multiple intercellular signalling pathways and control their adaptive immunity (Hanisch *et al.*, 2008). The pattern-recognition receptors are classified into:

1. lectin-type, mannose and β-glucan receptors (e.g. dectin-1);

2. nucleotide binding and oligomerisation domain (NOD)-like receptors;

3. receptors characterised by a RNA helicase domain and two caspase-recruitment domains (CARD), collectively known now as RIG-I-like receptors (RLR); and

4. the Toll-like receptors, or TLRs (Fritz *et al.*, 2006; Palm & Medzhitov, 2009).

Some of these receptors (and especially the Toll-like receptors) are also capable of recognising endogenous molecules associated with tissue damage, defined as *damage- or danger-associated molecular patterns* (DAMPs) or *alarmins* (Bianchi, 2007).

The Toll[2]-like receptors (of which 13 types are identified, TLR1 to TLR13) are particularly important for microglial function. These receptors are generally coupled to several intracellular signalling cascades, involving the adaptor protein MyD88 (with exception of TLR3) and finally converging on transcription factors Ap-1 or NF-kB (Hansson & Edfeldt, 2005). All Toll-like receptors are integral membrane glycoproteins, of which TLR1,2, 4, 5 and 6 are localised to the plasma membrane, and TLR3, 7, 8 and 9 are present in endosomes. In the CNS, Toll-receptors are predominantly expressed in microglia and astrocytes; microglial cells are in possession of TLR1 to 9 (see Kettenmann *et al.*, 2011 for extended referencing).

Different Toll receptors are activated by distinct pathogens. For example:

• TLR2 (which can oligomerise with TLR1 or TLR6) are sensitive to bacterial tri- and diacyl lipopeptides, lipoteichoic acid and peptidoglycan;

• TLR3 responds to virus-specific double-stranded RNA;

• TRP4 is sensitive to bacterial lypopolysaccharide (LPS);

---

[2] receptors were discovered in Drosophila; they control various aspects of embryogenesis and regulate immunne responses of this fly. The name *Toll receptors* was coined in the course of analysing the data by the discoverer, Christiane Nüsslein-Volhard, who exclaimed *'Das war ja toll!'* Hansson GK, Edfeldt K., 2005. Toll to be paid at the gateway to the vessel wall. Arterioscler Thromb Vasc Biol 25(6):1085-7.

- TLR5 is activated by bacterial flagellin;

- TLR7 and 8 are specific to viral single-stranded RNA;

- TLR9 are activated by bacterial and viral unmethylated CpG DNA (Aravalli *et al.*, 2007; Carpentier *et al.*, 2008).

In addition, Toll-like receptors can recognise numerous endogenous pathogens, such as various heat shock proteins.

Microglial Toll-like receptors directly control microglial activation in many types of neuropathologies, including infection, trauma, stroke, neurodegeneration and autoimmune diseases (Aravalli *et al.*, 2007; Okun *et al.*, 2009). Microglial activation, in turn, has a positive feedback on Toll-like receptor expression; the levels of microglial TLRs increase in pathological conditions.

## 7.4.8   Other receptor systems

Microglial cells express a wide variety of other receptor systems, which most likely increase their ability to monitor the status of surrounding tissue and tailor functional responses according to their immediate environment. Microglial cells can detect the anaphylotoxins, *complement fragments C3a and C5a*, by appropriate receptors. The *C3a* and *C5a receptors* are 7-transmembrane domain G-protein coupled metabotropic receptors linked to phosplipase C/InsP$_3$/ER Ca$^{2+}$ release and to K$^+$ channels (Moller *et al.*, 1997).

Microglia also express plasmalemmal *calcium receptor*, or *CaR*, which is another heptahelical G-protein coupled receptor sensitive to extracellular Ca$^{2+}$ concentrations. Activation of these receptors by an increase in extracellular Ca$^{2+}$ is linked to activation of various K$^+$ channels (Chattopadhyay *et al.*, 1999). Another important class of G-protein coupled receptors expressed in microglial cells is *proteinase-activated receptors* (*PARs*, which are activated by thrombin (PAR1,3 and 4) or by trypsin (PAR4). These receptors are activated when in contact with thrombin that may enter the CNS tissue following disruption of the blood-brain barrier. Activation of PAR receptors controls many different functions of microglia, including Ca$^{2+}$ signalling, stimulation of the release of NO, various cytokines and chemokines, and microglial activation (Moller *et al.*, 2006).

Microglial cells also express functional receptors to *cysteinyl leukotrienes*, or CysLTs. Stimulation of receptors of *CysLT1* and *CysLT2* types induces Ca$^{2+}$ signalling and promotes microglial release of ATP. The *Notch-1 receptors* in microglia may regulate production of cytokines and NO. The *macrophage colony-stimulating factor receptors* (*M-CSFRs*) are expressed only in activated microglia, and these receptors stimulate release of NO and cytokines, and promote phagocytosis. The *epidermal growth factor receptors* (*EGFRs*) are protein kinases, which positively modulate K$^+$ channels through G$_i$ proteins. The *CD200 receptors*, activated by surface glycoprotein CD200, are involved in regulation of phagocytosis. The *lysophosphatidic acid receptors* trigger microglial $Ca^{2+}$ signalling. Similarly, $Ca^{2+}$ signals are induced following stimulation of *formyl peptide receptors* by bacterial N-formylpeptides (see Kettenmann *et al.*, 2011 for details and references).

## 7.4.9   Microglial plasmalemmal transporters

Plasma membranes of microglial cells contain several types of ATP-dependent transporters and solute carriers (SLC) responsible for controlling ion gradients and regulating translocation of various molecules.

Substrate transport is mainly controlled by ABC-cassette transporters, glucose transporters and monocarboxylate transporters. The ABC-cassette transports in microglia were shown to mediate release of ATP and cysteinyl leukotrienes. These transporters are also involved in cholesterol transport and, hence, in lipid metabolism. Microglia specifically express *glucose transporter 5 (GLUT5)*, which is their main pathway for glucose accumulation. Activated microglial cells have relatively high levels of *monocarboxylate transporter 1* and 2 *(MCT1, 2)*, which may supply the cells with lactate.

Microglial cells participate in bi-directional glutamate transport. Resting microglia express low levels of glutamate transporters, but activation of microglia triggers significant up-regulation of expression of both *EAAT-1/GLAST* and *EAAT-2/GLT-1* transporters. High levels of these transporters have been detected in activated human microglia studied in post-mortem tissues affected by stroke or acute trauma. Similar increases in glutamate transporter expression have been found in microglia from HIV-1 patients and samples from different brain regions of patients affected by prion disease. Likewise, glutamate transporters were up-regulated in microglia isolated from animals subjected to various pathological insults, such as ischaemia or facial nerve axotomy.

The up-regulation of glutamate transporters is also observed *in vitro* after exposure of primary microglial cultures to activating stimuli, e.g. *Herpes simplex* virus or β-amyloid. Increase in expression of glutamate transporters by microglia is neuroprotective, as it contributes to the removal of excess of glutamate often accompanying neuropathological events, especially resulting from ischaemic or excitotoxic cell death.

Activated microglial cells, however, can also release glutamate, which occurs mainly through *glutamate-cystine antiporter Xc*, which exchanges glutamate for cystine. Cystine, in turn, is obligatory for formation of glutathione, the latter being at the core of microglial protection against reactive oxygen species. Increased glutamate release/cystine uptake in activated microglia is likely to be driven by massive demand for cystine/cysteine for replenishing glutathione needed to counteract ROS accumulation during oxidative bursts and phagocytosis (Barger & Basile, 2001).

Microglial cells have several types of ion transporters and solute carriers. Interestingly the $Na^+/K^+$ ATP-ase (sodium-potassium pump) are not functionally active in microglia, and intracellular $K^+$ concentration is mainly regulated by $H^+/K^+$ *ATP-ase* which, in addition, controls the flux of protons. Microglial cells have several $K^+/Cl^-$ *co-transporters (KCC1-4)*, which are activated during cell swelling and opening of swelling-activated $Cl^-$ channels. Cultured microglial cells express $Na^+/HCO_3^-$ *co-transporters* and $Na^+$-*dependent* $Cl^-/HCO_3^-$ *exchangers*, the latter being one of the main components in the regulation of intracellular pH. Another important molecule responsible for regulation of cytosolic pH is the $Na^+/H^+$ *exchanger (NHE-1* isoform), which is also linked to regulation of cytokine release.

## 7.5    Microglial migration and motility

Microglial cells are the most motile cells in the CNS. As has been already mentioned, the ramified (resting or survelliant) microglial cells constantly move processes which scan their territorial domains. In this kind of motility, only processes move and the cell body stays anchored. The amoeboid microglia (i.e. early invading microglial cells or activated microglia) show a very different type of movement when the entire cell moves through the nerve tissue. Precise mechanisms of process movements in resting microglia are unresolved. Local lesions, however, trigger rapid convergent movements of the processes towards injury, and this movement is activated mainly by $P2X_{12}$ purinoceptors (see Section 7.4.4).

The movement of amoeboid cells, which is a true cell migration, is regulated by multiple receptors and is mediated through water/ion transport and rearrangements of the cytoskeleton. In particular, $K^+$ channels, $Cl^-$ channels, $Na^+/H^+$ exchangers, $Cl^-/HCO_3^-$ exchangers, and $Na^+/HCO_3^-$ cotransporters are all involved in migration (Figure 7.9); they all also are linked to the actin cytoskeleton (for detailed account on mechanisms of cell migration see Schwab, 2001a, 2001b).

Migratory behaviour of amoeboid microglia is initiated and directed by various molecules. First, there are neurotransmitters, such as ATP, which is a potent chemoattractant for microglia (its action on cellular movement is mediated through $P2Y_{12}$ and adenosine receptors). Glutamate also triggers directed microglial migration through AMPA and metabotropic glutamate receptors. Similarly, migration is enhanced by adrenaline and dopamine.

A potent chemoattractant for microglia is represented by chemokines, which can be released by damaged cells. The chemokine CCL21, for example, triggers chemotaxic microglial migration, mediated through CXCR3 chemokine receptors and ultimately dependent on activation of $Cl^-$ channels. Microglial migration can be induced by stromal cell-derived factor-1$\alpha$ (SDF-1$\alpha$), acting through CXC chemokine receptor 4 (CXCR4).

Microglial migration is enhanced by: cannabinoids acting through $CB_2$ receptors; Lysophosphatidic acid, which acts through activation of $Ca^{2+}$-dependent $K^+$ channels; opioids, acting through mu receptors; bradykinin, which activates protein kinases and potentiates $Ca^{2+}$ entry through reverse mode of $Na^+/Ca^{2+}$ exchangers; and various growth factors.

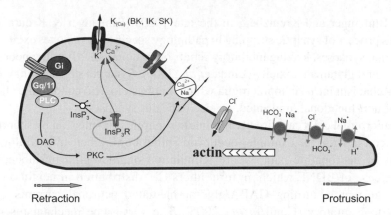

**Figure 7.9** Model summarising the role of ion channels and transporters in controlling micro-glial migration.

Cytosolic $Ca^{2+}$ signals, induced by activation of metabotropic receptors and $InsP_3$ cascade and/or by $Ca^{2+}$ entry through ionotropic receptors or reverse mode of $Na^+/Ca^{2+}$ exchanger, induces the retraction of the rear part of a migrating cell, which is paralleled by $K^+$ efflux via $Ca^{2+}$-dependent $K^+$ channels and shrinkage of the cell at the rear (retraction site). Transporters such as $Na^+/H^+$ and $Cl^-/HCO^{3-}$ exchangers at the front of migrating cells (protrusion site) are reported to contribute to the extension of the actin projection (lamellipodium) by mediating salt and osmotically obliged water uptake.

Modified from (Schwab 2001b) and reproduced from (Kettenmann et al. 2011).

# 7.6 Physiological functions of microglia: role in synaptic transmission and plasticity

For many years, microglial cells were considered to serve only a defensive role in the CNS – to identify the insult and provide an appropriate protective response. In recent years, however, evidence has accumulated indicating that microglia are actively involved in shaping neural networks and regulating various aspects of neuroplasticity (see Graeber & Christie, 2012; Tremblay & Majewska, 2011; Tremblay *et al.*, 2011 for recent detailed review).

First, microglial cells are involved in synaptogenesis. Early synaptogenesis in the embryonic CNS starts when astrocytes are not yet present (sometimes around embryonic day 14–15 in rodents). This first wave of embryonic synaptogenesis coincides with the first wave of CNS invasion by microglia. There is some evidence that microglial cells can assist, and even promote, synaptogenesis through secretion of growth factors and thrombospondins (Rigato *et al.*, 2011).

Second, microglial cells can remove redundant or malfunctioning synapses. In the healthy brain, microglial processes often contact synapses and, in certain conditions, these contacts are involved in synapse elimination. Microglia appear to scan the functional status of synapses and allow them to survive or perish (Wake *et al.*, 2009). This is very reminiscent of '*synaptic stripping*', discovered in post-traumatic nervous tissue by Blinzinger and Kreutzberg in the late 1960s (Blinzinger & Kreutzberg, 1968). This process of synaptic stripping in pathology specifically removes excitatory glutamatergic synapses, leaving inhibitory inputs operational, thus limiting neuronal excitability and glutamate toxicity (Linda *et al.*, 2000). Synaptic stripping may be a general mechanism intrinsic to microglia which, in physiological conditions, allows pruning of non-functional, unwanted, or else deficient synapses.

Third, microglial cells can directly modulate synaptic transmission by secreting various factors. This, for example, occurs in spinal cord, albeit in pathological conditions of neuropathic pain, where stimulation of microglial purinoceptors triggers release of BDNF which, in turn, alters $Cl^-$ distribution in neighbouring neurones, ultimately turning GABA/glycine-mediated neuronal currents from inhibitory to excitatory (Coull *et al.*, 2005). The very same mechanisms may operate in a physiological context. Microglial cells have the potential to influence homeostatic synaptic scaling, which entails uniform adjustments in the strength of all synapses on a cell – a mechanism distinct from long-term synaptic potentiation or depression. This scaling has been found to be mediated by microglia-derived TNFα (Stellwagen & Malenka, 2006). Similarly, interleukins secreted from microglia can modulate synaptic plasticity, for example by inhibiting long-term potentiation (Ross *et al.*, 2003). Synaptic strength and plasticity is also a subject of modulation by NO, which is synthesised and released by microglia.

Fourth, microglial processes can affect the morphology of the perisynaptic space, and possibly the synaptic cleft itself. For example, in the visual cortex of mice, microglial processes alter their morphology and synaptic contacts, depending on light stimulation (Tremblay *et al.*, 2010).

Fifth, microglial cells exert well-documented trophic effects through secretion of various neurotrophins, which may modulate the remodelling, growth and circuitry formation of neuronal networks (Kohsaka *et al.*, 1996; Morgan *et al.*, 2004).

Sixth, microglia affect neuronal connectivity, a phenomenon well known in post-lesioned CNS (Bessis *et al.*, 2007). For example, microglia control synaptic repair and reactive synaptogenesis following CNS insults (Moller *et al.*, 1996). It is also known that transplantation of microglia into lesioned CNS regions improves post-traumatic regeneration. The very same mechanisms could also act in the absence of pathology to shape neuronal rewiring.

Seventh, microglial cells can directly regulate adult neurogenesis in conjunction with environmental experience. For example, microglial cells from the hippocampi of animals subjected to running exercise acquired an ability to stimulate latent neuronal precursors *in vitro*, this effect being linked to chemokine signalling mediated by $CX_3CL1$ receptors (Vukovic *et al.*, 2012).

Finally, microglial cells can regulate behaviour. The first data supporting this role for microglia were obtained in experiments studying expression of the Hoxb8 gene. Deficits in functional expression of this gene in mice result in an obsessive grooming behaviour, a condition resembling the human pathology of compulsive hair pulling disorder, known as trichotillomania. It appears that this gene in the brain is expressed exclusively in microglia. Transplantation of bone marrow from wild-type animals into brains of Hox8b deficient mice inhibited compulsive hair removal. The effects of functionally expressed Hocb8 gene may be linked to secretion of cytokines (Chen *et al.*, 2010).

To conclude, microglial cells have the potential to regulate the development, structuring and function of neuronal networks. Furthermore, microglial cells are capable, at least potentially, of remodelling neuronal connectivity, and thus they may participate in physiological processes within neural networks.

## 7.7 Microglia in ageing

Microglial cells undergo several age-dependent changes, which in fact are more prominent compared to morphological senescence of neurones (for comprehensive review of the microglial ageing see Conde & Streit, 2006; Streit, 2006; Streit & Xue, 2010).

The total number of microglial cells increases with age ($\approx$65 per cent increase between 3 and 30 month old rats). Assuming that, during physiological senescence (i.e. in the absence of external insults or neurodegenerative pathology), there is very little (if any) myeloid cell invasion into the CNS, this increase in numbers most likely indicates the proliferation of endogenous microglia.

In the aged brain, microglial cells also undergo morphological and functional remodelling, manifested by decreased number and complexity of processes and slowing down of processes motility. All in all, microglia becomes less ramified and less dynamic (Damani *et al.*, 2012). The cell bodies of microglia in ageing increase in volume, mostly through accumulation of lipofuscin.

In addition, ageing microglia acquire a more prominent immunological profile by increasing various surface antigens. What is the nature and meaning of these ageing changes? Most likely, they represent defensive remodelling associated with neuro-protection. Most interestingly, atrophic changes in microglia which are observed in aged human brain generally signal the advent of pathology, as this microglial degeneration lessens neuroprotection and facilitates the development of neuro-degeneration (Streit *et al.*, 2008).

## 7.8 Concluding remarks

Microglial cells are the principal elements of CNS cellular and immune defence. Microglia invade the nervous system embryonically and disseminate throughout CNS parenchyma. When settling in the nervous system, microglial cells undergo fundamental changes in phenotype, acquiring a specific morphology and a complement of receptors that allow then to monitor the nervous system environment and detect pathological insults. When lesion occurs, microglial cells are activated and thus become a fundamental cellular element of neuropathology.

In addition, microglia participate in the physiology of the nervous system through regulation of development and connectivity of neural networks. Microglial cells therefore combine a defensive role with homeostatic and neuroprotective functions.

# References

Aravalli RN, Peterson PK, Lokensgard JR. (2007). Toll-like receptors in defense and damage of the central nervous system. *Journal of Neuroimmune Pharmacology* **2**(4), 297–312.

Barger SW, Basile AS. (2001). Activation of microglia by secreted amyloid precursor protein evokes release of glutamate by cystine exchange and attenuates synaptic function. *Journal of Neurochemistry* **76**(3), 846–54.

Bessis A, Bechade C, Bernard D, Roumier A. (2007). Microglial control of neuronal death and synaptic properties. *Glia* **55**(3), 233–8.

Bianchi ME. (2007). DAMPs, PAMPs and alarmins: all we need to know about danger. *Journal of Leukocyte Biology* **81**(1), 1–5.

Biber K, Neumann H, Inoue K, Boddeke HW. (2007). neuronal 'On' and 'Off' signals control microglia. *Trends In Neurosciences* **30**(11), 596–602.

Biber K, Vinet J, Boddeke HW. (2008). Neuron-microglia signaling: chemokines as versatile messengers. *Journal of Neuroimmunology* **198**(1–2) 69–74.

Blinzinger K, Kreutzberg G. (1968). Displacement of synaptic terminals from regenerating motoneurons by microglial cells. *Zeitschrift Fur Zellforschung und Mikroskopische Anatomie* **85**(2), 145–57.

Boddeke EW, Meigel I, Frentzel S, Gourmala NG, Harrison JK, Buttini M, Spleiss O, Gebicke-Harter P. (1999). Cultured rat microglia express functional beta-chemokine receptors. *Journal of Neuroimmunology* **98**(2), 176–84.

Bordey A, Spencer DD. (2003). Chemokine modulation of high-conductance $Ca^{2+}$-sensitive $K^+$ currents in microglia from human hippocampi. *European Journal of Neuroscience* **18**(10), 2893–8.

Boucsein C, Kettenmann H, Nolte C. (2000). Electrophysiological properties of microglial cells in normal and pathologic rat brain slices. *European Journal of Neuroscience* **12**(6), 2049–58.

Boucsein C, Zacharias R, Farber K, Pavlovic S, Hanisch UK, Kettenmann H. (2003). Purinergic receptors on microglial cells: functional expression in acute brain slices and modulation of microglial activation *in vitro*. *European Journal of Neuroscience* **17**(11), 2267–76.

Brockhaus J, Ilschner S, Banati RB, Kettenmann H. (1993). Membrane properties of ameboid microglial cells in the corpus callosum slice from early postnatal mice. *Journal of Neuroscience* **13**(10), 4412–21.

Brough D, Le Feuvre RA, Iwakura Y, Rothwell NJ. (2002). Purinergic P2X₇ receptor activation of microglia induces cell death via an interleukin-1-independent mechanism. *Molecular and Cellular Neurosciences* **19**(2), 272–80.

Burnstock G, Verkhratsky A. (2009). Evolutionary origins of the purinergic signalling system. *Acta Physiologica (Oxford)* **195**(4), 415–47.

Carpentier PA, Duncan DS, Miller SD. (2008). Glial toll-like receptor signaling in central nervous system infection and autoimmunity. *Brain, Behavior, and Immunity* **22**(2), 140–7.

Chattopadhyay N, Ye C, Yamaguchi T, Nakai M, Kifor O, Vassilev PM, Nishimura RN, Brown EM. (1999). The extracellular calcium-sensing receptor is expressed in rat microglia and modulates an outward $K^+$ channel. *Journal of Neurochemistry* **72**(5), 1915–22.

Chen SK, Tvrdik P, Peden E, Cho S, Wu S, Spangrude G, Capecchi MR. (2010). Hematopoietic origin of pathological grooming in Hoxb8 mutant mice. *Cell* **141**(5), 775–85.

Christensen RN, Ha BK, Sun F, Bresnahan JC, Beattie MS. (2006). Kainate induces rapid redistribution of the actin cytoskeleton in ameboid microglia. *Journal of Neuroscience Research* **84**(1), 170–81.

Collo G, Neidhart S, Kawashima E, Kosco-Vilbois M, North RA, Buell G. (1997). Tissue distribution of the P2X₇ receptor. *Neuropharmacology* **36**(9), 1277–83.

Conde JR, Streit WJ. (2006). Microglia in the aging brain. *J Neuropathol Experimental Neurology* **65**(3), 199–203.

Coull JA, Beggs S, Boudreau D, Boivin D, Tsuda M, Inoue K, Gravel C, Salter MW, De Koninck Y. (2005). BDNF from microglia causes the shift in neuronal anion gradient underlying neuropathic pain. *Nature* **438**(7070), 1017–21.

Damani MR, Zhao L, Fontainhas AM, Amaral J, Fariss RN, Wong WT. (2012). Age-related alterations in the dynamic behavior of microglia. *Aging Cell* **10**(2), 263–76.

Davalos D, Grutzendler J, Yang G, Kim JV, Zuo Y, Jung S, Littman DR, Dustin ML, Gan WB. (2005). ATP mediates rapid microglial response to local brain injury *in vivo*. *Nature Neuroscience* **8**(6), 752–8.

Del Rio-Hortega P. (1932). *Microglia*. In: Penfield W. (ed.). *Cytology and cellular pathology of the nervous system*. New York: Hoeber. p 482–534.

Eder C. (1998). Ion channels in microglia (brain macrophages). *American Journal of Physiology* **275**(2 Pt 1) C327–42.

Eder C, DeCoursey TE. (2001). Voltage-operated proton channels in microglia. *Progress In Neurobiology* **64**(3), 277–305.

Farber K, Kettenmann H. (2006). Purinergic signaling and microglia. *Pflugers Archiv* **452**(5), 615–21.

Farber K, Pannasch U, Kettenmann H. (2005). Dopamine and noradrenaline control distinct functions in rodent microglial cells. *Molecular and Cellular Neurosciences* **29**(1), 128–38.

Ferrari D, Villalba M, Chiozzi P, Falzoni S, Ricciardi-Castagnoli P, Di Virgilio F. (1996). Mouse microglial cells express a plasma membrane pore gated by extracellular ATP. *Journal of Immunology* **156**(4), 1531–9.

Ferrari D, Chiozzi P, Falzoni S, Hanau S, Di Virgilio F. (1997). Purinergic modulation of interleukin-1 b release from microglial cells stimulated with bacterial endotoxin. *Journal of Experimental Medicine* **185**(3), 579–82.

Feske S, Gwack Y, Prakriya M, Srikanth S, Puppel SH, Tanasa B, Hogan PG, Lewis RS, Daly M, Rao A. (2006). A mutation in Orai1 causes immune deficiency by abrogating CRAC channel function. *Nature* **441**(7090), 179–85.

Fritz JH, Ferrero RL, Philpott DJ, Girardin SE. (2006). Nod like proteins in immunity, inflammation and disease. *Nature Immunology* **7**(12), 1250–7.

Gebicke-Haerter PJ, Spleiss O, Ren LQ, Li H, Dichmann S, Norgauer J, Boddeke HW. (2001). Microglial chemokines and chemokine receptors. *Progress In Brain Research* **132**, 525–32.

Ginhoux F, Greter M, Leboeuf M, Nandi S, See P, Gokhan S, Mehler MF, Conway SJ, Ng LG, Stanley E.R. *et al.* (2010). Fate mapping analysis reveals that adult microglia derive from primitive macrophages. *Science* **330**(6005), 841–5.

Glees P. (1955). *Neuroglia Morphology and Function*. Oxford: Blackwell Scientific Publications.

Graeber MB. (2010). Changing face of microglia. *Science* **330**(6005), 783–8.

Graeber MB, Christie MJ. (2012). Multiple mechanisms of microglia: a gatekeeper's contribution to pain states. *Experimental Neurology* **234**(2), 255–61.

Graeber MB, Li W, Rodriguez ML. (2011). Role of microglia in CNS inflammation. *FEBS Letters* **585**(23), 3798–805.

Haas S, Brockhaus J, Verkhratsky A, Kettenmann H. (1996). ATP-induced membrane currents in ameboid microglia acutely isolated from mouse brain slices. *Neuroscience* **75**(1), 257–61.

Hanisch UK, Johnson TV, Kipnis J. (2008). Toll-like receptors: roles in neuroprotection? *Trends In Neurosciences* **31**(4), 176–82.

Hanisch UK, Kettenmann H. (2007). Microglia: active sensor and versatile effector cells in the normal and pathologic brain. *Nature Neuroscience* **10**(11), 1387–94.

Hansson GK, Edfeldt K. (2005). Toll to be paid at the gateway to the vessel wall. *Arteriosclerosis, Thrombosis, and Vascular Biology* **25**(6), 1085–7.

Haynes SE, Hollopeter G, Yang G, Kurpius D, Dailey ME, Gan WB, Julius D. (2006). The $P2Y_{12}$ receptor regulates microglial activation by extracellular nucleotides. *Nature Neuroscience* **9**(12), 1512–9.

Hoffmann A, Kann O, Ohlemeyer C, Hanisch UK, Kettenmann H. (2003). Elevation of basal intracellular calcium as a central element in the activation of brain macrophages (microglia): suppression of receptor-evoked calcium signaling and control of release function. *Journal of Neuroscience* **23**(11), 4410–9.

Ifuku M, Farber K, Okuno Y, Yamakawa Y, Miyamoto T, Nolte C, Merrino VF, Kita S, Iwamoto T, Komuro I. *et al.* (2007). Bradykinin-induced microglial migration mediated by $B_1$-bradykinin receptors depends on $Ca^{2+}$ influx via reverse-mode activity of the $Na^+/Ca^{2+}$ exchanger. *Journal of Neuroscience* **27**(48), 13065–73.

Inoue K. (2008). Purinergic systems in microglia. *Cellular and Molecular Life Sciences.*

Inoue K, Koizumi S, Kataoka A, Tozaki-Saitoh H, Tsuda M. (2009). $P2Y_6$-Evoked Microglial Phagocytosis. *International Review of Neurobiology* **85**, 159–63.

Kaindl AM, Degos V, Peineau S, Gouadon E, Chhor V, Loron G, Le Charpentier T, Josserand J, Ali C, Vivien D, Collingridge GL, Lombet A, Issa L, Rene F, Loeffler J P, Kavelaars A, Verney C, Mantz J, Gressens P. (2012). Activation of microglial N-methyl-D-aspartate receptors triggers inflammation and neuronal cell death in the developing and mature brain. *Annals of Neurology* **72**(4) 536–549.

Kershman J. (1939). Genesis of microglia in the human brain. *Archives of Neurology & Psychiatry* **41**, 24–50.

Kettenmann H, Hoppe D, Gottmann K, Banati R, Kreutzberg G. (1990). Cultured microglial cells have a distinct pattern of membrane channels different from peritoneal macrophages. *Journal of Neuroscience Research* **26**(3), 278–87.

Kettenmann H, Hanisch UK, Noda M, Verkhratsky A. (2011). Physiology of microglia. *Physiological Reviews* **91**(2), 461–553.

Kohsaka S, Hamanoue M, Nakajima K. (1996). Functional implication of secretory proteases derived from microglia in the central nervous system. *Keio Journal of Medicine* **45**(3), 263–9.

Krabbe G, Matyash V, Pannasch U, Mamer L, Boddeke HW, Kettenmann H. (2012). Activation of serotonin receptors promotes microglial injury-induced motility but attenuates phagocytic activity. *Brain, Behavior, and Immunity* **26**(3), 419–28.

Kuhn SA, van Landeghem FK, Zacharias R, Farber K, Rappert A, Pavlovic S, Hoffmann A, Nolte C, Kettenmann H. (2004). Microglia express $GABA_B$ receptors to modulate interleukin release. *Molecular and Cellular Neurosciences* **25**(2), 312–22.

Kuno R, Wang J, Kawanokuchi J, Takeuchi H, Mizuno T, Suzumura A. (2005). Autocrine activation of microglia by tumor necrosis factor-alpha. *Journal of Neuroimmunology* **162**(1–2) 89–96.

Laing KJ, Secombes CJ. (2004). Chemokines. *Developmental and Comparative Immunology* **28**(5), 443–60.

Lecca D, Trincavelli ML, Gelosa P, Sironi L, Ciana P, Fumagalli M, Villa G, Verderio C, Grumelli C, Guerrini U. *et al.* (2008). The recently identified P2Y-like receptor GPR17 is a sensor of brain damage and a new target for brain repair. *PLoS One* **3**(10), e3579.

Lee YB, Nagai A, Kim SU. (2002). Cytokines, chemokines, and cytokine receptors in human microglia. *Journal of Neuroscience Research* **69**(1), 94–103.

Linda H, Shupliakov O, Ornung G, Ottersen OP, Storm-Mathisen J, Risling M, Cullheim S. (2000). Ultrastructural evidence for a preferential elimination of glutamate-immunoreactive synaptic terminals from spinal motoneurons after intramedullary axotomy. *Journal of Comparative Neurology* **425**(1), 10–23.

Mastroeni D, Grover A, Leonard B, Joyce JN, Coleman PD, Kozik B, Bellinger DL, Rogers J. (2008). Microglial responses to dopamine in a cell culture model of Parkinson's disease. *Neurobiology of Aging* **30**(11), 1805–17.

McLarnon JG, Choi HB, Lue LF, Walker DG, Kim SU. (2005). Perturbations in calcium-mediated signal transduction in microglia from Alzheimer's disease patients. *Journal of Neuroscience Research* **81**(3), 426–35.

Milton RH, Abeti R, Averaimo S, DeBiasi S, Vitellaro L, Jiang L, Curmi PM, Breit SN, Duchen MR, Mazzanti M. (2008). CLIC1 function is required for beta-amyloid-induced generation of reactive oxygen species by microglia. *Journal of Neuroscience* **28**(45), 11488–99.

Moller JC, Klein MA, Haas S, Jones LL, Kreutzberg GW, Raivich G. (1996). Regulation of thrombospondin in the regenerating mouse facial motor nucleus. *Glia* **17**(2), 121–32.

Moller T, Nolte C, Burger R, Verkhratsky A, Kettenmann H. (1997). Mechanisms of C5a and C3a complement fragment-induced [Ca$^{2+}$]$_i$ signaling in mouse microglia. *Journal of Neuroscience* **17**(2), 615–24.

Moller T, Kann O, Verkhratsky A, Kettenmann H. (2000). Activation of mouse microglial cells affects P2 receptor signaling. *Brain Research* **853**(1), 49–59.

Moller T, Weinstein JR, Hanisch UK. (2006). Activation of microglial cells by thrombin: past, present, and future. *Seminars In Thrombosis and Hemostasis* **32** Suppl 1, 69–76.

Monif M, Reid CA, Powell KL, Smart ML, Williams DA. (2009). The P2X$_7$ receptor drives microglial activation and proliferation: a trophic role for P2X$_7$R pore. *Journal of Neuroscience* **29**(12), 3781–91.

Morgan SC, Taylor DL, Pocock JM. (2004). Microglia release activators of neuronal proliferation mediated by activation of mitogen-activated protein kinase, phosphatidylinositol-3-kinase/Akt and delta-Notch signalling cascades. *Journal of Neurochemistry* **90**(1), 89–101.

Nimmerjahn A, Kirchhoff F, Helmchen F. (2005). Resting microglial cells are highly dynamic surveillants of brain parenchyma *in vivo*. *Science* **308**(5726), 1314–8.

Noda M, Nakanishi H, Nabekura J, Akaike N. (2000). AMPA-kainate subtypes of glutamate receptor in rat cerebral microglia. *Journal of Neuroscience* **20**(1), 251–8.

Noda M, Kariura Y, Pannasch U, Nishikawa K, Wang L, Seike T, Ifuku M, Kosai Y, Wang B, Nolte C and others. (2007). Neuroprotective role of bradykinin because of the attenuation of pro-inflammatory cytokine release from activated microglia. *Journal of Neurochemistry* **101**(2), 397–410.

Norenberg W, Gebicke-Haerter PJ, Illes P. (1992). Inflammatory stimuli induce a new K$^+$ outward current in cultured rat microglia. *Neuroscience Letters* **147**(2), 171–4.

Norenberg W, Gebicke-Haerter PJ, Illes P. (1994). Voltage-dependent potassium channels in activated rat microglia. *Journal of Physiology* **475**(1), 15–32.

Ohana L, Newell EW, Stanley EF, Schlichter LC. (2009). The Ca$^{2+}$ release-activated Ca$^{2+}$ current (I$_{CRAC}$) mediates store-operated Ca$^{2+}$ entry in rat microglia. *Channels (Austin)* **3**(2), 129–39.

Okun E, Griffioen KJ, Lathia JD, Tang SC, Mattson MP, Arumugam TV. (2009). Toll-like receptors in neurodegeneration. *Brain Research Reviews* **59**(2), 278–92.

Palm NW, Medzhitov R. (2009). Pattern recognition receptors and control of adaptive immunity. *Immunological Reviews* **227**(1), 221–33.

Prinz M, Mildner A. (2011). Microglia in the CNS: immigrants from another world. *Glia* **59**(2), 177–87.

Prinz M, Hausler KG, Kettenmann H, Hanisch U. (2001). b-Adrenergic receptor stimulation selectively inhibits IL-12p40 release in microglia. *Brain Research* **899**(1–2), 264–70.

Ransohoff RM, Perry VH. (2009). Microglial physiology: unique stimuli, specialized responses. *Annual Review of Immunology* **27**, 119–45.

Rigato C, Buckinx R, Le-Corronc H, Rigo JM, Legendre P. (2011). Pattern of invasion of the embryonic mouse spinal cord by microglial cells at the time of the onset of functional neuronal networks. *Glia* **59**(4), 675–95.

Ross FM, Allan SM, Rothwell NJ, Verkhratsky A. (2003). A dual role for interleukin-1 in LTP in mouse hippocampal slices. *Journal of Neuroimmunology* **144**(1–2) 61–7.

Sanz JM, Chiozzi P, Ferrari D, Colaianna M, Idzko M, Falzoni S, Fellin R, Trabace L, Di Virgilio F. (2009). Activation of microglia by amyloid b requires P2X$_7$ receptor expression. *Journal of Immunology* **182**(7), 4378–85.

Sattayaprasert P, Choi HB, Chongthammakun S, McLarnon JG. (2005). Platelet-activating factor enhancement of calcium influx and interleukin-6 expression, but not production, in human microglia. *Journal of Neuroinflammation* **2**(1), 11.

Schlichter LC, Kaushal V, Moxon-Emre I, Sivagnanam V, Vincent C. (2010). The $Ca^{2+}$ activated SK3 channel is expressed in microglia in the rat striatum and contributes to microglia-mediated neurotoxicity *in vitro*. *Journal of Neuroinflammation* **7**(1), 4.

Schlichter LC, Sakellaropoulos G, Ballyk B, Pennefather PS, Phipps DJ. (1996). Properties of $K^+$ and $Cl^-$ channels and their involvement in proliferation of rat microglial cells. *Glia* **17**(3), 225–36.

Schwab A. (2001a). Function and spatial distribution of ion channels and transporters in cell migration. *American Journal of Physiology. Renal Physiology* **280**(5), F739–47.

Schwab A. (2001b). Ion channels and transporters on the move. *News in Physiological Sciences* **16**, 29–33.

Shytle RD, Mori T, Townsend K, Vendrame M, Sun N, Zeng J, Ehrhart J, Silver AA, Sanberg PR, Tan J. (2004). Cholinergic modulation of microglial activation by alpha 7 nicotinic receptors. *Journal of Neurochemistry* **89**(2), 337–43.

Stella N. (2010). Cannabinoid and cannabinoid-like receptors in microglia, astrocytes, and astrocytomas. *Glia* **58**(9), 1017–30.

Stellwagen D, Malenka RC. (2006). Synaptic scaling mediated by glial TNF-a. *Nature* **440**(7087), 1054–9.

Streit WJ. (2006). Microglial senescence: does the brain's immune system have an expiration date? *Trends In Neurosciences* **29**(9), 506–10.

Streit WJ, Xue QS. (2010). The Brain's Aging Immune System. *Aging & Disease* **1**(3), 254–261.

Streit WJ, Miller KR, Lopes KO, Njie E. (2008). Microglial degeneration in the aging brain –bad news for neurons? *Frontiers In Bioscience* **13**, 3423–38.

Syed H, Kennedy C. (2012). Pharmacology of P2X Receptors. *WIRES Membrane Transport and Signaling* **1**, 16–30.

Takenouchi T, Fujita M, Sugama S, Kitani H, Hashimoto M. (2009). The role of the $P2X_7$ receptor signaling pathway for the release of autolysosomes in microglial cells. *Autophagy* **5**(5), 723–4.

Toescu EC, Moller T, Kettenmann H, Verkhratsky A. (1998). Long-term activation of capacitative $Ca^{2+}$ entry in mouse microglial cells. *Neuroscience* **86**(3), 925–35.

Torres E, Gutierrez-Lopez MD, Borcel E, Peraile I, Mayado A, O'Shea E, Colado MI. (2010). Evidence that MDMA ('ecstasy') increases cannabinoid $CB_2$ receptor expression in microglial cells: role in the neuroinflammatory response in rat brain. *Journal of Neurochemistry* in press.

Tremblay ME, Majewska AK. (2011). A role for microglia in synaptic plasticity? *Communicative & Integrative Biology* **4**(2), 220–2.

Tremblay ME, Lowery RL, Majewska AK. (2010). Microglial interactions with synapses are modulated by visual experience. *PLoS Biology* **8**(11), e1000527.

Tremblay ME, Stevens B, Sierra A, Wake H, Bessis A, Nimmerjahn A. (2011). The role of microglia in the healthy brain. *Journal of Neuroscience* **31**(45), 16064–9.

Verkhratsky A, Krishtal OA, Burnstock G. (2009). Purinoceptors on neuroglia. *Molecular Neurobiology* **39**(3), 190–208.

Vukovic J, Colditz MJ, Blackmore DG, Ruitenberg MJ, Bartlett PF. (2012). Microglia modulate hippocampal neural precursor activity in response to exercise and aging. *Journal of Neuroscience* **32**(19), 6435–43.

Wake H, Moorhouse AJ, Jinno S, Kohsaka S, Nabekura J. (2009). Resting microglia directly monitor the functional state of synapses *in vivo* and determine the fate of ischemic terminals. *Journal of Neuroscience* **29**(13), 3974–80.

Yu Y, Ugawa S, Ueda T, Ishida Y, Inoue K, Kyaw Nyunt A, Umemura A, Mase M, Yamada K, Shimada S. (2008). Cellular localization of $P2X_7$ receptor mRNA in the rat brain. *Brain Research* **1194**, 45–55.

Zhang F, Vadakkan KI, Kim SS, Wu LJ, Shang Y, Zhuo M. (2008). Selective activation of microglia in spinal cord but not higher cortical regions following nerve injury in adult mouse. *Molecular Pain* **4**, 15.

# 8
# Peripheral Glial Cells

*Glial Physiology and Pathophysiology*, First Edition. Alexei Verkhratsky and Arthur Butt.
© 2013 by John Wiley & Sons, Ltd. Published 2013 by John Wiley & Sons, Ltd.

# 8.1    Peripheral nervous system

## 8.1.1    Basic structure

The *peripheral nervous system* (PNS) consists of the nerves and ganglia outside of the brain and spinal cord. The function of the PNS is to connect the CNS to the body (muscles, glands, sensory receptors) and its organs (e.g. skin, heart, lungs, gastro-intestinal (GI) tract), via the cranial nerves (excluding the optic nerve – cranial nerve II – which is part of the CNS) and the spinal nerves, which contain both sensory and motor fibres. Broadly speaking, the PNS is made up of the somatic (voluntary) and autonomic (involuntary, with sympathetic and parasympathetic divisions) nervous systems, as well as their associated sensory and autonomic ganglia, plus the enteric nervous system, which is the independent nervous system of the GI tract (Figure 8.1).

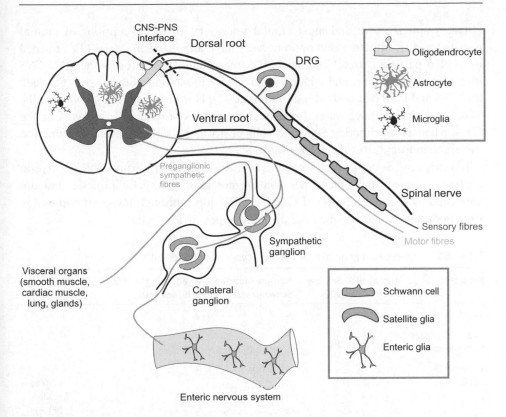

**Figure 8.1**   General structure of the peripheral nervous system.

The spinal cord and PNS connections are illustrated. The sensory neurones have their cell bodies in the dorsal root ganglia and extend axons through the dorsal root into the dorsal horn of the spinal cord. The somatic and autonomic neurones have somata in the ventral horn and extend their axons out through the ventral rootlet. Preganglionic sympathetic fibres synapse in the sympathetic ganglia, and postganglionic fibres innervate the organs. The main PNS glial cell types are the myelinating and non-myelinating Schwann cells of peripheral nerves, the satellite glial cells of the sensory and autonomic ganglia, and enteric glial cells that are located in the enteric nervous system of the gastrointestinal tract. Axons pierce a CNS-PNS interface, which marks the boundary between PNS glia and CNS glia (astrocytes, oligodendrocytes and microglia). (Full colour version in plate section.)

There are four major types of glia in the PNS:

1.  The *myelinating and non-myelinating Schwann cells*, which are associated with peripheral nerves (for review, see Jessen & Mirsky, 2005).

2.  The *satellite glial cells* (SGCs) found in sensory, parasympathetic and sympathetic ganglia (for review, see Hanani, 2010).

3.  *Enteric glial cells* (EGCs), which are localised within the ENS (for review, see Ruhl *et al.*, 2004).

4.  *Olfactory ensheathing cells* (OECs), which reside in both the PNS and CNS portions of the primary olfactory system (for review, see Su & He, 2010).

Every spinal nerve and most cranial nerves (with the exceptions of cranial nerves I and II, olfactory and optic nerves) have a *transitional zone* (TZ) formed by a glial partition stretching across the nerve bundle that forms the *PNS-CNS interface or boundary*, and which is pierced by the axons as they cross between the CNS and PNS (for review, see Fraher, 2002). Non-myelinating Schwann cells, SGCs, and EGCs have many functional properties similar to astrocytes in the CNS, whereas myelinating Schwann cells perform the same myelinating function as oligodendrocytes in the CNS (Table 8.1).

Myelinating Schwann cells can be identified by their expression of myelin proteins, whereas the other PNS glia do not express myelin proteins and are identified by their expression of GFAP and S100β, although levels of expression vary both within and between the different types of PNS glia.

**Table 8.1** Physiological properties of the main types of peripheral glia

| Property | Autonomic SGC | Sensory SGC | Non-myelinating Schwann cells | Myelinating Schwann cells | EGC | OEC |
|---|---|---|---|---|---|---|
| Sox10 | + | + | + | + | + | + |
| Neurotransmitter transporters | + | + | + | − | + | ? |
| Vimentin/S-100β | + | + | + | − | + | +/− (subset are S-100β+ /NPY+) |
| GFAP | + | + | + | − | + | +/− (subset) |
| p75$^{NTR}$ | ? | ? | + | − | ? | +/− (subset) |
| Glutamine synthetase | + | + | + | − | + | ? |
| Myelin protein | − | − | − | + | − | − |
| Gap Junctions | + | + | + | + | +++ | + |
| P2 receptors | P2Y$_{1, 6}$ | P2X$_7$ P2Y$_{1, 2, 4, 6, 12, 13}$ | P2X$_7$ P2Y$_{1, 2}$ | + | P2X$_7$ P2Y$_{2,4}$ | + |
| Calcium waves | ? | + | ? | + | + | + |
| Kir | K$_{ir}$4.1 | K$_{ir}$4.1 | + | + | + | + |
| Contact with blood vessels | − | − | − | − | + | ? |
| Phagocytosis | + | + | + | − | ? | ? |
| Cytokine expression | LIF | IL-1β, TNF-α | IL-1β, IL-10, TNF-α | ? | IL-1β, IL-6, TNF-α | ? |
| GluR | ? | ? | + | + | ? | + |

Three key physiological features appear to be common to most PNS glia, like their CNS counterparts:

1. They have strongly negative resting membrane potential predominated by potassium inward currents (dominated by $K_{ir}4.1$ in most PNS glia where it has been studied).

2. They are interconnected by gap junctions (with prominent roles for Cx32 in Schwann cells, and Cx43 in other PNS glia).

3. They exhibit $Ca^{2+}$ excitability (via ATP and P2 receptors).

In addition, where this has been studied, most PNS glia have been shown to express neurotransmitter transporters (glutamate and GABA) and also to express glutamine synthetase, although this depends on the neuronal environment. The physiological characteristics of PNS glia signify the importance of neurone-glial signalling in their behaviours and confirm the glial doctrine that they are homeostatic cells. In addition, PNS glial cells provide trophic support for neurones and are central to the injury response and the capacity for regeneration in the PNS. Nevertheless, the different kinds of PNS glia are phenotypically distinct, and it is important not to make too many generalisations in comparisons with each other or with CNS glia. One of the defining common characteristics of PNS glia is that they are derived from *neural crest cells*, whereas CNS glia are derived from the neuroepithelium of the neural tube (see Chapter 3). In addition, all PNS glial cells have in common that the transcription factor Sox10 plays a critical role in their development (Mollaaghababa & Pavan, 2003).

## 8.1.2 Development

*Neural crest cells* (NCCs) are an embryonic cell type, unique to vertebrates, that are pinched off from the dorsal neural tube. Pluripotent NCCs migrate throughout the embryo, at which stage they are often termed 'neural crest stem cells' (NCSCs) and give rise to PNS neurones and glia, together with other derivatives such as melanocytes and bone and cartilage of the skull (for review, see Le Douarin & Dupin, 2003). PNS glial cells are derived from distinct regions of the neural crest (Figure 8.2). The *vagal and sacral NCCs* form enteric neurones and glia, while Schwann cells and satellite glia come from *trunk NCCs*, which also give rise to the dorsal root ganglia and sympathetic ganglia, together with the sensory (dorsal root) and sympathetic neurones. OECs are derived from *cranial NCCs* that intermingle with ectodermally derived cells in the developing nasal placode that generate the olfactory system (Barraud *et al.*, 2010; Forni *et al.*, 2011). Thus, PNS glial cells have a common NCC origin.

*Vagal and sacral NCCs* enter the embryonic foregut (starting around E8.5–9 in the mouse) and migrate in a rostro-caudal direction to colonise almost the entire GI tract and give rise to most of the ENS. Sacral NCCs contribute to the ENS in the

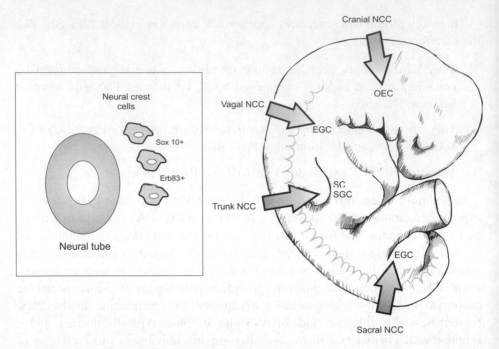

**Figure 8.2**  Peripheral glia have a neural crest origin.

Peripheral glia are derived from Sox10-expressing neural crest cells (NCC) that pinch off from the dorsal neural tube to migrate throughout the embryo and express receptors for endothelin 3. PNS glial cells are derived from distinct regions of the neural crest: vagal and sacral NCCs form enteric neurones and enteric glial cells (EGC); trunk NCCs form Schwann cells (SC), satellite glial cells (SGC), the dorsal root ganglia, sympathetic ganglia, and sensory and sympathetic neurones; and cranial NCCs give rise to olfactory ensheathing cells (OEC). Migratory and post-migratory NCCs express Sox10 and ErbB3 receptors (mediate effects of Neuregulin), which are essential for differentiation of PNS glia.

colon, and a region overlapping the most caudal vagal NCCs and most anterior trunk NCCs contribute to the ENS of the oesophagus and the anterior stomach. Differentiation of ENS cells from NCCs depends upon GDNF, acting via RET and GFRα1 receptors, and on the endothelin 3 (ET3)/endothelin receptor B pathway (for reviews, see Heanue & Pachnis, 2007; Sasselli *et al.*, 2012).

*Cranial NCCs* generate OEC that mingle with ectodermally derived cells in the developing nasal placode, from which olfactory sensory neurones are derived (starting around E10.5 in mouse) (for review, see Su & He, 2010). A cluster of cells called the migratory mass, which includes OEC progenitors and olfactory sensory neurones, leave the olfactory placode, often in contact with the developing olfactory nerve, and form the olfactory bulb. OECs provide essential growth and guidance for olfactory sensory axons. As in the developing ENS, it is likely that OEC precursors depend on GDNF/GFRα-1/Ret signalling.

*Trunk NCCs* give rise to dorsal root sensory neurones and autonomic neurones, together with SGC and Schwann cell precursors. Schwann cell and SGC precursors are intermingled with the early embryonic peripheral nerve trunks as they grow towards their targets (around E12/13 in mice) (for review, see Woodhoo & Sommer, 2008).

*Boundary cap* (BC) *cells* are another group of neural crest derivatives that feed a secondary wave of migration to the PNS after the major neural crest ventrolateral migratory stream (Maro *et al.*, 2004). BC cells form clusters at the surface of the neural tube, at entry and exit points of peripheral nerve roots, and they migrate along peripheral axons to colonise spinal nerve roots and the DRG. Fate-mapping studies have indicated that all Schwann cell precursors occupying the dorsal roots are derived from BC cells. In the DRG, BC-derived cells are the progenitors of both satellite glia and neurones, mainly nociceptive afferents. In addition, BC cells are involved in the formation of the CNS-PNS interface (see Section 8.3.1).

*The transcription factor Sox10* is expressed in virtually all migratory and post-migratory NCSCs and is required for development of PNS glia (Figure 8.3) (for review, see Mollaaghababa & Pavan, 2003). Sox10 is persistently expressed in most PNS glia, but is lost as NCSCs differentiate into neural precursors, and so Sox10 alone does not determine glial fate.

The factors regulating gliogenesis versus neurogenesis of NCSCs are not fully resolved, but it is known to involve interplay between bone morphogenetic proteins (BMP2 and BMP4) and Neuroregulin (NRG)1/2-ErbB signalling (for review, see Jessen & Mirsky, 2005). BMP2 induces the proneural gene Mash1, which interacts with BMP in a reciprocal manner to promote neurogenesis. BMP neurogenic activity inhibits the gliogenic effect of neuregulin-ErbB3, which in turn suppresses neuronal differentiation and directs NCSCs to a glial fate. The expression of ErbB3, like that of Sox10, is initiated in NCSCs and is maintained in PNS glia, but it is down-regulated in other derivatives of NCSCs. Sox10 controls expression of ErbB3 in NCSCs, and down-regulation of ErbB3 in Sox10 knockout mice accounts for many of the observed changes in glial development (Britsch *et al.*, 2001).

Differentiation of the final neuronal and glial cell types depends on the local environment. In developing DRG, SGC are specified through activation of Notch receptors by Delta/Jagged on neuronal precursors. SGCs can be distinguished from Schwann cells by expression of the Ets-domain transcription factor Erm and lack of dependence on NRG1. The transcription factor Krox20 is of pivotal importance for development of the myelinating Schwann cell phenotype, and Sox10 is central to Krox20 induction and activation of myelin genes. In adults, the SGC phenotype is probably maintained by the repression of Krox-20 and other genes. *In vitro*, however, SGCs can up-regulate Schwann cell markers such as myelin proteins and Krox-20, and can down-regulate SGC specific markers such as Erm.

## 8.1.3 The CNS-PNS interface

**(i) Structure of the CNS-PNS interface**  Motor axons and sensory axons enter and exit the CNS at the transitional zone (TZ), which delimits the territories of astrocytes and oligodendrocytes in the CNS and Schwann cells in the PNS

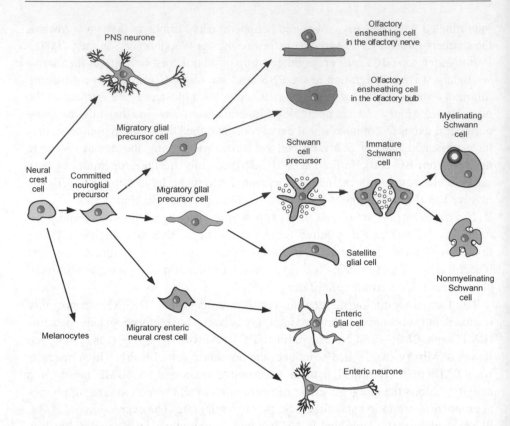

**Figure 8.3**   Lineage of peripheral glia.

Neural crest cells (NCC) generate peripheral neurones and glia, together with other derivatives such as melanocytes. The transcription factor Sox10 is expressed in virtually all migratory and post-migratory NCSCs and is required for development of PNS glia. Sox10 is lost as NCSCs differentiate into neural precursors. On entering the gut, NCCs are termed enteric neural crest cells, and these give rise to all the neurones and glial cells of the enteric nervous system. Olfactory ensheathing cells are derived from NCC that mingle with ectodermally derived cells in the developing nasal placode, from which olfactory sensory neurones are derived. A range of OEC phenotypes have been described, defined mainly as those ensheathing olfactory nerve axons and those located in the olfactory nerve. Migratory glial precursors entering the developing peripheral nerves and ganglia generate both satellite glia and Schwann cell precursors. Schwann cell precursors develop into immature Schwann cells, which generate both myelinating and non-myelinating Schwann cells by a process of radial sorting.

(Figure 8.4; Fraher, 2002). The interface consists of a mosaic of astrocyte processes that form a central glia limitans, which in turn is covered by a basal lamina that is continuous with that around the PNS axons. The myelinating cells, oligodendrocytes and Schwann cells, meet at a transitional node of Ranvier, which has features of both central and peripheral nodes. Myelinating Schwann cells are separated from astrocytes by the basal lamina.

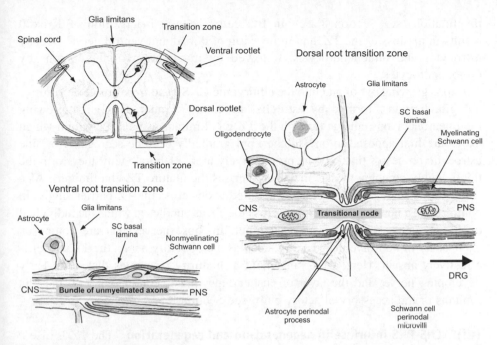

**Figure 8.4**   The CNS-PNS interface.
Diagrammatic transverse section of spinal cord with ventral and dorsal roots, showing the extents and levels of the dorsal and ventral rootlet transitional zones (TZ). The dorsal and ventral root transition zones are illustrated in greater detail in the larger diagrams. The diagram of the dorsal root TZ shows an individual myelinated sensory axon crossing from the PNS to the CNS, demarcated by a transitional node circumscribed by the oligodendrocyte myelin sheath on the CNS side and Schwann cell myelin sheath on the PNS side, separated by the astroglial glia limitans barrier and basal lamina of the Schwann cell. The diagram of the ventral root transition zone illustrates the transition of non-myelinated axons, which cross the CNS-PNS interface as bundles, enwrapped on the PNS side by non-myelinating Schwann cells that are directly apposed to astrocyte processes over a short distance at the entry zone. (Full colour version in plate section.)

Where it occurs, the closest apposition is of Schwann cell microvilli and astrocyte perinodal processes at the transitional node gap. By contrast, at the transitions of non-myelinated axon bundles, non-myelinating Schwann cells are directly apposed to astrocyte processes over a short distance. Thus, myelination seems to be associated with the greatest degree of repulsion between astrocytes and Schwann cells.

**(ii)   Development of the CNS-PNS interface**   As noted above, CNS and PNS glia have different embryonic origins – the neural tube and the neural crest, respectively. During the embryonic period, the CNS/PNS interface is populated by another neural crest derivative, the boundary cap (BC) cells (Maro *et al.*, 2004). These cells are clustered at the entry and exit points of peripheral nerve roots and are essential for the development and maintenance of the integrity of the CNS-PNS interface, involving the transcription factor Krox20 (Coulpier *et al.*, 2011). Krox20 is expressed by BC and Schwann cells. In Schwann cells, Krox20 constitutes a master regulatory gene for myelination (see Section 8.2.2). In BC cells, genetic inactivation of Krox20 results in the loss of the TZ, and in invasion of dorsal and ventral nerve roots by astrocytes and oligodendrocytes, followed by myelination of their axons by oligodendrocytes.

Axons growing out of and into the embryonic CNS have to penetrate a primitive TZ glia limitans, formed by astroglial processes (Fraher, 2002). Outgrowing motoneurone axons emerge through the TZ glia limitans as bundles, within which axons are first apposed to one another, but gradually become segregated by fine astrocytic processes that become progressively more elaborate until they form the thick, highly complex mosaic that characterises the mature TZ glia limitans. As a result of the segregation process, myelinated axons cross the TZ barrier singly. In contrast, most non-myelinated axons cross the TZ as bundles in which the individual axons are not segregated from each other. In those nerves that are composed exclusively of non-myelinated axons, such as the olfactory nerve, the TZ barrier is effectively absent. Here, the arrangement at maturity resembles that of an early developing nerve, and the layer of ensheathing glia is continuous with the glia limitans of the accessory olfactory bulb (see Section 8.5.1).

**(iii)   CNS-PNS interface in degeneration and regeneration**   The TZ is also a glial barrier to axon regeneration across the CNS-PNS interface (Fraher, 2000). Following damage, PNS axons re-grow through the endoneurial tube formed by Schwann cells, whereas CNS axons attempt to re-grow, as in the PNS, but the regenerative sprouts are largely unsuccessful, because of the lack of an endoneurial tube and because the glial scar inhibits axon re-growth (see Chapter 9, Section 9.3). Notably, following transection, motoneurone axons can regenerate through the CNS scar tissue and grow out through the ventral TZ for long distances into the ventral rootlets and PNS. The reasons for this selective regeneration are unresolved.

In contrast, there is no regeneration through the mature dorsal rootlet TZ by axons of primary afferent sensory neurones. Here, following transection, regenerating PNS sensory axons are prevented from growing into the CNS by the astroglial scar at the TZ. The astrocytic outgrowth extends distally into the dorsal root for a considerable distance.

## 8.2   Schwann cells

Schwann cells are of fundamental importance in the PNS, because of their myelinating function and their role in nerve pathology and repair. The two types of Schwann cells, myelinating and non-myelinating, are equally numerous. Non-myelinating Schwann cells can be subdivided into Remak cells, which ensheath unmyelinated axons along their length (Remak fibres), and terminal or perisynaptic Schwann cells, which are located on axon terminals at the neuromuscular junction (Figure 8.5). Myelinating Schwann cells perform the same myelinating function as oligodendrocytes in the CNS, while non-myelinating Schwann cells have many of the same homeostatic properties as astrocytes.

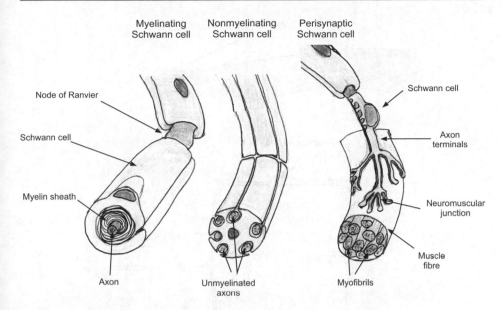

**Figure 8.5**   Schwann cell subtypes.
There are equal numbers of myelinating and non-myelinating Schwann cells in the PNS. Myelinating Schwann cells myelinate a single axon above a critical diameter of 1 μm. Non-myelinating Schwann cells ensheath multiple unmyelinated axons which are smaller than the critical diameter of 1 μm. Perisynaptic Schwann cells ensheath terminal axon branches and synaptic boutons at the neuromuscular junction.

The divergence of myelinating and non-myelinating Schwann cells is determined by the diameter of the axons they associate with, axons above a critical diameter of 1 μm becoming myelinated by a process termed *radial sorting*, while smaller axons remain unmyelinated. In addition, Schwann cells display many aspects of dynamic neurone-glial signalling seen in astrocytes (Rousse & Robitaille, 2006) and are known to contribute to the inflammatory response that can change the nociceptive thresholds following nerve injury (Martini *et al.*, 2008).

An important difference between CNS glia and Schwann cells is their response to axonal injury. Schwann cells support regeneration and subsequent remyelination of PNS axons, whereas astrocytes and oligodendrocytes (CNS myelin) inhibit regeneration in the CNS. These properties of Schwann cells have made them promising candidates for cell-based therapies for CNS regeneration and remyelination (Oudega, 2007; Woodhoo *et al.*, 2007).

## 8.2.1   Schwann cell subtypes

*Myelinating Schwann cells* have a 1:1 relationship with axons, whereby each cell myelinates a single axon, which has a critical diameter above 1 μm (Figure 8.6). Myelinating Schwann cells are distinguished by a complex structural framework of caveolae, which depends on caveolin-1 localised in the outer/abaxonal myelin

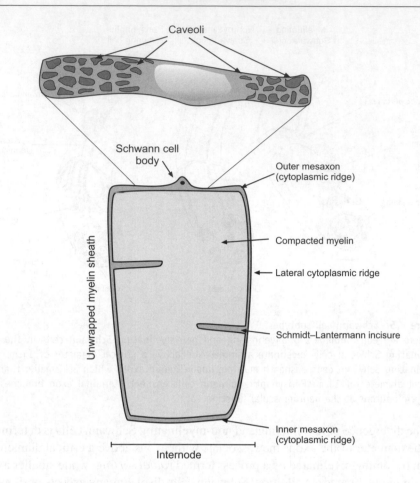

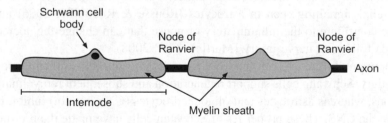

**Figure 8.6**  Myelinating Schwann cell.

There is a 1:1 relationship between a myelinating Schwann cell and the axon it myelinates. Myelinating Schwann cells display a complex structural framework of caveolae in the outer/abaxonal myelin membranes and cytoplasmic compartments. Each myelin sheath, if unwrapped, would be an extremely large trapezoid sheet comprising compacted myelin surrounded by a continuous cytoplasmic rim, and numerous Schmidt-Lantermann incisures that extend into the compacted myelin. Consecutive Schwann cell myelin internodes are separated by nodes of Ranvier, the site of action potential propagation.

membranes and cytoplasmic compartments (Mikol *et al.*, 2002). Caveolins have been implicated in the regulation of cellular transport processes, particularly cholesterol trafficking, which is essential for myelination (Saher *et al.*, 2011).

As with oligodendrocytes, Schwann cells exhibit a strict 1: 10 g-ratio (axon diameter to number of lamellae), and approximate 1: 100 ratio of axon diameter to internodal length, which vary up to 1,000 $\mu$m, depending on axon diameter. Hence, a single Schwann cell myelinating an axon of 10 $\mu$m diameter supports a volume of myelin of 100,000 $\mu$m$^3$ which, if unwrapped, would be visible to the naked eye. Following injury, myelinating Schwann cells dedifferentiate to become a class of non-myelinating Schwann cell, which is critical for the regenerative and remyelinating capacity of the PNS.

*Non-myelinating Schwann cells* surround bundles of small-diameter (0.5–1.5 $\mu$m) unmyelinated axons, including postganglionic sympathetic fibres and nociceptive C fibres (Remak fibres; see Griffin & Thompson, 2008). Non-myelinating Schwann cells serve multiple functions, physically supporting and separating unmyelinated axons with fine processes as well as providing trophic support (e.g. GDNF) and ion homeostasis (e.g. potassium regulation), and preventing ephaptic transmission between axons (Robert & Jirounek, 1994).

Mature non-myelinating Schwann cells express a number of surface molecules characteristic of immature Schwann cells that are not found on mature myelinating Schwann cells, including the neural cell adhesion molecule L1. Non-myelinating Schwann cells specifically express $\alpha1\beta1$ and $\alpha7\beta1$ integrins, which are essential for interactions with laminin in the basal lamina; in their absence, Schwann cells do not develop and there are decreased C-fibre sensory neurones (Yu *et al.*, 2009b). More strikingly, NRG1-ErbB signalling mediates reciprocal interactions between non-myelinating Schwann cells and unmyelinated sensory axons and is essential for their survival (Chen *et al.*, 2003).

Following injury, Schwann cells provide essential guidance and trophic support for regenerating axons, and non-myelinating Schwann cells can adopt a myelinating phenotype which is essential for remyelination of regenerated axons following injury. Schwann cells transplanted into the CNS in demyelinated lesions will remyelinate axons and, following injury, will promote axon regeneration, which does not normally occur in the CNS (Oudega, 2007; Woodhoo *et al.*, 2007).

*Perisynaptic (terminal) Schwann cells* ensheath terminal axonal branches and synaptic boutons at neuromuscular junctions and some sensory transducers, such as Pacinian and Meissner's corpuscles (Griffin & Thompson, 2008). Perisynaptic Schwann cells are covered by a basal lamina that fuses with that of the muscle fibre and motor endplate, and they play essential roles in synaptic function, maintenance, development and regeneration (Figure 8.7; Feng *et al.*, 2005). In addition, perisynaptic Schwann cells respond to nerve activity by increased intracellular $Ca^{2+}$ and regulate the efficacy of synaptic transmission and neurotransmitter release by modulating perisynaptic ions and $Ca^{2+}$ concentration (Rousse & Robitaille, 2006).

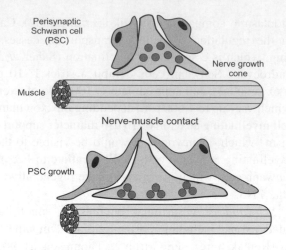

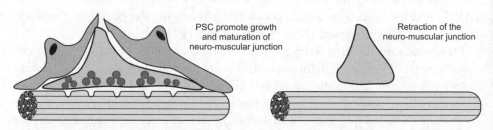

**Figure 8.7** Functions of perisynaptic Schwann cells at the neuromuscular junction.

Perisynaptic Schwann cells (PSC) guide nerve terminal sprouts to neuromuscular junctions during development and during regeneration following axon transection. Nerve terminals grow along the perisynaptic Schwann cells. In addition, perisynaptic Schwann cells induce the aggregation of post-synaptic acetylcholine receptors and are essential for maturation of the neuromuscular junction. Axons regenerating after nerve injury trigger perisynaptic Schwann cells to sprout and these, in turn, guide regenerating nerve terminals, as they do during development. Ablation of perisynaptic Schwann cells causes widespread nerve terminal retraction and synapse loss

Adapted from Feng *et al.*, 2005.

During development, perisynaptic Schwann cells contribute to the maturation and extension of the motor endplate and they stabilise post-synaptic ACh receptor aggregation (Griffin & Thompson, 2008). Furthermore, in regeneration, perisynaptic Schwann cells guide the growth of regenerating pre-synaptic nerve terminals and play an important role in the re-establishment of neuromuscular junctions and recovery of function.

## 8.2.2    Development of Schwann cells

**(i)    Stages of Schwann cell differentiation**    *Schwann cell precursors* (SCPs) are derived from neural crest cells generate under the influence of Delta/Notch, neuregulin 1 (NRG-1)-ErbB3 and the transcription factor SOX10. SCPs then

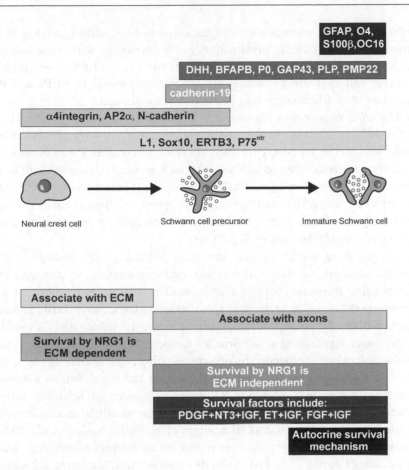

**Figure 8.8** Markers of Schwann cell development.
Transitional stages in Schwann cell development can be defined by their molecular profile, signalling responses and gene expression

Adapted from Jessen & Mirsky, 2005.

develop into immature Schwann cells, which generate both myelinating and non-myelinating Schwann cells (Woodhoo & Sommer, 2008). A set of markers have been developed to distinguish the stages of Schwann cell development (Figure 8.8; see review by Jessen & Mirsky, 2005). NCC express Sox10 and ErbB3, as well as p75$^{NTR}$ and the neural cell adhesion molecule L1, whereas SCP are distinguished by their expression of myelin genes, such as P0, but without losing the aforementioned markers.

*In embryonic nerves*, SCPs surround large groups of axons and are intricately associated with growth cones at nerve fronts. As the axons reach their targets and establish the first synaptic connections (E14 and onwards in the mouse), SCPs differentiate into immature Schwann cells and form 'axon–Schwann cell families', consisting of axons grouped together in small bundles by Schwann cells inter-connected by gap junctions. Expression of the gap junctional proteins connexins is developmentally regulated in Schwann cells (Li *et al.*, 2007). Cx43 is expressed from NCC onwards, whereas Cx29 appears first in SCP, and expression of Cx32 commences with the onset of myelination. Early developing nerves are maintained by extensive SCP–SCP contact, mediated by the cell-adhesion molecules N-cadherin and cadherin-19, which are strongly expressed in SCPs and down-regulated as they differentiate into immature Schwann cells.

*As SCP differentiate into immature Schwann cells*, they up-regulate S100 and GFAP. A striking difference between SCP and immature Schwann cells is the latter's absolute dependence on NRG1 for their survival, whereas SCP can maintain their own survival by autocrine mechanisms. As well as survival, axonal NRG1 is the major axonally derived mitogen for Schwann cells (Garratt *et al.*, 2000) Besides NRG, Schwann cell survival and proliferation depend on laminin (Yang *et al.*, 2005), and a variety of mitogens are also important in controlling proliferation division, including TGF-β (D'Antonio *et al.*, 2006).

*By a process of radial sorting*, immature Schwann cells undergo profound phenotypic changes as they differentiate into myelinating or non-myelinating Schwann cells. Immature Schwann cells send processes into groups of axons, progressively defasciculating them. Larger diameter axons, above a critical diameter of 1 μm, undergo the process of radial sorting until a 1:1 relationship is established with individual myelinating cells. Smaller diameter axons are destined to remain unmyelinated and are surrounded by non-myelinating cells. Radial sorting is dependent on interactions between laminins present in the basal lamina surrounding Schwann cells and their receptors, β1 integrins present on Schwann cell outer membranes. The Rho family GTPase Rac1 has been identified as the downstream molecule involved in this process (Benninger *et al.*, 2007; Nodari *et al.*, 2007).

*Non-myelinating Schwann cells* express many of the markers of immature Schwann cells, including L1, p75[NTR], GFAP and S100. Interestingly, immature Schwann cells express NG2 which, in CNS, is specifically expressed by NG2-glia, or oligodendrocyte progenitors (see Chapter 6). NG2 is down-regulated when immature Schwann cells up-regulate myelin genes, although a subpopulation of non-myelinating Schwann cells retain NG2 expression in the adult (Schneider *et al.*, 2001).

*Differentiation of myelinating Schwann cells* proceeds with up-regulation of genes associated with myelination and down-regulation of most of the antigens associated with immature Schwann cells (Jessen & Mirsky, 2005). Accordingly, myelinating Schwann cells can be identified by their expression of the transcription factor Krox20, as well as the myelin proteins PLP, PMP-22, P0 and MBP (although these are expressed at low levels in earlier Schwann cells). The promyelination factors Sox10, Krox20 and Oct-6 have integral functions in up-regulation of myelin genes (see below).

**(ii)  Regulation of Schwann cell differentiation**  The generation of Schwann cells from their precursors is controlled by the transcription factor AP2α, which is sharply down-regulated at the SCP/SC transition, and its overexpression in SCPs *in vitro* delays Schwann cell generation (Stewart *et al.*, 2001). Subsequently, development of the myelinating phenotype is controlled by the transcription factor

Krox-20. Sox10 is required for inducing Krox20 and requires cooperation with Oct6 (Reiprich *et al.*, 2010). Krox20 expression is regulated by axoglial interactions, a key one being NRG1-ErbB2 signalling, which has critical roles during myelination (Birchmeier & Nave, 2008). Thus, NRG-1 is involved in all stages of Schwann cell development and is the major axon-derived mitogen, survival factor and regulator of myelination (Jessen & Mirsky, 2005).

**(iii) Control of myelination** Krox20, in cooperation with Oct6 and Sox10, induces the myelin proteins P0, PMP22, Cx32, periaxin and MBP (Jessen & Mirsky, 2005). In humans, Krox20 (Egr2, early growth response 2) and Sox10 mutations are associated with variants of Charcot-Marie-Tooth (CMT) disease, an inherited demye-linating disease of the PNS, which also involves mutations in P0, PMP22, Cx32, and periaxin (Scherer & Wrabetz, 2008). P0 is the major component of PNS myelin and is essential for the spiralling of the myelin sheath and adhesion of the myelin lamellae (see Section 8.2.4). Binding of Krox20 to a highly conserved element within the first intron of the P0 (Mpz) gene acts synergistically with Sox10 to activate this intron element and mediate the large increase in P0 expression found in myelinating Schwann cells (LeBlanc *et al.*, 2006). NRG1-ErbB2 signalling induces expression of P0, and disruption of ErbB signalling in Schwann cells results in delayed onset of myelination, thinner myelin, shorter internodal lengths and smaller axonal calibre (Chen *et al.*, 2006).

The switch of NRG1 from a proliferative signal to a myelin differentiation signal in Schwann cells depends on Krox20 and cAMP (Arthur-Farraj *et al.*, 2011). In addition, there are numerous negative regulators of myelination, such as Notch signalling, which has complex and extensive regulatory functions in Schwann cells, promoting differen-tiation of SCP but inhibiting myelination by opposing Krox20 (Woodhoo *et al.*, 2009). Similarly, c-Jun inhibits myelin gene activation by Krox-20 or cAMP, and drives myelinating Schwann cells back to the immature state in transected nerves; c-Jun and Krox-20 show a cross-antagonistic functional relationship (Parkinson *et al.*, 2008).

Laminins present in the basal lamina and their integrin receptors on Schwann cells have critical roles during myelination (Chernousov *et al.*, 2008), and Schwann cells lacking laminins do not ensheath or myelinate axons (Yu *et al.*, 2009a). Trophic factors have also been shown to regulate myelination, including TGFβ. The steroid hormone progesterone has been shown to up-regulate P0 and PMP22; it increases the rate of myelination and is a potential treatment in CMT disease (Meyer zu Horste *et al.*, 2006).

## 8.2.3 Axoglial interactions and myelination

During development, Schwann cells gradually invest smaller and smaller bundles of axons until a 1 : 1 relationship is established. Myelin formation is by the progression of the inner cytoplasmic ridge or lip, which spirals under the compacted myelin. Schwann cells then undergo substantial longitudinal growth to establish the incipient internodal segment at an early stage, and subsequent growth depends on the developmental lengthening of the nerve. Interdependent radial growth of the axon and myelin sheath continues until adult dimensions are achieved.

Schwann cells exert a profound influence on axon radial growth, in part through MAG-mediated neurofilament phosphorylation (de Waegh *et al.*, 1992). In addition, Schwann cells are essential for the development of nodes of Ranvier and the separation of voltage-operated Na$^+$ and K$^+$ channels at nodes, involving Caspr-contactin-Neurofascin interactions that are essential for the integrity of the paranode (Scherer & Arroyo, 2002). Schwann cell-axon units continue to be mutually interdependent functional units, and the disastrous consequences of demyelination on axon degeneration explains the serious long-term disabilities in demyelinating diseases of the PNS, such as CMT disease (Sherman & Brophy, 2005).

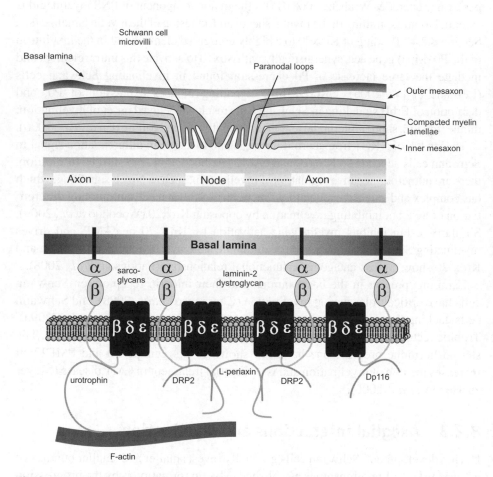

**Figure 8.9**  The Schwann cell basal lamina.

Schwann cells extend microvilli from their outer myelin sheath lamella to fill the nodal gap, and the Schwann cell basal lamina completely covers PNS nodes and internodes, to form a tube along the axon. Interactions between laminin-2 in the basal lamina and α6β4 integrin-dystroglycan complexes at the adaxonal Schwann cell membrane are essential for Schwann cell integrity and myelination.

**(i)  The Schwann cell basal lamina**  The basal lamina of myelinating Schwann cells contains laminin-2 and, on their outer membranes, Schwann cells express the laminin-2 receptors α6β4 integrin and dystroglycan (Figure 8.9). Dystroglycan binds to a macromolecular complex comprising utrophin, a short dystrophin isoform (Dp116), and dystroglycan-related protein 2 (DRP2). Utrophin is linked to the actin cytoskeleton, while DRP2 binds to periaxin, a PDZ domain protein associated with the cell membrane. Periaxin-null mice develop a demyelinating neuropathy, and recessive PRX mutations in humans cause inherited demyelinating neuropathy (Masaki & Matsumura, 2010).

**(ii)  Organisation of nodes of Ranvier in the PNS**  The clustering and segregation of voltage operated sodium and potassium channels at nodes of Ranvier is dependent on the complex developmental organisation of the Schwann cell paranodes and juxtaparanodes (see Figure 5.6; Scherer & Arroyo, 2002). The juxtaparanodal axonal membrane contains the $K^+$ channels $K_v1.1$ and $K_v1.2$ and their associated β2 subunits, and their clustering in the axolemma depends on the axon proteins, Caspr and contactin, and their glial partner neurofascin 155 (NF155). The clustering of $Na^+$ channels at nodes requires the axonal adhesion proteins, NrCAM and NF186 and the axon cytoskeletal proteins ankG and βIV spectrin.

Developmentally, ion channel clustering at nodes is triggered by direct cell-cell contact by Schwann cells, and the first event is the clustering of NrCAM and NF186, followed closely by clustering of $Na^+$ channels. As the myelin sheath becomes compacted, the lateral cytoplasmic ridges stack upon each other to form the paranodal septate-like junctions, via Caspr/contactin/NF155 complexes. The importance of Schwann cells in the development of nodes of Ranvier is demonstrated in mice deficient in the main PNS myelin protein P0, which is essential for myelination (see Section 8.2.4). In the absence of P0, abnormal myelin formation and compaction is associated with immature nodal cluster types of $Na^+$ channels (Ulzheimer et al., 2004). Most strikingly in this study, P0-deficient motor nerves displayed an ectopic nodal expression of the $Na_v1.8$ isoform, where it is co-expressed with the ubiquitous $Na_v1.6$. Furthermore, the $K^+$ channel $K_v1.2$ and Caspr2 were not confined to juxtaparanodes, but were often protruding into the paranodes.

Formation of the Caspr-contactin-NF155 complex depends on the myelin galactolipids, most likely through lipid rafts (Poliak et al., 2001). Genetic ablation of contactin in mutant mice disrupts Caspr and NF155, and $K_v1.1$, $K_v1.2$ become relocated to nodal axolemma, resulting in altered conduction of myelinated fibres (Boyle et al., 2001). In Neurofascin-null mice, neither paranodal adhesion junctions nor nodal complexes are formed (Sherman et al., 2005). Expression of NF155 in the myelinating glia of Neurofascin-null nerves rescues the axoglial adhesion complex by recruiting the axonal proteins Caspr and contactin to the paranodes. However, in the absence of NF186, sodium channels remain diffusely distributed along the axon.

**(iii)  Schwann cell perinodal microvilli**  The outer lamellae of the Schwann cell myelin sheath extend cytoplasmic microvilli into the nodal gap, similar to those formed by astrocytes and NG2-glia in the CNS (Figure 8.9). Interestingly, NG2 is expressed in a restricted manner to the nodal gap in the PNS and is absent from the paranodal or juxtaparanodal region (Martin *et al.*, 2001). NG2 is present in membrane fractions that contain high levels of Na$_V$, Caspr and neurone-glia related cell adhesion molecules, suggesting that NG2 may be involved in the clustering of Na$^+$ channels in the nodal axolemma. Dystroglycan-Laminin2 interactions are also essential for nodal architecture and Na$^+$ channel clustering at nodes in the PNS (Occhi *et al.*, 2005). In addition, gliomedin is specifically expressed by myelinating Schwann cells and is a glial ligand for neuronal NF186 and NrCAM at nodes; disruption of gliomedin abolishes node formation (Eshed *et al.*, 2005). In P0 deficient mice, enlarged nodal gaps and poorly developed nodal Schwann cell microvilli are associated with sensory deficits in the absence of profound myelin degeneration in the sensory nerves of these mutants (Samsam *et al.*, 2002).

## 8.2.4  PNS myelin structure and biochemistry

The general structure and biochemistry of myelin has been described in Chapter 5, Section 5.2.4; here we will focus on the specific aspects of PNS myelin (Figure 8.10).

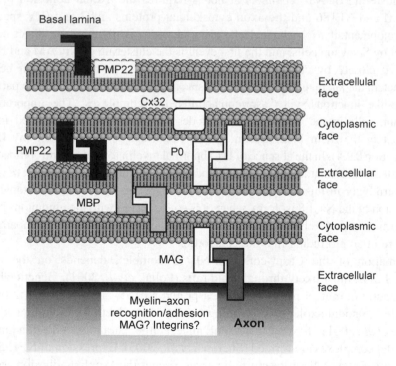

**Figure 8.10**  PNS myelin composition.
  The myelin sheath comprises layer upon layer of Schwann cell membrane with most of the cytoplasm extruded. The major proteins are P0 and PMP22, which function to stabilise and fuse the myelin lamella. In addition, PNS myelin contains gap junction protein connexin 32, which is essential for myelin formation, and myelin associated glycoprotein (MAG), which is important for axon-glial interactions.

The myelin sheath consists of tightly compacted expansions of the Schwann cell plasmalemmal membrane, and hence it is made up mainly of lipids, which provide the insulating properties, together with a number of specific proteins that maintain myelin integrity through interactions between the myelin lamellae and axoglial junctions at paranodes. Many of the proteins in PNS and CNS myelin are similar, but there are some very important differences, and peripheral myelin protein zero (P0), peripheral myelin protein 22 kDa (PMP22), peripheral nerve P2 protein and periaxin are specific to PNS myelin (Patzig *et al.*, 2011).

PNS myelin is characterised by prominent Schmidt-Lantermann incisures, which form a series of cytoplasmic channels connecting with the inner and outer cytoplasmic ridges (mesaxons) and the lateral cytoplasmic ridges that form the paranodal loops. Membranes of these Schmidt-Lantermann incisures and paranodal loops contain myelin-associated glycoprotein (MAG), Connexin-32 and E-cadherin, which (along with its binding partner, β-catenin) is involved in forming adherens junctions between adjacent loops of membrane at the paranode (Scherer & Arroyo, 2002). Mutations in the P0 gene, together with PMP22 and Cx32, are responsible for most CMT neuropathies, and genetic manipulation of these genes has led to the development of animal models of peripheral neuropathies.

**(i)   Lipids**   Myelin is highly enriched in glycosphingolipids and cholesterol. The specific galactolipids found in PNS myelin are largely the same as those in CNS myelin, such as GalC, although some glycolipids (e.g. sulphated glucoronyl paragloboside and its derivatives) are specific for PNS myelin. Cholesterol has emerged as the only integral myelin component that is essential and rate-limiting for the development of myelin. Experiments with conditional mouse mutants that lack cholesterol biosynthesis show that protein trafficking and myelin compaction depend on cholesterol in Schwann cells (Saher *et al.*, 2011). Schwann cell caveolae are involved in the intracellular trafficking of cholesterol.

**(ii)   Proteins**   *P0* is highly specific to PNS myelin and is its major structural element (>50 per cent of PNS myelin). P0 acts as a homotypic adhesion molecule that binds the extracellular leaflets of PNS compact myelin membranes by transbinding between cis-linked P0 tetramers to form the intraperiod line. As such, it serves the same function as PLP in CNS myelin.

Interestingly, the evolutionary replacement of P0 with PLP has bestowed a neuroprotective function of myelin in CNS myelin (Yin *et al.*, 2006). Furthermore, the extracellular domain of P0 is larger than that of PLP and, as a result, the interlamellar spacing is ≈20 Å greater in PNS, compared to CNS myelin. Thus, the switch from P0 to PLP in CNS myelin, in addition to providing a greater degree of neuroprotection, reduced the thickness of myelin, providing further miniaturisation in the CNS (see Chapter 5, Section 5.4).

P0 is involved, either directly or indirectly, in the regulation of both myelin gene expression and myelination. In the absence of P0, mice develop a severe dysmyelinating neuropathy (Giese *et al.*, 1992). Initiation of myelination in these mice is normal, but P0 is essential for subsequent spiralling and compaction, as well as for subsequent maintenance of myelin and axonal integrity. P0 is essential for the development of Schmidt-Lantermann incisures, which are absent in P0-null mice (Yin *et al.*, 2008) and, as noted above, Caspr2 and ion channel segregation are disrupted in P0-deficient motor nerves (Ulzheimer *et al.*, 2004). Furthermore, in the absence of P0, E-cadherin and β-catenin are dislocated from the paranodes to small puncta throughout the cell, although the formation of paranodal axoglial junctions appears normal (Menichella *et al.*, 2001).

*PMP22* is a tetraspan membrane glycoprotein that regulates the initiation of myelination as well as the determination of myelin thickness, and it is essential for the maintenance of myelin and axonal integrity. Point mutations in the PMP22 gene, such as those in the trembler mouse, result in PNS-specific dysmyelination, with phenotypes comparable to P0 knockout mice. Mice lacking PMP22 develop focal hypermyelination followed by myelin degeneration and axonal atrophy (Adlkofer *et al.*, 1995). In addition, studies in PMP22 knockout mice indicate that it is a binding partner for β4 integrin in the integrin/laminin complex and is involved in mediating the interaction of Schwann cells with the basal lamina (Amici *et al.*, 2006).

Defects at the PMP22 locus are associated with CMT disease type 1A (CMT1A), in which there is 1.5-fold overexpression of PMP22, due to a partial duplication of human chromosome 17. An equivalent increase in PMP22 gene dosage in mice results in demyelination, secondary axonal loss, and neurogenic muscle atrophy. Progesterone increases PMP22 expression in Schwann cells, and treatment with progesterone receptor antagonists can reduce PMP22 overexpression and clinical severity in a CMT1A rat model (Meyer zu Horste *et al.*, 2006).

*P2* is a basic protein and a member of the fatty acid binding protein family, with a high affinity for oleic acid, retinoic acid and retinol. P2 is expressed on the cytoplasmic side of compacted myelin and may be involved in intracellular fatty acid transport. P2 induces experimental allergic neuritis in animals, and is used as a model for the PNS demyelinating disease, Guillain-Barré syndrome.

*MBP* is present in PNS myelin, but it does not appear to play a major role in myelin compaction as it does in the CNS. MBP disruption in shiverer mice results in severe hypomyelination in the CNS, but PNS myelin appears normal. MBP function in PNS myelin may be interchangeable with P0.

*PLP/DM20* is found in Schwann cells and PNS myelin, but its function is unclear. PNS myelin appears normal in PLP knockout mice and most mutations.

*MAG* is located in the periaxonal Schwann cell membrane, the internal and external mesaxons, the paranodal loops and the Schmidt-Lantermann incisures. MAG has the same function in PNS and CNS myelin, participating in axonal recognition, adhesion and maintenance of myelin integrity. However, the function of MAG appears more related to axonal integrity than to myelin integrity (Yin *et al.*, 1998). MAG somehow provides trophic support to axons; in adult MAG-null sciatic nerves, axonal pathology is restricted to axonal regions directly beneath paranodes and incisures.

*Cx32* is found mainly in the paranodal regions and Schmidt-Lantermann incisures. Cx32 gap junctions interconnect paranodal loops and link the partially compacted second layer of myelin to the non-compact outer tongue. The presence of mutations in the X-linked Cx32 gene in CMT disease type X indicates a role for Cx32 in formation and maintenance of PNS myelin (Neuberg & Suter, 1999). Mice lacking Cx32 have a similar phenotype to CMT disease type X and develop late-onset demyelination and peripheral neuropathy. Although oligodendrocytes also express Cx32, the loss of this connexin causes demyelination only in the PNS. In the CNS, this may be due in part to compensation by other connexins, such as Cx29. In the PNS, Cx29 expression precedes that of Cx32 and declines to lower levels than Cx32 in adulthood. In adult sciatic nerve, Cx29 has been found to be primarily localised to the innermost aspects of the myelin sheath, the paranode, the juxtaparanode and the inner mesaxon (Altevogt *et al.*, 2002).

*Periaxin* is a PNS-specific glycoprotein representing about five per cent of total myelin protein. There are two isoforms, S- and L-periaxin, and the latter is a constituent of the dystroglycan-dystrophin-DRP2 complex linking the Schwann cell cytoskeleton to the basal lamina (Scherer & Arroyo, 2002). The expression of periaxin is developmentally regulated, being first concentrated in the adaxonal membrane as Schwann cells first ensheath axons; but, as myelin sheaths mature, periaxin becomes predominately localised to the abaxonal Schwann cell membrane apposing the basal lamina.

Mutations in the periaxin gene cause autosomal recessive Dejerine-Sottas neuropathy and the severe demyelinating CMT disease known as CMT4F (Guilbot *et al.*, 2001). Periaxin knockout mice myelinate normally, but they develop a demyelinating peripheral neuropathy due to disruption of the DRP2-dystroglycan complex and destabilisation of the SC-axon unit (Sherman *et al.*, 2001). In addition, mice lacking functional periaxin display extensive pre-terminal branching at neuromuscular junctions, due to segmental demyelination near the neuromuscular synapse, and this results in asynchronous failure of action potential transmission at high stimulation frequencies (Court *et al.*, 2008).

## 8.2.5 Physiology of Schwann cells

**(i) Ion channels and neurotransmitter receptors** *Electrophysiological studies* have identified functional $K^+$ channels, $Cl^-$ channels, $Na^+$ channels and $Ca^{2+}$ channels in Schwann cells (Table 8.2; see review by Baker, 2002). The molecular and biophysical characteristics of Schwann cell ion channels are closely similar or identical to those in astrocytes (see Chapter 4).

Most physiological studies have been on cultured Schwann cells, which have an immature or dedifferentiated phenotype, and ion channel and neurotransmitter expression (e.g. P2R, $Ca^{2+}$ channels and $K_{ir}$) could have a particular function in controlling cell proliferation in these cells. Nonetheless, histological studies have identified the expression and localisation of some of these ion channels *in vivo* in

**Table 8.2**   Ion channels in Schwann cells

| Ion channel | Molecular identity | Localisation | Function |
| --- | --- | --- | --- |
| Potassium channels | | | |
| Inward rectifier potassium channels | $K_{ir}1.1$, $K_{ir}3.1$ | Myelin terminal loops and soma | $K^+$ regulation? |
| Fast delayed rectifier $K^+$ channels | $K_v3.1b$, $K_v3.2$ | | In neurones, fast repolarisations and after hyperpolarisations. |
| Slow delayed rectifier $K^+$ channels | $K_v1.1$, $K_v 1.2$ $K_v1.3$, and $K_v1.5$  $K_v2.1$ | 1.1 expressed strongly  1.2 in embryo | Setting RMP. In neurones, regulate neuronal excitability. |
| Rapidly inactivating A-type potassium currents ($K_A$) | $K_v 1.4$ | Soma, may form heteromers | In neurones, regulation of the fast repolarising phase of action potentials. |
| $Ca^{2+}$-dependent $K^+$ channels | Maxi-K | Soma | |
| Sodium channels | TTX-sensitive ($Na_v1.7$) TTX-resistant NaG ($Na_x$) | Soma; related to proliferative state? | |
| Calcium channels | L- and T-type | Soma | |
| Chloride channels | Voltage-operated, high conductance | Soma, myelin | |
| ATP receptors | P2X | Paranodal loops, soma, low sensitivity to ATP | |

myelinating Schwann cells, particularly $K^+$ channels, which may have a special function in $K^+$ homeostasis (Figure 8.11).

Schwann cells also express P2X receptors, which may regulate their development in response to ATP released by electrically active axons (Figure 8.12; Fields & Stevens, 2000). In addition, perisynaptic Schwann cells express G-protein coupled muscarinic ACh and adenosine A1 receptors, which are activated by neurotransmitters released by the motor nerve terminals (Rochon *et al.*, 2001). Perisynaptic Schwann cells may be exceptional in this respect, and myelinating Schwann cells may not have the same dynamic responses to axonal activity (Baker, 2002).

*Potassium channels*: although no ion channels appear to exist in the greater part of the myelin sheaths, Schwann cells express voltage-dependent $K^+$ channels and inwardly rectifying $K^+$ channels at nodes of Ranvier, the site of axonal $K^+$ release

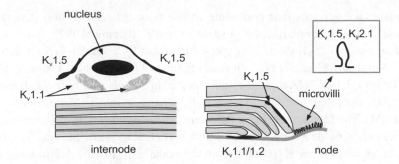

**Figure 8.11**  Localisation of inward rectifying potassium channels in myelinating Schwann cells. The localisation of Kir2.1 and Kv1.5 on perinodal microvilli suggests a role in the uptake of $K^+$ extruded from axons during electrical excitation.

during action potential propagation (Figure 8.11). $K_{ir}2.1$ and $K_{ir}2.3$, together with $K_v1.5$, are localised at the outer Schwann cell surfaces and perinodal microvilli, whereas $K_v1.1$ appear to remain cytoplasmic. It has been suggested that the Kir channels are responsible for the uptake of $K^+$ extruded from axons during electrical excitation, and that $K_v1.5$ extrudes $K^+$ to the extracellular solution. Schwann cells maintained in culture, or following nerve transection, are reported to lose functional Kir channels and maintain Kv, which may related to cell proliferation.

*Anion channels*: high-conductance anion channels which operate over the range $-60$ to $+60\,mV$ with a linear current-membrane potential relation have been reported in cultured Schwann cells, and it is suggested that they are involved in electrically balancing $K^+$ uptake. Schwann cells in culture also generate voltage-

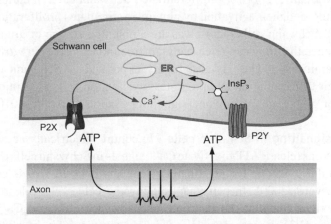

**Figure 8.12**  Axoglial signalling in myelinating Schwann cells. Release of ATP from axons during action potential propagation activates P2X and P2Y receptors on Schwann cells to mediate $Ca^{2+}$ signals. P2X7 receptors in myelinating Schwann cells may mediate $Ca^{2+}$ signals at perinodal microvilli

dependent Cl$^-$ currents that contribute to the outward rectification generated in response to a step depolarisation positive to 0 mV (Ritchie, 1992).

*Sodium channels*: Schwann cells express functional TTX-sensitive (Na$_v$1.2, Na$_v$1.3) and TTX-resistant (Na$_v$1.7) Na$^+$ channels (Chiu, 1991). The Na$^+$ channel sub-type Na$_x$ (NaG/Na$_v$2.1/SCN7A) has also been reported in Schwann cells; these channels are not voltage-operated, but are activated by changes in the extracellular [Na$^+$] ($\approx$150 mM). The function of Na$_v$ in Schwann cells is unknown. It has been suggested that they may provide a route for Na$^+$ influx sufficient to prime the Na$^+$/K$^+$-ATPase which is responsible for K$^+$ uptake from the nodal gap (Robert & Jirounek, 1994).

*Calcium channels*: Schwann cells in culture express Ca$^{2+}$ channels with properties of L-type and T-type channels. The expression and physiological role of Ca$^{2+}$ channels in myelinating Schwann cells *in vivo* are unknown. Transmembrane Ca$^{2+}$ fluxes through L-type Ca$^{2+}$ channels occur in perisynaptic Schwann cells in response to axonal activity, but Ca$^{2+}$ channels do not appear to mediate Ca$^{2+}$ influx in myelinating or non-myelinating Schwann cells during normal impulse activity.

*ATP purinoceptors*: Schwann cells express P2X and P2Y receptors *in vitro* and *in situ*. The P2X subtypes have not been fully characterised, but they generally display low sensitivity to ATP and they have pharmacological properties of the P2X$_7$ subtype, which have been localised by immunocytochemistry in cultured Schwann cells (Colomar & Amedee, 2001). Confocal Ca$^{2+}$ imaging has indicated that P2X$_7$ receptors are localised to paranodal loops of myelinating Schwann cells in isolated rat spinal roots (Grafe *et al.*, 1999). Presynaptic Schwann cells express P2X and P2Y receptors, and adenosine-driven P1 receptors (Rousse & Robitaille, 2006).

*Other neurotransmitters*: Schwann cells have been reported to express both GABA$_A$ and GABA$_B$ receptors (Magnaghi *et al.*, 2006). In addition, activation of muscarinic ACh receptors has been shown to elevate Ca$^{2+}$ levels in perisynaptic glia (Rousse & Robitaille, 2006). De-differentiated Schwann cells in culture appear to express mGluR, and their activation by glutamate stimulates proliferation (Saitoh & Araki, 2010). Schwann cells themselves are a potential source of glutamate, since there is evidence that they can release glutamate (and D-serine) *in vitro* (Wu *et al.*, 2005). Glutamine synthetase is also highly expressed in Schwann cells, and it regulates their differentiation and promotes myelination following injury, suggesting a role for glutamate cycling and signalling (Saitoh & Araki, 2010).

**(ii)  Ca$^{2+}$ signalling in Schwann cells**  In culture, electrically active premyelinated DRG axons release ATP to activate Ca$^{2+}$ signals in Schwann cells (Figure 8.12), although similar evidence for myelinating Schwann cells *in vivo* is contradictory (Fields & Stevens, 2000). In perisynaptic Schwann cells, ATP released by axons during synaptic activity at the neuromuscular junction induces Ca$^{2+}$ responses through P2X and P2Y receptors, and also through the action of its breakdown product adenosine on A1 receptors (Rousse & Robitaille, 2006). In addition, activation of muscarinic ACh receptors in perisynaptic Schwann cells elevates intracellular Ca$^{2+}$ via transmembrane Ca$^{2+}$ fluxes through ligand- and voltage-operated channels and release from intracellular stores. Notably, perisynaptic Schwann cells also modulates the release of neurotransmitters from motor terminals and increases synaptic efficacy at the frog neuromuscular junction.

**(iii)   Schwann cells and pain**   There is evidence that Schwann cells have a direct role in the generation and maintenance of neuropathic pain (Campana, 2007), by the secretion of pro-inflammatory cytokines such as TNF-α, which sensitise nocicep-tors and function as chemoattractants for immune cells. At the same time, Schwann cells produce factors that counterbalance the pro-inflammatory cytokines, including IL-10 and erythropoietin (Epo), which facilitates recovery from chronic pain states.

# 8.3   Satellite glial cells

## 8.3.1   Organisation of sensory and autonomic ganglia

The sensory and autonomic ganglia are clusters of neuronal cell bodies and their closely associated satellite glia (Figure 8.13; for review, see Hanani, 2010). The main types of sensory ganglia are the dorsal root ganglia (DRG; also trigeminal ganglia, etc.), which innervate most of the body and internal organs and contain

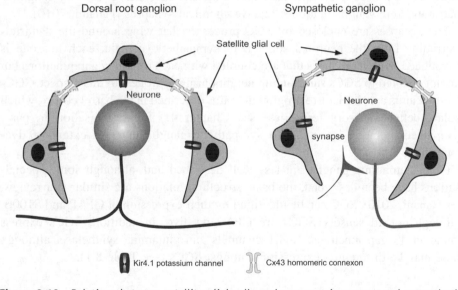

**Figure 8.13**   Relations between satellite glial cells and neurones in sensory and sympathetic ganglia.

The sensory and autonomic ganglia contain clusters of neuronal cell bodies and their closely associated satellite glia. A notable difference between sensory and autonomic ganglia is that neurones in the latter receive chemical synapses, and these are enclosed by satellite glial cells. Satellite glial cells surrounding a particular neurone are extensively dye-coupled to each other via Cx43 gap junctions. Satellite cells express Kir4.1 channels, which are believed to be important for uptake of $K^+$ released by electrically active neurones, and they play an important role in pain (see text for details) neuronal cell bodies of sensory afferent nerves (mechano-, thermo-, noci- and proprioception). In addition, there are nodose ganglia, which receive sensory inputs from internal organs such as heart, respiratory tract and stomach.

The autonomic ganglia serve as junctions between autonomic nerves originating from the CNS and autonomic nerves innervating their target organs in the periphery. The sympathetic ganglia consist of the paravertebral ganglia (which form a bilateral chain alongside the vertebral column), and the prevertebral ganglia (which include the ciliary, ceoliac, and mesenteric ganglia). Parasympathetic ganglia are near or within the organs they innervate (e.g. heart, trachea, urinary bladder), and they receive preganglionic inputs from the vagus nerves and also from the sacral region of the spinal cord.

## 8.3.2    Satellite glia in sensory and autonomic ganglia

Satellite glial cells (SGC) are the main glial cell type in sensory ganglia, which also contain myelinating and non-myelinating Schwann cells. Each sensory neurone is completely enclosed by its own SGC sheath, consisting of several SGCs, which are laminar cells and do not have true processes (Hanani, 2005). Sensory neurones send numerous fine processes (microvilli) into invaginations of SGCs, which may facilitate the exchange of chemicals. Sympathetic and parasympathetic ganglion neurones are also covered with SGCs, but a notable difference to sensory ganglia is that autonomic ganglia neurones receive chemical synapses (Hanani, 2010).

The synapses are enclosed by SGC processes that wrap around the dendrites protruding from the neuronal somata. In sympathetic ganglia, each neurone is surrounded by several SGCs that are coupled with each other via gap junctions but are not coupled to SGCs surrounding neighbouring neurones. In this respect, SGC-neurone units are similar to astroglial domains described in the barrel cortex, which isolate defined sensory territories (see Chapter 4). The organisation in para-sympathetic ganglia is similar to sympathetic ganglia, but the extent of dye-coupling is less.

Other autonomic ganglia are less well described and, although some special-isations have been described, the basic structural relations are similar (for review, see Hanani, 2010). SGC can be identified by their expression of GFAP and S100$\beta$, although not all sensory SGCs are GFAP positive. In addition, SGCs express connexin 43 gap junctions, $K_{ir}$4.1 channels and glutamine synthetase, although there may be differential expression amongst SGCs (see Table 8.1).

## 8.3.3    Physiology of satellite glia

(i) Electrical properties    SGCs have strongly negative resting membrane potential ($-90$ mV) and low input resistance ($<10$ M$\Omega$) due to high $K^+$ conduct-ance and cell coupling. In sensory ganglia, they respond to preganglionic stimula-tion by slow evoked potentials, most likely mediated by $K^+$.

**(ii)   Homeostatic function**   $K_{ir}4.1$ is the principal $K_{ir}$ channel type in SGCs, generating the main $K^+$ conductance in SGC membranes, and it seems likely that they are involved in the uptake of $K^+$ released by electrically active ganglion neurones (Tang *et al.*, 2010). In sensory ganglia, SGC express glutamate transporters as well as glutamine synthetase, which mediate the glutamate-glutamine shuttle, as in astrocytes (see Chapter 4) – although it has not been shown that glutamate is released by sensory neurones within the ganglia. Sensory SGCs also contain glutamate dehydrogenase and pyruvate carboxylase, and they can convert glutamate to lactate, which suggests they may supply energy to the sensory neurones. Parasympathetic SGCs have also been shown to express glutamine synthetase, but sympathetic RGCs have not been examined in this respect. For sympathetic ganglia, only GABA uptake by SGCs has been reported. The source of GABA appears to be preganglionic nerves and, when glial uptake of GABA is inhibited, the electrophysiological actions of GABA on neurones is enhanced, apparently due to GABA accumulation in the extracellular space.

**(iii)   $Ca^{2+}$ signalling**   The mechanisms of intercellular $Ca^{2+}$ signalling in SGCs involve Cx43 gap junctions and purinergic signalling. SGCs express P2 receptors (with evidence for $P2Y_{1/2/4/6}$ and $P2X_{2/3/7}$) and ecto-nucleotidases (NTPDase2), and they possess mechanisms for the release of ATP (Suadicani *et al.*, 2010). In DRG sensory ganglia, neurones have been shown to release ATP to activate $P2X_7$ receptors in SGC, stimulating them to release TNF-$\alpha$, which in turn potentiates $P2X_3$ receptor-mediated responses and increases the excitability of DRG neurones (Figure 8.14; Zhang *et al.*, 2007). Purinergic signalling in sensory SGCs is increased under pathological conditions, involving a switch from P2Y to P2X receptors (Ceruti *et al.*, 2008; Kushnir *et al.*, 2011).

**(iv)   Other receptors in SGCs**   SGC in DRG express group III mGluR8, with minimal staining for group I (mGluR1) and II (mGluR2/3). The functional relevance of mGluR expression in DGCs is unclear, but they reflect the high expression mGluR8 in DRG (which also express group II mGluR2/3 and, to a very small extent, group I mGluR1$\alpha$), although the source of glutamate in DRG is unclear (Carlton & Hargett, 2007). DRG neurones express the vesicular acetylcholine transporter and presumed synaptic vesicles containing ACh, and they may release this neurotransmitter to act on SRC, which express muscarinic ACh receptors. Even less is known about autonomic SGCs, although there is evidence that they express nicotinic ACh receptor $\alpha7$ subunit and noradrenaline $\beta$ receptors.

**(v)   Neurotrophic function of SGC**   SGCs contain BDNF and the truncated form of BDNF receptor, and DRG neurones and SGCs both possess the low affinity p75 and high affinity trkA NGF receptors.

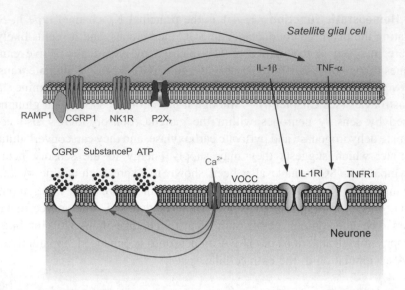

**Figure 8.14**   Intraganglionic neuroglial signalling.
   Activated neurones release neurotransmitters into the extracellular space within the sensory ganglia, such as calcitonin gene-related peptide (CGRP), substance P and ATP, which also activate satellite glia via specific receptors. Activated satellite glial cells release cytokines such as interleukin (IL)-1β and tumour necrosis factor α (TNFα), which can potentiate neuronal excitability

Adapted from Takeda *et al.*, 2009.

## 8.3.4   Injury response of satellite glia

SGCs in sensory ganglia undergo structural changes following peripheral injury, akin to reactive astrogliosis in the CNS, including proliferation and up-regulation of GFAP (Ohara *et al.*, 2009). EM studies show that, following axotomy, SGC processes in sympathetic ganglia become interposed between the retracting terminals and the post-synaptic cells and play a role in 'synaptic stripping'. An important point is that changes in SGCs are often secondary to, and driven by, active signalling mechanisms between the injured neurone and/or the central or peripheral part of the axon (Ohara *et al.*, 2009).

A large number of chemicals are released from injured neurones, including NO, TNF-α and ATP. DRG neurones contain nNOS and SGCs contain the enzyme guanylate cyclase, which is activated by NO to catalyze cGMP formation. The NO-cGMP pathway has a neuroprotective role in DRG and may contribute to nociception. In addition, augmented SGC sensitivity to ATP appears to be a general functional outcome of peripheral nerve injury and inflammation, and it also contributes to nociception (see Section 8.3.5).

SGCs express a number of cytokines and chemokines and their receptors (e.g. TNF-α and TNF-α type I receptor, IL-6, IL-1β, and IL-1 type 1 receptor, bradykinin, LIF, endothelin), and they can synthesise prostaglandins (PGs), which are increased following injury. Following axotomy, SGCs are the main source of the neurotrophic factors TGFβ and FGF2 in sensory and sympathetic ganglia. BMP, NGF and NT3 released from SGCs are likely to be major contributors to neuronal sprouting following injury, and they can contribute to the recovery of injured neurones following axotomy.

## 8.3.5 Sensory satellite glia and pain

*Activation of SGCs in sensory ganglia* may play a role in the increased responses to pain caused both by noxious stimuli (hyperalgesia) and by normally innocuous stimuli (allodynia) following peripheral tissue injury/inflammation (Hanani, 2005; Ohara *et al.*, 2009; Takeda *et al.*, 2009).

*ATP signalling mechanisms* are increased in peripheral injury and inflammation. Purinergic signalling in SGCs is also altered under pathological conditions in trigeminal sensory ganglia, whose hyperactivation leads to the development of migraine pain, with a marked potentiation of $P2X_3$ receptors and augmented P2Y-mediated ($P2Y_6$) $Ca^{2+}$ responses in SGC (Ceruti *et al.*, 2008). Following inflammation, trigeminal ganglion SGC have also been shown to display a marked increase in sensitivity to ATP due to a shift from P2Y to P2X receptors, largely due to $P2X_2$ and/or $P2X_5$ receptors (Kushnir *et al.*, 2011). $P2X_7$ receptors are expressed only by SGCs in DRGs, and they are activated by ATP released from DRG neurones, stimulating SGCs to release TNF-α, which potentiates $P2X_3$ receptor-mediated responses and excitability in DRG neurones (Zhang *et al.*, 2007). Incongruently, activation of $P2X_7$ receptors in DRG SGC also appears to evoke their release of ATP. This acts on neuronal $P2Y_1$ receptors to tonically inhibit their expression of $P2X_3Rs$, which contributes to reduced allodynia after inflammation (Chen *et al.*, 2008).

These studies indicate a complex role for neurone-SGC ATP signalling in regulating the excitability of primary afferent neurones, which may contribute to chronic pain states via autocrine and/or paracrine mechanisms.

*$K_{ir}4.1$ in sensory ganglia* are expressed specifically by SGCs, and knockdown of $K_{ir}4.1$ expression in trigeminal ganglia leads to neuronal hyperexcitability and heightened nociception (Vit *et al.*, 2008). Furthermore, $K_{ir}4.1$ appear to be essential for the full effect of analgesic drugs, although this was studied in the context of their expression in the periaqueductal gray matter (Smith *et al.*, 2008). In addition, reducing the expression of GLAST in the trigeminal ganglia increases evoked pain, in the form of facial allodynia, suggesting that glutamate uptake by SGCs is important for maintaining neuronal excitability (Ohara *et al.*, 2009). Thus, SGC emerge as key regulators of neuronal excitability in sensory ganglia.

*Gap junctional communication* between SGCs is dramatically increased in DRG following inflammation, as is neurone-neurone coupling, contributing to neuronal hyperexcitability, which in turn contributes to visceral pain (Huang *et al.*, 2010).

*Increased production of PGs, cytokines and chemokines* by SGC may also contribute to neuronal sensitisation following injury. Activated SGCs have been shown to modulate the excitability of nociceptive DRG neurones via an IL-1β paracrine mechanism, and up-regulation of IL1-RI in the soma may be a part of the mechanism underlying inflammatory hyperalgesia (Takeda *et al.*, 2009). The release of LIF from SGCs (and/or Schwann cells) stimulates a large increase in the synthesis of VIP in sympathetic ganglion neurones after axotomy. Endothelin and bradykinin receptors on SGCs may also have a role in increased sympathetic excitability and in the transmission of pain signals in sensory ganglia.

## 8.4   Enteric glia

### 8.4.1   Organisation of the enteric nervous system

The ENS is comprised of an outer myenteric plexus and inner submucosal plexus (Figure 8.15).

*The myenteric plexus* is situated between the circular and longitudinal muscle layers and controls the motility of the GI tract, in addition to receiving and transmitting signals between the submucosal plexus and the autonomic nervous system.

*The submucosal plexus* is responsible for coordinating secretion and absorption, as well as controlling the submucosal muscle layer (muscularis mucosa), and it has

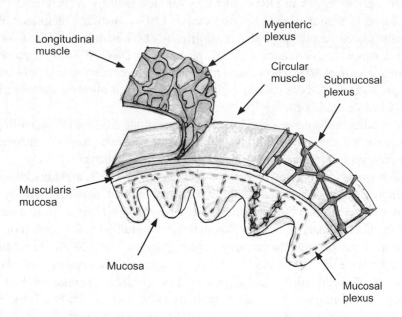

**Figure 8.15** Organisation of the enteric nervous system.
The ENS is comprised of an outer myenteric plexus, situated between the circular and longitudinal muscle layers, and an inner submucosal plexus which, together with the mucosal plexus, connects the epithelial lining and the submucosal plexus

multiple functions in signalling from the mucosal sensory nerve endings, regulating blood flow, maintaining the mucosal barrier and signalling with the immune system.

In addition, the mucosal layer contains delicate nerve networks that form the *mucosal plexus*, which connects the epithelial lining and the submucosal plexus. The mucosal plexus is in close contact with neuroendocrine cells that release transmitters to act on neighbouring epithelial cells and the ENS. Enteric glial cells accompany neurones at all levels throughout the ENS.

## 8.4.2 Development of enteric glia

Both enteric glia and neurones originate from common neural crest cells that migrate into the GI tract embryonically (see Section 8.1.2; Sasselli *et al.*, 2012). Migratory NCC express SOX10, endothelin receptor B and p75$^{NTR}$ and, on entering the gut, they express the transcription factor Phox2B and the receptor tyrosine kinase RET and are termed enteric neural crest cells (ENCCs). Upon commitment to neurogenic and gliogenic precursor cells, Mash1 expression is up-regulated. Subsequently, cells that differentiate into neurones down-regulate Sox10, Mash1 and p75 but maintain RET expression, and up-regulate the neural marker TUJ1 and other neuronal subtype-specific markers. In contrast, cells that differentiate into glia maintain Sox10 and p75 expression, down-regulate RET and Mash1, and up-regulate glial markers such as S100 and GFAP.

Upon deletion of Sox10 or RET/GDNF, enteric ganglia fail to form, demonstrating critical roles for these factors in ENS development. RET/GDNF is a strong proliferative signal for ENCC, whereas endothelin 3 (ET-3) signalling promotes ENCC migration and inhibits their differentiation into neurones. Sox10 is required for glial fate acquisition, and its inhibition is a prerequisite for neuronal specification, involving GDNF and BMPs (Bondurand *et al.*, 2006). Gliogenesis is positively regulated by neuregulin/ErbB3 signalling; mice with a targeted deletion of ErbB3 lack enteric glia. The neurotrophin NT-3 also promotes enteric glial development. The transcriptional cofactor HIPK2 (homeodomain interacting protein kinase 2) is an important transcriptional cofactor that regulates the BMP signalling pathway, which promotes gliogenesis, and mice lacking HIPK2 display a progressive loss of enteric neurones and an increase in enteric glia (Chalazonitis *et al.*, 2011).

## 8.4.3 Structure of enteric glia

Enteric glia can be identified by their expression of GFAP, S-100, Ran-2 and glutamine synthetase. The morphology of EGCs differs in the myenteric and submucosal plexuses (Figure 8.16).

Neurones and glia are tightly packed within the ganglia, which are interconnected by nerve fibre bundles containing the axons of intrinsic (enteric) as well as extrinsic (sympathetic, parasympathetic, primary afferent) neurones. Glial cells located

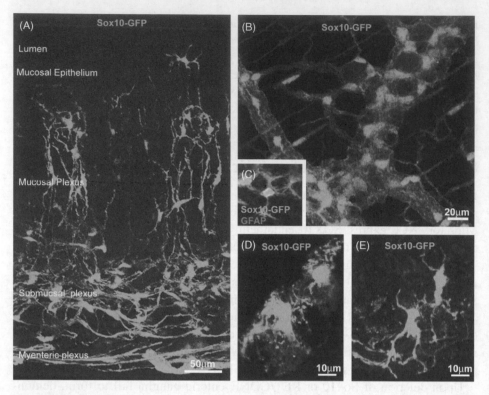

**Figure 8.16**  Enteric glia.
Sections through the small intestine of transgenic mice in which the enteric glial transcription factor Sox10 drives expression of enhanced green fluorescent protein.

A.  Enteric glia form a continuous chain extending from the mucosal epithelium lining the gut lumen to the myenteric plexus, circumnavigating the outer layer of the gut.

B.  In the myenteric plexus, neurones and glia are tightly packed within the ganglia, interconnected by nerve fibre bundles containing axons and enteric glia.

C.  Enteric glia co-express GFAP and Sox10.

D, E.  The morphology of enteric glia differs in the myenteric (D) and mucosal plexuses (E). (Full colour version in plate section.)

within the ganglia have small somata and extend very short, irregularly branched processes that encapsulate neurones (Hanani & Reichenbach, 1994). In contrast, glial cells within the interganglionic fibre tracts extend long processes that branch infrequently and run parallel to the fibre tracts.

In the submucosal and mucosal plexuses, EGCs extend a small number of long, fine unbranching processes that ensheath axons, and others that terminate at the mucosal epithelium. There are no neuronal somata in the 'mucosal plexus', which is aganglionic, so EGCs are the sole neural cell type in the area beneath the epithelium. EGCs form several endfeet on blood vessels and at neuronal synapses/varicosities (Gabella, 1981) and are responsive to neuronal activity (Gulbransen & Sharkey,

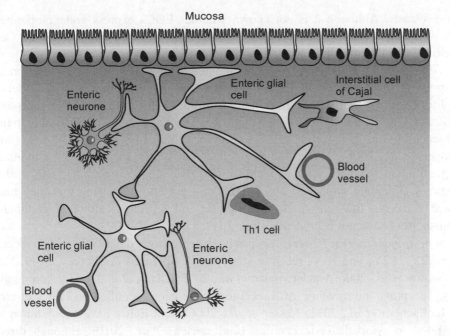

**Figure 8.17**   Connections of enteric glia.
  Enteric glia are extensively dye-coupled and form a functional chain from the mucosal epithelial layer to the myenteric plexus, interconnecting the sensory and motor neurones, blood vessels, the mucosal barrier and the immune system.

2009). In addition, EGCs are extensively coupled by gap junctions, so that they form a continuous chain from the mucosal epithelial layer to the myenteric plexus, interconnecting the sensory and motor neurones, blood vessels, the mucosal barrier and the immune system, akin to astrocytes in the CNS (Figure 8.17).

## 8.4.4   Physiology of enteric glia

**(i)   Electrical properties**   Enteric glia are characterised by a resting membrane potential of around −55 mV, low input resistances (≤100 MΩ) – at least partly a result of extensive gap junctional coupling – and mostly 'passive' currents, with characteristics of delayed-rectifier and inwardly rectifying currents (Hanani *et al.*, 2000). ENGs also display TTX-sensitive sodium currents, although calcium currents and glutamate-gated currents have not been demonstrated (Broussard *et al.*, 1993).

**(ii)   Ion channels and neurotransmitter receptors**   $K_v$ and $K_{ir}$ channels are indicated by electrophysiological studies in ECGs, and immunohistochemical studies have confirmed expression of $K_v1.1$ and $K_v1.2$ in EGC throughout the ENS (Costagliola *et al.*, 2009). Immunohistochemical analysis of $K_{ir}$ expression is lacking, but electrophysiological findings are consistent with a role for ECGs in $K^+$

homeostasis. Although it is not known whether EGCs express voltage-operated $Ca^{2+}$ channels, they do exhibit raised $Ca^{2+}$ in response to a variety of stimuli (see below), and they display capacitative $Ca^{2+}$ entry (Sarosi et al., 1998).

*Glutamate receptors* have been demonstrated in EGCs. There is widespread expression of mGluR5 by EGCs, and expression was reduced in an animal model of colitis (Nasser et al., 2007). In primary culture, EGCs express AMPA receptors (GluA1, GluA3, and GluA4), which might be expected to be $Ca^{2+}$-permeable in the absence of GluA2, as well as NMDA receptor subunits (GluN1, GluN2A/B) (von Boyen et al., 2006). These studies suggest that EGCs are targets of glutamate signalling in the ENS, although physiological evidence is lacking. EGCs also express glutamine synthetase and GABA transporters, suggesting that they may have a role in the neurotransmitter uptake and recycling, although glutamate transporters have not been demonstrated (Fletcher et al., 2002).

*A prominent role for P2 receptors* has been demonstrated in EGCs, with evidence for $P2Y_2$, $P2Y_4$ and $P2X_7$ receptor subtypes (Gulbransen & Sharkey, 2009; Van Nassauw et al., 2006; Vanderwinden et al., 2003; Zhang et al., 2003). Adrenergic $\alpha_{2A}$ receptors and nicotinic ACh receptors have been identified on EGCs *in vivo* (MacEachern et al., 2011; Nasser et al., 2006), and EGCs have been shown to respond to sympathetic innervation (Gulbransen et al., 2010), although direct adrenergic and cholinergic signalling onto EGCs has not been demonstrated.

**(iii)   $Ca^{2+}$ signalling**   Enteric glial cells respond to neuronally released ATP with increased $[Ca^{2+}]_i$ *in situ*, mediated via $P2Y_4$ receptors (Gulbransen & Sharkey, 2009). Autonomic control of colonic function is mediated by intrinsic (enteric) and extrinsic (sympathetic, parasympathetic, primary afferent) neural pathways. Gulbransen and colleagues provide evidence that glial $[Ca^{2+}]_i$ responses are selectively elicited by ATP released from active sympathetic fibres (Figure 8.18), whereas intrinsic neurones did not activate glial $[Ca^{2+}]_i$ responses (Gulbransen et al., 2010). Sympathetic fibres in the ENS release ATP as a co-transmitter with norepinephrine, and release of NE and ATP would act on adrenergic $\alpha_{2A}$ receptors and P2 receptors on EGCs, which enclose the sympathetic varicosities.

The physiological consequences of neurone-glial signalling in the ENS are unknown. However, most excitatory neurotransmission in the myenteric plexus is cholinergic, and nicotinic stimulation elicits small $Ca^{2+}$ responses in enteric glia and results in the release of nitric oxide (NO) from both neurones and enteric glia to modulate epithelial ion transport, a key component of homeostasis and innate immunity (MacEachern et al., 2011).

## 8.4.5   Functions of EGCs

**(i)   Homeostatic functions**   Loss of EGCs results in the loss of enteric neurones, indicating that EGCs are essential for neuronal integrity. The mechanisms are unknown, but they may take the form of homeostatic functions, such as $K^+$ regulation, or trophic

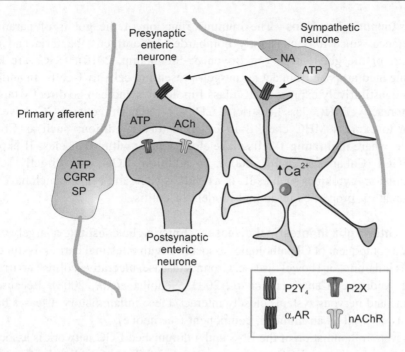

**Figure 8.18**  Neuroglial signalling in enteric glia.
Sympathetic fibres in the ENS release ATP as a co-transmitter with norepinephrine, and enteric glial cells respond to neuronally released ATP with increased $[Ca^{2+}]_i$, mediated via P2Y$_4$ receptors

Adapted from Gulbransen *et al.*, 2010.

support, since EGCs produce neuroprotective factors GDNF and NT-3, as well as S-nitrosoglutathione (GSNO). In addition, EGCs release cytokines and chemokines, including IL-6, endothelins and TGF-β1 (von Boyen & Steinkamp, 2010).

**(ii)  Barrier function**  The mucosal epithelium forms a crucial barrier that provides constant protection from bacteria and other contents of the gut lumen (Savidge *et al.*, 2007). The functional components of the barrier are the epithelial cells, immune cells, nerve fibres and EGCs (Figure 8.18). Indeed, the 'mucosal plexus' is aganglionic, so EGCs are the main ENS entity directly beneath the epithelium and their processes are in contact with both epithelial cells and immune cells. Targeted ablation of EGCs caused a complete breakdown of the mucosal barrier, with characteristics of inflammatory bowel disease (Bush *et al.*, 1998).

Enteric glia are the main sources of TGFβ and GSNO (see above), which promote barrier function and up-regulation of the expression of tight junction proteins in epithelial cells. In addition, wound healing of the gastrointestinal mucosa is essential for gut integrity, and EGCs play a major role in enhancing repair processes. This involves, at least in part, proEGF as a secreted glial mediator leading to consecutive activation of epidermal growth factor receptor and focal adhesion kinase signalling pathways in intestinal epithelial cells (Van Landeghem *et al.*, 2011).

**(iii)   Immune functions**   The immune function of the gut is of paramount importance, since it is constantly bombarded by antigens, bacteria and other contents of the gut lumen (von Boyen & Steinkamp, 2010). EGCs are likely immune mediators and can act as antigen-presenting cells to T-cells. In addition, EGCs constitutively express MHC class I molecules and can be directly targeted by autoreactive MHC class I-restricted CD8+ T-cells. Moreover, EGCs have been shown to express MHC class II in inflammatory conditions such as Crohn's disease, where infiltrating T-cells make close contact with MHC class II-expressing EGCs (Cabarrocas *et al.*, 2003). In addition, EGCs can directly secrete inflammatory cytokines such as IL-6, as well as NGF and NT-3, which have anti-inflammatory properties in animal models of colitis.

**(iv)   Enteric glia in intestinal diseases**   Enteric glia constitute a largely unrecognised component of GI pathologies associated with intestinal barrier dysfunction, such as inflammatory bowel disease, Crohn's disease, ulcerative colitis and irritable bowel syndrome (Cabarrocas *et al.*, 2003; Neunlist *et al.*, 2008). Because the immune and nervous systems closely interact, these inflammatory diseases have a nervous, as well as an immune, component (see above).

A severe inflammation of the ENS and a diminished EGC network is associated with Chrone's disease. EGC markers such as S-100β and GFAP are differentially altered in Crohn's disease and ulcerative colitis, with a decrease in EGC density in the former and a gliosis-like phenomenon in the latter. Altered expression of EGC markers such as S-100β has also been shown in colonic adenocarcinoma, suggesting that these cells could also be involved in carcinogenesis.

# 8.5   Olfactory ensheathing cells (OECs)

## 8.5.1   Organisation and structure of OECs

Olfactory receptor neurones in the olfactory epithelium extend their axons through the lamina propria to the olfactory bulb, and they project through the olfactory nerve layer to the glomerular layer, where they synapse onto mitral cells (Figure 8.19). The somata of mitral neurones are located in the mitral layer, and they extend their primary dendritic arborisations to the glomeruli and their axons to the pyriform cortex. Olfactory neurone axons are accompanied along their length to the glomerulus by OECs, which extend very fine processes that enclose large numbers of unmyelinated olfactory axons (Barnett & Chang, 2004; Raisman, 2001; Rieger *et al.*, 2007; Ruitenberg *et al.*, 2006).

A range of OEC phenotypes has been described, defined mainly by high or low expression of p75$^{NTR}$ (Barnett & Chang, 2004). Most OECs in the olfactory nerve and bulb express S100β, with S100β+ cells ensheathing the olfactory receptor neurones up to the olfactory nerve layer intensely expressing p75$^{NTR}$ and low levels of GFAP, whereas those in the olfactory bulb express low levels of p75$^{NTR}$ and high levels of GFAP. Microarray characterisation of OECs, subdivided according to

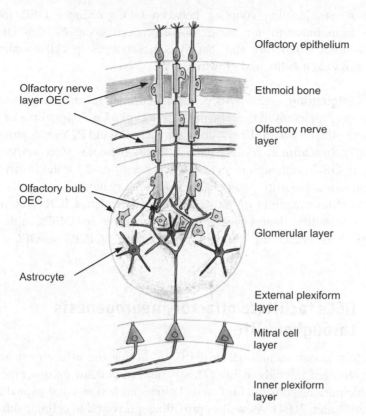

Olfactory epithelium

Olfactory nerve
layer OEC

Ethmoid bone

Olfactory nerve
layer

Olfactory bulb
OEC

Glomerular layer

Astrocyte

External plexiform
layer

Mitral cell
layer

Inner plexiform
layer

**Figure 8.19**   Organisation of the olfactory system.

Olfactory ensheathing cells accompany olfactory neurone axons along their length from the olfactory epithelium to the glomerulus of the olfactory bulb, where the axons synapse onto mitral cells. Olfactory ensheathing cells intermingle with CNS astrocytes within the glomerulus. (Full colour version in plate section.)

p75$^{NTR}$ expression, indicated that OECs with a high level of p75$^{NTR}$ overexpress genes involved in regulation of the inflammatory response and axonal guidance, whereas OECs with a low level of p75$^{NTR}$ overexpress genes implicated in the modulation of the extracellular matrix and cell sorting, suggesting that the two OEC subtypes have specific roles during neurogenesis (Honore *et al.*, 2012). Lamina propria OECs express additional developmentally important markers.

## 8.5.2   Physiology of OECs

**(i)   Electrical properties**   OECs express high levels of Cx43, and Lucifer yellow injections revealed selective dye coupling among small subgroups of OECs, which determines their electrophysiological properties, with either:

1.  low input resistance, linear current profiles, and frequently dye coupling; or

2.  high input resistance, nonlinear current profiles and infrequent dye coupling (Rela *et al.*, 2010).

The loss of gap junction coupling between OECs changes OEC membrane properties from linear to non-linear. These properties suggest that OECs may play a role in $K^+$ buffering and that dynamic changes in cell coupling could influence axon excitability and growth.

**(ii)   $Ca^{2+}$ signalling**   Activity-dependent neuronal release of glutamate and ATP from receptor axons in the olfactory nerve evoke $Ca^{2+}$ signalling of OECs in acute mouse olfactory bulb slices, acting via mGluR1 and $P2Y_1$ receptors (Rieger *et al.*, 2007). In addition, cooling induced $InsP_3$-mediates store-activated $Ca^{2+}$ signalling in OECs, although no evidence has been found for the involvement of known temperature-sensitive ion channels such as ryanodine receptors, TRPM8 and TRPA1 (Stavermann *et al.*, 2012). $InsP_3R$-dependent CICR is an important pathway to amplify ligand-evoked $Ca^{2+}$ signalling in OECs, although the physiological relevance of temperature-dependent CICR in OECs remains obscure.

## 8.5.3   OECs facilitate olfactory neurogenesis throughout life

The olfactory system is unusual in the CNS, in that the olfactory neurones are regularly renewed throughout life. This is due, in part, to unique properties of OECs, which are responsible for fasciculation, cell sorting, and axonal targeting (Barnett & Chang, 2004). As well as providing a favourable cellular substrate for axon growth (e.g. laminin and fibronectin), OECs release diffusible factors that regulate proliferation and differentiation of neural progenitor cells (e.g. FGF2, IGF1, inhibitors of Wnt and Notch signalling; Su & He, 2010). Interestingly, olfactory axonal outgrowth *in vivo* is dependent on tight junctions interconnecting OECs, which form a micro-compartment that is beneficial for axonal growth (Wolburg *et al.*, 2008).

OECs accompany receptor axons in the olfactory nerve and promote axonal growth into the CNS. In this respect, OECs are unique amongst glia, in that they exist within both the CNS and the PNS. Within the glomeruli, OECs mingle with astrocytes to ensheath the synapses between olfactory sensory neurones and the mitral dendritic arborisation (Figure 8.20).

In addition to facilitating olfactory nerve growth into the glomerulus, the OECs that encapsulate glomeruli may also be involved in regulating synaptic function (Rieger *et al.*, 2007). The glomerulus also contains neural precursors (NPs) that migrate to the olfactory bulb along the rostral migratory stream (RMS) from the subventricular zone (SVZ) and differentiate into granule and periglomerular cells of the olfactory bulb. The migration of NPs in the RMS depends on chemoattractive factors derived from the olfactory bulb, and there is evidence that OECs attract NPs through the release of diffusible factors (Su & He, 2010).

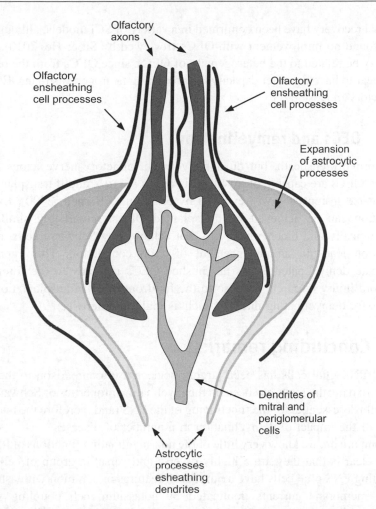

Olfactory
axons

Olfactory
ensheathing
cell processes

Olfactory
ensheathing
cell processes

Expansion
of astrocytic
processes

Dendrites of
mitral and
periglomerular
cells

Astrocytic
processes
esheathing
dendrites

**Figure 8.20**   Olfactory ensheathing cells interact closely with astrocytes in the olfactory bulb. Olfactory ensheathing cells are unique amongst peripheral glia, in that they are found within the CNS and they interact closely with astrocytes without causing a reactive astrogliosis. Within the glomerulus of the olfactory bulb, olfactory ensheathing cells surround the incoming olfactory axons as they synapse with the mitral cell dendrites which, in turn, are enwrapped by astroglial processes

Adapted from Raisman, 2001. (Full colour version in plate section.)

## 8.5.4   OECs and regeneration

The ability of OECs to support neuronal growth and intermingle with astrocytes without inducing astroglial reactivity have made OECs one of the most promising candidates for cell-based therapies for CNS repair (for reviews, see Barnett & Chang, 2004; Raisman, 2001; Su & He, 2010). Raisman and colleagues first showed that implantation of OECs can promote repair after spinal cord injury (SCI) (Li *et al.*, 1997), and the beneficial effects of OEC on axonal regeneration and functional recovery have been confirmed in a variety of SCI models, although some studies found no improvement with OECs (reviewed by Su & He, 2010). Differences may be related to the heterogeneity of OECs, since OECs from the olfactory bulb appear to have a greater capacity for promoting neurogenesis than OECs from the olfactory mucosa.

### 8.5.5   OECs and remyelination

OECs normally ensheath, but do not myelinate, olfactory nerve axons *in vivo*. However, OECs are capable of myelinating axons *in vitro*, and if transplanted into demyelinated lesions *in vivo* (reviewed by Franklin & Barnett, 2000). Extensive myelination can be achieved by transplanted OECs, remarkably similar both morphologically and biochemically to that achieved by Schwann cells, and this myelination leads to an enhancement of axon conduction. This capacity to remyelinate demyelinated axons has pushed OECs not only to the forefront of spinal cord injury research, but also to the forefront of cell transplantation-based therapies for demyelinating diseases such as multiple sclerosis.

## 8.6   Concluding remarks

Study of PNS glial cells has been largely neglected in comparison to their CNS cousins. To date, the focus has been on the myelinating properties of Schwann cells, because this is essential for the functioning of the PNS (and therefore the body), and because of the impact of demyelination in a number of diseases.

By comparison, we know very little of the non-myelinating functions of PNS glia. What is clear is that they are a highly diverse and versatile group of cells. Non-myelinating PNS glial cells have a number of features in common with astrocytes, such as membrane currents dominated by potassium, cell coupling via gap junctions, and many express glutamine synthetase. This has led to direct comparisons with the $K^+$ and glutamate homeostatic functions of astrocytes. However, there is little indication that local $K^+$ and glutamate homeostasis are major functions of PNS glia.

It is important to move away from generalised comparisons between PNS glia and astrocytes. The needs of the PNS are markedly different than those of the tightly controlled and privileged CNS. A striking feature of PNS glia is their $Ca^{2+}$ excitability, which signifies the potential importance of neurone-glial signalling in regulating their functions. We now need to determine what these functions are. Satellite glia, for example, have been shown to have a role in pain transmission.

In addition, the sheer size and complexity of the enteric glial network signifies their importance in co-ordinating GI tract function in health and disease. Indeed, enteric glia have a clear role in the inflammatory response and immune defences of the gut. Moreover, enteric glia have the capacity to generate neurones in the adult, which makes them a target for regeneration.

These diverse functions of PNS glia will surely open up new avenues of research. In the case of olfactory ensheathing cells, research will almost certainly continue to be largely limited to their use as potential therapies for CNS regeneration and remyelination. However, we would argue that we will never learn the causes or find effective treatments for diseases of the PNS and gut unless we begin to concentrate some of our energies upon answering fundamental questions about the cell biology and normal functions of PNS glia.

# References

Adlkofer K, Martini R, Aguzzi A, Zielasek J, Toyka KV, Suter U. (1995). Hypermyelination and demyelinating peripheral neuropathy in Pmp22-deficient mice. *Nature Genetics* **11**(3), 274–80.

Altevogt BM, Kleopa KA, Postma FR, Scherer SS, Paul DL. (2002). Connexin29 is uniquely distributed within myelinating glial cells of the central and peripheral nervous systems. *Journal of Neuroscience* **22**(15), 6458–70.

Amici SA, Dunn WA, Jr., Murphy AJ, Adams NC, Gale NW, Valenzuela DM, Yancopoulos GD, Notterpek L. (2006). Peripheral myelin protein 22 is in complex with alpha6beta4 integrin, and its absence alters the Schwann cell basal lamina. *Journal of Neuroscience* **26**(4), 1179–89.

Arthur-Farraj P, Wanek K, Hantke J, Davis CM, Jayakar A, Parkinson DB, Mirsky R, Jessen KR. (2011). Mouse schwann cells need both NRG1 and cyclic AMP to myelinate. *Glia* **59**(5), 720–33.

Baker MD. (2002). Electrophysiology of mammalian Schwann cells. *Progress In Biophysics and Molecular Biology* **78**(2-3) 83–103.

Barnett SC, Chang L. (2004). Olfactory ensheathing cells and CNS repair: going solo or in need of a friend? *Trends In Neurosciences* **27**(1), 54 60.

Barraud P, Seferiadis AA, Tyson LD, Zwart MF, Szabo-Rogers HL, Ruhrberg C, Liu KJ, Baker CV. (2010). Neural crest origin of olfactory ensheathing glia. *Proceedings of The National Academy Of Sciences Of The United States Of America* **107**(49), 21040–5.

Benninger Y, Thurnherr T, Pereira JA, Krause S, Wu X, Chrostek-Grashoff A, Herzog D, Nave KA, Franklin RJ, Meijer D. *et al.* (2007). Essential and distinct roles for cdc42 and rac1 in the regulation of Schwann cell biology during peripheral nervous system development. *Journal of Cell Biology* **177**(6), 1051–61.

Birchmeier C, Nave KA. (2008). Neuregulin-1, a key axonal signal that drives Schwann cell growth and differentiation. *Glia* **56**(14), 1491–7.

Bondurand N, Natarajan D, Barlow A, Thapar N, Pachnis V. (2006). Maintenance of mammalian enteric nervous system progenitors by SOX10 and endothelin 3 signalling. *Development* **133**(10), 2075–86.

Boyle ME, Berglund EO, Murai KK, Weber L, Peles E, Ranscht B. (2001). Contactin orchestrates assembly of the septate-like junctions at the paranode in myelinated peripheral nerve. *Neuron* **30**(2), 385–97.

Britsch S, Goerich DE, Riethmacher D, Peirano RI, Rossner M, Nave KA, Birchmeier C, Wegner M. (2001). The transcription factor Sox10 is a key regulator of peripheral glial development. *Genes and Development* **15**(1), 66–78.

Broussard DL, Bannerman PG, Tang CM, Hardy M, Pleasure D. (1993). Electrophysiologic and molecular properties of cultured enteric glia. *Journal of Neuroscience Research* **34**(1), 24–31.

Bush TG, Savidge TC, Freeman TC, Cox HJ, Campbell EA, Mucke L, Johnson MH, Sofroniew MV. (1998). Fulminant jejuno-ileitis following ablation of enteric glia in adult transgenic mice. *Cell* **93**(2), 189–201.

Cabarrocas J, Savidge TC, Liblau RS. (2003). Role of enteric glial cells in inflammatory bowel disease. *Glia* **41**(1), 81–93.

Campana WM. (2007). Schwann cells: activated peripheral glia and their role in neuropathic pain. *Brain, Behavior, and Immunity* **21**(5), 522–7.

Carlton SM, Hargett GL. (2007). Colocalization of metabotropic glutamate receptors in rat dorsal root ganglion cells. *Journal of Comparative Neurology* **501**(5), 780–9.

Ceruti S, Fumagalli M, Villa G, Verderio C, Abbracchio MP. (2008). Purinoceptor-mediated calcium signaling in primary neuron-glia trigeminal cultures. *Cell Calcium* **43**(6), 576–90.

Chalazonitis A, Tang AA, Shang Y, Pham TD, Hsieh I, Setlik W, Gershon MD, Huang EJ. (2011). Homeodomain interacting protein kinase 2 regulates postnatal development of enteric dopaminergic neurons and glia via BMP signaling. *Journal of Neuroscience* **31**(39), 13746–57.

Chen S, Rio C, Ji RR, Dikkes P, Coggeshall RE, Woolf CJ, Corfas G. (2003). Disruption of ErbB receptor signaling in adult non-myelinating Schwann cells causes progressive sensory loss. *Nature Neuroscience* **6**(11), 1186–93.

Chen S, Velardez MO, Warot X, Yu ZX, Miller SJ, Cros D, Corfas G. (2006). Neuregulin 1-erbB signaling is necessary for normal myelination and sensory function. *Journal of Neuroscience* **26**(12), 3079–86.

Chen Y, Zhang X, Wang C, Li G, Gu Y, Huang LY. (2008). Activation of P2X7 receptors in glial satellite cells reduces pain through downregulation of P2X3 receptors in nociceptive neurons. *Proceedings of The National Academy Of Sciences Of The United States Of America* **105**(43), 16773–8.

Chernousov MA, Yu WM, Chen ZL, Carey DJ, Strickland S. (2008). Regulation of Schwann cell function by the extracellular matrix. *Glia* **56**(14), 1498–507.

Chiu SY. (1991). Functions and distribution of voltage-operated sodium and potassium channels in mammalian Schwann cells. *Glia* **4**(6), 541–58.

Colomar A, Amedee T. (2001). ATP stimulation of P2X(7) receptors activates three different ionic conductances on cultured mouse Schwann cells. *European Journal of Neuroscience* **14**(6), 927–36.

Costagliola A, Van Nassauw L, Snyders D, Adriaensen D, Timmermans JP. (2009). Voltage-operated delayed rectifier K v 1-subunits may serve as distinctive markers for enteroglial cells with different phenotypes in the murine ileum. *Neuroscience Letters* **461**(2), 80–4.

Coulpier F, Decker L, Funalot B, Vallat JM, Garcia-Bragado F, Charnay P, Topilko P. (2011). CNS/PNS boundary transgression by central glia in the absence of Schwann cells or Krox20/Egr2 function. *Journal of Neuroscience* **30**(17), 5958–67.

Court FA, Brophy PJ, Ribchester RR. (2008). Remodeling of motor nerve terminals in demyelinating axons of periaxin-null mice. *Glia* **56**(4), 471–9.

D'Antonio M, Droggiti A, Feltri ML, Roes J, Wrabetz L, Mirsky R, Jessen KR. (2006). TGFbeta type II receptor signaling controls Schwann cell death and proliferation in developing nerves. *Journal of Neuroscience* **26**(33), 8417–27.

de Waegh SM, Lee VM, Brady ST. (1992). Local modulation of neurofilament phosphorylation, axonal caliber, and slow axonal transport by myelinating Schwann cells. *Cell* **68**(3), 451–63.

Eshed Y, Feinberg K, Poliak S, Sabanay H, Sarig-Nadir O, Spiegel I, Bermingham JR, Jr., Peles E. (2005). Gliomedin mediates Schwann cell-axon interaction and the molecular assembly of the nodes of Ranvier. *Neuron* **47**(2), 215–29.

Feng Z, Koirala S, Ko CP. (2005). Synapse-glia interactions at the vertebrate neuromuscular junction. *Neuroscientist* **11**(5), 503–13.

Fields RD, Stevens B. (2000). ATP: an extracellular signaling molecule between neurons and glia. *Trends In Neurosciences* **23**(12), 625–33.

Fletcher EL, Clark MJ, Furness JB. (2002). neuronal and glial localization of GABA transporter immunoreactivity in the myenteric plexus. *Cell and Tissue Research* **308**(3), 339–46.

Forni PE, Taylor-Burds C, Melvin VS, Williams T, Wray S. (2011). Neural crest and ectodermal cells intermix in the nasal placode to give rise to GnRH-1 neurons, sensory neurons, and olfactory ensheathing cells. *Journal of Neuroscience* **31**(18), 6915–27.

Fraher J. (2002). Axons and glial interfaces: ultrastructural studies. *Journal of Anatomy* **200**(4), 415–30.

Fraher JP. (2000). The transitional zone and CNS regeneration. *Journal of Anatomy* **196**(Pt 1), 137–58.

Franklin RJ, Barnett SC. (2000). Olfactory ensheathing cells and CNS regeneration: the sweet smell of success? *Neuron* **28**(1), 15–8.

Gabella G. (1981). Ultrastructure of the nerve plexuses of the mammalian intestine: the enteric glial cells. *Neuroscience* **6**(3), 425–36.

Garratt AN, Britsch S, Birchmeier C. (2000). Neuregulin, a factor with many functions in the life of a schwann cell. *Bioessays* **22**(11), 987–96.

Giese KP, Martini R, Lemke G, Soriano P, Schachner M. (1992). Mouse P0 gene disruption leads to hypomyelination, abnormal expression of recognition molecules, and degeneration of myelin and axons. *Cell* **71**(4), 565–76.

Grafe P, Mayer C, Takigawa T, Kamleiter M, Sanchez-Brandelik R. (1999). Confocal calcium imaging reveals an ionotropic P2 nucleotide receptor in the paranodal membrane of rat Schwann cells. *Journal of Physiology* **515**(Pt 2), 377–83.

Griffin JW, Thompson WJ. (2008). Biology and pathology of nonmyelinating Schwann cells. *Glia* **56**(14), 1518–31.

Guilbot A, Williams A, Ravise N, Verny C, Brice A, Sherman DL, Brophy PJ, LeGuern E, Delague V, Bareil C. *et al.* (2001). A mutation in periaxin is responsible for CMT4F, an autosomal recessive form of Charcot-Marie-Tooth disease. *Human Molecular Genetics* **10**(4), 415–21.

Gulbransen BD, Sharkey KA. (2009). Purinergic neuron-to-glia signaling in the enteric nervous system. *Gastroenterology* **136**(4), 1349–58.

Gulbransen BD, Bains JS, Sharkey KA. (2010). Enteric glia are targets of the sympathetic innervation of the myenteric plexus in the guinea pig distal colon. *Journal of Neuroscience* **30**(19), 6801–9.

Hanani M. (2005). Satellite glial cells in sensory ganglia: from form to function. *Brain Research Brain Research Reviews* **48**(3), 457–76.

Hanani M. (2010). Satellite glial cells in sympathetic and parasympathetic ganglia: in search of function. *Brain Research Reviews* **64**(2), 304–27.

Hanani M, Reichenbach A. (1994). Morphology of horseradish peroxidase (HRP)-injected glial cells in the myenteric plexus of the guinea-pig. *Cell and Tissue Research* **278**(1), 153–60.

Hanani M, Francke M, Hartig W, Grosche J, Reichenbach A, Pannicke T. (2000). Patch-clamp study of neurons and glial cells in isolated myenteric ganglia. *American Journal of Physiology. Gastrointestinal and Liver Physiology* **278**(4), G644–51.

Heanue TA, Pachnis V. (2007). Enteric nervous system development and Hirschsprung's disease: advances in genetic and stem cell studies. *Nature Reviews Neuroscience* **8**(6), 466–79.

Honore A, Le Corre S, Derambure C, Normand R, Duclos C, Boyer O, Marie JP, Guerout N. (2012). Isolation, characterization, and genetic profiling of subpopulations of olfactory ensheathing cells from the olfactory bulb. *Glia* **60**(3), 404–13.

Huang TY, Belzer V, Hanani M. (2010). Gap junctions in dorsal root ganglia: possible contribution to visceral pain. *European Journal of Pain* **14**(1), 49e1–11.

Jessen KR, Mirsky R. (2005). The origin and development of glial cells in peripheral nerves. *Nature Reviews Neuroscience* **6**(9), 671–82.

Kushnir R, Cherkas PS, Hanani M. (2011). Peripheral inflammation upregulates P2X receptor expression in satellite glial cells of mouse trigeminal ganglia: a calcium imaging study. *Neuropharmacology* **61**(4), 739–46.

Le Douarin NM, Dupin E. (2003). Multipotentiality of the neural crest. *Current Opinion In Genetics and Development* **13**(5), 529–36.

LeBlanc SE, Jang SW, Ward RM, Wrabetz L, Svaren J. (2006). Direct regulation of myelin protein zero expression by the Egr2 transactivator. *Journal of Biological Chemistry* **281**(9), 5453–60.

Li J, Habbes HW, Eiberger J, Willecke K, Dermietzel R, Meier C. (2007). Analysis of connexin expression during mouse Schwann cell development identifies connexin29 as a novel marker for the transition of neural crest to precursor cells. *Glia* **55**(1), 93–103.

Li Y, Field PM, Raisman G. (1997). Repair of adult rat corticospinal tract by transplants of olfactory ensheathing cells. *Science* **277**(5334), 2000–2.

MacEachern SJ, Patel BA, McKay DM, Sharkey KA. (2011). Nitric oxide regulation of colonic epithelial ion transport: a novel role for enteric glia in the myenteric plexus. *Journal of Physiology* **589**(Pt 13) 3333–48.

Magnaghi V, Ballabio M, Consoli A, Lambert JJ, Roglio I, Melcangi RC. (2006). GABA receptor-mediated effects in the peripheral nervous system: A cross-interaction with neuroactive steroids. *Journal of Molecular Neuroscience* **28**(1), 89–102.

Maro GS, Vermeren M, Voiculescu O, Melton L, Cohen J, Charnay P, Topilko P. (2004). Neural crest boundary cap cells constitute a source of neuronal and glial cells of the PNS. *Nature Neuroscience* **7**(9), 930–8.

Martin S, Levine AK, Chen ZJ, Ughrin Y, Levine JM. (2001). Deposition of the NG2 proteoglycan at nodes of Ranvier in the peripheral nervous system. *Journal of Neuroscience* **21**(20), 8119–28.

Martini R, Fischer S, Lopez-Vales R, David S. (2008). Interactions between Schwann cells and macrophages in injury and inherited demyelinating disease. *Glia* **56**(14), 1566–77.

Masaki T, Matsumura K. (2010). Biological role of dystroglycan in Schwann cell function and its implications in peripheral nervous system diseases. *Journal of Biomedicine and Biotechnology* 2010, 740403.

Menichella DM, Arroyo EJ, Awatramani R, Xu T, Baron P, Vallat JM, Balsamo J, Lilien J, Scarlato G, Kamholz J. *et al.* (2001). Protein zero is necessary for E-cadherin-mediated adherens junction formation in Schwann cells. *Molecular and Cellular Neurosciences* **18**(6), 606–18.

Meyer zu Horste G, Prukop T, Nave KA, Sereda MW. (2006). Myelin disorders: Causes and perspectives of Charcot-Marie-Tooth neuropathy. *Journal of Molecular Neuroscience* **28**(1), 77–88.

Mikol DD, Scherer SS, Duckett SJ, Hong HL, Feldman EL. (2002). Schwann cell caveolin-1 expression increases during myelination and decreases after axotomy. *Glia* **38**(3), 191–9.

Mollaaghababa R, Pavan WJ. (2003). The importance of having your SOX on: role of SOX10 in the development of neural crest-derived melanocytes and glia. *Oncogene* **22** (20), 3024–34.

Nasser Y, Ho W, Sharkey KA. (2006). Distribution of adrenergic receptors in the enteric nervous system of the guinea pig, mouse, and rat. *Journal of Comparative Neurology* **495** (5), 529–53.

Nasser Y, Keenan CM, Ma AC, McCafferty DM, Sharkey KA. (2007). Expression of a functional metabotropic glutamate receptor 5 on enteric glia is altered in states of inflammation. *Glia* **55**(8), 859–72.

Neuberg DH, Suter U. (1999). Connexin32 in hereditary neuropathies. *Advances In Experimental Medicine and Biology* **468**, 227–36.

Neunlist M, Van Landeghem L, Bourreille A, Savidge T. (2008). Neuro-glial crosstalk in inflammatory bowel disease. *Journal of Internal Medicine* **263**(6), 577–83.

Nodari A, Zambroni D, Quattrini A, Court FA, D'Urso A, Recchia A, Tybulewicz VL, Wrabetz L, Feltri ML. (2007). Beta1 integrin activates Rac1 in Schwann cells to generate radial lamellae during axonal sorting and myelination. *Journal of Cell Biology* **177**(6), 1063–75.

Occhi S, Zambroni D, Del Carro U, Amadio S, Sirkowski EE, Scherer SS, Campbell KP, Moore SA, Chen ZL, Strickland S. *et al.* (2005). Both laminin and Schwann cell dystroglycan are necessary for proper clustering of sodium channels at nodes of Ranvier. *Journal of Neuroscience* **25**(41), 9418–27.

Ohara PT, Vit JP, Bhargava A, Romero M, Sundberg C, Charles AC, Jasmin L. (2009). Gliopathic pain: when satellite glial cells go bad. *Neuroscientist* **15**(5), 450–63.

Oudega M. (2007). Schwann cell and olfactory ensheathing cell implantation for repair of the contused spinal cord. *Acta Physiologica (Oxford)* **189**(2), 181–9.

Parkinson DB, Bhaskaran A, Arthur-Farraj P, Noon LA, Woodhoo A, Lloyd AC, Feltri ML, Wrabetz L, Behrens A, Mirsky R. *et al.* (2008). c-Jun is a negative regulator of myelination. *Journal of Cell Biology* **181**(4), 625–37.

Patzig J, Jahn O, Tenzer S, Wichert SP, de Monasterio-Schrader P, Rosfa S, Kuharev J, Yan K, Bormuth I, Bremer J. *et al.* (2011). Quantitative and integrative proteome analysis of peripheral nerve myelin identifies novel myelin proteins and candidate neuropathy loci. *Journal of Neuroscience* **31**(45), 16369–86.

Poliak S, Gollan L, Salomon D, Berglund EO, Ohara R, Ranscht B, Peles E. (2001). Localization of Caspr2 in myelinated nerves depends on axon-glia interactions and the generation of barriers along the axon. *Journal of Neuroscience* **21**(19), 7568–75.

Raisman G. (2001). Olfactory ensheathing cells – another miracle cure for spinal cord injury? *Nature Reviews Neuroscience* **2**(5), 369–75.

Reiprich S, Kriesch J, Schreiner S, Wegner M. (2010). Activation of Krox20 gene expression by Sox10 in myelinating Schwann cells. *Journal of Neurochemistry* **112**(3), 744–54.

Rela L, Bordey A, Greer CA. (2010). Olfactory ensheathing cell membrane properties are shaped by connectivity. *Glia* **58**(6), 665–78.

Rieger A, Deitmer JW, Lohr C. (2007). Axon-glia communication evokes calcium signaling in olfactory ensheathing cells of the developing olfactory bulb. *Glia* **55**(4), 352–9.

Ritchie JM. (1992). Voltage-operated ion channels in Schwann cells and glia. *Trends In Neurosciences* **15**(9), 345–51.

Robert A, Jirounek P. (1994). Uptake of potassium by nonmyelinating Schwann cells induced by axonal activity. *Journal of Neurophysiology* **72**(6), 2570–9.

Rochon D, Rousse I, Robitaille R. (2001). Synapse-glia interactions at the mammalian neuromuscular junction. *Journal of Neuroscience* **21**(11), 3819–29.

Rousse I, Robitaille R. (2006). Calcium signaling in Schwann cells at synaptic and extra-synaptic sites: active glial modulation of neuronal activity. *Glia* **54**(7), 691–9.

Ruhl A, Nasser Y, Sharkey KA. (2004). Enteric glia. *Neurogastroenterology and Motility* **16** (Suppl 1), 44–9.

Ruitenberg MJ, Vukovic J, Sarich J, Busfield SJ, Plant GW. (2006). Olfactory ensheathing cells: characteristics, genetic engineering, and therapeutic potential. *Journal of Neurotrauma* **23**(3–4), 468–78.

Saher G, Quintes S, Nave KA. (2011). Cholesterol: a novel regulatory role in myelin formation. *Neuroscientist* **17**(1), 79–93.

Saitoh F, Araki T. (2010). Proteasomal degradation of glutamine synthetase regulates schwann cell differentiation. *Journal of Neuroscience* **30**(4), 1204–12.

Samsam M, Frei R, Marziniak M, Martini R, Sommer C. (2002). Impaired sensory function in heterozygous P0 knockout mice is associated with nodal changes in sensory nerves. *Journal of Neuroscience Research* **67**(2), 167–73.

Sarosi GA, Barnhart DC, Turner DJ, Mulholland MW. (1998). Capacitative $Ca^{2+}$ entry in enteric glia induced by thapsigargin and extracellular ATP. *American Journal of Physiology* **275**(3 Pt 1) G550–5.

Sasselli V, Pachnis V, Burns AJ. (2012). The enteric nervous system. *Developmental Biology* **366**(1), 64–73.

Savidge TC, Sofroniew MV, Neunlist M. (2007). Starring roles for astroglia in barrier pathologies of gut and brain. *Laboratory Investigation* **87**(8), 731–6.

Scherer SS, Arroyo EJ. (2002). Recent progress on the molecular organization of myelinated axons. *Journal of the Peripheral Nervous System* **7**(1), 1–12.

Scherer SS, Wrabetz L. (2008). Molecular mechanisms of inherited demyelinating neuropathies. *Glia* **56**(14), 1578–89.

Schneider S, Bosse F, D'Urso D, Muller H, Sereda MW, Nave K, Niehaus A, Kempf T, Schnolzer M, Trotter J. (2001). The AN2 protein is a novel marker for the Schwann cell lineage expressed by immature and nonmyelinating Schwann cells. *Journal of Neuroscience* **21**(3), 920–33.

Sherman DL, Brophy PJ. (2005). Mechanisms of axon ensheathment and myelin growth. *Nature Reviews Neuroscience* **6**(9), 683–90.

Sherman DL, Fabrizi C, Gillespie CS, Brophy PJ. (2001). Specific disruption of a schwann cell dystrophin-related protein complex in a demyelinating neuropathy. *Neuron* **30**(3), 677–87.

Sherman DL, Tait S, Melrose S, Johnson R, Zonta B, Court FA, Macklin WB, Meek S, Smith AJ, Cottrell DF and others. (2005). Neurofascins are required to establish axonal domains for saltatory conduction. *Neuron* **48**(5), 737–42.

Smith SB, Marker CL, Perry C, Liao G, Sotocinal SG, Austin JS, Melmed K, Clark JD, Peltz G, Wickman K. *et al.* (2008). Quantitative trait locus and computational mapping identifies Kcnj9 (GIRK3) as a candidate gene affecting analgesia from multiple drug classes. *Pharmacogenetics and Genomics* **18**(3), 231–41.

Stavermann M, Buddrus K, St John JA, Ekberg JA, Nilius B, Deitmer JW, Lohr C. (2012). Temperature-dependent calcium-induced calcium release via InsP(3) receptors in mouse olfactory ensheathing glial cells. *Cell Calcium* **52**(2), 113–123.

Stewart HJ, Brennan A, Rahman M, Zoidl G, Mitchell PJ, Jessen KR, Mirsky R. (2001). Developmental regulation and overexpression of the transcription factor AP-2, a potential regulator of the timing of Schwann cell generation. *European Journal of Neuroscience* **14**(2), 363–72.

Su Z, He C. (2010). Olfactory ensheathing cells: biology in neural development and regeneration. *Progress In Neurobiology* **92**(4), 517–32.

Suadicani SO, Cherkas PS, Zuckerman J, Smith DN, Spray DC, Hanani M. (2010). Bidirectional calcium signaling between satellite glial cells and neurons in cultured mouse trigeminal ganglia. *Neuron Glia Biology* **6**(1), 43–51.

Takeda M, Takahashi M, Matsumoto S. (2009). Contribution of the activation of satellite glia in sensory ganglia to pathological pain. *Neuroscience and Biobehavioral Reviews* **33**(6), 784–92.

Tang X, Schmidt TM, Perez-Leighton CE, Kofuji P. (2010). Inwardly rectifying potassium channel Kir4.1 is responsible for the native inward potassium conductance of satellite glial cells in sensory ganglia. *Neuroscience* **166**(2), 397–407.

Ulzheimer JC, Peles E, Levinson SR, Martini R. (2004). Altered expression of ion channel isoforms at the node of Ranvier in P0-deficient myelin mutants. *Molecular and Cellular Neurosciences* **25**(1), 83–94.

Van Landeghem L, Chevalier J, Mahe MM, Wedel T, Urvil P, Derkinderen P, Savidge T, Neunlist M. (2011). Enteric glia promote intestinal mucosal healing via activation of focal adhesion kinase and release of proEGF. *American Journal of Physiology. Gastrointestinal and Liver Physiology* **300**(6), G976–87.

Van Nassauw L, Costagliola A, Van Op den Bosch J, Cecio A, Vanderwinden JM, Burnstock G, Timmermans JP. (2006). Region-specific distribution of the P2Y4 receptor in enteric glial cells and interstitial cells of Cajal within the guinea-pig gastrointestinal tract. *Autonomic Neuroscience* **126–127**, 299–306.

Vanderwinden JM, Timmermans JP, Schiffmann SN. (2003). Glial cells, but not interstitial cells, express P2X7, an ionotropic purinergic receptor, in rat gastrointestinal musculature. *Cell and Tissue Research* **312**(2), 149–54.

Vit JP, Ohara PT, Bhargava A, Kelley K, Jasmin L. (2008). Silencing the Kir4.1 potassium channel subunit in satellite glial cells of the rat trigeminal ganglion results in pain-like behavior in the absence of nerve injury. *Journal of Neuroscience* **28**(16), 4161–71.

von Boyen G, Steinkamp M. (2010). The role of enteric glia in gut inflammation. *Neuron Glia Biology* **6**(4), 231–6.

von Boyen GB, Steinkamp M, Adler G, Kirsch J. (2006). Glutamate receptor subunit expression in primary enteric glia cultures. *Journal of Receptor and Signal Transduction Research* **26**(4), 329–36.

Wolburg H, Wolburg-Buchholz K, Sam H, Horvat S, Deli MA, Mack AF. (2008). Epithelial and endothelial barriers in the olfactory region of the nasal cavity of the rat. *Histochemistry and Cell Biology* **130**(1), 127–40.

Woodhoo A, Sommer L. (2008). Development of the Schwann cell lineage: from the neural crest to the myelinated nerve. *Glia* **56**(14), 1481–90.

Woodhoo A, Sahni V, Gilson J, Setzu A, Franklin RJ, Blakemore WF, Mirsky R, Jessen KR. (2007). Schwann cell precursors: a favourable cell for myelin repair in the Central Nervous System. *Brain* **130**(Pt 8), 2175–85.

Woodhoo A, Alonso MB, Droggiti A, Turmaine M, D'Antonio M, Parkinson DB, Wilton DK, Al-Shawi R, Simons P, Shen J. *et al.* (2009). Notch controls embryonic Schwann cell differentiation, postnatal myelination and adult plasticity. *Nature Neuroscience* **12**(7), 839–47.

Wu SZ, Jiang S, Sims TJ, Barger SW. (2005). Schwann cells exhibit excitotoxicity consistent with release of NMDA receptor agonists. *Journal of Neuroscience Research* **79**(5), 638–43.

Yang D, Bierman J, Tarumi YS, Zhong YP, Rangwala R, Proctor TM, Miyagoe-Suzuki Y, Takeda S, Miner JH, Sherman L.S. *et al.* (2005). Coordinate control of axon defasciculation and myelination by laminin-2 and -8. *Journal of Cell Biology* **168**(4), 655–66.

Yin X, Crawford TO, Griffin JW, Tu P, Lee VM, Li C, Roder J, Trapp BD. (1998). Myelin-associated glycoprotein is a myelin signal that modulates the caliber of myelinated axons. *Journal of Neuroscience* **18**(6), 1953–62.

Yin X, Baek RC, Kirschner DA, Peterson A, Fujii Y, Nave KA, Macklin WB, Trapp BD. (2006). Evolution of a neuroprotective function of central nervous system myelin. *Journal of Cell Biology* **172**(3), 469–78.

Yin X, Kidd GJ, Nave KA, Trapp BD. (2008). P0 protein is required for and can induce formation of schmidt-lantermann incisures in myelin internodes. *Journal of Neuroscience* **28**(28), 7068–73.

Yu WM, Chen ZL, North AJ, Strickland S. (2009a). Laminin is required for Schwann cell morphogenesis. *Journal of Cell Science* **122**(Pt 7), 929–36.

Yu WM, Yu H, Chen ZL, Strickland S. (2009b). Disruption of laminin in the peripheral nervous system impedes nonmyelinating Schwann cell development and impairs nociceptive sensory function. *Glia* **57**(8), 850–9.

Zhang W, Segura BJ, Lin TR, Hu Y, Mulholland MW. (2003). Intercellular calcium waves in cultured enteric glia from neonatal guinea pig. *Glia* **42**(3), 252–62.

Zhang X, Chen Y, Wang C, Huang LY. (2007). neuronal somatic ATP release triggers neuron-satellite glial cell communication in dorsal root ganglia. *Proceedings of The National Academy Of Sciences Of The United States Of America* **104**(23), 9864–9.

# 9
# General Pathophysiology of Neuroglia

## 9.1   Neurological disorders as gliopathologies

All diseases, including neurological diseases, can be broadly defined as homeostatic failures. Glia are the principal homeostatic cells of the nervous system and, accordingly, they are integral to homeostatic failures in all neurological diseases. Indeed, neuroglia as a major element of neuropathological processes was already understood by Rudolf Virchow, who was convinced that *Nervenkitt/Neuroglia* is central for neuropathology: '*This very interstitial tissue of the brain and spinal marrow is one of the most frequent seats of morbid change*' (Virchow, 1858).

For a long time, our perception of brain pathology has naturally focused on neurones and on their survival or death. This perception is now being challenged, and neuroglia are beginning to be recognised as a central element of neurological diseases (De Keyser *et al.*, 2008; Giaume *et al.*, 2007; Verkhratsky *et al.*, 2012). Indeed, brain pathology is, to a very great extent, glial pathology, since the failure of

*Glial Physiology and Pathophysiology*, First Edition. Alexei Verkhratsky and Arthur Butt.
© 2013 by John Wiley & Sons, Ltd. Published 2013 by John Wiley & Sons, Ltd.

glia to function properly determines the degree of neuronal death and the scale of neurological deficit.

Neurological disorders reflect several levels of compromised tissue homeostasis, and the pathological response of glia determines the *degree* of homeostatic loss. Acute insults (trauma, stroke or toxic attack) compromise brain homeostasis on many levels, from organ (disruption of the blood-brain barrier), and metabolic (shutting down brain energetics), to molecular (loss of neurotransmitter homeostasis with subsequent excitotoxicity). Specific homeostatic failures operate in many forms of chronic pathology, such as when down-regulation of glutamate transporters induces neuronal death in Wernicke encephalopathy. In many neuropathologies, homeostatic failures progress and multiply – for example, when initial disruption of protein catabolism triggers inflammatory reactions, initiates cytotoxicity and compromises the blood brain barrier (which happens in various neurodegenerative processes).

Neuroglia are protective and, in the face of disruption, they attempt to maintain tissue and cellular homeostasis. Glia can also be destructive but, again, this should be considered as an overall homeostatic function in which severely compromised neural elements are cleared up (e.g. neurones, synapses, injured axons, blood vessels, oligodendrocytes). This latter homeostatic function of glia serves to limit the spread of destruction and protect the surrounding uncompromised cells/tissue. Finally, glia are entirely responsible for the recovery of homeostasis, by promoting vascularisation, reformation of the blood-brain barrier, producing neurotrophic factors, stimulating synapse formation and providing for remyelination. In fact, it is when glial homeostatic functions are compromised that severe neurodegeneration and neurological diseases occur.

Neuroglia are responsible for neuronal well-being and provide multiple lines of defence for nervous tissue (Figure 9.1). Astrocytes are key to the preservation of tissue homeostasis, and their fundamental function is neuroprotection. In addition, astrocytes are fundamental elements of CNS defence, whereby every insult to the nervous tissue invariably triggers reactive astrogliosis, the ancient and conserved astroglial defence reaction. NG2-glia are a further homeostatic element of the nervous tissue, and they react to pathological attacks by launching a classical gliogenesis. Oligodendroglia and Schwann cells ensure proper function of axons, and damaging oligodendrocytes and Schwann cells triggers Wallerian degeneration, another conserved defensive reaction. Massive death of oligodendrocytes, which often happens in ischaemia, signals the demise of white matter, with the gravest consequences for the nervous tissue. Finally, microglia are the only system of specific immune and cellular defence in the CNS.

Malfunction of glia is fatal for the nervous system. Neurones cannot function correctly or survive in the absence of glia, whereas glial cells do survive and operate in the presence of dead or dying neurones. At the same time, glia are endowed with an inherent dichotomy – they protect the nervous tissue as long as possible, but act as natural killers in order to save the whole at the expense of the part.

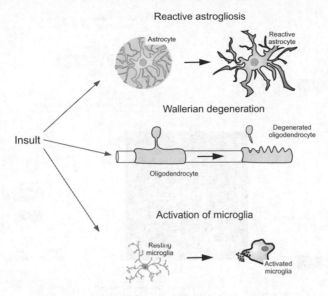

Reactive astrogliosis

Astrocyte → Reactive astrocyte

Wallerian degeneration

Degenerated oligodendrocyte

Oligodendrocyte

Activation of microglia

Resting microglia → Activated microglia

Insult

**Figure 9.1**   Neuroglial responses to pathological insults.

# 9.2   Reactive astrogliosis

Astrocytes form the brain defence system by virtue of many homeostatic mechanisms, through which they contain damage and sustain neuronal survival. One of many examples is represented by the astroglial maintenance of brain metabolism following ischaemia/hypoglycaemia, when astrocytes break down their glycogen stores to produce lactate that they transfer to adjacent neurones, which use it aerobically as fuel (Suh *et al.*, 2007).

In conditions of severe insult, however, the very same homeostatic molecular cascades can assume damaging and toxic proportions (Figure 9.2). For example, aquaporins expressed in astroglia are critical for water movements through brain tissue, but they can also be instrumental in mediating oedema in pathology. Similarly, $K^+$ channels responsible for potassium buffering can, when under pathological stress, add to the accumulation of extracellular $K^+$ and mediate spreading depression. The connexins, which connect astrocytes into multicellular syncytia, can become the passages for death signals underlying the spread of necrosis through ischaemic penumbra. Depolarisation and $Na^+$ accumulation in astroglia triggers reversal of glutamate transporters, which increases glutamate excitotoxicity (see Verkhratsky *et al.*, 2012 for details and references).

In addition to general neuroprotection offered by astroglial homeostatic systems, astrocytes are capable of mounting a specific defensive reaction. All types of brain insults, regardless of aetiology, trigger a complex astroglial response, which is generally manifested by astrocyte hypertrophy and proliferation. This glial response is defined as *reactive astrogliosis* (Figures 9.3, 9.4, 9.5; and see Bringmann *et al.*,

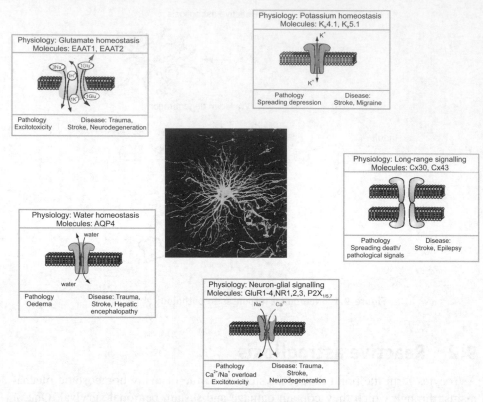

**Figure 9.2**  Pathological potential of astroglial homeostatic cascades.

The homeostatic cascades expressed in astrocytes control various aspects of CNS homeostasis, including extracellular ion homeostasis ($K^+$ buffering via $K_{ir}$ channels, $Na^+/K^+$ pumps and $K^+$ transporters), regulating movements and distribution of water (via aquaporins and connexins), control of extracellular concentration of neurotransmitters (by dedicated transporters) and providing the main reactive-oxygen species scavenging system. In pathological conditions, the very same systems may contribute to brain damage. Failure in water transport triggers brain oedema, reversal of neurotransmitter transporters contributes to glutamate excitotoxicity, inadequate $K^+$ buffering promotes over-excitation of neural cells and spreading depression, and connexins become a conduit for death signals.

Reproduced with permission from Verkhratsky, A. (2012) Neurotransmitters and Integration in Neuronal-Astroglial Networks. Neurochemical Research © Springer Publishing.

2009; De Keyser *et al.*, 2008; Pekny and Nilsson, 2005; Robel *et al.*, 2011; Sofroniew, 2009; Sofroniew and Vinters, 2010 for references and detailed coverage). As with many other aspects of glial biology, a generally accepted definition of reactive astrogliosis has not been developed. Importantly, the perception of astrogliosis as a purely deleterious and negative process is an oversimplification and is factually wrong. Similarly, the widely popularised definition of astrogliosis as 'astroglial inflammation' is not correct.

### Isomorphic (i.e. preserving morphology) astrogliosis
**Astroglial domain structure is preserved**
In astrocytes experiencing lesser insult or distal to the lesion site, the reactive changes are much milder and, although astroglial cells modify their appearance and undergo multiple biochemical and immunological changes, they do not distort the normal architecture of CNS tissue, but rather permit growth of neurites and synaptogenesis, thus facilitating the remodelling of neuronal networks.

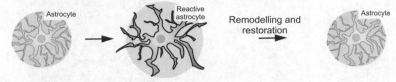

### Anisomorphic (i.e. changing the morphology) astrogliosis
**Astroglial domain structure is disrupted**
Astrocytes subjected to strong insult undergo a robust hypertrophy and proliferation, which ultimately ends up in complete substitution of previously existing tissue architecture with a permanent glial scar

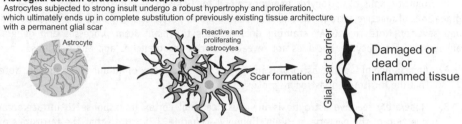

**Figure 9.3**   Isomorphic and anisomorphic reactive astrogliosis.

Reactive astrogliosis can be defined as a *constitutive, graded, multi-stage and evolutionary conserved defensive astroglial reaction.* Michael Sofroniew (2009) provided an expanded definition of reactive astrogliosis as integrating four inter-dependent key features:

1. Reactive astrogliosis is a spectrum of changes in astrocytes that occur in response to all forms and severities of CNS injury and disease including subtle perturbations.

2. The changes undergone by reactive astrocytes vary with the nature and severity of the insult along a gradated continuum of progressive alterations in molecular expression, progressive cellular hypertrophy and, in severe cases, proliferation and scar formation.

3. The changes of astrogliosis are regulated in a context-specific manner by specific signalling events that have the potential to modify both the nature and degree of those changes.

4. The changes undergone during reactive astrogliosis have the potential to alter astrocyte activities through both gain and loss of functions that can impact both beneficially and detrimentally on surrounding neural and non-neural cells.

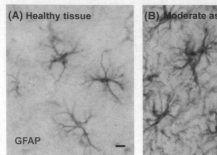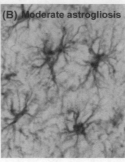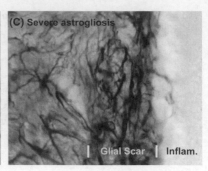

**Figure 9.4**  Graded severity of reactive astrogliosis.

Photomicrographs of astrocytes immunostained for GFAP in healthy tissue and of different gradations of reactive astrogliosis and glial scar formation after tissue insults of different types and severity. Note that GFAP staining demonstrates the main stem processes and general appearance of astrocytes, but does not reveal all of the fine branches and ramifications.

A.  Appearance of 'normal' astrocytes in healthy cerebral cortex of an untreated mouse. Note that the territories of astrocyte processes do not overlap.

B.  Moderately reactive astrogliosis in mouse cerebral cortex in response to intracerebral injection of the bacterial antigen, lipopolysaccharide (LPS). Note that the territories of moderately reactive astrocyte processes also do not overlap.

C.  Severely reactive astrogliosis and glial scar formation adjacent to a region of severe traumatic injury and inflammation (Inflam.) in the cerebral cortex. Note the extensive overlap and interdigitations of processes of severely reactive and scar-forming astrocytes. Scale bar = 8 μm.

Reproduced with permission from Sofroniew, M. V. (2009) Molecular dissection of reactive astrogliosis and glial scar formation. Trends in Neurosciences 32:12, pp. 638–647 © Elsevier Ltd. (Full colour version in plate section.)

Functionally, astrogliosis is aimed at:

1.  increased neuroprotection and trophic support of insult-stressed neurones;

2.  isolation of the damaged area from the rest of the CNS tissue;

3.  reconstruction of the compromised blood-brain barrier;

4.  facilitation of the remodelling of brain circuits in areas surrounding the lesioned region.

Within the framework of remodelling the neural circuits, reactive astrocytes may acquire properties of stem cells (Robel *et al.*, 2011). The overall result of these functional reactions is clearly beneficial for the nervous tissue, since experimental removal of reactive astrocytes greatly increases the degree of tissue damage and neuronal death (Robel *et al.*, 2011; Sofroniew and Vinters, 2010).

Reactive astrogliosis can be classified according to (a) morphological appearances, and (b) severity. According to morphological criteria (Figure 9.3), astrogliosis can be

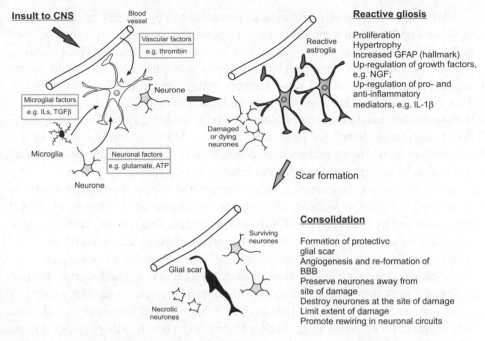

**Figure 9.5**   Initiation and progression of reactive astrogliosis.

Insults to the CNS trigger release of numerous factors that interact with astroglial cells and subsequently trigger reactive astrogliosis, which is generally represented by hypertrophy and proliferation of astrocytes. Astrogliosis ultimately ends up in the complete substitution of previously existing tissue architecture with a permanent *glial scar* (see the text for detailed explanation)

classified into *isomorphic* (i.e. preserving morphology) and *anisomorphic* (i.e. changing the morphology).

In *isomorphic gliosis*, astroglial cells became hypertrophic, increase expression of GFAP and vimentin, and undergo multiple biochemical and immunological changes. However, they do not distort the normal architecture of CNS tissue and do not alter astroglial domain organisation, but rather they permit growth of neurites and synaptogenesis, thus facilitating the remodelling of neuronal networks. With waning of the pathological process, astrocytes return to their previous normal state.

In *anisomorphic gliosis*, astrocytes undergo a robust hypertrophy associated with up-regulation of GFAP and vimentin expression. These reactive astrocytes start to proliferate and they lose their domain organisation. Reactive astrocytes in aniso-morphic gliosis produce chondroitin and keratin, which inhibit axonal regeneration and thus prevent nerve processes from entering the damaged zone. Reactive astroglia also release quantities of mucopolysaccharides, which cement the areas of damage. Anisomoprhic gliosis ultimately ends up in complete substitution of previously existing tissue architecture, with a permanent *glial scar*.

Another classification ranges astrogliotic changes according to their severity (Figure 9.4) (Sofroniew, 2009; Sofroniew and Vinters, 2010).

*Mild to moderate reactive astrogliosis* is manifested by an array of changes (up- or down-regulation) in gene expression, hypertrophy of cell body and processes and up-regulation of GFAP expression and increased cytoskeleton. These changes proceed without affecting astroglial territorial domains, and with little or no astrocyte proliferation (all of these features being similar to isomorphic gliosis). This type of astrogliosis is observed in mild non-penetrating and non-contusive trauma, diffuse innate immune activation (viral infections, system bacterial infections) and areas distant to focal CNS lesions. Because there is little or no reorganisation of tissue architecture, resolution of the pathology prompts full restoration of astroglia to their normal healthy phenotype.

*Severe diffuse reactive astrogliosis* also begins with multiple changes (up- or down-regulation) in gene expression, with rather prominent up-regulation of GFAP expression and hypertrophy of cell body and processes. This type of gliotic response also involves astrocyte proliferation and disruption of astroglial territorial domains, with substantive intermingling and overlapping of neighbouring astrocyte processes. These changes can result in long-lasting reorganisation of tissue architecture that can extend diffusely over substantive areas. This type of response is generally found in areas surrounding severe focal lesions, infections or areas responding to chronic neurodegenerative lesions (e.g. senile plaques and chronic MS plaques). Tissue reorganisation becomes permanent, and the ability of full restoration back to a healthy astroglial phenotype is much reduced.

*Severe reactive astrogliosis with compact glial scar formation* similarly demonstrates changes in gene expression, prominent cellular hypertrophy and GFAP synthesis, and astrocyte proliferation. Astroglial territorial domains are completely disrupted, and astroglial profiles form compact borders around areas of severe tissue damage, necrosis, infection or autoimmune-triggered inflammatory infiltration. The glial scar border includes other cell types – in particular, activated microglia, NG2-glia and fibromeningeal cells, and deposited collagenous extracellular matrix that contains molecular factors that inhibit axonal and cellular migration. This type of gliosis is observed in penetrating trauma, severe contusive trauma, invasive infections or abscess formation, neoplasm, some forms of chronic neurodegeneration, or systemically triggered inflammatory attacks. Formation of the glial scar leads to substantive tissue reorganisation and structural changes that persist even after termination of the initial pathological process.

The primary signals that trigger astrogliosis derive from damaged cells at the core of the insult (Figure 9.5), and they are represented by neurotransmitters (most importantly glutamate and ATP), cytokines, adhesion molecules, growth factors and blood factors (serum, thrombin etc.). The actual combination of these 'damage signals' and their relative concentrations most likely determines the type of astrogliosis in different regions surrounding the initial insult zone.

It is still unclear how normal mature astrocytes are turned into reactive ones. Several sources for reactive astrocytes are implicated. First, mature protoplasmic astrocytes can, under the influence of damage-associated signals, dedifferentiate and enter a proliferative state. Alternatively, the reactive astrocytes may arise from astroglial precursors, diffusely dispersed throughout the brain parenchyma, or even from multipotent NG2-expressing precursors and astroglial stem cells. The main evidence from genetic fate-mapping studies has identified mature protoplasmic astrocytes as the main origin of reactive astrocytes in response to traumatic injury (stab wound) to the murine brain (Buffo *et al.*, 2008). Nonetheless, the considerable heterogeneity displayed by reactive astroglial cells may indicate that several routes may be involved in astroglial metamorphosis.

Reactive astrocytes in the areas of isomorphic astrogliosis produce and release several types of growth factors (e.g. NGF and FGF) and cytokines (e.g. interleukins). These factors are important for neuroprotection and preservation of neurones. At the same time, reactive astrocytes synthesise numerous recognition molecules (e.g. extracellular matrix molecules, cell adhesion molecules, etc.) which promote neurone-astrocyte interactions and help axonal growth. In contrast, in the areas of anisomorphic astrogliosis and glial scar barrier, astrocytes produce factors that inhibit axonal growth. Therefore, reactive astroglia may either inhibit axonal entry by forming a non-permissive scar around the necrotic areas, or assist axonal growth and neuronal remodelling in areas distant to the site of initial insult.

Another important property of reactive astrocytes is their proliferative activity. In severe astrogliosis, reactive astrocytes rapidly (in 3–5 days after initial insult) up-regulate expression of proteins characteristic for neural progenitors and radial glia, which include the intermediate filament nestin, proteoglycan DSD1 or RNA-binding protein Musashi-1. Moreover, about half of reactive astrocytes re-enter the cell cycle and become proliferative (Robel *et al.*, 2011).

# 9.3 Wallerian degeneration

The severance of an axon from the nerve cell body initiates a series of coordinated events, which produce the disintegration of the distal axonal segment, removal of myelin and remodelling of myelinating cells, and finally nerve fibre regeneration, by axonal growth from the proximal stump. This process of nerve degeneration was discovered by Augustus Volney Waller (1856–1922) in 1850 and is generally known as Wallerian degeneration (Waller, 1850).

The term 'Wallerian degeneration' (for details and references, see Coleman and Freeman, 2010; Gaudet *et al.*, 2011; Koeppen, 2004; Rotshenker, 2011; Vargas and Barres, 2007) is currently used to describe axonal degeneration in both CNS and PNS, although the properties and underlying processes can be entirely different (Figures 9.6 and 9.7).

In the PNS, mechanical disruption of the axon triggers demyelination of its distal segment, which begins from the point of the trauma. This demyelination commences within 24–48 hours after the insult and proceeds rather rapidly, with a rate varying between 50 μm per 24 hours for the thickest axons, to 250 μm per 24 hours for the thinnest ones. The degenerating axon is rapidly cleared by phagocytes

Wallerian Degeneration in PNS

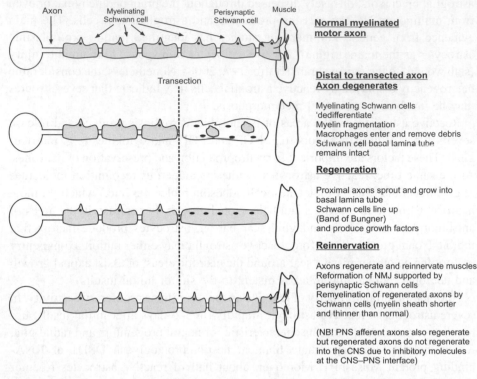

**Figure 9.6**   General scheme of Wallerian degeneration in the peripheral nervous system.

arriving from neighbouring tissue or blood. By the time the degenerated axon is removed, the Schwann cells have undergone dedifferentiation and proliferation, and are prepared to receive the sprouts of regenerating axons and to begin their myelination. This particular arrangement underlies the remarkable regeneration potential of the PNS (Figure 9.6).

Regeneration of neuromuscular synapses is regulated by perisynaptic Schwann cells. Following muscle denervation, the latter send processes which link the denervated endplates to the regenerating axons (see Chapter 8: Figure 8.6 and Section 8.2.1).

In the CNS, axonal degeneration after injury proceeds in a different way (Figure 9.7). First, its course is much slower than in the PNS, although the rate of degeneration depends on phyological and developmental age, being much faster in the phylogenetically oldest vertebrates (e.g. fish and amphibia) and in very young mammals. Second, there is no specific reaction from the myelinating cells. After the myelin sheath of the degenerating axon disintegrates, oligodendrocytes do not show any signs of plastic changes or proliferation; instead, this is a specialised function of NG2-glia (see Chapter 6). In addition, activation of microglia and invading

## Wallerian Degeneration in CNS

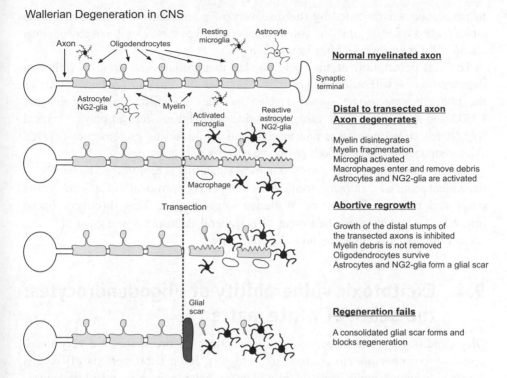

**Figure 9.7**   General scheme of Wallerian degeneration in the central nervous system.

macrophages is incomplete, and myelin debris is not effectively removed. Furthermore, reactive astrocytes and NG2-glia migrate to the site of axonal damage and replace the remnants of the nerve fibres with the glial scar. These multiple factors determine the regeneration failure in damaged CNS axonal fibres.

The ability of Schwann cells to provide essential guidance and trophic support for regenerating axons has led to them being used as a potential treatment for CNS injury. Transplantation of Schwann cells into the CNS following injury promotes axon regeneration. However, Schwann cells do not interact well with astrocytes, which form a glia limitans around Schwann cells to isolate them from surrounding CNS tissue, reminiscent of the CNS-PNS interface transition zone (see Chapter 8, Section 8.1). In contrast, olfactory ensheathing cells have become promising candidates for cell-based transplantation therapies for CNS regeneration, because they naturally support neuronal growth and are able to intermingle with astrocytes without inducing astroglial reactivity (see Chapter 8, Section 8.5).

For many years, axonal degeneration following transection was considered to be due to the cessation of support from the cell body. Recently, however, it has become obvious that Wallerian degeneration is a specialised active process that involves activation of localised signals in both axons and surrounding glial cells. This change in perception was initiated by the discovery of a spontaneously mutated mouse strain (called $Wld^S$ or '*ola*'), in which peripheral nerves survive without any obvious changes for many weeks after transection.

The full description of the local signals that initiate and control Wallerian degeneration is still wanting, yet it is clear that the enzyme system known as the ubiquitin-proteasome system (which includes ubiquitin regulatory enzyme UFD2 and the nicotinamide mononucleotide adenylyltransferase) plays a critical role. It has been found that pharmacological inhibition of proteasomes delayed Wallerian degeneration in both peripheral nerves and optic nerve.

Another important player involved in local signalling is represented by the $Ca^{2+}$-dependent proteases, calpains; inhibition of calpains or removal of $Ca^{2+}$ delays the onset and reduces the rate of Wallerian degeneration. This discovery opens important perspectives for treatment of peripheral neuropathies, e.g. in diabetes, some forms of HIV infection and chemotherapy.

## 9.4   Excitotoxic vulnerability of oligodendrocytes: the death of white matter

Oligodendrocytes, and in particular oligodendroglial precursors are very much sensitive to ischaemia (in contrast to astroglia). Even short periods of oxygen deprivation cause rapid death of oligodendroglial precursors and oligodendrocytes. This, in turn, triggers severe damage to the white matter with serious neurological consequences. Ischaemia-induced death of cells of the oligodendroglial lineage is mainly mediated through glutamate excitotoxicity. Excess glutamate activates AMPA, kainate and NMDA receptors present in oligodendrocytes, which induces rapid $Ca^{2+}$ overload and necrotic/apoptotic cell death (for detailed overview of excitotoxic damage to white matter, see Karadottir and Attwell, 2007; Matute, 2010; Matute, 2011; Matute *et al.*, 2007; Stys and Lipton, 2007; Volpe *et al.*, 2011).

Substantial $Ca^{2+}$ influx into oligodendroglial cells can also be mediated by $P2X_7$ purinoceptors. A central event in this process is accumulation of $Ca^{2+}$ within mitochondria, which leads to the depolarisation of this organelle, increased production of oxygen free radicals and release of pro-apoptotic factors which activate caspases (Figure 9.8). Glutamate can also cause oligodendroglial damage by several indirect pathways, for example by inducing the release of toxic agents from microglia that can potentiate glutamate toxicity through inhibition of glutamate uptake. Glutamate at relatively low concentrations may also sensitise oligodendrocytes to complement attack.

Substantial oligodendroglial death with subsequent damage to white matter occurs in stroke, traumatic injury, neurodegenerative diseases and multiple sclerosis, as well as in psychiatric diseases (Matute *et al.*, 2006; see Chapter 10). Particularly severe damage to white matter occurs in perinatal ischaemia, which

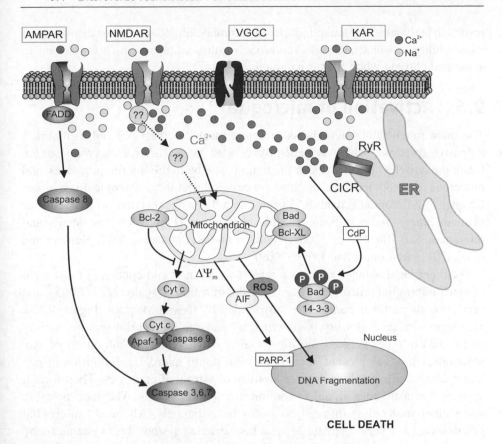

**Figure 9.8** Signalling cascades triggered by activation of glutamate receptors induce oligo-dendrocyte death.

Selective activation of AMPA receptors (AMPAR) and kainate receptors (KAR) leads to $Na^+$ and $Ca^{2+}$ influx through the receptor channel complex. Subsequent depolarization activates voltage-operated $Ca^{2+}$ channels (VGCC), which contributes to the rise in $[Ca^{2+}]_i$. $Ca^{2+}$ overload induces rapid uptake by mitochondria, which results in attenuation of the mitochondrial potential and an increase in the production of reactive oxygen species (ROS). Cytochrome c (Cyt c) is released from depolarized mitochondria, interacts with apoptotic protease activating factor 1 (Apaf-1) and activates caspases. Other pro-apoptotic factors include apoptosis-inducing factor (AIF) which activates poly(ADP-ribose)polimerase-1 (PARP-1). In oligodendrocytes, insults channelled through KAR activate caspases 9 and 3, whereas those activating AMPAR induces apoptosis by recruiting caspase 8, which truncates Bid, caspase 3 and PARP-1, or cause necrosis. In addition, $Ca^{2+}$ influx triggered by KAR stimulation but not by AMPAR activates calcineurin (CdP), which dephosphorylates Bad and facilitates apoptosis. Finally, activation of NMDA receptors (NMDAR) also initiates oligodendrocyte death, which is entirely dependent on $Ca^{2+}$ influx; however, the molecular mechanisms activated by these receptors are not yet known.

Abbreviations: FADD, Fas-associated death domain; 14-3-3, phosphoserine-binding protein 14-3-3.

Reproduced with permission from Giaume *et al.*, 2007.

results in periventricular leukomalacia. In summary, oligodendrocytes display great vulnerability to ischaemic and excitotoxic insults, a feature which is relevant to acute and chronic white matter pathology.

## 9.5   Activation of microglia

The main function of microglia is to detect insults to the CNS and to mount a defensive response, which is generally defined as the *activation of microglia*. Resting microglia constantly scan the brain tissue by highly motile processes, and numerous receptors localised on these processes detect the pathological insult (see Chapter 7). Microglial activation is primarily a defensive reaction, which develops in many stages and results in multiple phenotypes (Figure 9.9; for details and references, see Biber *et al.*, 2007; Hanisch and Kettenmann, 2007; Kettenmann *et al.*, 2011; Ransohoff and Perry, 2009).

Focal neuronal damage induces a rapid ($\approx$1.5 $\mu$m/s) and concerted movement of many microglial processes towards the site of lesion (Davalos *et al.*, 2005), and very soon the latter is completely surrounded by these processes (Figure 9.10). This injury-induced motility is governed by activation of purinoceptors, mainly of the $P2Y_{12}$ type. Process motility is also sensitive to the inhibition of gap junctions, which are present in astrocytes but not in microglia. Inhibition of gap junctions also affects physiological motility of astroglial processes. Therefore, it appears that astrocytes signal to the microglia by releasing ATP (and possibly some other molecules) through connexin hemichannels. All in all, microglial processes act as a very sophisticated and fast scanning system. This system can, by virtue of receptors residing in the microglial cell plasmalemma, immediately detect injury and initiate the active response process, which represents the first stage in microglial activation.

When a brain insult is detected by microglial cells, they launch a specific pro-gramme that results in the gradual transformation of resting microglia into a phagocyte; this process is generally referred to as 'microglial activation' and proceeds through several steps (Figure 9.9). The first stage of microglial activation produces 'normally' activated or reactive microglia. During this transition, resting microglia retract their processes, which become fewer and much thicker, increase the size of their cell bodies, change the expression of various enzymes and receptors and begin to produce immune response molecules. At this activated stage, some microglial cells enter into a proliferative mode and microglial numbers around the lesion site start to multiply. Finally, microglial cells became motile and, using amoeboid-like movements, they gather around sites of insult. If the damage persists and CNS cells begin to die, microglial cells undergo further transformation and become phagocytes.

This is, naturally, a rather sketchy account of the complex and highly coordinated changes that occur in microglial cells. The process of activation is gradual and, most likely, many sub-states exist on the way from resting to phagocytic microglia.

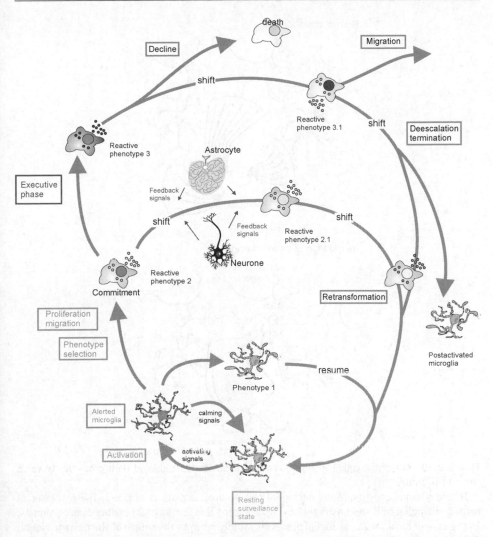

**Figure 9.9**  Microglial activity states throughout an activation process.

'Resting' microglia constantly and actively scan their environment for exogenous or endogenous signals indicating a threat to the homeostasis. The sudden appearance of 'activating' signals, or a loss of constitutively 'calming' inputs, can then trigger transitions to alerted and activated states. Cells can commit to distinct reactive phenotypes, depending on the stimuli and context. Initial response profiles may further shift as instructed by additional influences; not only resident CNS cells, but also invading immune cells, would exert such modulating influences. Initial reactive phenotypes with a defence orientation may convert to repair-orientated activity profiles. Cells may eventually return to a resting state or stay 'experienced'. 'Experienced' microglia could exhibit altered responsiveness and exert distinct responses upon re-challenge.

Reproduced with permission from Kettenmann *et al.*, 2011. (Full colour version in plate section.)

Normal conditions

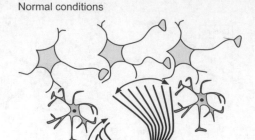

Initial stage of brain damage

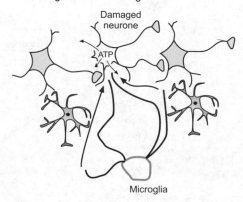

**Figure 9.10**  Microglial cells constantly scan their territories and send their processes towards the site of injury.

In the resting condition, every microglial cell occupies a distinct territory. The processes of resting microglial cells are constantly moving, scanning this territory for possible damage signals. In the case of local insult, microglial processes rapidly move to the source of the damage signal; the latter is most likely represented by ATP that stimulates microglial process movement through activation of metabotropic P2Y purinoreceptors.

Furthermore, activated microglial cells may display quite heterogeneous properties in different types of pathology and in different parts of the brain.

The precise nature of the initial signals that trigger the process of microglial activation is not fully understood. The current concept postulates the existence of two groups of chemical signals, generally referred to as 'on-signals' and 'off-signals' (Biber *et al.*, 2007; Hanisch and Kettenmann, 2007; van Rossum and Hanisch, 2004). The 'on-signals' are chemicals which are absent in the healthy tissue and appear only in association with pathological insult. These signals can be represented by infectious pathogens (e.g. fragments of bacterial cell walls, viral envelopes or their respective DNAs and/or RNAs), or by intracellular proteins released following cell damage, or by factors coming from blood which signals disruption of blood-brain barrier. The 'on-signals' can also be represented by substances normally present in the brain environment that achieve pathologically high concentrations following insults, the best example being the massive release of ATP that invariably accompanies cell damage. It might well be that different molecules can activate various sub-programmes, thus regulating the speed, degree and peculiar features of microglial activation.

The 'off-signals' are associated with withdrawal of some molecules which are normally present in the CNS. These molecules normally suppress microglial activation, and their disappearance signals damage. Most neurotransmitters (especially GABA, acetylcholine and adenosine) act as 'off-signals'; their presence in the CNS microenvironment generally indicates healthy conditions, while disruption of synaptic transmission signals abnormalities.

Some molecules can carry both 'off-' and 'on-' signals. For example, low concentrations of ATP may be indicative of normal ongoing synaptic activity, whereas high concentrations signal cell damage. Microglia are also capable of sensing disturbances in brain metabolism. For example, accumulation of ammonia, which follows grave metabolic failures (e.g. during hepatic encephalopathy) can activate microglial cells either directly or via intermediates such as NO or ATP.

The 'off-signals' that may indicate deterioration in neural networks are not yet fully characterised. A good example of this type of communication is represented by neuronal firing, depression of which affects neighbouring microglia, turning them into an 'alerted' state, if not quite activated. Microglial cells start to up-regulate several immunocompetent molecules in response to blockade of neuronal activity. In fact, these 'off-signals' can be defensively important, as they allow microglia to sense some disturbance even if the nature of the damaging factor cannot be identified.

Astrocytes are also capable of releasing a variety of molecules that can activate microglia. This is especially characteristic of activated astroglia, which can up-regulate the synthesis and release of biologically active molecules. Microglial cells can also be activated by signals released from their sister cells that have already undergone activation. An important activator signal is conveyed by molecules arriving with infectious agents, e.g. by lypopolysaccharides forming the bacterial cellular wall, by prions, or by viral components, such as g120 protein from HIV. Finally, microglia can be activated by a number of molecules that can infiltrate the brain following damage to the blood-brain barrier, e.g. coagulation factors, immunoglobulins, albumin, thrombin, etc.

Intracellularly, most of the 'on' signals produce elevations in $[Ca^{2+}]_i$, the amplitude and shape of which can vary significantly, depending on the type and concentration of molecule/receptor complex involved. Most likely, these variabilities of the $Ca^{2+}$ signals are instrumental for information encoding, although the precise nature of this type of informational processing remains unknown.

Activation that follows the recognition of damage signals can be a very rapid process indeed. The initial changes in cellular biochemistry occur within minutes after the presenting signal, and the full activation of microglial cells can follow within several hours. Activated microglial cells change their physiological and biochemical properties considerably. First, activated microglia start to up-regulate potassium channels, initially $K_{ir}$ and then delayed $K^+$ channels. Second, activated microglia can change the repertoire and levels of expression of numerous receptors, e.g. by down-regulating 'neuronal' receptors and up-regulating the 'immunocompetent' ones. Furthermore, activated microglial cells alter their biochemistry by stimulating the synthesis of numerous enzymes. Finally, micro-glial cells change their motility as they gather at the site of damage, first by sending their processes, then by migration of their somata.

All of these changes allow the execution of the primary function of microglia – defence. This function requires the ability to attack and kill the invader rapidly. Subsequently, the remnants of the aggressor, its victims and the collateral damage must be effectively removed. Thus, activated microglial cells are fully equipped with cytotoxic tools, such as reactive oxygen species or NO (most notably, the NO system is absent in human microglia, although it is fully operative in rodents) or, indeed, the cytokines and chemokines. Not only do activated microglial cells aim to destroy the foreign cells, they also assist neurones in overcoming the damage. In line with this, microglial cells express and release various growth factors (NGF, BDNF, NT-3, NT-4 etc.).

Microglial activation often leads to high expression of glutamate transporters (GLT-1), which assists in clearing the excess of glutamate. It has been suggested that microglial cells, after arriving at the site of damage, can selectively remove excitatory glutamatergic synapses (so-called 'synaptic stripping'), which further limits glutamate release into compromised brain regions.

In addition, microglial cells produce an incredible array of immunocompetent molecules, which include numerous interleukins (IL-1$\alpha$/$\beta$; IL-3, IL-6, IL-8, IL-10, IL-12, IL-15, IL-18), TNF $\alpha$, interferon inducing factor (IGIF), inflammatory proteins, transforming growth factor TGF$\beta$, etc. All these molecules regulate the inflammatory processes and control the immune response of the brain. Many of these, such as TGF$\beta$, are also important regulators of astrogliosis and are important in the orchestration of glial scar formation.

Microglial activation is a reversible process (except for the final, phagocytic, stage), which occurs when the pathological factor is defeated. The nature of the signals regulating the deactivation of microglia is unknown. Most likely, the waning of pathological stimulation may be sufficient, although some active 'terminating' message is not excluded. Some *in vitro* experiments have shown the existence of certain astrocyte-derived factors that may initiate deactivation of microglia.

The final transmutation from activated microglia into a phagocytic stage is also initiated by factors released from dying or already dead neurones or astrocytes. The nature of these 'death signals' is not very clear. It seems likely that vanishing cells can release certain chemoattractants (e.g. phosphatidylserine and lysophosphati-dylcholine), which can initiate the ultimate transformation of microglial cells into phagocytes. These then engulf and devour the remnants of the dying cells that induced them. Importantly, the actual killing of neurones by microglia is confined to the damaged area, and it does not extend normally to undamaged areas. When this constraint fails, however, activated microglia may assume the role of 'brain destroyer', which does happen in certain pathological conditions.

Microglial phagocytosis is also regulated by many factors – for example, pharmacological inhibition of the intracellular chloride channel (CLIC1) or down-regulation of its expression by small interfering RNA impairs phagocytic activity. The growth factor ciliary neurotrophic factor (CNTF) increases microglial phagocytosis through a $Ca^{2+}$-mediated pathway. Similarly, GDNF and macrophage colony-stimulating factor (M-CSF) increase the phagocytotic capability of microglia. Substrate-bound complement component C1q has been shown to enhance both FcR-and CR1-mediated phagocytosis two- to four-fold.

The metabotropic $P2Y_6$ receptor controls microglial phagocytosis. $P2Y_6$ receptors are up-regulated when neurones are damaged and function as a sensor/trigger for phagocytosis. At the same time, activation of $P2X_7$ receptors in cultured rat microglia suppresses phagocytosis in a $Ca^{2+}$-independent manner, and inhibition of $P2X_7$ expression restores phagocytic activity (see Kettenmann et al., 2011).

## 9.5.1  Pathological potential of activated microglia

As is the case for macrophages in many body systems, microglia are capable of providing both protection and destruction. The exaggerated or prolonged activation of microglial cells can be detrimental to the brain. In certain cases, the pathological activation of microglia may have a decisive input. This may happen, for example, in infectious diseases, in particular in certain types of bacterial infection or in prion diseases (see Chapter 10). Similarly, chronic neurodegenerative diseases (e.g. Alzheimer's or Parkinson's disease – Chapter 10) may underlie the long-lasting over-activation of microglial cells, which subsequently may produce neuronal or astroglial death.

## 9.6  Concluding remarks

Neuroglial cells are a major component of pathogenesis of neurological diseases. Their fundamental role in neuropathology is yet to be fully appreciated, but nonetheless it is becoming increasingly clear that every disease of the nervous system critically depends on neuroglial reactions. Simply put, the pathological response of glia largely determines the outcome and scale of neurological diseases.

The function of neuroglia is neuroprotection. In neurological diseases, glia attempt to maintain tissue and cellular homeostasis. However, glia can also be neurodestructive, which serves to clean up the compromised tissue and protect the surrounding uncompromised cells/tissue.

Finally, without glia there can be no recovery from neural injury. Diseases of the nervous system are the most difficult to handle and to cure. The therapeutic advances in neurology are, at best, modest when compared to other branches of medicine. The reason is simple – the singular complexity of the human brain and of its connections, both morphological and functional. A further reason is that, with few exceptions, the central role of glial cells in neurological diseases is overlooked. This must change in the future if we hope to find effective therapies for neurological diseases.

# References

Biber K, Neumann H, Inoue K, Boddeke HW. (2007). neuronal 'On' and 'Off' signals control microglia. *Trends In Neurosciences* **30**(11), 596–602.

Bringmann A, Iandiev I, Pannicke T, Wurm A, Hollborn M, Wiedemann P, Osborne NN, Reichenbach A. (2009). Cellular signaling and factors involved in Muller cell gliosis: neuroprotective and detrimental effects. *Progress in Retinal and Eye Research* **28**(6), 423–51.

Buffo A, Rite I, Tripathi P, Lepier A, Colak D, Horn AP, Mori T, Gotz M. (2008). Origin and progeny of reactive gliosis: A source of multipotent cells in the injured brain. *Proceedings of The National Academy Of Sciences Of The United States Of America* **105**(9), 3581–6.

Coleman MP, Freeman MR. (2010). Wallerian degeneration, wld(s), and nmnat. *Annual Review of Neuroscience* **33**, 245–67.

Davalos D, Grutzendler J, Yang G, Kim JV, Zuo Y, Jung S, Littman DR, Dustin ML, Gan WB. (2005). ATP mediates rapid microglial response to local brain injury *in vivo*. *Nature Neuroscience* **8**(6), 752–8.

De Keyser J, Mostert JP, Koch MW. (2008). Dysfunctional astrocytes as key players in the pathogenesis of central nervous system disorders. *Journal of The Neurological Sciences* **267**(1–2), 3–16.

Gaudet AD, Popovich PG, Ramer MS. (2011). Wallerian degeneration: gaining perspective on inflammatory events after peripheral nerve injury. *Journal of Neuroinflammation* **8**, 110.

Giaume C, Kirchhoff F, Matute C, Reichenbach A, Verkhratsky A. (2007). Glia: the fulcrum of brain diseases. *Cell Death & Differentiation* **14**(7), 1324–35.

Hanisch UK, Kettenmann H. (2007). Microglia: active sensor and versatile effector cells in the normal and pathologic brain. *Nature Neuroscience* **10**(11), 1387–94.

Karadottir R, Attwell D. (2007). Neurotransmitter receptors in the life and death of oligodendrocytes. *Neuroscience* **145**(4), 1426–38.

Kettenmann H, Hanisch UK, Noda M, Verkhratsky A. (2011). Physiology of microglia. *Physiological Reviews* **91**(2), 461–553.

Koeppen AH. (2004). Wallerian degeneration: history and clinical significance. *Journal of The Neurological Sciences* **220**(1–2), 115–7.

Matute C. (2010). Calcium dyshomeostasis in white matter pathology. *Cell Calcium* **47**(2), 150–7.

Matute C. (2011). Glutamate and ATP signalling in white matter pathology. *Journal of Anatomy* **219**(1), 53–64.

Matute C, Domercq M, Sanchez-Gomez MV. (2006). Glutamate-mediated glial injury: mechanisms and clinical importance. *Glia* **53**(2), 212–24.

Matute C, Alberdi E, Domercq M, Sanchez-Gomez MV, Perez-Samartin A, Rodriguez-Antiguedad A, Perez-Cerda F. (2007). Excitotoxic damage to white matter. *Journal of Anatomy* **210**(6), 693–702.

Pekny M, Nilsson M. (2005). Astrocyte activation and reactive gliosis. *Glia* **50**(4), 427–34.

Ransohoff RM, Perry VH. (2009). Microglial physiology: unique stimuli, specialized responses. *Annual Review of Immunology* **27**, 119–45.

Robel S, Berninger B, Gotz M. (2011). The stem cell potential of glia: lessons from reactive gliosis. *Nature Reviews Neuroscience* **12**(2), 88–104.

Rotshenker S. (2011). Wallerian degeneration: the innate-immune response to traumatic nerve injury. *Journal of Neuroinflammation* **8**, 109.

Sofroniew MV. (2009). Molecular dissection of reactive astrogliosis and glial scar formation. *Trends In Neurosciences* **32**(12), 638–47.

Sofroniew MV, Vinters HV. (2010). Astrocytes: biology and pathology. *Acta Neuropathologica* **119**(1), 7–35.

Stys PK, Lipton SA. (2007). White matter NMDA receptors: an unexpected new therapeutic target? *Trends In Pharmacological Sciences* **28**(11), 561–6.

Suh SW, Bergher JP, Anderson CM, Treadway JL, Fosgerau K, Swanson RA. (2007). Astrocyte glycogen sustains neuronal activity during hypoglycemia: studies with the glycogen phosphorylase inhibitor CP-316,819 ([R-R*,S*]-5-chloro-N-[2-hydroxy-3-(methoxymethylamino)-3-oxo-1-(phenylmet hyl)propyl]-1H-indole-2-carboxamide). *Journal of Pharmacology and Experimental Therapeutics* **321**(1), 45–50.

van Rossum D, Hanisch UK. (2004). Microglia. *Metabolic Brain Disease* **19**(3–4), 393–411.

Vargas ME, Barres BA. (2007). Why is Wallerian degeneration in the CNS so slow? *Annual Review of Neuroscience* **30**, 153–79.

Verkhratsky A, Sofroniew MV, Messing A, Delanerolle NC, Rempe D, Rodriguez JJ, Nedergaard M. (2012). Neurological diseases as primary gliopathies: a reassessment of neurocentrism. *ASN Neuro* **4**(3), e00082.

Virchow R. (1858). *Die Cellularpathologie in ihrer Begründung auf physiologische und pathologische Gewebelehre. Zwanzig Vorlesungen gehalten während der Monate Februar, März und April 1858 im pathologischen Institut zu Berlin*. Berlin: August Hirschwald. 440 p.

Volpe JJ, Kinney HC, Jensen FE, Rosenberg PA. (2011). The developing oligodendrocyte: key cellular target in brain injury in the premature infant. *International Journal of Developmental Neuroscience* **29**(4), 423–40.

Waller A. (1850). Experiments on the Section of the Glossopharyngeal and Hypoglossal Nerves of the Frog, and Observations of the Alterations Produced Thereby in the Structure of Their Primitive Fibres. *Philosophical Transactions of The Royal Society Of London* **140**, 423–429.

# 10

# Neuroglia in Neurological Diseases

*Glial Physiology and Pathophysiology*, First Edition. Alexei Verkhratsky and Arthur Butt.
© 2013 by John Wiley & Sons, Ltd. Published 2013 by John Wiley & Sons, Ltd.

# 10.1   Introduction

Neurological diseases are disorders of the brain, spinal cord and the nerves. There are more than 600 neurologic diseases, and the major types include:

1.  genetic diseases, such as Huntington's disease;

2.  developmental disorders, such as cerebral palsy and spina bifida;

3.  degenerative diseases, such as Alzheimer's disease and Parkinson's disease;

4.  cerebrovascular diseases, such as stroke;

5.  physical injuries to the brain, spinal cord or nerves;

6.  seizure disorders, such as epilepsy;

7.  brain tumours, such as gliomas;

8.  infections, such as meningitis;

9.  mental disorders, such as affective and personality disorders (e.g. bipolar disorder and schizophrenia), sleep disorders (e.g. insomnia), and addictive disorders (e.g. alcoholism).

Glial cells are involved in all neurological diseases, although they are not always the primary targets. In its broadest sense, the function of glia is homeostasis – maintaining a state of equilibrium both metabolically within neural cells, the nervous tissue and the body as a whole, as well as psychologically within the individual. Thus, altered glial homeostatic function invariably contributes to CNS neurological diseases, sometimes as a principal element, but often secondary to neural or environmental changes. In fact, the picture is rarely clear cut, and what are most often considered neuronal diseases actually have a significant, and often primary, glial component. It is more meaningful to consider glia and neurones as functional partners, as it is inconceivable that dysfunction in one element would not cause dysfunction in the other.

This concept is exemplified by a number of neurological diseases in which glia are the primary target. For example, glial cells are the primary targets in genetic disorders grouped under the leukodystrophies (from the Greek *leuko*, white, *dys*, lack of, and *troph*, growth). These include Alexander disease (caused by mutations in the *Gfap* gene located on chromosome 17q21), Krabbe disease (caused by mutations in the *Galc* gene located on chromosome 14q31) and Pelizaeus-Merbacher disease (caused by mutations of the *Plp1* gene located on the X-chromosome (Xq21-22), usually resulting in duplications of the entire *Plp1* gene).

In addition, myelin destruction in the CNS and PNS are the hallmarks of the metabolic leukodystrophies (e.g. metachromatic leukodystrophy and adrenoleukodystrophy), and the genetic disorder Charcot-Marie Tooth disease, which is specific to PNS myelin (most commonly caused by duplication in the *Pmp22* gene located on chromosome 17p12). Furthermore, oligodendrocytes and Schwann cells are the specific targets of the autoimmune demyelinating diseases multiple sclerosis and Guillian-Barré syndrome, respectively.

## 10.2    Genetic astrogliopathology: Alexander disease

*Alexander disease* (AxD) is the only known example of primary astrogliopathology, being caused by the mutation of astroglia-specific gene, encoding GFAP (for review, see Messing *et al.*, 2010, 2012). The disease bears the name of Stewart Alexander, a Scottish neuropathologist (Alexander, 1949). This is a rare and fatal disease (with a prevalence of 1 in 2.7 million people, according to a study of Japanese population (Yoshida *et al.*, 2011)) that strikes infants and young adults.

From a clinical perspective, Alexander disease belongs to the leukodystrophies, being manifested (especially in young patients) by serious deficits in white matter (Figure 10.1). The current classification of AxD is based on the age of onset – infantile, juvenile, and adult (Li *et al.*, 2005).

Infantile AxD usually becomes manifest at around six months of age and the symptoms include head enlargement, convulsions, pyramidal symptoms, and muscle weakness. The early symptoms in young patients are generally associated with forebrain lesions and include psychomotor delays and frequent seizures. The juvenile form, with onset around nine years, is characterised by progressive paresis, gait disturbances, bulbar signs or autonomic dysfunction, which are mostly associated with lesions in the hindbrain, sometimes including atrophy of the

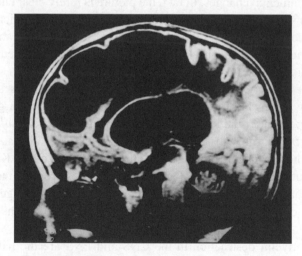

**Figure 10.1**  Image of a child with infantile Alexander disease.
This female patient had an R416W mutation; disease onset was at three months and death at eight years.
T1-weighted MRI of the patient at seven years, showing cystic degeneration
in the frontal lobes, enlarged ventricles, and some atrophy of the vermis.

Reproduced with permission from Johnson, 1996.

medulla and cervical spinal cord. Notwithstanding the difference in neurological symptoms, both forms of AxD are rapidly progressive, with median survivals at 3.6 years for the early onset group, and eight years for the juvenile group. Very rarely, AxD can be diagnosed in adults.

Another, slightly more recent, classification divides the disease into two groups, Types 1 and 2. Type I AxD is characterised by early onset, seizures, megalencephaly or macrocephaly, motor delay, encephalopathy, failure to thrive, paroxysmal deterioration and typical leukodystrophic morphology. Type II has later onset, autonomic dysfunction, ocular movement abnormalities, bulbar symptoms and atypical morphology (Prust *et al.*, 2011).

The precise pathogenesis of AxD remains somewhat obscure, although it is an initial dysfunction of astrocytes that instigates a cascade of events, ultimately affecting the whole CNS. The histological hallmark of AxD is the presence of *Rosenthal fibres* in astrocytes, which are cytoplasmic inclusions, formed by GFAP in association with stress proteins (such as α- and β-crystallin and heat shock protein 27).

Many of the GFAP mutations causing AxD have been characterised. Most are heterozygous single base pair changes within the coding region that translates into single amino acid changes in the protein. In some cases, the AxD associated mutations involve in-frame deletions or insertions. All the mutations are heterozygous, genetically dominant and have almost 100 per cent penetrance. Very rarely, patients with AxD-like pathology do not have identifiable coding region mutations, which suggests possible occurrence of other types of alterations at the GFAP locus, such as promoter mutations or gene duplication. Most mutations occur *de novo* and remain unique; however, some patients with late onset can reach reproductive age and convey the mutation through generations with typical autosomal dominant inheritance pattern. Most surprisingly, 71 known single acid mutations in the GFAP protein, which contains 432 amino acids, cause the same clinically defined disease. Some mutations have been reported to be associated with late onset AxD, but these indications are still rather speculative.

The GFAP mutations cause overexpression/increase in function of the protein, which assumes toxic proportions and possibly triggers disease progression. At a biochemical level, increased GFAP expression decreases its solubility, which may underlie the formation of Rosenthal fibres. Overexpression of normal non-mutated GFAP in genetically modified animals reproduces symptoms of AxD and triggers formation of Rosenthal fibres.

There is evidence that the pathogenesis of AxD involves an overall malfunction of astrocytes, resulting in permanent disruption of the blood-brain barrier (Rosenthal fibres tend to accumulate in endfeet, both in perivascular and pial zones), as well as increased autophagy, apoptosis and oxidative stress. In addition, reduction of glutamate uptake by pathologically modified astrocytes can account for both seizures and neuronal death in AxD.

A marked decrease in EAAT2 (GLT-1) immunoreactivity in CA1/CA2 hippocampal areas has been demonstrated in AxD post-mortem tissues. This decrease correlated with severe neuronal loss observed in the CA1 region, although neuronal numbers in the CA2 region remained unchanged. Notably, overexpression of GFAP in knock-in mice or in cultured astrocytes leads to a decrease in expression and activity of EAAT2. Indeed, astrocytes expressing mutant GFAP lose the ability to protect neurones against glutamate toxicity when grown together in co-cultures. The therapeutic strategies for treating AxD need to be aimed at reducing accumulation of GFAP, and the first screenings using an *in vitro* primary culture model have been started (Cho *et al.*, 2010).

## 10.3 Stroke and ischaemia

It is a truth generally acknowledged that disruption of blood flow in the brain causes considerable damage and death of neuronal cells. The disruption of blood flow can be caused either by blood vessel rupture, which results in *haemorrhage*, or by a restriction of blood supply to the brain or parts of the brain, commonly referred to as *brain ischaemia*, due to vascular occlusion (because of thrombosis or embolism) or to a systemic decrease in blood supply (e.g. associated with heart failure). As a consequence, brain ischaemia can be either global or focal, the latter corresponding to a *stroke*. Stroke is one of the main causes of death and disabilities in the developed world, affecting many millions every year. Numerous clinical trials testing a wide variety of neuroprotective agents have generally failed and the pharmacological containment of stroke remains largely unavailable.

Global ischaemia develops as a consequence of transient heart arrest. This leads to an almost immediate cessation of the cerebral blood flow from a normal $\approx 8$ ml/g/min to zero. About 10–15 seconds of global brain ischaemia results in loss of consciousness, while electrical activity of the brain disappears 30–40 seconds after the beginning of circulatory arrest. Global ischaemia lasting for more than ten minutes at normal temperature is lethal for humans. On a cellular level, short periods of global ischaemia trigger delayed selective neuronal death while, at least initially, astrocytes survive and become activated.

Focal ischaemia triggers local cell death, the site and volume of the damage being determined by anatomical location of vessel occlusion. Often, the conditions of focal ischaemia are transient, as the blood flow can be restored when the vessel blockage is removed. In this case, restored blood flow results in *reperfusion* of the damaged area, which itself is potentially damaging because of the production of reactive oxygen species (ROS) and secondary ion disbalances. The pathogenesis of ischaemia is associated with the limitation of oxygen supply (hypoxia or anoxia), as well as restrictions in supply of metabolic substrates.

The development of focal ischaemic damage to brain tissue has complex kinetics. The cessation of, or considerable decrease in, local cerebral blood flow triggers the onset of infarction. The *core* (Figure 10.2) of the infarction zone (where blood flow rates are reduced below 1 ml/g/min) is the region of pan-necrosis, which rapidly kills all cells, including neurones and glia. The infarction core is surrounded by a

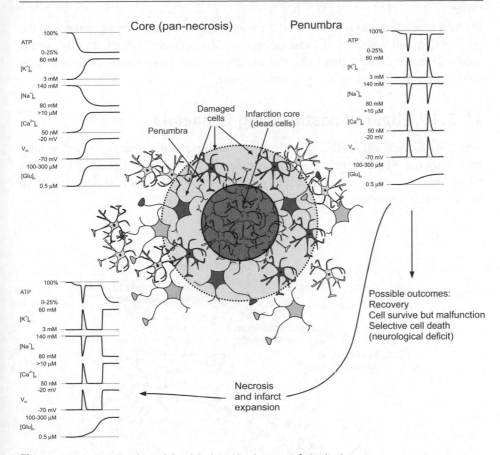

**Figure 10.2**  Organisation of focal ischaemic damage of the brain.

Focal ischaemic damage (or stroke) comprises the central zone of the infarction core, where all the cells are dead, and a much larger surrounding zone, the penumbra, which contains partially damaged cells. The progression of the penumbra and increase of the infarction core may take several days and is mainly determined by the balance between defensive capabilities of astrogliosis and microglial activation versus glia-related neurotoxicity and propagation of death signals through the astroglial syncytium.

Changes in ATP production, ion concentrations and membrane potential of cells in different regions of the ischaemic lesion are schematically presented (redrawn from Rossi *et al.*, 2007; full colour version in plate section)

zone of reduced circulation (with rates 2–4 ml/g/min) known as the '*ischaemic penumbra*' (Figure 10.2). This contains viable cells, albeit with compromised metabolism and function. The infarction core is formed very rapidly, within minutes and hours after initiation of the stroke. This is followed by a much slower process of expansion of the infarction zone through the penumbra, developing over many hours and even days.

Glial cells are intimately involved in the CNS response to ischaemia (see Takano *et al.*, 2009; Vangeison & Rempe, 2009; Yenari *et al.*, 2010; Zhao & Rempe, 2010 for further reading and references). To a very large extent, astrocytes determine the progression and outcome of focal ischaemia. Importantly, astroglial cells have a dual role, as they may either reduce or exacerbate neuronal damage, depending on the depth and duration of the ischaemic insult.

## 10.3.1   Glial cell death during ischaemia

The cells located within the infarction core region rapidly lose their intracellular energy source ATP and undergo an anoxic depolarisation (Rossi *et al.*, 2007). As a result, neurones cease to be electrically excitable and all cells lose their ability to maintain transmembrane ion gradients (Figures 10.2, 10.3).

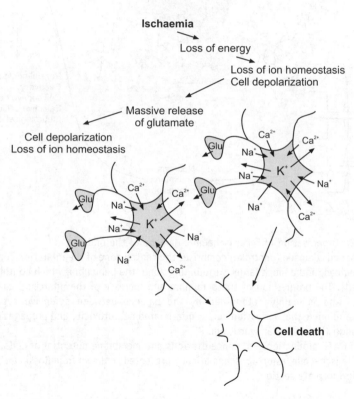

**Figure 10.3**  Mechanisms of ischaemic cell death.

Ischaemic cell death is initiated by compromised energy production which, in turn, triggers loss of ion homeostasis and depolarization of the injured neural cell. This depolarization leads to a massive release of glutamate, which further depolarizes the injured cells and the cells in their immediate vicinity; this induces additional glutamate release, thus establishing the vicious circle of glutamate excitotoxicity. Opening of NMDA glutamate receptors and depolarization induces uncontrolled $Ca^{2+}$ entry in the cytosol, which: (a) further compromises mitochondria and ATP production; and (b) activates numerous proteolytic enzymes and caspase-dependent cell death pathways. This results in necrotic cell death, cell disintegration and release of cellular contents into the brain parenchyma, which acts as a damage signal for neighbouring neurones and glia.

This induces considerable $Na^+$ and $Ca^{2+}$ influx into the cells, accompanied by a substantial $K^+$ efflux, so that very soon (within minutes), extracellular ion concentrations deteriorate severely. For example, in the grey matter, $[K^+]_o$ rises to 40–80 mM, whereas $[Na^+]_o$ and $[Ca^{2+}]_o$ decline to 60 mM and 0.2–0.5 mM, respectively (Figure 10.2). Massive $Ca^{2+}$ influx increases cytosolic $Ca^{2+}$ concentration to tens of $\mu M$ and, in neurones, this triggers release of glutamate from synaptic terminals, which further amplifies the vicious circle by '*glutamate excitotoxicity*' (Figure 10.4). Simultaneously, the extracellular milieu becomes acidic as pH drops to 6.5.

These events almost immediately kill neurones and glial cells located in the core. In the penumbra, the extent of cellular changes is much less pronounced. Neurones lose electrical excitability, yet all the cells retain their ion homeostasis and continue

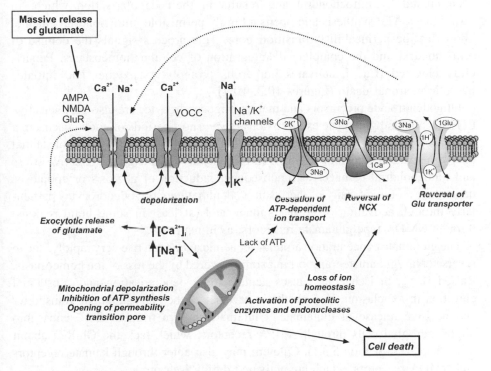

**Figure 10.4** The 'vicious cycle' of glutamate excitotoxicity.
Massive release of glutamate opens glutamate receptors, which depolarise the cellular membrane and activate voltage-operated channels that further depolarise the cell. This results in $Ca^{2+}$ influx and sustained increase in cytosolic $Ca^{2+}$ concentration. Cytosolic $Ca^{2+}$ ions are accumulated by mitochondria and the overload of the latter with $Ca^{2+}$ stops ATP production, which further compromises ion homeostasis. Increased intracellular $Ca^{2+}$ triggers additional release of glutamate, which further activates glutamate receptors. Cell depolarisation and energy deficit also underlie the increase in cytosolic $Na^+$ concentration. This eventually reverses the glutamate transporter, which produces additional glutamate release. Finally, sustained increase in intracellular $Ca^{2+}$ activates proteolytic enzymes, endonucleases and other death pathways, which results in cell demise.

to survive, although their cytosol is often acidified, they swell, and protein synthesis and general metabolism are inhibited. Ion homeostasis and ATP synthesis are also compromised, but this occurs in an oscillating fashion, interspersed by relatively long periods of 'normality' (Figure 10.2). Cells in the penumbra may either recover or die, which determines the final size of ischaemic damage.

Neurones, oligodendrocytes and oligodendroglial precursor cells are the most vulnerable and sensitive to ischaemic shock, whereas astrocytes are considered to be generally more resilient. The initial cell death that follows the stroke is associated with glutamate excitotoxicity, due to a massive release of glutamate in the core region. In neurones, this leads to the sustained activation of NMDA receptors, resulting in $Ca^{2+}$ influx, and simultaneously, neuronal depolarisation opens voltage-operated $Ca^{2+}$ channels, which adds to the $Ca^{2+}$ entry. Ultimately, neurones become overloaded with $Ca^{2+}$. A substantial part of the $Ca^{2+}$ is accumulated by mitochondria and results in their depolarisation which, in turn, blocks ATP synthesis and opens a highly permeable mitochondrial channel known as the permeability transition pore. This process signals the demise of mitochondria and the complete disintegration of cellular homeostasis. Persistently elevated $[Ca^{2+}]_i$ activates numerous proteolytic enzymes and initiates necrotic neuronal death (Figures 10.3, 10.4).

Oligodendrocyte precursors and mature oligodendrocytes are also very sensitive to ischaemia and glutamate excitotoxicity. Even short periods of anoxia/ischaemia cause complete loss of oligodendroglial ion homeostasis and a very substantial $[Ca^{2+}]_i$ elevation. Calcium overload in oligodendrocytes triggers oxidative stress and mitochondrial damage, with subsequent induction of necrosis or apoptosis, depending on the intensity of the insult. Calcium enters oligodendrocytes particularly through activation of AMPA/kainate and (at least in some brain regions) through NMDA type glutamate receptors, as in neurones.

The glutamate concentration around ischaemic axons can rise very rapidly, due to reversed $Na^+$/glutamate transport in axons triggered by the loss of ion homeostasis. Raised $[K^+]_o$ in ischaemia causes acute axonal depolarisation and substantial elevation in axoplasmic $Na^+$ results in reversal of the $Na^+$/glutamate transporter and massive release of glutamate. Glutamate in turn triggers $Ca^{2+}$ entry into oligodendroglial cells through AMPA receptors, which lack the GluR2 subunit (see Chapter 5, Section 5.3.1). Calcium may also enter through kainate receptors and NMDA receptors, which are activated during ischaemia.

Oligodendrocyte precursors and immature oligodendrocytes, which have particularly high levels of AMPA/kainate receptor expression, appear most vulnerable to glutamate toxicity, and this is considered to be a major cause of oligodendrocyte loss in cerebral palsy. In addition, exposure to glutamate can directly destroy the myelin sheath, involving $Ca^{2+}$ influx through NMDA receptors that are apparently localised to myelin sheaths. In contrast, ionotropic AMPA receptors appear to be localised to the cell bodies and may mediate cell death. Indeed $Ca^{2+}$ influx into the compact myelin subjected to ischaemia has been directly demonstrated in imaging experiments; treatment with NMDA receptors antagonists prevented ischaemia-induced deterioration of myelin.

Another important pathway for $[Ca^{2+}]_i$ elevation is associated with $Ca^{2+}$ release from the ER store activated by depolarisation of oligodendrocyte membrane. This results from acute elevation in extracellular $[K^+]$ triggered by ischaemia that evokes depolarisation-induced $Ca^{2+}$ release through ryanodine receptors.

Astrocytes generally are less sensitive to glutamate excitotoxicity. Astroglial cultures readily survive relatively prolonged periods (up to several hours) of oxygen and/or glucose deprivation. *In vivo,* however, astrocyte sensitivity to ischaemic insults seems to be much higher. Many, but not all, astroglial cells in hippocampus survive brief ($\approx 10\,min$) periods of ischaemia (which is enough to kill a very significant number of neurones), yet longer cessation of blood flow causes prominent astrocytic death. White matter astrocytes seem to be even more vulnerable, and astroglial cells in the optic nerve begin to die within 10–20 minutes after the onset of ischaemia.

Nonetheless, astroglial cells can survive for long periods of time in the penumbra, where the reduced blood flow still delivers relatively high amounts of glucose, which can be utilised by astrocytes through anaerobic glycolysis. This produces lactate which can be used to support neuronal metabolism through the lactate shuttle. However, increase in lactate production also results in acidosis.

Importantly, astroglia are rather sensitive to acidification of their environment. Lowering of pH to $\approx 6.6$ completely inhibits astroglial ATP production and very rapidly (in about 15 minutes *in vitro*) kills astrocytes. Interestingly, hyperglycaemia exacerbates growth of the infarction core, most likely through intensifying anaerobic glycolysis and increasing acidosis. At the same time, astrocytes are also vulnerable to ROS, which can be produced in large quantities during reperfusion; ROS induce cell death through mitochondrial depolarisation and opening of the permeability transition pore. One of the early consequences of astroglial injury is the disruption of their distal processes, a phenomenon described a century ago by Alzheimer and Ramón y Cajal as *clasmatodendrosis* ('fragmentation of dendrites' from the Greek 'clasmato' 'κλασματο'– fragment, piece broken off).

## 10.3.2  Astroglia protect the brain against ischaemia

Astrocytes are the most ischaemia-resistant elements of neural circuits, as they are able to survive in conditions of limited blood supply and protect the brain against injury (Figure 10.5).

First and foremost, astrocytes form the main barrier against glutamate excitotoxicity. Astroglial cells, by virtue of numerous transporters expressed in their membrane, act as the main sink for the glutamate in the CNS (see Chapter 4). Furthermore, the astroglial ability to maintain anaerobic ATP production allows sustained ion and glutamate transport in hypoxic conditions. Astroglial protection against glutamate excitotoxicity became very obvious from *in vitro* experiments, in which withdrawal of astrocytes from neuronal cultures led to a 100-times increase

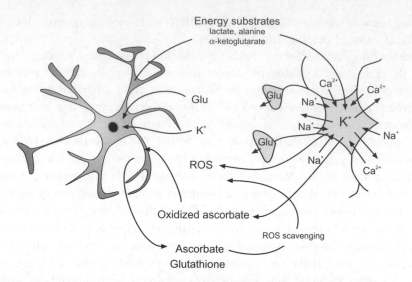

**Figure 10.5** Mechanisms of astroglia-dependent neuroprotection. Astroglial cells act as the main sink for glutamate, buffer extracellular potassium, provide neurones with energy substrates and serve as the main source of reactive oxygen species (ROS) scavengers.

in the vulnerability of neurones to glutamate. Similarly, genetic down-regulation of glial glutamate transporters exacerbates brain ischaemic damage *in vivo*.

Second, astrocytes are powerful scavengers of ROS, one of the main mediators of ischaemic brain injury. Astrocytes contain high concentrations of glutathione and ascorbate, which are the principal antioxidants in the brain. Ascorbate is a component of neuronal-astroglial exchange, as neurones release oxidised ascorbate, which is accumulated by astrocytes and is subsequently converted into ascorbate, ready for a new cycle of ROS scavenging. The ability of astrocytes to protect neurones against ROS has been clearly demonstrated *in vitro*, where neuronal-astroglial cultures were found to be much more resistant to injury produced by superoxide or hydrogen peroxide, compared to purified neuronal cultures.

Third, anaerobic metabolism sustained by astrocytes in hypoxic conditions produces several intermediate substrates, such as lactate, alanine and α-ketoglutarate, which can be fed to neurones and support energy production in conditions of glucose deprivation.

Fourth, astrocytic networks are involved in potassium buffering (see Chapter 4) which, by removing the excess of potassium in ischaemia, may slow down neuronal depolarisation and depolarisation-induced glutamate release.

Fifth, ischaemia induces astroglial release of a number of neuroprotective factors, including erythropoietin, vascular endothelial growth factor (VEGF) and glial-derived neurotrophic factor, all of which may either reduce ischaemic neuronal damage or improve functional recovery following stroke.

Finally, in later stages of infarction, the process of reactive astrogliosis leads to the formation of a protective astroglial barrier which isolates the damaged area. Subsequently, the reactive astrocytes produce a scar that fills the necrotic core.

## 10.3.3 Astrocytes may exacerbate brain damage in ischaemia

Astrocytes, however, may act not only as protectors of the brain. In certain conditions, and especially upon severe insults, astroglial cells exacerbate the cell damage, contributing to several vicious cycles triggered by the stroke. First of all, the astroglial involvement in controlling brain glutamate concentration is double-edged. The ability of astrocytes to remove glutamate from the extracellular space leads to glutamate accumulation in their cytosol in very high concentrations, especially in conditions of excessive glutamate release. Upon severe hypoxic/hypoglycaemic conditions, astroglial cells may turn from being the sink for glutamate to being the main source of the latter.

Astrocytes can release glutamate by several mechanisms, which are potentially triggered in ischaemia:

1.  Reversal of glutamate transporters can be caused by an increase in intracellular $Na^+$ concentration and cell depolarisation, due to elevation of extracellular $K^+$.

2.  Elevation of $[Ca^{2+}]_i$ in astrocytes, which follows the ischaemic insult, may trigger the exocytotic release of glutamate stored in vesicles.

3.  Acidosis and lowering of extracellular $Ca^{2+}$ concentration can open glutamate-permeable hemichannels.

4.  ATP, released in high concentrations by dying and disintegrating neurones, can open astroglial $P2X_7$ purinoceptors, which also allow glutamate release.

5.  Brain oedema can activate volume-sensitive channels, which allow passage of glutamate. Similar mechanisms can also produce release of ATP that may further exacerbate excitotoxicity.

The second important pathological role of astrocytes is associated with a progression of the infarction core through the penumbra. This expansion of the death zone is a slow process, which may proceed for several days after the initial insult. The progression of damage implicates specific signalling processes propagating from the infarction core towards the surrounding tissue. Signalling through the neuronal network can be excluded, as neuronal excitability is lost after even a mild reduction of cerebral blood flow.

The alternative route for propagation of death signals likely involves the astroglial syncytium. This scenario begins with the generation of aberrant $[Ca^{2+}]_i$ waves in

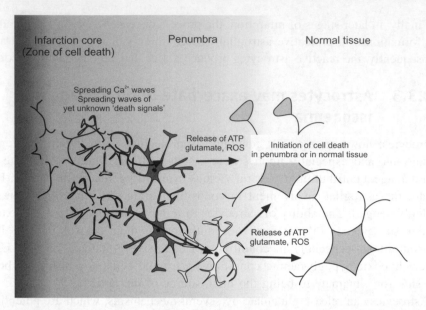

Infarction core
(Zone of cell death)

Penumbra

Normal tissue

Spreading Ca²⁺ waves
Spreading waves of
yet unknown 'death signals'

Release of ATP
glutamate, ROS

Initiation of cell death
in penumbra or in normal tissue

Release of ATP
glutamate, ROS

**Figure 10.6** Astrocytes may exacerbate infarction progression through the penumbra by propagating $Ca^{2+}$ waves or by propagating 'death signals'.
Death signals may travel through the astroglial syncytium, injuring cells distant to the site of the infarction. See the text for detailed explanation.

astrocytes, which may, in turn, evoke the distant release of glutamate from astrocytes beyond the ischaemic focus. Thus, a propagating wave of glutamate release from astrocytes can contribute to the extension of infarction (Figure 10.6).

Another route for infarction expansion is associated with spreading depression, which often occurs in the penumbra (see also Section 10.3). Spreading depression waves originate at the very border between the necrotic core and the ischaemic penumbra, and these waves are initiated by high extracellular $K^+$ concentration present around the core. The spreading depression wave occurs as often as every 10–15 minutes, which is determined by the refractory period of the cells in the penumbra.

There is a fundamental difference between spreading depression in normal brain tissue and in the compromised ischaemic penumbra. The ion homeostasis in cells in penumbra is compromised, and therefore each wave of spreading depression results in further imbalance between the energy requirement of the depolarised tissue and the energy supply; this imbalance promotes cell death. As a result, there is a direct correlation between the number of spreading depression waves and the spread of necrotic area into the penumbra. Metabolic imbalance also determines the longer duration and longer recovery of spreading depression in ischaemic penumbra. The spreading depression waves propagate from the ischaemic region to the healthy tissue, causing some functional disturbances, although this does not result in any cell death outside the borders of the ischaemic tissue.

The expansion of the necrotic zone through the penumbra may demarcate the primary extension of astroglial failure, which, in turn, depends on a variety of factors. For example, the extent of the circulation breakdown would determine the relative activity of glycolysis and, hence, production of lactate and accumulation of protons in the extracellular space. Profound extracellular acidification will, in turn, induce astrocytic collapse. This process can be further exacerbated by accumulation of extracellular $K^+$ ions and subsequent depolarisation, accompanying, for example, the wave of spreading depression.

At the same time, release of glutamate by astrocytes in the penumbra can kill neighbouring neurones and produce even further accumulation of $K^+$ and secondary release of glutamate and ATP. Alongside this, increases in $[K^+]_o$ initiate astroglial swelling, which will reduce the extracellular space, hence further increasing concentrations of $K^+$ and glutamate in the latter and further obstructing circulation.

In other words, the very same mechanisms that protect neurones during ischaemic stress may also participate in extending the damage. This happens when the astroglial capacity for survival in ischaemic conditions is exhausted which, in turn, activates several vicious positive feedback loops that result in cell death and extension of the necrotic zone through the ischaemic penumbra. All in all, the clinical deficits in stroke are due to neuronal loss, but it should never be considered a primary neuronal disease, since the outcome of focal brain ischaemia is directly determined by astroglial performance.

### 10.3.4   Oligodendrocytes and microglia in stroke

Death of oligodendrocytes leads to axonal disintegration. As mentioned above, oligodendroglia are particularly vulnerable to focal ischaemia. Strokes located in the white matter may therefore trigger particularly dangerous disruptions of nerve fibres and lead to severe functional disabilities (e.g. focal insults to the internal capsule). Microglial cells are also activated during brain ischaemia, and their activation is associated with the release of numerous immunocompetent molecules, which can have either beneficial or detrimental effects. Profound activation of microglial cells may turn them into phagocytes, which can launch a direct attack on neural cells, thus contributing to the expansion of the necrotic zone.

## 10.4   Migraine and spreading depression

One of the mechanisms of migraine is represented by a specific wave of cortical depolarisation known as spreading depression, which is also linked to the aura preceding migraine attack. The link between migraine and spreading depression has recently been demonstrated in mice carrying mutant human W887R gene associated with aberrant $\alpha2$ subunit of $Na^+/K^+$ ATPase associated with familial hemiplegic migraine type 2. These animals had significantly increased susceptibility to spreading depression with decreased threshold and increases speed of depression propagation (Leo *et al.*, 2011).

The spreading depression of electric activity in the cerebral cortex, initially described by Aristide Leão (1944), is a wave of cellular depolarisation that travels through the grey matter at a velocity of about 1.5 to 7.5 mm/min (for further reading and references, see Dreier, 2011; Eikermann-Haerter & Ayata, 2010; Grafstein, 2011). This propagating wave of depolarisation can be triggered by local massive increases in extracellular $K^+$ and/or glutamate, which are the consequences of exaggerated focal electrical activity or mechanical or ischaemic injury.

The most striking features of spreading depression are the rapid propagating elevation of extracellular $K^+$ concentration up to 80 mM, a dramatic (about ten times) decrease in extracellular $Ca^{2+}$ concentration, and propagating shrinkage of the extracellular space by up to 50 per cent. These changes have complex kinetics, and they begin with an initial slight elevation in $[K^+]_o$, followed by a regenerative steep increase in $[K^+]_o$, a decrease in $[Ca^{2+}]_o$ and shrinkage of the extracellular space. During this period of excessive rise in $[K^+]_o$, there is an entry into cells of $Na^+$, $Ca^{2+}$ and $Cl^-$, which rapidly inhibits neuronal excitability. Meanwhile, astroglial cells become alkaline, most likely due to the activity of bicarbonate transporters. Elevation of $[K^+]_o$ lasts for one to two minutes, after which the cells repolarise and all ion gradients are normalised (the recovery period). Neurones regain their excitability within the subsequent three to five minutes, and the whole wave of spreading depression can be repeated after another ten minutes (which reflects the refractory period).

Spreading depression waves in normal tissue do not result in any cell damage, although repetitive incidences of spreading depression may activate microglia and induce reactive astrogliosis in its mild form; both processes seem to be fully reversible. In conditions of brain ischaemia, however, spreading depression may increase the area of cellular damage (see Section 10.3).

There is much evidence linking the development of spreading depression with astroglial networks. Particularly important are the demonstration of the effective inhibition of spreading depression by pharmacological inhibition of gap junctions (Nedergaard *et al.*, 1995), and the discovery of circulating currents passing through the glial syncytium during a course of spreading depolarisation (Sugaya *et al.*, 1975).

An apparent similarity between propagating astroglial calcium waves and the propagation of spreading depression led to the hypothesis of a triggering role for the former. However, this remains controversial as, in mouse neocortex for example, it is possible to pharmacologically dissociate astroglial calcium waves and spreading depression. Nevertheless, the leading role played by astrocytes in the development of spreading depression remains firm, although the underlying mechanisms require further elaboration.

The already mentioned familial hemiplegic migraine type 2 mutant W887R gene encodes the α2 subunit of $Na^+/K^+$ ATPase, which is expressed almost exclusively in astrocytes. Aberrant astroglial $Na^+/K^+$ pumps affect $K^+$ and glutamate clearance by astrocytes, which can contribute to the development of spreading depression (Leo *et al.*, 2011). Similarly relevant could be astroglial energetics, whereby compromised astroglial energy metabolism increases the susceptibility of neural tissue to spreading depression, while astroglial glycogen stores may affect spreading depression kinetics (Seidel & Shuttleworth, 2011).

Spreading depression also affects microglia. Depressed synaptic activity triggers a kind of microglial activation associated with the release of cytokines and increased microglial motility. Restoration of synaptic connectivity at the end of spreading depression relaxes microglial cells, which return into their survelliant resting mode (Grinberg *et al.*, 2011).

## 10.5   CNS oedema

Homeostatic regulation of brain volume and water content is of paramount importance for its function. Brain size is limited by the skull, and therefore increases in brain volume lead to an increase in intracranial pressure and compression damage of neural tissue. Water redistribution between brain compartments compromises the extracellular space with similarly grave consequences. Brain oedema (Ayata & Ropper, 2002; Simard *et al.*, 2007) is, in essence, a collapse of brain volume/water regulation, which exists in two forms – *vascular* and *cellular* (also known as *cytotoxic*). Vascular oedema is a consequence of disruption of the blood-brain barrier, which triggers water flow into the tissue, whereas cellular oedema is a redistribution of water into cellular compartments, which does not necessarily affect total volume of the brain parenchyma.

Astrocytes form the main system of water homeostasis in the CNS by specifically expressing the water channels aquaporins (see Chapter 4). Astroglia are capable of rapidly responding to changes in extracellular osmotic pressure by an initial swelling and subsequent regulatory volume decrease, determined by ion and water movements. In pathology, these mechanisms are compromised, which hampers the ability of astrocytes to maintain water homeostasis (for references, see Saadoun & Papadopoulos, 2010; Wright *et al.*, 2010).

Cellular oedema is primarily astroglial pathology, as astrocytes are capable of large volume changes due to water fluxes. Indeed, many brain insults, such as ischaemia or acute trauma, result in rapid swelling of astrocytes, which is accompanied by a significant increase in astroglial surface area. Astroglial swelling can trigger numerous secondary effects, which exacerbate the brain damage (Figure 10.7). In particular, swelling of perivascular astrocytes and astrocyte endfeet may compress brain vessels and limit circulation. This compression, for example, accounts for incomplete filling of brain vessels during reperfusion following focal ischaemia – known as the *no-reflow* phenomenon.

Swelling of astrocytes can result in opening of volume-regulated ion channels, permeable to glutamate and other excitatory amino acids, whose release can induce or exacerbate excitotoxic cell death. Prominent swelling of astrocytes can severcly

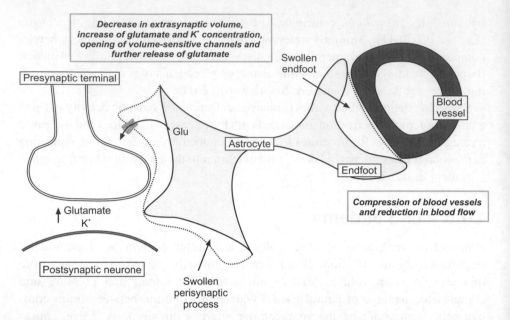

**Figure 10.7**  Pathological potential of astroglial swelling.

Astroglial swelling decreases extracellular volume, hence increasing concentration of neuro-transmitters and damage signals in the interstitium, and compresses brain capillaries further, compromising circulation in the damaged area.

reduce the extracellular space volume, with obvious consequences in terms of increased concentration of extracellular glutamate and $K^+$ ions, which can rise to excitotoxic levels during a several-fold reduction in the extracellular space.

## 10.5.1   Traumatic oedema

Post-traumatic astroglial swelling occurs within 30–40 minutes after trauma, and mechanistically this is very similar to ischaemic swelling (see below), with extracellular increases in glutamate and $K^+$ concentration taking the lead pathological roles. Post-traumatic oedema is complicated, however, by the presence of a strong vascular component, which underlies water influx into the brain through a compromised blood-brain barrier.

## 10.5.2   Ischaemic oedema

Astroglial swelling becomes apparent within 30 minutes of the onset of focal ischaemia. This swelling is quite prominent, and water redistribution into the astroglial cells may reduce the total extracellular volume by 50–75 per cent. The initiation of astrocyte swelling upon ischaemia is most likely associated with increased levels of glutamate and $K^+$, which, being taken up into astrocytes, trigger osmotic overload. This activates water influx through aquaporins, abundantly expressed in astrocyte membranes, and results in the dramatic increase in their volume.

### 10.5.3 Oedema in hepatic encephalopathy

Brain oedema frequently accompanies liver failure and represents cytotoxic, cellular oedema in its pure form. As a consequence of intoxication, astrocytes are primarily affected, and they are the only cells which show prominent morphological changes in post-mortem analysis. Astroglial swelling is proportional to the blood levels of ammonia (which increases following liver breakdown) and results from intracellular accumulation of organic osmolytes, with subsequent collapse of volume-regulating mechanisms.

### 10.5.4 Hyponatremia

Decreases in plasma sodium levels below 120 mM, which occur following disruption of kidney electrolyte handling, result in the rapid development of brain oedema, which is the main cause of mortality. Disruption of electrolyte secretion/reuptake in kidneys can be triggered by a variety of clinical factors, including endocrine pathology (e.g. hypothyroidism or overproduction of antidiuretic hormone), heart failure, HIV infection, etc. Hypernatremia induces hypo-osmotic shock in the brain tissue which, in turn, triggers prominent swelling of astrocytes and neuronal dendrites. In mild cases, transport of electrolytes and osmolytes may fully compensate for disruption of osmotic gradients.

## 10.6 Metabolic disorders

### 10.6.1 Hepatic encephalopathy

Mental disorders associated with liver failure and, specifically, with inability of the latter to process ammonium, are known as a *hepatic encephalopathy*. This type of encephalopathy essentially reflects the poisoning of the nervous tissue by excess of ammonium in conditions when the liver fails to absorb ammonia from the blood. The causal role of ammonia in hepatic encephalopathy was identified in 1930s (van Caulaert & Deviller, 1932), and its pathogenic role is now generally accepted. Clinically, hepatic encephalopathy is characterised by neuropsychiatric symptoms ranging from a state of confusion, forgetfulness and irritability to severe alterations of consciousness, represented by lethargy, somnolence and, in the terminal stages, coma.

Ammonia in the nervous tissue either derives from the blood or is produced endogenously from amino-acid catabolism. This ammonia can be utilised by enzymatic conversion into glutamate or glutamine, the reactions being carried out by neuronal glutamate dehydrogenase and astroglial glutamine synthetase, respectively (Cooper & Plum, 1987).

The glutamate synthetase pathway (in which ammonia ion is used for formation of glutamine from glutamate) is the most important. Glutamine synthetase in the CNS is expressed predominantly in astrocytes, which carry the task of ammonia detoxification, and which are primarily injured in the hepatic encephalopathy (for detailed overview and references, see Brusilow *et al.*, 2010; Butterworth, 2010, 2011). Hepatic encephalopathy is, in essence, a toxic astrogliopathology. Increased activity of glutamine synthetase in hyperammonemia overloads astrocytes with glutamine, which results in osmotic shock and cell swelling.

Enlarged astrocytes with watery, swollen nuclei and cytosol (so-called *Alzheimer's type II cells*) represent the main histopathological hallmark of hepatic encephalopathy and hyperammonemia. In contrast, there are little, if any, changes in neurones. In mild cases of hepatic encephalopathy, compromised glutamate uptake by stressed astrocytes contributes to neuropsychiatric symptoms. In severe cases of hyperammonemia, astrocytes contribute to brain oedema by excessive swelling through ion and water redistribution into astroglia (the phenomenon known as *osmotic gliopathy*), and this oedema represents the leading pathological phenomenon. In acute hepatic encephalopathy, brain oedema, often resulting in brain herniation, is the leading cause of death.

## 10.6.2   Congenital glutamine deficiency with glutamine synthetase mutations

Congenital glutamine synthetase deficiency arises from mutations to the gene encoding glutamine synthetase, and it is manifested by malformation of the brain, with severe white matter deficiency and abnormal gyration. This disease results in prenatal malformation of various organs and is generally incompatible with life; most infants with this condition die shortly after birth. The brain pathology is related most likely to the inability of astrocytes to conduct glutamine metabolism (Haberle *et al.*, 2005).

## 10.6.3   Pyruvate carboxylase deficiency

Pyruvate carboxylase is involved in the gluconeogenesis and anaplerotic (i.e. producing intermediates for metabolic chains such as Krebs cycle) metabolic pathways. In the CNS, pyruvate carboxylase is predominantly expressed in astrocytes. Pyruvate carboxylase deficiency represents an autosomal recessive disorder, characterised by impaired metabolism. The disease is generally manifested by retardation of mental development, recurrent seizures and metabolic acidosis. There are three clinically distinct forms:

- Type A, or the infantile form, in which children die in early years.

- Type B, or severe neonatal form, with many neurological signs, including pyramidal symptoms, in which babies die within three months after birth.

- Type C, or the benign form, which is characterised by mild neurological developmental deficits.

The cellular pathogenesis remains largely unknown, but it is probably linked to reduced astroglial homeostatic function, such as glutamate buffering and regulation of angiogenesis (Brun *et al.*, 1999; De Keyser *et al.*, 2008).

## 10.6.4   Niemann-Pick type C disease

Niemann-Pick type C disease is a progressive, usually fatal, neurodegenerative disease associated with hepatosplenomegaly. It is characterised as an autosomal recessive lysosomal storage disease associated with loss of function mutations of genes encoding NPC- or NPC-2 proteins (Rosenbaum & Maxfield, 2011). In the CNS, these proteins are localised in astroglial perisynaptic processes and may be involved in regulation of cholesterol transport and, hence, synaptogenesis or synaptic maintenance (Patel *et al.*, 1999). There is also evidence of a possible contribution for NPC-1 protein in calcium homeostasis and signalling.

## 10.6.5   Aceruloplasminemia

Ceruloplasmin (or ferroxidase) is an important component of iron metabolism. In the nervous tissue, this enzyme is synthesised almost exclusively in perivascular astrocytes and is involved in nervous tissue protection against iron-associated lipid peroxidation and formation of hydroxyl radicals. Loss of function mutation of the ceruloplasmin gene causes the autosomal recessive disease known as *aceruloplasminemia*. This disease is characterised by primary lesions to astrocytes, which substantially distorts their morphology, manifested by an appearance of foamy, spheroid bodies at the vascular endfeet (Oide *et al.*, 2006). The neurodegenerative changes also include neuronal death and appearance of iron deposition.

# 10.7   Toxic encephalopathies

## 10.7.1   Methylmercury toxic encephalopathy

Poisoning by methylmercury or *Minamata*[1] *disease* is clinically represented by visual abnormalities, sensory lesions, cerebellar ataxia, hearing loss, weakness, tremor and cognitive decline. Methylmercury primarily accumulates in astroglia, where it inhibits glutamate and cystine transporters. This leads to reduced glutamate uptake, which promotes excitotoxic neuronal death and reduced astroglial capacity

---

[1] So-named from the city of Minamata, where the disease was first described in 1956. See McAlpine & Araki, 1958.

to buffer reactive oxygen species, due to decreased glutathione synthesis (De Keyser *et al.*, 2008; Yin *et al.*, 2007). These two mechanisms cause the progression of neurodegeneration.

## 10.7.2    Lead toxic encephalopathy

Lead poisoning causes acute neurodegeneration. In the CNS, lead accumulates in astroglia (De Keyser *et al.*, 2008), where it impairs glutamate transport (mainly via down-regulation of EAAT-2 transporter expression), increases astroglial production of vascular endothelial growth factor, and affects astroglial water homeostatic performance by increasing the water permeability of aquaporin 4 (Gunnarson *et al.*, 2005). These last two mechanisms contribute to the development of cytotoxic and vascular brain oedema in lead poisoned patients.

## 10.7.3    Manganese neurotoxicity

Acute exposure to toxic concentrations of manganese induces acute psychosis, whereas chronic manganese neurotoxicity is manifested by parkinsonism. Astroglia express the high capacity manganese transport system and exposure of primary cultured astrocytes to manganese inhibits glutamate uptake and promotes apoptosis (De Keyser *et al.*, 2008); both these mechanisms are potentially relevant for pathogenic development of manganese neurotoxicity.

## 10.7.4    Aluminium toxic encephalopathy

Aluminium toxic encephalopathy is clinically characterised by speech alterations, seizures, flapping wrist tremor (asterixis) and cognitive impairments. Exposure of cultured astrocytes to aluminium induces swelling, destruction of the cytoskeleton, reduction in gap junctional connectivity, inhibition of glutamate uptake and increased astroglial apoptosis. Compromised astrocytic glutamate transport has been shown to be responsible for neuronal death in neuronal-glial co-cultures (Struys-Ponsar *et al.*, 2000; Suarez-Fernandez *et al.*, 1999).

## 10.8    Neurodegenerative diseases

Neurodegeneration is a chronic process that results in a progressive loss of function, structure and number of neural cells, leading to generalised atrophy of the brain and profound cognitive deficit. The neurodegenerative diseases are rather specific to humans, being generally absent in animal species. Indeed, no animal naturally develops Parkinson's or Alzheimer's disease, and very rarely do animals show signs of senile dementia. However, neurodegenerative pathologies can profoundly affect the life of humans, as nothing can be more fearsome than loss of intellect and ultimate fading of humanness into a helpless body.

The causes of neurodegenerative diseases are many, from traumatic or infectious attacks, to intrinsic processes associated with genetic predispositions or the accumulation of sporadic errors of yet unknown origins. The neurodegenerative process affects the connectivity of neural networks that are critical for information processing and cognitive power. The early events occurring at the onset of various neurodegenerative diseases are generally unknown, yet we may safely suggest that it all begins with altered synaptic transmission, synaptic weakness and imbalance of neurotransmission, all of which affect information processing by neural networks. These initial functional abnormalities grow deeper with disease progression, leading to the loss of synapses, alteration of cellular structure and, eventually, to cell death. Brain atrophy resulting from massive death of neural cells represents the final, irreversible stage of the neurodegenerative process, where the volume of the nervous tissue shrinks and neurological functions are severely affected (Heneka *et al.*, 2010; Knight & Verkhratsky, 2010; Palop & Mucke, 2010; Terry, 2000).

The pathological potential of neuroglia in neurodegeneration began to be explored only very recently because, for a long time, neurodegenerative diseases were considered as a primary neuronal pathology. However, if we view neuro-degeneration as a chronic and progressive failure of brain homeostasis, then clearly neuroglia are fundamentally involved (for a detailed overview of the role of glia in neurodegenerative diseases and comprehensive bibliography, see Heneka *et al.*, 2010; Parpura *et al.*, 2012; Rodriguez & Verkhratsky, 2011; Verkhratsky *et al.*, 2010, 2012).

Indeed, all the evidence indicates that neuroglia are invariably affected at the early stages of neurodegenerative processes; neuroglial alterations determine to a large extent the progression and severity of these diseases. Several investigations have discovered atrophic changes in astroglia that appear at the very early stages of different models of neurodegenerative diseases. Atrophic changes in astrocytes may lie at the very core of initial disruption of neural circuitry, as reduced astroglial support affects synaptic maintenance and strength.

At the later stages of the neurodegenerative process, the appearance of specific lesions (e.g. senile plaques or Lewy bodies) initiates astrogliosis, whereby reactive astrocytes try to seal the lesioned area and drive the neuroinflammatory process (Figure 10.8). In addition, altered myelination by oligodendroglia, which is essential for rapid inter-neuronal connections, inevitably affects cognitive function. Finally, microglia (in concert with astrocytes) orchestrate the brain immune defence and neuroinflammation, the balance of these two fundamental processes defining cell survival and death, and hence progression of neurodegenerative pathology.

## 10.8.1   Post-stroke dementia

*Post-stroke dementia* (PSD) is currently defined as any dementia occurring after a stroke. The overall statistic is striking, as the incidence of stroke doubles the risk of dementia. There is also a direct link between stroke and development of

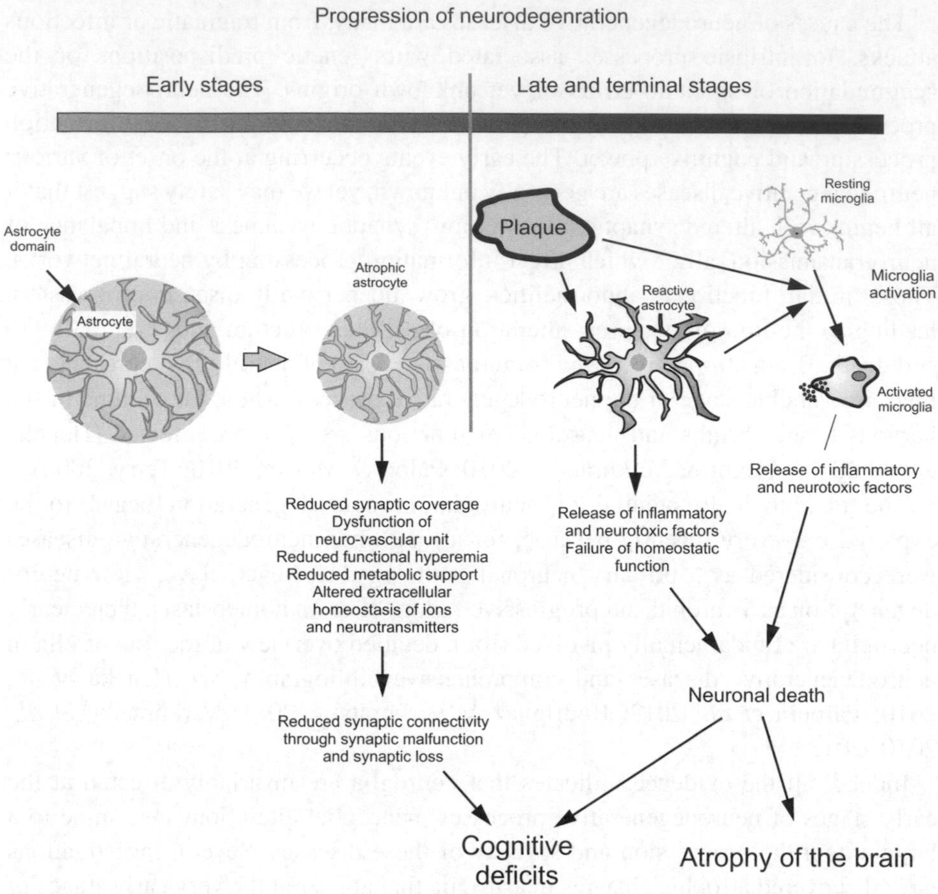

**Figure 10.8**  Neuroglial hypothesis of neurodegenerative disease.

The initial impairments of brain connectivity and synaptic transmission observed in neuro-degenerative diseases can result from generalised atrophy of astrocytes. Atrophy of astroglia may cause reduced synaptic coverage, affect homeostasis of ions and neurotransmitters, alter neuro-vascular unit performance and reduce metabolic support to neurones. These factors can contribute to synaptic malfunction and synaptic loss, thus causing early cognitive deficits. At the later stages of AD, appearance of disease-specific lesions (e.g. senile plaques in Alzheimer's disease) presents a strong pro-gliotic signal which triggers activation of both astrocytes and microglia. Reactive astrocytes further reduce synaptic support and may exacerbate microglial activation. Reactive glia release inflammatory and neurotoxic factors, which induce neuronal death and brain atrophy, thus causing severe dementia.

Reproduced with permission from Verkhratsky et al., 2010.

Alzheimer's disease. As noted above, brain defects that develop after stroke are directly associated with glial cells; both astrocytes and microglia determine the size of the infarction and, through permissive astrogliosis, they determine post-traumatic remodelling and regeneration of brain regions that were not put to death by infarction (see Chapter 9). Therefore, new therapeutic strategies aimed at glial cells may significantly affect the functional outcome and prevalence of PSD.

A particular type of post-stroke dementia is represented by *Binswanger's disease* (or *subcortical dementia*; Libon *et al.*, 2004), a form of vascular dementia, characterised by diffuse white matter lesions, that leads to progressive loss of memory, cognition and behavioural adaptation. The infarct occurring in white matter triggers progressive death of oligodendrocytes, activation of microglia and degeneration of axons. The primary pathological steps most likely are associated with ischaemic death of oligodendrocytes.

Another relatively frequent and grim outcome of brain ischaemia-related disease is represented by *periventricular leucomalacia* (Blumenthal, 2004), a condition that causes diffuse cerebral white matter injury. This occurs mostly in prematurely ($<32$ weeks) born infants – an especially high incidence (up to 20 per cent) of periventricular leucomalacia is observed among those born with very low weight ($<1500\,g$).

The roots of this pathology can be found in:

1.  poor vascularisation of white matter in premature infants; and

2.  prevalence of oligodendrocyte progenitors and immature oligodendrocytes, which are particularly sensitive to ischaemia, reactive oxygen species and glutamate excitotoxicity.

Thus, periods of even comparatively mild ischaemia result in profound damage to white matter and the demise of many oligodendrocyte progenitors. This, in turn, leads to defective myelination, with further defects in cerebral cortex development and impairment of pyramidal tracts, and subsequent neurological disorders, including cerebral palsy and cognitive defects.

## 10.8.2 Amyotrophic lateral sclerosis

Amyotrophic lateral sclerosis (ALS; in the USA, also known as 'Lou Gehrig's disease', after the baseball player who suffered and died from this pathology) was described by Jean-Martin Charcot in 1869 (Charcot, 1881; Charcot & Joffroy, 1869). ALS is a specific degeneration of motor neurones located in the cortex, in the brain stem and in the spinal cord. Clinically, ALS appears in the form of progressive paralysis and muscle atrophy, which ends in respiratory failure causing death. ALS exists in both familial and sporadic forms. About 20 per cent of cases are associated with dominant mutations in the gene coding for Cu-Zn superoxide dismutase or *SOD1*. This mutated gene has been used for generating several animal models of ALS (Turner & Talbot, 2008).

ALS is associated with astrogliosis and microglial activation, which was described in both humans and transgenic animals (see Rossi *et al.*, 2008; Rossi & Volterra, 2009, for further details and references). The astrogliosis, however, is preceded by astroglial degeneration and atrophy, which occur before neuronal death and the appearance of clinical symptoms in the hSOD1$^{G93A}$ transgenic mouse. Reactive astroglia appear at later stages of the disease, although atrophic astrocytes are also present close to lesion sites. Astrocytes specifically expressing SOD1 mutant gene have been found to acquire vulnerability to glutamate excitotoxicity, which was mediated by mGluR5 receptors. These astrocytes also released several neurotoxic factors and, somehow, trigger activation of microglia. Selective silencing of the SOD1 mutant gene in astrocytes significantly slowed the progression of ALS in transgenic mice (Yamanaka *et al.*, 2008). In humans suffering from ALS, a profound astrocytic proliferation has been found in PET imaging studies.

Another important pathogenic factor in ALS is represented by deficient glutamate clearance, which promotes excitotoxic neuronal damage. Reduced glutamate clearance is associated with a disappearance of astroglial glutamate transporter EAAT2 in the affected brain areas. Genetic deletion of EAAT2 (GLT-1) in mice leads to a pronounced loss of motor neurones, thus mimicking ALS. The disappearance of EAAT2 in human astroglia in sporadic ALS is the consequence of gene failure and may result from aberrant RNA splicing, exon skipping and intron retention. In the hereditary form of ALS, the down-regulation of glutamate transporter can result from oxidative damage associated with malfunction of superoxide dismutase. In addition to deficient glutamate clearance, astrocytes may participate in neuronal damage through increased glutamate release. Patients with ALS are reported to have increased levels of cyclooxygenase 2 (COX2), which produces prostaglandin E2, a potent activator of glutamate release from astrocytes.

Astrocytes can be considered as central players in ALS pathology. At the initial stages, glutamate induces gliotoxicity, which results in astroglial atrophy. The atrophic astrocytes in turn reduce synaptic coverage and fail to perform their homeostatic and neurone-supportive functions. This initiates neurodegeneration, which triggers reactive gliosis. Reactive astrocytes release neurotoxic factors and stimulate microglial activation, thus initiating the vicious cycle of neurodegeneration.

ALS, especially at later stages, is associated with microglial activation, which, for example has been found in the prefrontal and motor cortex, in the thalamus and the pons of ALS patients (Turner *et al.*, 2004). Similarly, microglial activation has been detected in mice overexpressing mutant SOD1. In this disease model, activation of microglia developed before appearance of neuronal lesions and disease symptoms.

Microglial activation may be important, therefore, for disease progression through mounting the neuroinflammatory response. Indeed, selectively silencing mutant SOD1 genes in microglial cells from the disease model animals increases the survival rate, indicating that the presence of mutant SOD1 in microglial cells is fundamental for their detrimental effect on motor neurone integrity. Likewise, progression of ALS in an animal model can be delayed by transplanting wild-type bone marrow cells (Beers *et al.*, 2006; Boillee *et al.*, 2006). The development of ALS in the SOD1 animal model can also be delayed by anti-inflammatory treatment with inhibitors of COX2 (celecoxib or nimesulide) or broad spectrum blockers of microglia-mediated neuroinflammation such as minocycline or pioglitazone (see Heneka *et al.*, 2010 for details).

## 10.8.3   Wernicke encephalopathy

Wernicke encephalopathy (also known as Wernicke-Korsakoff syndrome) is the combination of ataxia, ophthalmoplegia and mental confusion, which, in terminal stages, is manifested by Korsakoff psychosis (ante- and retrograde amnesia, apathy and confabulation). This disease reflects profound neuronal loss, with deep thalamo-cortical lesions caused by a deficiency of thiamine (the disease mostly affects alcoholics). It was initially described by Carl Wernicke (Wernicke, 1881–1883); whereas the psychotic component was described by Sergei Korsakoff in 1889 (Korsakoff Корсаков, 1889).

Wernicke encephalopathy is caused by functional atrophy of astroglial glutamate uptake. Levels of astroglial transporters EAAT1 and EAAT2 in cortical samples from human tissues obtained from confirmed cases of the disease are reduced by 60–70 per cent. A similar profound decrease in astroglial glutamate transporters has been found in the rat thiamine deficiency model of the disease (Hazell, 2009; Hazell *et al.*, 2009). The failure of astroglial glutamate uptake causes severe neuronal excitotoxicity and subsequent tissue lesions. In addition, a significant decrease in expression of GFAP, astrocytic glutamine synthetase and astrocytic GAT-3 GABA transporter, all indicative of astroglial dystrophy, have been observed in the thalamus of thiamine deficient rats (Hazell, 2009; Hazell *et al.*, 2009).

## 10.8.4   Fronto-temporal, thalamic, HIV-associated and other non-Alzheimer's type dementias

Astrocytes are pathologically affected in several types of dementia of 'non-Alzheimer's type'. Depending on the type and stage of the disease, both astroglial atrophy and astrogliosis are observed; these two processes can also develop in parallel. In *fronto-temporal dementia* (the clinical definition covering several types of familial and sporadic non-Alzheimer type cognitive disruptions which include, for example *Pick's disease* and *fronto-temporal lobar degeneration* (Josephs, 2008)), early and profound apoptotic death and dystrophy of astrocytes, as well as astrogliosis, are observed. The degree of glial atrophy displays direct correlation with the severity of dementia (Broe *et al.*, 2004; Kersaitis *et al.*, 2004).

Early, prominent and disease-specific astrogliosis also accompanies *thalamic dementia*. In this form of pathology, a specific proliferation of perivascular and perineuronal astroglial processes are observed. These changes in astroglia are considered to be the primary pathological change, and this can produce dementia even in the absence of severe neuronal loss (Potts & Leech, 2005).

Various types of non-AD dementias (e.g. *progressive supranuclear palsy*, *corticobasal degeneration* and *Pick's disease*) are associated with the appearance of tau protein inclusions in astroglial cells, which normally express very little (if any) tau protein (Komori, 1999). This astro-taupathology seems to be specific for each type of disease, with distinct morphological manifestations (Komori, 1999). Targeted expression of FTDP-17 tau protein (the FTDP-17 gene is associated with fronto temporal dementia and parkinsonism linked to chromosome 17) into astrocytes in a transgenic mouse model triggered age-dependent neurodegeneration, thus directly indicating that astroglia can indeed be a primary cause of a chronic neurodegenerative disease (Forman *et al.*, 2005).

Astrocytes and microglia also play a primary neurotoxic role in immuno-deficiency virus-1 (HIV-1) associated dementia, or HAD (Kaul *et al.*, 2001), in which significant astrogliosis and an increase in GFAP expression is observed in the entorhinal cortex and the hippocampus. The progression of HAD also promotes a significant astroglial cell loss through apoptosis, which is specifically prominent in subjects with rapidly progressing cognitive deficits (Thompson *et al.*, 2001). The HIV-1 virus infects exclusively microglia in the CNS, although the dementia progresses due to NMDA-receptor mediated neuronal death through necrosis or apoptosis.

Glutamate excitotoxicity can result from TNF-$\alpha$ release from infected and activated microglia. This triggers a massive release of glutamate from astrocytes, following TNF-$\alpha$-mediated activation of chemokine receptors of the CXCR4 type expressed in astroglial membranes. Incidentally, the same CXCR4 receptors can also be activated by the isoform of HIV-1 coat protein gp120$_{IIIB}$, implicated in HAD pathology. Neurotoxicity can also be exacerbated by the release of additional inflammatory and death factors from both astrocytes and activated microglia.

## 10.8.5   Alzheimer's disease (AD)

*Alzheimer's disease* (AD), together with multi-infarct post-stroke dementia, is the main cause of senile dementia. Named after Alois Alzheimer, who was the first to describe this pathology in 1907 (Alzheimer, 1907), it is characterised by profound neuronal loss throughout the brain, which compromises memory and results in severe impairment of cognitive functions. Histological hallmarks of AD are represented by the formation of deposits of *β-amyloid protein* (Aβ) in the walls of blood vessels, accumulation of Aβ plaques (also known as *senile plaques*) in the grey matter and intra-neuronal accumulation of abnormal tau-protein filaments in the form of neuronal tangles.

The pathological remodelling of neuroglial cells in demented brains was initially observed by Alois Alzheimer himself, who had found glial cells abundantly populating neuritic plaques and associated with damaged neurones (Figure 10.9; Alzheimer, 1910). These pathologically remodelled cells are activated microglia

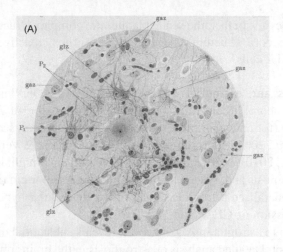

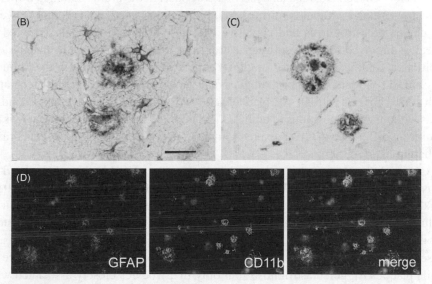

**Figure 10.9**   Activation of glial cells at sites of β-amyloid deposition in human brain and in APP transgenic mice.

A.   Neuritic plaques as seen and drawn by Alois Alzheimer (Alzheimer, 1910). The plaque is surrounded by activated astrocytes, and activated microglia are present at the peripheral region. Abbreviations: P1 – the central part of the plaque (amyloid deposition); P2 – periphery of the plaque; gaz – neurone; glz – glial cell (Full colour version in plate section).

B.   Double immunostaining of a human brain section derived from a 70-year-old Alzheimer's disease patient reveals GFAP positive astrocytes (blue) surrounding 6E10 positive β-amyloid deposits (brown).

C.   Double-staining for β-amyloid (brown) and CD68-positive microglia cells. Scale bar = 50 μm.

D.   Double immunostaining of GFAP and CD11b in a cortical section of a 12-month-old APP23 transgenic mouse shows a focal and close association of both markers for astro- and microglial reactivity.

Reproduced with permission from Verkhratsky et al., 2010

and reactive astrocytes. In fact, the senile plaques are complex structures formed by Aβ deposits (the core structure), degenerating neurites, reactive astroglia and activated microglial cells.

**(i)   Astrogliosis and astroglial degeneration in AD**   Our knowledge about modifications of neuroglia and their roles in the progression of AD remains, at best, fragmentary (for review of modern theories and references, see Heneka *et al.*, 2010; Nagele *et al.*, 2004; Rodriguez *et al.*, 2009; Rodriguez & Verkhratsky, 2011; Verkhratsky *et al.*, 2010). It is generally accepted that the main glial reaction to AD is profound astrogliosis and, indeed, many studies of post-mortem tissues from AD patients found generalised astrogliosis, manifested by cellular hypertrophy and an increase in expression of GFAP and S100β.

A closer look into astroglia in AD, however, reveals substantial digressions from the general concept. Detailed analysis of astrogliosis in the brains obtained from old patients (with and without confirmed AD) has demonstrated a correlation between the degree of astrogliosis and cognitive decline, but the same analysis failed to reveal a direct correlation between astrogliotic changes and senile plaques. In addition, a significant decrease in GFAP expression was observed in the brain of very old AD patients. The morphological data showed reactive astrocytes associated with some, but not with all Aβ plaques, and astrogliotic fields were also found in areas without Aβ depositions in both AD and non-AD brains. Moreover, there is no significant difference in GFAP expression in demented versus non-demented brains (Wharton *et al.*, 2009).

Astroglial degeneration/atrophy at the early stages of AD was discovered in transgenic animal models (Olabarria *et al.*, 2010; Rodriguez & Verkhratsky, 2011; Verkhratsky *et al.*, 2010). Astroglial atrophy was found in several brain regions including hippocampus, prefrontal and entorhinal cortex, and was persistent through all ages. In contrast, Aβ plaques started to accumulate in the brains of these transgenic AD animals only at the more advanced ages. The appearance of senile plaques triggered astrogliosis, but only in astrocytes closely associated with these plaques whereas astroglial cells localised distantly to the plaques (more than 50 μm) were atrophic. The astrogliotic reaction in AD animals was not uniform in brain regions: astrogliosis was prominent in the hippocampus and was absent in entorhinal cortex (Yeh *et al.*, 2012). This is of interest because, in AD, the first senile plaques appear in the entorhinal cortex, and its specific vulnerability may be associated with a defective astroglial defensive response.

Reactive astrogliosis in AD is triggered by several factors, with β-amyloid peptide being a disease-specific signal; exposure of cultured astrocytes to Aβ rapidly induces astrogliosis. Extracellular Aβ also induces spontaneous $[Ca^{2+}]_i$ signals and $[Ca^{2+}]_i$ oscillations, which contribute to astroglial neurotoxicity *in vitro*. These abnormal, spontaneous $Ca^{2+}$ oscillations and $Ca^{2+}$ waves have also been observed *in vivo* in astrocytes associated with neuritic plaques (Kuchibhotla *et al.*, 2009). Astrocytes in Aβ overexpressing transgenic mice demonstrate increased coupling in neocortical regions and elevated expression of AMPA/kainate glutamate receptors. At the same time, Aβ reduces expression of astroglial glutamate transporters, which compromises glutamate uptake.

**(ii)  Astroglia and β-amyloid**  The role of astroglia in Aβ processing and metabolism remains controversial. Reactive astrocytes in AD have been suggested to participate in the clearance and degradation of β-amyloid (for review, see Nagele *et al.*, 2004). Indeed, activated astrocytes located in the close vicinity to Aβ plaques formed in the brains of transgenic APP mice have been found to express neprilysin, the amyloid-degrading enzyme. Accumulation of Aβ has been observed in astrocytes from entorhinal cortex of AD patients, although it has rarely been found in astrocytes from various AD model mice. Functional experiments have also demonstrated the ability of astrocytes to phagocytose and degrade β-amyloid deposits *in vitro*. These experiments, however, also demonstrated that only astrocytes isolated from healthy brains sequestered β-amyloid, while astrocytes obtained from APP transgenic mice were ineffective. This latter difference is another indication of astroglial functional dysfunction in AD.

Remarkably, AD results in a selective increase of the neuronal type of nicotinic acetylcholine receptor (α7nAChRs) in astroglial cells (Aβ has a very high affinity for α7nAChRs, which possibly explains the high vulnerability of cholinergic neurones to AD). It may well be that increased astroglial expression of α7nAChRs contributes to the scavenging of Aβ.

AD pathology may also affect the ability of astrocytes to produce Aβ. Astrocytes are not equipped with β-secretase, which is the central enzyme for Aβ production (this enzyme is also known as β-site APP-cleaving enzyme 1, or BACE 1). In the healthy brain, β-secretase is expressed exclusively in neurones. However, in conditions of AD-like pathology, or even under chronic stress, astrocytes start to express BACE 1, thus acquiring Aβ producing ability. Astroglial BACE 1 has been detected in activated astrocytes surrounding Aβ plaques in several transgenic AD mice models. Various brain insults that triggered astrogliosis (e.g. immunological or ischaemic attack) also triggered astrocytic expression of BACE 1 (Rossner *et al.*, 2005). Similarly, increased APP production has been detected in a rat model of chronic neocortical astrogliosis, induced by grafting foetal cortical tissue in the midbrain of neonatal animals; chronically activated astrocytes were immunopositive for APP, as well as for another AD-related marker, ApoE (see Heneka *et al.*, 2005; Rossner *et al.*, 2005 for details).

**(iii)  The neuro-vascular unit in AD: role for astrocytes**  Vascular impairment represents an important factor in the pathology of AD. A significant reduction in brain blood flow is well documented in humans suffering from AD. Similarly, morphological analysis found pronounced vascular pathology in nervous tissue affected by AD.

As has been described in Chapter 4, the elementary component of brain microcirculation is represented by a neuro-vascular unit, in which astrocytes integrate neurones, brain endothelium, pericytes and vascular smooth muscle cells into a functional entity. In AD, the neurovascular unit is specifically affected because Aβ plaques often encompass brain capillaries, which may deregulate microcirculation and possibly alter vascular clearance of Aβ. There are also indications that primary vascular pathology (e.g. atherosclerosis) may contribute to the production of Aβ through as yet unknown mechanisms (see Bell & Zlokovic, 2009 for details).

Control of the neurovascular unit, local cerebral circulation and functional hyperaemia are functions of astroglia. In addition, astrocytes contribute to transport of water and electrolytes, as well as utilisation of glucose and providing neurones with energy substrates. Astroglial changes that occur in AD (astroglial atrophy and astrogliosis) may therefore compromise the neuro-vascular unit and contribute to cognitive abnormalities.

**(iv)   Metabolic remodelling of astroglia in AD**   The AD-affected human brain shows signs of metabolic stress, manifested by progressive decrease in glucose utilisation, measured by functional imaging, from the very early stages of the disease (Mosconi *et al.*, 2008). Exposure of primary astroglial cultures to Aβ affects glucose metabolism and increases ROS production, although these data remain controversial, since both decreased and increased astroglial glucose utilisation have been found following Aβ treatment (see, for example, Allaman *et al.*, 2010, for details). Similarly, in post-mortem analysis, both decreased and increased activity of glucose metabolism enzymes have been detected (see Verkhratsky *et al.*, 2010, for details and references). Furthermore, co-culturing neurones with astrocytes pre-treated with Aβ significantly decreases neuronal survival, compared with co-culturing with naïve astrocytes (Allaman *et al.*, 2010). These discrepancies may reflect opposite cell-specific changes in glucose metabolism developing at different stages of AD (Allaman *et al.*, 2010).

**(v)   Microglia in AD**   The activation of microglia and neuroinflammatory response is considered to be the third (after plaques and tangles) fundamental component of AD (see Heneka *et al.*, 2010; Solito & Sastre, 2012; Wyss-Coray & Rogers, 2012, for relevant references). The formation of senile plaques triggers activation of microglia, which (depending on the stage of the disease) occurs both locally in the vicinity of the plaques and diffusely throughout the brain parenchyma. Activated microglia surround the plaques and participate in their formation. Microglial cells have been suggested to associate specifically with certain amyloid plaque types, indicating that plaque development and the degree of microglial reaction may be interrelated.

It is unclear whether it is the senile plaque or soluble Aβ that represents the microglia-activating signal. For example, in APP V717I transgenic mice, where the plagues appear at about 10–12 months of age, focal microglial activation is observed much earlier, and can be seen already at three months (Heneka *et al.*, 2005). In contrast, *in vivo* confocal imaging has demonstrated that microglial activation starts only after the plaque has been formed (Meyer-Luehmann *et al.*, 2008). In another animal model of the disease, 3xTg-AD transgenic mice, an early increase in the density of resting microglia has been detected; the number of resting microglial cells is almost doubled compare to the controls, as if preparing for the subsequent activation, which became apparent after the appearance of senile plaques (Rodriguez *et al.*, 2010).

Activation of microglia by Aβ proceeds through several pathways which, in particular, include TLR4 receptors, $P2X_7$ receptors and intracellular $Ca^{2+}$ signalling (see Chapter 4). Activated microglia contribute to AD progression and the balance of neuronal survival and death through the release of multiple factors, including complement factors, chemokines and cytokincs. There have been numerous suggestions that activated microglia may participate in Aβ clearance, which has been observed *in vitro* in microglial cultures treated with Aβ, but this has not been universally confirmed *in vivo*. Similarly, treatment of AD patients with anti-inflammatory drugs has not shown beneficial effects in discase progression (Streit, 2010). Finally, there are indications of microglial dystrophy (manifested with cell fragmentation), which coincide with the appearance of tangles and may prompt AD-related neurodegeneration (Streit *et al.*, 2009).

## 10.8.6   Parkinson's disease

*Parkinson's disease* (PD) was described by James Parkinson at the beginning of the 19th century (Parkinson, 1817). It is characterised by a progressive degeneration of dopaminergic midbrain neurones in the substantia nigra (SN) and becomes clinically apparent when more than 50 per cent of SN neurones have been lost. Astrogliosis and activation of microglia have been found in the (post-mortem) brain areas affected by the disease (see McGeer & McGeer, 2008; Mena & Garcia de Yebenes, 2008 for further details and references). In particular, a rather prominent gliosis is observed in the substantia nigra, which contains the cell bodies of neurones forming the nigrostriatal pathway. At the same time, the substantia nigra has a low density of astrocytes compared to other brain regions, and early astroglial atrophy may have a pathological significance – astrodegeneration can result in diminished support of dopaminergic neurones, thus increasing their vulnerability. Experiments *in vitro* in neuronal-glial co-cultures have demonstrated that astrocytes protect dopaminergic neurones. Furthermore, astrocytes prevent direct neurotoxicity of L-DOPA and thus are required for L-DOPA substitute therapy (Mena *et al.*, 1996).

Microglial activation has been found in tissues from PD patients and in all animal models of the disease (see Heneka *et al.*, 2010 for references). The SN neurones appear to be particularly vulnerable to attack by activated microglia, and this observation initiated the hypothesis of microglia-mediated neurodegeneration and cell death as instrumental for PD pathogenesis. Indeed, anti-inflammatory therapies and treatment with the general inhibitor of microglial activation, minocycline, has been found to reduce loss of dopaminergic neurones.

## 10.8.7   Huntington's disease

*Huntington's disease* (HD), so named after George Huntington, who described this pathology in 1872, is an autosomal dominant neurodegenerative disease, characterised by death of neurones in the cortex and striatum (Huntington, 1872). This neuronal loss causes numerous movement disorders and dementia. The gene concerned is known as *Huntington* or *Htt*; this gene is expressed by neurones and neuroglia, as well as by many peripheral cells.

HD post-mortem tissues show prominent astrogliosis and activation of microglia. The primary astroglial pathology in HD is, however, associated with a decrease in expression of glutamate transporters and, hence, impaired glutamate homeostasis (see Estrada-Sánchez & Rebec, 2012, for recent review). In addition, HD-affected astrocytes have decreased ability to produce and release glutathione and ascorbic acid, which substantially reduces their neuroprotection through ROS scavenging.

Transgenic mice specifically expressing mutant *Htt* gene in astrocytes display many symptoms of HD, clearly demonstrating that selective insult to astrocytes is fundamentally relevant for HD pathology. In post-mortem HD tissues, aggregates of mutated Htt protein were also found in microglia, and activation of microglia can be seen at the early, pre-symptomatic stages of this disease.

## 10.8.8   Infantile neuroaxonal dystrophy

*Infantile neuroaxonal dystrophy*, also known as *Seitelberger disease*, is an inherited degenerative nervous system disorder characterised by abnormalities in CNS and PNS axons. These are caused by mutations in the PLA2G6 gene, which encodes a $Ca^{2+}$-independent phospholipase A2. Clinically, this disease manifests in progressive movement abnormalities and early dementia. In genetically modified animal models carrying mutant genes, severe abnormalities in astroglial $Ca^{2+}$ signalling have been described, caused by suppressed store-operated $Ca^{2+}$ entry (Strokin *et al.*, 2012). How these astroglial abnormalities relate to disease progression, however, remains unknown.

## 10.8.9   Nasu-Hakola disease: microglial pre-senile dementia

Nasu-Hakola disease is an autosomal recessive disorder characterised by progressive pre-senile dementia and bone cysts; this disease is also known as polycystic lipomembranous osteodysplasia with sclerosing leukoencephalopathy (Bianchin *et al.*, 2004). The disease starts in middle age, and death follows several years after onset. At the early stages of the disease, a peculiar neuropsychiatric sympatomatology, with emotional abnormalities, silly, euphoric, facetious and unrestrained behaviour, together with social inhibition, may complicate diagnostics. The primary event in Nasu-Hakola disease seems to be associated with prominent activation and loss of function of microglia in the cerebral white matter. It is suggested that impaired microglia massively release neurotoxic factors that trigger region-specific neuronal death and dementia (Bianchin *et al.*, 2010). This theory, however, is not universally accepted (Satoh *et al.*, 2011).

# 10.9 Leukodystrophies

## 10.9.1 Megalencephalic leukoencephalopathy with subcortical cysts

Megalencephalic leukoencephalopathy with subcortical cysts (MLC) is an autosomal recessive disease of the white matter, accompanied by the appearance of subcortical cysts in the anterior-temporal and frontoparietal cortex (De Keyser *et al.*, 2008). Clinically, it is represented by macrocephaly, which can either be present at birth or may develop during the first year of life. Neurological symptoms include cerebellar ataxia and mild spasticity.

This disease is caused by mutations of a gene that encodes the MLC1 protein, which is specifically present in astroglial processes. MLC1 encodes an integral membrane protein with low and questionable homology to ion channels. It has been proposed that MLC1 is related to the activation of the volume-regulated chloride channel. GlialCAM was recently identified as a second MLC gene, and the GlialCAM protein helps target MLC1 and the Cl⁻ channel ClC-2 to astrocyte-astrocyte junctions and to their perivascular endfeet. Unlike MLC1, GlialCAM is also detected in myelin and axons (Jeworutzki *et al.*, 2012; Lopez-Hernandez *et al.*, 2011). These studies indicate that disruption of volume-regulated chloride transport is of primary importance to the pathology of MLC.

## 10.9.2 Vanishing white matter disease

Vanishing white matter disease (VWM) is one of the most frequent inherited childhood white-matter disorders (van der Knaap *et al.*, 2006), and it was described in 1962 by Werner Eicke (Eicke, 1962). VWM is caused by mutations in any of the five genes encoding the subunits of eukaryotic translation initiation factor eIF2B, and it is manifested by chronic progressive neurological deterioration, with cerebellar ataxia and mild mental decline. eIF2B is a Guanine nucleotide exchange factor which is required for the exchange of the GDP in eIF2 for a GTP, in order for the ternary complex to reform for a new round of translation initiation.

The disease usually reveals itself at an early age (2–6 years), and most of the patients die within several years after diagnosis. VWM disease stems from a severe deterioration of white matter, which shows myelin loss, malformation of myelin sheaths, and vacuolation. The white matter degenerates and appears cystic, and cavities are often observed (van der Knaap *et al.*, 2006). Around these cavities, a pronounced loss of oligodendrocytes is detected, and many oligodendrocytes also have an abnormal morphological appearance. Astrocytes are dysmorphic, with blunt, broad processes rather than their typical delicate arborisations. There is no specific treatment for VWM.

## 10.10   Epilepsy

Epilepsy manifests in the appearance of recurrent seizures. Epilepsy results from abnormal synchrony in the neuronal networks, when many nerve cells start to fire simultaneously. These discharges can be visualised on the EEG, which reveals cortical spikes and sharp waves. The cellular substrate of epilepsy is a slow depolarisation of neurones, which occurs without any apparent provocation and develops synchronously in virtually all nerve cells within the epileptic foci. This slow neuronal depolarisation is known as *paroxysmal depolarisation shift*, or PDS.

The PDS results from large excitatory post-synaptic potentials, which develop slower than normal EPSPs, triggered by electrical excitation of incoming synaptic terminals; usually, the PDS lasts from 50–200 ms. The synaptic potential underlying the PDS is mediated by glutamate receptors of AMPA and NMDA types and is caused by simultaneous glutamate release around many neurones comprising epileptic foci. When the PDS fails to terminate, the prolonged synchronous depolarisation of many neurones results in seizures, which are the hallmarks of epilepsy.

Reactive gliosis and appearance of a gliotic scar have been long recognised as a specific feature in human epilepsy (Penfield & Humphreys, 1940). Astrocytes are involved in the pathogenesis of epilepsy at very early stages of the disease; they become reactive, are hypertrophied, change their shape and increase in number. This reactive astrogliosis occurs before any neurodegenerative changes, and even before the appearance of fully developed seizures (for detailed overview and relevant references, see Aronica *et al.*, 2012; Carmignoto & Haydon, 2012; Coulter & Eid, 2012; Heinemann *et al.*, 2012; Seifert *et al.*, 2010; Seifert & Steinhauser, 2011; Steinhauser *et al.*, 2012; Tian *et al.*, 2005; Verkhratsky *et al.*, 2012). An important change in astrocytes in epileptic brain tissue is the loss of their domain organisation (Oberheim *et al.*, 2008), which has been observed both in post-mortem human samples and in brain tissue from animal models of the disease.

Epilepsy also remodels physiological properties of astrocytes. Astroglial cells from epileptic tissues demonstrate increased expression of ionotropic and metabotropic glutamate receptors and voltage-operated $Na^+$ channels. In contrast, expression of inward rectifying $K^+$ channels and aquaporin AQP4 water channels in perivascular endfeet are decreased. Also, epileptic astrocytes have reduced glutamine synthetase, which may signal impaired glutamate homeostasis and turnover. Remodelling of membrane channel expression makes some of the epileptic astrocytes electrically excitable and, additionally, most astrocytes have increased amplitudes of $Ca^{2+}$ signals in response to glutamate stimulation.

Astrocytes have been shown to assume a leading role in the generation of epileptic status in several animal models, such as the epileptic (EL) mouse, or transgenic mice with astroglia-specific deletion of the Tsc1 gene. In both models, astrocytes become reactive, with morphological hypertrophy and increased GFAP expression, together with decreased expression of glutamate transporters, resulting in impaired glutamate uptake. In Tsc1 deficient mice, astrocytes also have lower expression of inward rectifying $K^+$ channels, resulting in an imbalance in glutamate and $K^+$ homeostasis, which are likely to be instrumental in affecting neuronal excitability and development of seizures.

Physiologically, neuronal PDS and seizures lead to depolarisation of astrocytes surrounding the epileptic zone. Recently, it has become apparent that PDS can still develop in conditions of synaptic isolation – i.e. when neuronal firing is completely blocked by tetrodotoxin, which effectively poisons $Na^+$ channels. Moreover, it has also been shown that local stimulation of astroglial $[Ca^{2+}]_i$ signals in brain slices prepared from hippocampus can trigger release of glutamate, which in turn initiates PDS and epileptiform discharges in neighbouring neurones. Glial $[Ca^{2+}]_i$ waves always preceded spontaneous PDS in the brains of animals experimentally made epileptic (Tian et al., 2005).

This new knowledge about the role of astrocytes in producing neuronal epileptiform activity will considerably change our understanding of epilepsy pathogenesis. In fact, the introduction of astrocytes into the epileptic circuit (Figure 10.10) may be instrumental in describing the most enigmatic property of the epileptic brain – i.e. the precise synchronisation between many neurones. This synchronisation may result, for example, from abnormal glutamate release from an individual astrocyte, which, in humans, can reach up to two million synapses within the astroglial domain virtually simultaneously. Furthermore, several astroglial cells can work as a single unit, being synchronised through gap junctions, and then the number of neurones affected by one simultaneous glutamate discharge can be much greater.

These new insights into the pathology of epilepsy may also modify the quest for new therapeutic strategies considerably, as astroglial cells may well be the primary target. Incidentally, several anti-epileptic drugs, including valproate, gabapentin and phenytoin, are able to inhibit astroglial $Ca^{2+}$ signalling, and this may, at least in part, account for their anticonvulsant potency.

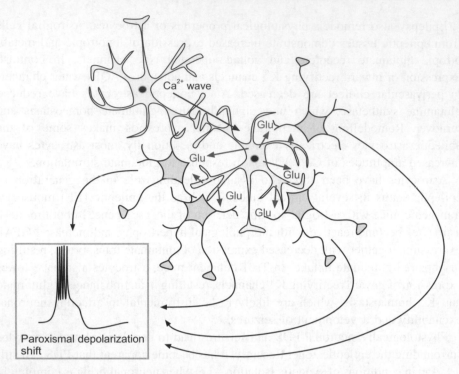

**Figure 10.10**  Astroglia and epileptic seizures.
  Astroglial calcium waves may trigger synchronous release of glutamate which, in turn, may act simultaneously on many neurones and trigger the specific depolarization – the paroxysmal depolarization shift – considered to be the electrical correlate of epileptic seizure.

## 10.11   Psychiatric diseases

All three major psychiatric disorders – schizophrenia, bipolar disorder and major depressive disorder – affect brain cytoarchitecture. Along with numerous histopathological signs of neuronal malfunction (e.g. reduction in neuronal size, dendritic length and dendritic spines density), these diseases also affect glial cells (see Bernstein *et al.*, 2009 for recent review).

Notably, these diseases are not associated with an astrogliotic reaction. On the contrary, there are indications for loss of astrocytes and GFAP expression in schizophrenia, bipolar disorder and major depressive disorder. In bipolar and major depressive disorders, significant decreases in the numbers and volume of astroglial cells have been detected in prefrontal and orbital cortex (Rajkowska & Miguel-Hidalgo, 2007).

Schizophrenia is more and more regarded as a disease resulting from compromised connectivity in neuronal networks and neurotransmission imbalance. Atrophy of astroglial cells would result in widespread discoordination of synaptic transmission and, therefore, may be a key pathological step in the development of psychiatric diseases.

In addition, major psychiatric disorders are associated with profound degeneration of oligodendrocytes and reduction in myelin in cortical areas, which may substantially affect brain connectivity (Davis *et al.*, 2003; Segal *et al.*, 2007). There is also evidence for microglial activation in psychiatric disorders. Moreover, microglial activation has been proposed to be associated with suicidal behaviour (Bernstein *et al.*, 2009), but this remains a daring speculation.

# 10.12   Autistic disorders

## 10.12.1   Autism

Autism (derived from the Greek *autos* (αυτοσ), which means *self*), is generally defined as a neurodevelopmental disorder characterised by aberrant social interactions, deficient communicative skills, and fixed and restricted behavioural patterns. This form of pathology was described by Leo Kanner in 1943 (Kanner, 1943). The term 'autism' incorporates various neurodevelopmental pathologies, including pervasive developmental disorders, autism-spectrum disorders, Rett's syndrome, Asperger's syndrome, childhood disintegrative disorder, etc. Not much is known about the role of neuroglia in autistic development. However, considering the importance of glia for neurogenesis and development of the nervous system, they can, conceivably, play a key role. In particular, various forms of autism can be connected to neuro-inflammation and chronic activation of microglia, induced, for example, by perinatal infections (Tetreault *et al.*, 2012).

## 10.12.2   Fragile X syndrome

Fragile X syndrome, also known as Martin-Bell syndrome or Escalante's syndrome, is the most common single-gene cause of autism and mental retardation. This disease is associated with the expression of Fragile X mental retardation protein, which is found in both neurones and astrocytes, and it has been suggested that changes in astroglia may be relevant for development of this type of pathology, through affecting the proper development of neuronal connections (Jacobs *et al.*, 2012).

## 10.12.3   Rett syndrome

Rett syndrome is another genetic form of autistic disorder linked to the X chromosome. It is caused by a loss of function mutation of the MECP2 gene, which encodes a methyl-CpG-binding protein. Elimination of this gene in astrocytes has been shown to affect their ability to support normal development of dendrites in neurones *in vitro*. In contrast, expression of wild-type MECP2 gene in astrocytes from animals in which this gene was deleted, removed the disease symptoms (altered locomotion and increased anxiety), increased lifespan and restored normal dendritic morphology (Lioy *et al.*, 2011). Furthermore, microglial cells without the MECP2 gene were also affected and had a deficient immune response and decreased phagocytic capacity. Transplantation of wild-type microglia into MECP2 deficient mice ameliorated the symptoms of the disease (Derecki *et al.*, 2012).

## 10.13  Neuropathic pain

Peripheral neuropathic chronic pain is a severe and debilitating pathological condition which affects many millions of people. Neuropathic pain is a consequence of either neurotrophic infections (most notably HIV) or injuries of peripheral nerves, which may occur following trauma, nerve compression or diabetes. The mechanisms of neuropathic pain are poorly understood, and existing therapy is often ineffective.

Very recently, the role of glial cells, particularly microglia and, to lesser extent astroglia, as primary mediators of chronic pain, has begun to be considered, and this has gained substantial experimental support (for references and detailed discussion, see Gao & Ji, 2010; Inoue & Tsuda, 2009, 2012; Kettenmann *et al.*, 2011; Tsuda *et al.*, 2005).

It is now firmly established that injury to peripheral nerve causes rapid and significant activation of microglia in the dorsal horn of the spinal cord, on the side of the peripheral nerve entry (Figure 10.11). Activated microglial cells in the spinal cord express pain-related signalling molecules – $P2X_4$ purinoreceptors and p38 mitogen-activated protein kinase (p38 MAPK). The activation of $P2X_4$ receptors is necessary and sufficient to produce allodynia (pain arising from stimuli which are normally not painful), which is a very common symptom of chronic pain. Direct injection of $P2X_4$ stimulated microglia into rat spinal cord triggers allodynia; conversely, pharmacological inhibition of $P2X_4$ receptors reverses allodynia following experimental peripheral nerve injury. Similarly, microglial p38 MAPK is rapidly activated following nerve injury, and pharmacological inhibition of p38 MAPK attenuates neuropathic pain symptoms.

The second important pathway is associated with $P2Y_{12}$ purinoceptors, which in the spinal cord are confined exclusively to microglia, and are critically involved in the genesis of neuropathic pain. Spinal nerve injury triggers a significant up-regulation of $P2Y_{12}$ receptors at both mRNA and protein levels, and activation of these receptors is instrumental in inducing tactile allodynia and thermal hyperalgesia. Genetic deletion or pharmacological inhibition of $P2Y_{12}$ receptors significantly reduces symptoms of neuropathic pain following peripheral nerve lesioning.

How microglia affect spinal cord sensory neurones and increase their excitability is a matter of intensive investigation. One mechanism involves ATP-stimulated release of brain-derived neurotrophic factor (BDNF) from activated microglia. In turn, BDNF suppresses neuronal potassium/chloride exporter KCC-2, thus

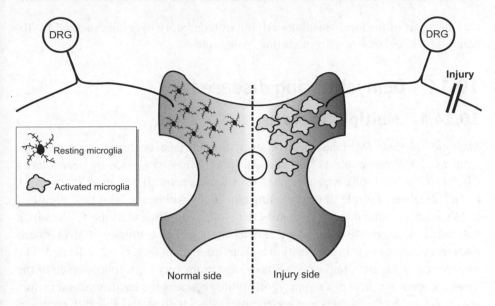

**Figure 10.11**   Activation of microglia as a mediator of neuropathic pain.

Injury to peripheral nerves triggers activation of microglia in the ipsilateral side of the dorsal horn. This activation is mediated through P2X$_4$ ionotropic purinoceptors and contributes to the development of chronic pain.

Redrawn from Tsuda *et al.*, 2005.

increasing intra-neuronal concentration of Cl$^-$ ions. As a result, GABA/glycine-mediated currents change their direction and become excitatory, thereby increasing the overall excitability of spinal neurones (Coull *et al.*, 2005). Furthermore, BDNF may also increase the availability of NMDA receptors, which also increase neuronal excitability. Finally, the third purinergic pathway involved in neuropathic pain is mediated through P2X$_7$ receptors (see Kettenmann *et al.*, 2011, for details).

Spinal cord astrocytes also demonstrate signs of reactive gliosis following peripheral nerve injury. These astrocytes express some receptors related to pain, most notably vanilloid receptors type 1 (also known as capsaicin receptors – activated by obnoxious heat and chilli pepper) and cannabinoid receptors type 1. Peripheral nerve injury increases the synthesis of growth factors (e.g. FGF2) and cytokines in astroglial cells in the spinal cord. The precise role played by astrocytes in chronic pain remains to be discovered.

There is evidence that Schwann cells and satellite glial cells also have direct roles in the generation and maintenance of neuropathic pain (Campana, 2007; Takeda *et al.*, 2009). Schwann cells and satellite glia secrete pro-inflammatory cytokines such as TNF-$\alpha$, which potentiates P2X$_3$ receptor-mediated responses and excitability in DRG nociceptor neurones. At the same time, Schwann cells and satellite glia produce both pro- and anti-inflammatory cytokines, including IL-1$\beta$, which may be a part of the mechanism underlying inflammatory hyperalgesia, and IL-10, which facilitates recovery from chronic pain states.

# 10.14   Demyelinating diseases

## 10.14.1   Multiple sclerosis

*Multiple sclerosis* (MS) has been known through past centuries as *paraplegia* (Murray, 2009), although its first classical description was made by Jean Martin Charcot (Charcot, 1868), who also gave this disease a name. It was also Charcot who, in 1877, realised the role of disrupted myelin in the pathogenesis of this disease.

MS is an autoimmune inflammatory demyelinating disease of the CNS, which culminates in progressive neurological deterioration. The aetiology of MS remains elusive, as both genetic predisposition and environmental factors are indicated. The importance of genetic predisposition is evident from very high concordance of the disease occurrence between monozygotic twins, whereas the environmental factors are implicated by the existence of geographical areas with remarkable differences in MS prevalence (generally, MS is significantly more frequent in northern rather than in southern parts of the world).

The general theory regards MS aetiology as an infection which presents the immune system with an antigen similar to CNS myelin. Numerous viruses that display homology to myelin components, such as MBP, are implicated and proposed as the infective trigger, such as hepatitis B virus and the herpes viruses, Epstein-Barr virus, herpes simplex virus, and cytomegalovirus (CMV), as well as influenza viruses and papillomaviruses. The resulting antibodies eventually attack CNS myelin and cause demyelination. This theory, however, is very broad and imprecise, as MS can cover several aetiologically distinct diseases with similar pathological endpoint and clinical features. Indeed, the pathogenesis of MS shows several distinct demyelinating patterns (Compston & Coles, 2008).

The first type of MS has a relapse-remitting time-course, and lesions are characterised by preferential destruction of myelin, complemented by local inflammation, most likely resulting from an autoimmune reaction. This type of MS is characterised by well-pronounced remyelination manifested by clinical remissions. NG2-glia (adult OPCs) are considered the source of remyelinating cells in MS (see Chapters 5 and 6).

The second type of MS is *primary progressive*, which is associated with oligodendrocyte death and severe neurological deterioration, and the disease does not show any relapses. In most cases, relapse-remitting MS ultimately develops a *secondary progressive* pathology, characterised by degenerative changes and poor recovery.

In both types of disease pathogenesis, the areas of demyelination always show the signs of inflammatory processes and are rich in activated T lymphocytes (Lassmann, 2005). The latter cross the blood-brain barrier and attack the antigen-presenting tissues which, in the case of MS, are myelin components or some parts of oligodendrocytes, or both. The target antigen/s in MS are uncertain, but *myelin oligodendrocyte glycoprotein* (MOG) is a prime candidate, because it is CNS-specific, and antigens to MOG can induce the animal model of MS, *experimental autoimmune encephalomyelitis* or *EAE*.

Other CNS myelin autoantigens in the development of autoimmune demyelinating disease include OSP/claudin-11, which is specific to CNS myelin/oligodendrocytes. Although myelin proteins have been the favoured candidates for initiation of MS, other factors have been implicated, including antibodies against neurofascin, which may mediate axonal injury in MS.

MS can be considered a disease of oligodendrocytes, but all neural cell types are involved (Compston & Coles, 2008). The pathological hallmark of MS is the white matter lesion, caused by loss of myelin and oligodendrocytes, but, in addition, there is axon degeneration and loss of grey matter neurones. Moreover, microglia play the central role in the immune and inflammatory response in MS, releasing pro- and anti-inflammatory cytokines and chemokines. Ultimately, there is marked loss of oligodendrocytes and axons/neurones, with shrinkage of grey matter. Chronic lesions are largely acellular and are filled by the inhibitory astroglial scar. Remyelination is a major aspect of MS, but remyelination ultimately fails, for unresolved reasons, which are most likely numerous.

Based on MRI and studies in animal models, it is generally believed that in MS CNS inflammatory activity might precede clinical symptoms by many years. MRI has shown that there are approximately ten new plaques in each clinical episode, and this is accepted as a clinical threshold, below which there are no clinical signs due to compensatory mechanisms.

The first event in MS is lymphocyte-driven inflammation, seen histologically as perivascular cuffing and on gadolinium brain scans as 'hotspots', corresponding to areas of blood-brain barrier opening. The accumulation of T and B lymphocytes, as well as other plasma cells and macrophages, and the release of pro-inflammatory cytokines, recruits naive microglia, which is key step in the amplification and local spread of the inflammatory response. Activated microglia contribute to inflammation by the release of cytokines, with destructive roles, e.g. TNFα and IFNγ, and with roles in repair and remyelination, e.g. IL-10. Microglia are also important in repair by removal of myelin debris, which is otherwise inhibitory for remyelinating NG2-glia (OPCs).

Action potential conduction is impeded by demyelination and also by inflammatory mediators, such as nitric oxide. Remyelination is dependent on the recruitment, proliferation and differentiation of NG2-glia, which is stimulated by factors such as PDGF-AA, FGF2, CNTF, LIF and IL-6 present within lesions. Chronic activation of microglia leads to neuronal loss in later stages of the disease and, in response to chronic tissue injury, there is astrogliosis and scar formation, which can act as a mechanical and biochemical barrier for repair. In addition, disruption of normal homeostatic functions in scar astrocytes can promulgate neuronal and oligodendrocyte degeneration. The astroglial scar contains factors that inhibit remyelination, including elements of Wnt and Notch signalling (see Chapter 5). Notably, in primary progressive MS, there is significant axonal degeneration, which can occur with or without a preceding inflammatory phase.

The precise mechanisms that determine the progression of MS, and the role of different cellular elements in it, remains unresolved. Particularly interesting is the question of the initiation of oligodendroglial death, which can involve the $Ca^{2+}$ toxic route. There are some indications that incubation of oligodendrocytes with antibodies to MOG may trigger $[Ca^{2+}]_i$ elevations and activation of intracellular kinases. Moreover, both ATP- and glutamate-mediated $Ca^{2+}$ dependent excitoxicity are implicated in oligodendrocyte loss in MS (Matute, 2011). Oligodendroglial $P2X_7$ and $P2Y_{12}$ receptors are implicated in MS.

Although MS is a white matter disease, the incidence of demyelination and axonal injury is prominent also in gray matter. Analysis of post-mortem samples demonstrates that decreased expression of $P2Y_{12}$ receptors is directly correlated with the extent of demyelination found in all types of gray matter cortical plaques and subcortical white matter.

## 10.14.2 Neuromyelitis optica

Neuromyelitis optica (NMO) or Devic's disease (Thornton *et al.*, 2011), is an inflammatory demyelinating disease that lesions the optic nerves and spinal cord. This disease is characterised by an appearance of the so-called NMO immuno-globulin G autoantibody (NMO-IgG) in blood. This antibody selectively binds to the astroglial water channel aquaporin-4, AQP4 (see Chapter 4). Indeed, the AQP4 channel is absent from neuromyelitis optica affected nerve tissues and, therefore, this disease may reflect autoimmune astrogliopathology (see De Keyser *et al.*, 2008, for review and references).

## 10.15 Infectious diseases

### 10.15.1 Bacterial and viral infections

Bacterial and viral infections of brain parenchyma invariably trigger reactive astrogliosis and activation of microglia. These processes may be local (e.g. in the case of brain abscesses) or diffuse (e.g. upon encephalitis). Reactive astrogliosis and activation of microglia are components of the brain's defence reaction and, in fact, their success very much determines the outcome of infection.

Glial reactions can be acute (e.g. in the case of acute meningitis or encephalitis) or chronic (e.g. upon infections evoked by *Toxoplasma gondii*, which persists in neurones). Sometimes, glial reactions can be the first step in pathogenesis of the disease, which often happens upon viral infections such as HIV (see below) or Borna virus. In the latter case, reactive astrogliosis occurs prior to the onset of encephalitis, and astrocytes begin to produce many inflammatory proteins, including interferon-γ-inducible protein and inflammatory protein-10, which are important for further development of the disease.

It is quite possible that astrocytes become infected by Borna viruses early in the progression of the disease, and the virus-stimulated secretion of chemokines and cytokines, as well as inflammatory proteins, is important for the attraction of invading T lymphocytes able to cope with viral infection. In particular, astroglial synthesis and release of inflammatory protein-10 is a possible general reaction of astroglia to viruses, as similar changes have been observed during CNS infections with hepatitis virus, adenovirus and lymphocytic choriomeningitis virus. Inflammatory protein-10 also has a direct antiviral effect against herpes simplex virus.

Bacterial infections usually affect the subarachnoid space and result in meningitis without affecting the brain parenchyma. Therefore, as a rule, glial reactions are relatively mild. Bacterial meningitis results in activation of numerous immunological responses, including activation of the complement system and release of C3a and C5a anaphylatoxins. The reactive glial cells are concentrated in brain layers located closely to the meninges, and may participate in local defensive and immune reactions. Certain bacterial infections, such as infections with gram-positive *Streptococcus pneumonia,* may trigger over-activation of microglia (indeed, the pneumococcal cell walls are extremely efficient microglia activators), which may, in turn, be involved in diffuse brain damage. Microglial activation may be a reason for the exceptionally high mortality and treatment resistance of gram-positive brain infections.

## 10.15.2  Human immunodeficiency virus (HIV) infection

Brain damage is a frequent outcome of acquired immunodeficiency syndrome (AIDS), the pathology manifesting in a form of *HIV-encephalitis* (*HIVE*). The latter progresses through cognitive impairments, psychomotor abnormalities (including ataxia), towards severe *HIV-associated dementia* (*HAD*). In addition to HAD, AIDS also produces HIV-related sensory neuropathies. The combined prevalence of HIV-associated dementia and sensory neuropathies can reach up to 50 per cent in patients.

Microglia and perivascular macrophages are the principal targets for HIV infection of the brain; the virus essentially cannot infect neurones. To infect the cells, the HIV uses surface receptors for chemokines (e.g. CD4 or CCR5) which, in the brain parenchyma, are mostly associated with microglia. The virus can invade the brain very soon after infection, yet at the latent stages it does not result in any productive infection. There are some indications that, during this latent stage, the virus can survive in the brain within the microglial cells, the latter serving as a reservoir (a so-called Trojan horse) for HIV, which can re-infect the periphery. This is particularly important in the targeting of antiviral drug therapies. This long-lasting presence of HIV in the brain parenchyma may explain the appearance of

CNS-specific strain variances. Viral HAD commences only after onset of AIDS, and then the production of virus in the CNS is very significant.

Histopathologically, HAD is manifested by prominent neuronal death (usually through the apoptotic pathway) – most prominent in the basal ganglia. The histological hallmark of HIVE/HAD is the appearance of *multinucleated giant cells*, which represent fused infected microglia/macrophages. Astroglial cells show fewer changes. In fact, astrocytes (which also contain surface chemokine receptors) can be readily infected by HIV *in vitro*, but their infection *in vivo* is much less documented.

The neurotoxicity in HIVE results from two principal sources: from viral products and from activated microglia/macrophages. The cytotoxic viral components are glycoprotein 120 (gp120, which assists virus binding to plasmalemmal receptors and entry into the cell), *tat* protein, which acts as a viral transactivator, and Vpr protein.

Gp120 kills neurones both *in vitro* (after being added to culture media) and *in vivo* (when gp120 was delivered by intra-hippocampal injection). Direct induction of astroglial expression of gp120 in transgenic mice resulted in the development of brain damage similar to HIVE. The actual neurotoxic action of gp120 is mediated through disruption of neuronal $Ca^{2+}$ homeostasis and $Ca^{2+}$ excitotoxicity. Gp120 can cause both sustained $Ca^{2+}$ entry and massive $Ca^{2+}$ release from the ER stores, and the combination of the two causes $Ca^{2+}$ overload and cell death.

*Tat* protein also induces neuronal apoptosis, which can be initiated through $Ca^{2+}$ dyshomeostasis. *Tat* protein was reported to induce substantial increases in neuronal $[Ca^{2+}]_i$ through activation of NMDA receptors, which led to neuronal death, and both $Ca^{2+}$ increase and cell demise can be prevented by NMDA receptor blockers. *Tat* is also able to trigger $Ca^{2+}$ signals in microglia through CCR3 chemokine receptors, which may assist in spreading the microglial activation. Finally, *tat* may also stimulate reactive astrogliosis.

The Vpr protein triggers apoptotic neuronal death *in vitro* through yet unknown mechanisms.

The second important source of neuronal death is associated with neurotoxic agents released by activated microglia, which fully realises its pathological potential in the case of HIVE. In fact, the relative HIV production in the brain is not dramatic; it is much less, for example, than production of other neurotrophic viruses such as herpes simplex or arboviruses. Therefore, the activated microglia and macrophages may be the leading players in mediating neuronal cell death in HIVE/HAD.

## 10.15.3   Human T-lymphotropic virus type-1

Human T-lymphotropic virus type-1 (HTLV-1), which belongs to retroviruses, leads to a progressive myelopathy, manifested with demyelination and axonal loss. This virus infects astrocytes, which leads to a specific alteration of glutamate homeostasis. Infected astrocytes have reduced glutamate uptake and reduced expression/activity of glutamine synthetase. This is believed to induce excitotoxicity in oligodendrocytes, with subsequent damage to white matter (De Keyser *et al.*, 2008).

### 10.15.4  Human herpes virus-6

Human herpes virus is the cause of encephalitis which may be complicated with convulsions and epileptiform seizures especially in young children. The virus infects astrocytes and decreases expression of the glutamate transporter EAAT-1/GLAST. Reduced astroglial glutamate uptake is believed to be primarily responsible for the pathogenetic process (De Keyser *et al.*, 2008).

## 10.16  Peripheral neuropathies

### 10.16.1  Hereditary neuropathies

There are several hereditary peripheral neuropathies, associated with mutation of genes encoding either myelin- or Schwann cell-specific proteins. These genetic pathologies of Schwann cells include *Charcot-Marie-Tooth disease* (CMT), *hereditary neuropathy with liability to pressure palsies* (HNPP), *Roussy-Levy syndrome* and *congenital hypomyelinating neuropathy* (CHN).

Charcot-Marie-Tooth disease, also known as peroneal muscular atrophy, covers several disorders characterised by progressive deterioration of peripheral innervation (Berger *et al.*, 2006). At least some of the incidences of CMT disease are the autosomal-recessive demyelinating neuropathies caused by transmission of mutated gene(s) encoding the so-called *ganglioside-induced differentiation-associated protein 1* (or GDAP1), which is believed to be involved in permanent bridging of Schwann cells and axons. Other variants of CMT are associated with duplication of a large region of chromosome 17, that includes the gene PMP22. The disease is characterised by rapidly developing demyelination and axonal degradation, which trigger paralysis and early death. Additionally, some versions of CMT result from mutations in connexin 32, the main gap junctional protein in PNS myelin.

*Roussy-Levy syndrome* is a variant of CMT, which is manifested by tremor and weakness in upper limbs, sensory loss and ataxia. It may arise from the mutation of the gene encoding P0, which is involved in adhesion of compact myelin (see Chapter 5), or from chromosomal disorders, e.g. partial duplication of chromosome 17.

Hereditary neuropathy with liability to pressure palsies results from deletion of point mutation in the same chromosome 17. This affects the gene encoding PMP22, which stabilises the myelin sheath. HNPP pathology stems from dys-myelination, as numerous redundant layers, loops or folds of myelin (known as tomaculae) are produced. This altered myelin production eventually results in prominent axonal death.

Finally, congenital hypomyelinating neuropathy can be caused by various mutations which affect the production of myelin. In particular, CHN can be associated with mutations in the gene encoding periaxin, which is important for Schwann cell-axonal interactions. Alternatively, hypomyelination syndromes can result from mutations in the dystrophin gene.

## 10.16.2   Acquired inflammatory neuropathies

Acquired peripheral neuropathies are broadly classified into acute and chronic inflammatory demyelinating neuropathies (AIDP and CIDP, respectively). Clinical forms of these neuropathies are many, and all of them proceed with sensory abnormalities or motor weaknesses, or with a combination of both. Inflammatory neuropathies are autoimmune diseases.

The actual neuropathy usually follows viral infection, triggering an immune response, which turns into an autoimmune reaction aimed at myelin or protein components of Schwann cells. Important roles are played by antibodies against viral oligosaccharide components, which are, incidentally, identical to gangliosides (GM1 or GD1a) of the peripheral nerve. As a result, antibodies produced against viruses attack the body's own tissue. In addition, certain infections may produce antibodies against myelin proteins, most frequently against PMP22.

The autoreactive T-cells, bearing the autoantibodies, migrate towards the peripheral nerve and recruit macrophages (by release of cytokines and chemokines), which attack both Schwann cells and myelin sheaths. Initially, macrophages form infiltrations within the peripheral nerve and destroy the myelin. Subsequently, they phagocytose the remnants of the glial cells and demyelinated axons.

## 10.16.3   Diabetic neuropathies

Diabetic neuropathies are the most frequent complications of diabetes mellitus, which affect about 50 per cent of all patients. Clinically, the sensory neuropathies dominate and motor weakness develops rather rarely. The primary cause of nerve damage is associated with blood glucose levels; aggressive glycaemic control substantially reduces the prevalence of neuropathies. The primary target of the impaired glucose homeostasis is, however, debatable.

Traditionally, the leading aetiological factor was considered to be abnormalities in neurovascular circulation which, indeed, suffers remarkably. According to these theories, the nerve damage was a direct consequence of poor circulation, ischaemia and oxidative injury. Yet, in many cases, neuropathies develop without any obvious degradation in neurocirculation.

An alternative theory stresses the pathogenetic importance of Schwann cells, which are particularly sensitive to hyperglycaemia and undergo damage through oxidative stress. Indeed, diabetes is associated with significant morphological abnormalities of Schwann cells and high incidence of their apoptotic death. The obvious consequence of the demise of Schwann cells is demyelination and reduced nerve conductance velocity, which is the most common symptom of diabetic neuropathy.

## 10.16.4 Leprosy

Leprosy is the primary infectious disease of Schwann cells. The infectious agent, *Mycobacterium leprae*, specifically invades the Schwann cells, where it multiplies with impunity, being protected by organism-specific host immunity. The infected Schwann cells eventually die, thus triggering powerful immune reactions, which in turn destroy myelin and kill the axons, hence producing profound nerve damage. This nerve damage defines the clinical signature of the disease, which progresses as an acute neuropathy, resulting initially in anaesthetic skin patches and, later, in trophic and motor abnormalities. The pathogenic involvement of autoimmune components is important for therapeutic strategy, which currently relies on a combination of immunosuppression and anti-mycobacterial therapy.

# 10.17 Gliomas

Gliomas are tumours of the nervous system that develop from glial cells, and they account for the majority of primary brain neoplasias. Clinically, gliomas are classified, according to their malignancy (the WHO classification), into four grades. Grade I covers benign tumours (e.g. pilocytic astrocytoma), while grades II to IV are malignant neoplasias, which differ in their aggressiveness – the most violent being glioblastoma, which belongs to group IV. Histopathologically, the gliomas are divided into *astrocytomas*, *oligodendrocytomas* and *glioblastomas*, although this division mostly relates to the morphological similarity of the tumour to the respective types of microglia. However, the exact origin of the different kinds of glial tumours cannot be determined (Chen *et al.*, 2012).

Biologically, the gliomas are very different from other neoplasias, as they express several systems which adapt them to malignant growth within the CNS environment (Westphal & Lamszus, 2011). A key property of the CNS environment, compared to most tissues, is the lack of free space into which the tumour can grow and the existence of firm boundaries (skull for the brain, vertebrae for spinal cord), which present additional restraints for neoplasia expansion. The second complication of the CNS architecture, from the point of view of cancerous growth, is a very complicated structure of parenchyma, formed by extremely narrow and low volume clefts. These prevent free dissemination of malignant cells through the tissue, which is so characteristic for tumour expansion in non-brain organs. Therefore, in order to grow, gliomas must clear the space by actively eliminating the surrounding healthy cells, and actively propagating neoplasmic cells though the brain matter.

Malignant gliomas produce the room for their expansion by actively killing neurones in their vicinity. One mechanism by which this is achieved is by secretion of high amounts of glutamate which, in turn, triggers excitotoxic, NMDA- and $[Ca^{2+}]_i$-dependent neuronal death (de Groot & Sontheimer,

2011). This glutamate-induced neuronal death also results in seizures, which often accompany malignant gliomas. The amount of glutamate synthesised and released by glioma cells is truly impressive; for example, cultured glioma cells can increase glutamate concentration in their media from 1 μM to 100 μM within 5–6 hours.

Release of glutamate is mediated through an electroneutral amino acid transporter, which exchanges cystine for glutamate; this transporter is specifically expressed only in glioma cells (Figure 10.12). Glutamate excitotoxicity is critical for glioma expansion, and inhibition of the cystine/glutamate transporter (which can be blocked by 4-carboxyphenylglycine) has been shown to significantly retard their growth. Cystine brought into the glioma cells is converted into glutathione, which increases the resistance of tumour cells to oxidative stress.

The second important peculiarity of gliomas is represented by their active propagation through the nervous tissue (Claes *et al.*, 2007). Glioma cells are able to travel through the brain, for example easily migrating from one hemisphere to another. As a consequence, gliomas almost invariably disseminate through the whole brain. The mechanisms of glioma cell migration are several.

First, they express a number of metalloproteinases, which assist in breaking down the extracellular matrix, and produce migrating tunnels.

Second, glioma cells are able to undergo substantial shrinkage, which helps them to attain an elongated shape and thus penetrate into narrow interstitial compartments. This loss of glioma cell volume is supported by several families of Cl⁻ channels, which are activated by voltage or changes in osmolarity; in addition, glioma cells express Cl⁻ permeable GABA$_A$ receptors (see Cuddapah & Sontheimer, 2011). Glioma cells have a high concentration of cytoplasmic Cl⁻, which

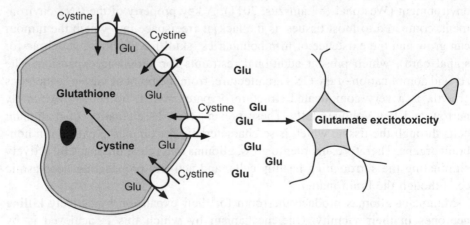

**Figure 10.12**  Glioma induced glutamate excitotoxicity and neuronal death.
Glioma cells express a high density of glutamate/cystine transporters; glutamate released by this transporter triggers excitotoxic neuronal death, thus clearing space for glioma invasion.

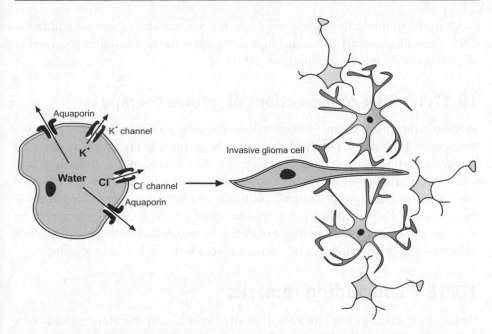

**Figure 10.13** Chloride and potassium channels assist glioma cell shrinkage; decrease in glioma cell volume greatly facilitates their invasive capabilities.

To shrink, glioma cells release $K^+$ and $Cl^-$ through ion channels, which induce water to leave the cells through aquaporins. The maintenance of $K^+$ and $Cl^-$ concentration in glioma is accomplished by the activity of the NKCC $Cl^-$ transporter and the $Na^+$-$K^+$ ATPase.

Redrawn from McFerrin & Sontheimer, 2006.

sets the $Cl^-$ reversal potential at levels more positive than the resting potential (-40 mV). Activation of $Cl^-$ channels therefore leads to $Cl^-$ efflux, which in turn drives water out of the cell, reducing its volume (Figure 10.13). Inhibition of $Cl^-$ channels arrests the motility of glioma cells.

Third, glioma migration is also driven by cytosolic $Ca^{2+}$ oscillations, which results from the activation of $Ca^{2+}$-permeable AMPA receptors. Inhibition of $Ca^{2+}$ permeability of AMPA receptors suppresses glioma dissemination and limits the tumour growth.

Finally, gliomas remodel brain defensive systems and utilise them for expansion. Indeed, gliomas tumour tissues contain unusually high density of microglia (up to 30 per cent). These microglial cells, however, do not attack glioma cells, but rather facilitative their expansion; experimental ablation of microglia substantially slows down growth of glioma tumours. These microglial effects are mediated most likely through specific expression of membrane type 1 matrix metalloprotease stimulated by glioma-derived signalling factors (Charles *et al.*, 2012; Markovic *et al.*, 2011).

All in all, glioma cells utilise several specific mechanisms to expand within the CNS. These mechanisms also render high malignancy and rapid clinical progression of glial-derived tumours (Sontheimer, 2003).

## 10.17.1    Glial complications of glioma therapy

Irradiation therapy of gliomas often results in cognitive and memory decline of a yet undiscovered nature. One of the current hypotheses highlights the role of activated hippocampal microglia, which may interfere with neurogenesis. Indeed, it was found that irradiation of the brain causes activation of microglia and inhibition of neurogenesis, and a very similar result was obtained after intra-hippocampal injections of LPS, which is a powerful microglial activator. Neurogenesis can be restored, and activation of microglia placated, by anti-inflammatory drugs such as indomethacin, or by inhibitors of microglial activation such as minocycline.

# 10.18    Concluding remarks

Neurological diseases are almost universally defined, and therefore treated, as a malfunction of neurones. This neurocentric view is being challenged by the wealth of recent data indicating the primary role of neuroglia in homeostasis and defence of nervous tissue. Indeed, neuroglial cells contribute to initiation and development of many (if not all) neuropathological processes.

The specific reactions of neuroglial cells to various diseases are multifaceted and most likely pathology-specific. Yet, to a very large extent, glial responses determine the progression and outcome of neuropathological process. The majority of therapeutic approaches currently in clinical use target neurones, but it seems likely that future therapeutic efforts may benefit by a stronger focus on neuroglia.

# References

Alexander WS. (1949). Progressive fibrinoid degeneration of fibrillary astrocytes associated with mental retardation in a hydrocephalic infant. *Brain* **72**(3), 373–381.

Allaman I, Gavillet M, Belanger M, Laroche T, Viertl D, Lashuel HA, Magistretti PJ. (2010). Amyloid-b aggregates cause alterations of astrocytic metabolic phenotype: impact on neuronal viability. *Journal of Neuroscience* **30**(9), 3326–38.

Alzheimer A. (1907). Über eine eigenartige Erkrankung der Hirnrinde. *Allg Z Psychiat Psych-Gericht Med* **64**, 146–148.

Alzheimer A. (1910). *Beiträge zur Kenntnis der pathologischen Neuroglia und ihrer Beziehungen zu den Abbauvorgängen im Nervengewebe*. In: *Nissl F, Alzheimer A, editors. Histologische und histopathologische Arbeiten über die Grosshirnrinde mit besonderer Berücksichtigung der pathologischen Anatomie der Geisteskrankheiten*. Jena: Gustav Fischer. p 401–562.

Aronica E, Ravizza T, Zurolo E, Vezzani A. (2012). Astrocyte immune responses in epilepsy. *Glia* **60**(8), 1258–1268.

Ayata C, Ropper AH. (2002). Ischaemic brain oedema. *Journal of Clinical Neuroscience* **9**(2), 113–24.

Beers DR, Henkel JS, Xiao Q, Zhao WH, Wang JH, Yen AA, Siklos L, McKercher SR, Appel SH. (2006). Wild-type microglia extend survival in PU.1 knockout mice with familial amyotrophic lateral sclerosis. *Proceedings of The National Academy Of Sciences Of The United States Of America* **103**(43), 16021–16026.

Bell RD, Zlokovic BV. (2009). Neurovascular mechanisms and blood-brain barrier disorder in Alzheimer's disease. *Acta Neuropathologica* **118**(1), 103–13.

Berger P, Niemann A, Suter U. (2006). Schwann cells and the pathogenesis of inherited motor and sensory neuropathies (Charcot-Marie-Tooth disease). *Glia* **54**(4), 243–57.

Bernstein HG, Steiner J, Bogerts B. (2009). Glial cells in schizophrenia: pathophysiological significance and possible consequences for therapy. *Expert Review of Neurotherapeutics* **9**(7), 1059–71.

Bianchin MM, Capella HM, Chaves DL, Steindel M, Grisard EC, Ganev GG, da Silva Junior JP, Neto Evaldo S, Poffo MA, Walz R. *et al.* (2004). Nasu-Hakola disease (polycystic lipomembranous osteodysplasia with sclerosing leukoencephalopathy-PLOSL): a dementia associated with bone cystic lesions. From clinical to genetic and molecular aspects. *Cellular and Molecular Neurobiology* **24**(1), 1–24.

Bianchin MM, Martin KC, de Souza AC, de Oliveira MA, Rieder CR. (2010). Nasu-Hakola disease and primary microglial dysfunction. *Nature Reviews Neurology* **6**(9), 2 p following 523.

Blumenthal I. (2004). Periventricular leucomalacia: a review. *European Journal of Pediatrics* **163**(8), 435–42.

Boillee S, Yamanaka K, Lobsiger CS, Copeland NG, Jenkins NA, Kassiotis G, Kollias G, Cleveland DW. (2006). Onset and progression in inherited ALS determined by motor neurons and microglia. *Science* **312**(5778), 1389–1392.

Broe M, Kril J, Halliday GM. (2004). Astrocytic degeneration relates to the severity of disease in frontotemporal dementia. *Brain* **127**(Pt 10), 2214–20.

Brun N, Robitaille Y, Grignon A, Robinson BH, Mitchell GA, Lambert M. (1999). Pyruvate carboxylase deficiency: prenatal onset of ischemia-like brain lesions in two sibs with the acute neonatal form. *American Journal of Medical Genetics* **84**(2), 94–101.

Brusilow SW, Koehler RC, Traystman RJ, Cooper AJ. (2010). Astrocyte glutamine synthetase: importance in hyperammonemic syndromes and potential target for therapy. *Neurotherapeutics* **7**(4), 452–70.

Butterworth RF. (2010). Altered glial-neuronal crosstalk: cornerstone in the pathogenesis of hepatic encephalopathy. *Neurochemistry International* **57**(4), 383–8.

Butterworth RF. (2011). Hepatic encephalopathy: a central neuroinflammatory disorder? *Hepatology* **53**(4), 1372–6.

Campana WM. (2007). Schwann cells: activated peripheral glia and their role in neuropathic pain. *Brain, Behavior, and Immunity* **21**(5), 522–7.

Carmignoto G, Haydon PG. (2012). Astrocyte calcium signaling and epilepsy. *Glia* **60**(8), 1227–1233.

Charcot JM. (1868). Histologie de la sclerose en plaques. *Gazette des hopitaux Paris* **41**, 554–555.

Charcot JM. (1881). *Amyotrophic lateral sclerosis: symptomatology. Lectures on diseases of the nervous system*. London: New Sydenham Society. p 192–204.

Charcot JM, Joffroy A. (1869). Deux cas d'atrophie musculaire progressive avec lesions de la substance grise et de faisceaux anterolateraux de la moelle epiniere. *Arch Physiol Norm Pathol* **1**, 354–367.

Charles NA, Holland EC, Gilbertson R, Glass R, Kettenmann H. (2012). The brain tumor microenvironment. *Glia* **60**(3), 502–14.

Chen J, McKay RM, Parada LF. (2012). Malignant glioma: lessons from genomics, mouse models, and stem cells. *Cell* **149**(1), 36–47.

Cho W, Brenner M, Peters N, Messing A. (2010). Drug screening to identify suppressors of GFAP expression. *Human Molecular Genetics* **19**(16), 3169–78.

Claes A, Idema AJ, Wesseling P. (2007). Diffuse glioma growth: a guerilla war. *Acta Neuropathologica* **114**(5), 443–58.

Compston A, Coles A. (2008). Multiple Sclerosis. *The Lancet* **372**, 25–31.

Cooper AJ, Plum F. (1987). Biochemistry and physiology of brain ammonia. *Physiological Reviews* **67**(2), 440–519.

Coull JA, Beggs S, Boudreau D, Boivin D, Tsuda M, Inoue K, Gravel C, Salter MW, De Koninck Y. (2005). BDNF from microglia causes the shift in neuronal anion gradient underlying neuropathic pain. *Nature* **438**(7070), 1017–21.

Coulter DA, Eid T. (2012). Astrocytic regulation of glutamate homeostasis in epilepsy. *Glia* **60**(8), 1215–1226.

Cuddapah VA, Sontheimer H. (2011). Ion channels and transporters [corrected] in cancer. 2. Ion channels and the control of cancer cell migration. *American Journal of Physiology. Cell Physiology* **301**(3), C541–9.

Davis KL, Stewart DG, Friedman JI, Buchsbaum M, Harvey PD, Hof PR, Buxbaum J, Haroutunian V. (2003). White matter changes in schizophrenia: evidence for myelin-related dysfunction. *Archives of General Psychiatry* **60**(5), 443–56.

de Groot J, Sontheimer H. (2011). Glutamate and the biology of gliomas. *Glia* **59**(8), 1181–9.

De Keyser J, Mostert JP, Koch MW. (2008). Dysfunctional astrocytes as key players in the pathogenesis of central nervous system disorders. *Journal of The Neurological Sciences* **267**(1–2), 3–16.

Derecki NC, Cronk JC, Lu Z, Xu E, Abbott SB, Guyenet PG, Kipnis J. (2012). Wild-type microglia arrest pathology in a mouse model of Rett syndrome. *Nature* **484**(7392), 105–9.

Dreier JP. (2011). The role of spreading depression, spreading depolarization and spreading ischemia in neurological disease. *Nature Medicine* **17**(4), 439–47.

Eicke WJ. (1962). Polycystische Umwandlung des Marklagers mit progredientem Verlauf. *European Archives of Psychiatry and Clinical Neuroscience* **203**, 599–609.

Eikermann-Haerter K, Ayata C. (2010). Cortical spreading depression and migraine. *Current Neurology and Neuroscience Reports* **10**(3), 167–73.

Eng LF, Lee YL, Kwan H, Brenner M, Messing A. (1998). Astrocytes cultured from transgenic mice carrying the added human glial fibrillary acidic protein gene contain Rosenthal fibers. *Journal of Neuroscience Research* **53**(3), 353–60.

Estrada-Sánchez AM, Rebec GV. (2012). Corticostriatal dysfunction and glutamate transporter 1 (GLT1) in Huntington's disease: Interactions between neurons and astrocytes. Basal Ganglia in press.

Forman MS, Lal D, Zhang B, Dabir DV, Swanson E, Lee VM, Trojanowski JQ. (2005). Transgenic mouse model of tau pathology in astrocytes leading to nervous system degeneration. *Journal of Neuroscience* **25**(14), 3539–50.

Gao YJ, Ji RR. (2010). Targeting astrocyte signaling for chronic pain. *Neurotherapeutics* **7**(4), 482–93.

Grafstein B. (2011). Subverting the hegemony of the synapse: complicity of neurons, astrocytes, and vasculature in spreading depression and pathology of the cerebral cortex. *Brain Research Reviews* **66**(1–2), 123–32.

Grinberg YY, Milton JG, Kraig RP. (2011). Spreading depression sends microglia on Levy flights. *PLoS One* **6**(4), e19294.

Gunnarson E, Axehult G, Baturina G, Zelenin S, Zelenina M, Aperia A. (2005). Lead induces increased water permeability in astrocytes expressing aquaporin 4. *Neuroscience* **136**(1), 105–14.

Haberle J, Gorg B, Rutsch F, Schmidt E, Toutain A, Benoist JF, Gelot A, Suc AL, Hohne W, Schliess F. *et al.* (2005). Congenital glutamine deficiency with glutamine synthetase mutations. *New England Journal of Medicine* **353**(18), 1926–33.

Hazell AS. (2009). Astrocytes are a major target in thiamine deficiency and Wernicke's encephalopathy. *Neurochemistry International* **55**(1–3), 129–35.

Hazell AS, Sheedy D, Oanea R, Aghourian M, Sun S, Jung JY, Wang D, Wang C. (2009). Loss of astrocytic glutamate transporters in Wernicke encephalopathy. *Glia* **58**, 148–156.

Heinemann U, Kaufer D, Friedman A. (2012). Blood-brain barrier dysfunction, TGFβ signaling, and astrocyte dysfunction in epilepsy. *Glia* **60**(8), 1251–1257.

Heneka MT, Sastre M, Dumitrescu-Ozimek L, Dewachter I, Walter J, Klockgether T, Van Leuven F. (2005). Focal glial activation coincides with increased BACE1 activation and precedes amyloid plaque deposition in APP[V717I] transgenic mice. *Journal of Neuroinflammation* **2**(1), 22.

Heneka MT, Rodriguez JJ, Verkhratsky A. (2010). Neuroglia in neurodegeneration. *Brain Research Reviews* in press.

Huntington G. (1872). On chorea. *Med Surg Rep (Philadelphia)* **26**, 317–321.

Inoue K, Tsuda M. (2009). Microglia and neuropathic pain. *Glia* **57**(14), 1469–79.

Inoue K, Tsuda M. (2012). Purinergic systems, neuropathic pain and the role of microglia. *Experimental Neurology* **234**(2), 293–301.

Jacobs S, Cheng C, Doering LC. (2012). Probing astrocyte function in fragile X syndrome. *Results and Problems In Cell Differentiation* **54**, 15–31.

Jeworutzki E, Lopez-Hernandez T, Capdevila-Nortes X, Sirisi S, Bengtsson L, Montolio M, Zifarelli G, Arnedo T, Muller CS, Schulte U. *et al.* (2012). GlialCAM, a protein defective in a leukodystrophy, serves as a ClC-2 Cl( ) channel auxiliary subunit. *Neuron* **73**(5), 951–61.

Johnson AB. (1996). Alexander disease. In: Moser HW. (ed.). *Handbook of clinical neurology.* Amsterdam: Elsevier. p 701–710.

Josephs KA. (2008). Frontotemporal dementia and related disorders: deciphering the enigma. *Annals of Neurology* **64**(1), 4–14.

Kanner L. (1943). Autistic disturbances of affective contact. *Nervous Child* **2**, 217–250.

Kaul M, Garden GA, Lipton SA. (2001). Pathways to neuronal injury and apoptosis in HIV-associated dementia. *Nature* **410**(6831), 988–94.

Kersaitis C, Halliday GM, Kril JJ. (2004). Regional and cellular pathology in frontotemporal dementia: relationship to stage of disease in cases with and without Pick bodies. *Acta Neuropathologica* **108**(6), 515–23.

Kettenmann H, Hanisch UK, Noda M, Verkhratsky A. (2011). Physiology of microglia. *Physiological Reviews* **91**(2), 461–553.

Knight RA, Verkhratsky A. (2010). Neurodegenerative diseases: failures in brain connectivity? *Cell Death & Differentiation* **17**(7), 1069–70.

Komori T. (1999). Tau-positive glial inclusions in progressive supranuclear palsy, corticobasal degeneration and Pick's disease. *Brain Pathology* **9**(4), 663–79.

Korsakoff SS, Корсаков СС. (1889). Психическое расстройство в сочетании с множественным невритом (psychosis polineuritica, s. cerebropathia psychica toxaemica). English translation: Korsakoff, SS. Psychic disorder in conjunction with multiple neuritis,

Translated from Russian by Victor, M. and Yakovlev, Neurology (1955), 5, 394–406. *Мед обозр* **32**, 3–18.

Kuchibhotla KV, Lattarulo CR, Hyman BT, Bacskai BJ. (2009). Synchronous hyperactivity and intercellular calcium waves in astrocytes in Alzheimer mice. *Science* **323**(5918), 1211–5.

Lassmann H. (2005). Multiple sclerosis pathology: evolution of pathogenetic concepts. *Brain Pathology* **15**(3), 217–22.

Leão AAP. (1944). Spreading depression of activity in the cerebral cortex. *Journal of Neurophysiology* **7**, 359–390.

Leo L, Gherardini L, Barone V, De Fusco M, Pietrobon D, Pizzorusso T, Casari G. (2011). Increased susceptibility to cortical spreading depression in the mouse model of familial hemiplegic migraine type 2. *PLoS Genetics* **7**(6), e1002129.

Li R, Johnson AB, Salomons G, Goldman JE, Naidu S, Quinlan R, Cree B, Ruyle SZ, Banwell B, D'Hooghe M. *et al.* (2005). Glial fibrillary acidic protein mutations in infantile, juvenile, and adult forms of Alexander disease. *Annals of Neurology* **57**(3), 310–26.

Libon DJ, Price CC, Davis Garrett K, Giovannetti T. (2004). From Binswanger's disease to leuokoaraiosis: what we have learned about subcortical vascular dementia. *The Clinical Neuropsychologist* **18**(1), 83–100.

Lioy DT, Garg SK, Monaghan CE, Raber J, Foust KD, Kaspar BK, Hirrlinger PG, Kirchhoff F, Bissonnette JM, Ballas N. *et al.* (2011). A role for glia in the progression of Rett's syndrome. *Nature* **475**(7357), 497–500.

Lopez-Hernandez T, Ridder MC, Montolio M, Capdevila-Nortes X, Polder E, Sirisi S, Duarri A, Schulte U, Fakler B, Nunes V. *et al.* (2011). Mutant GlialCAM causes megalencephalic leukoencephalopathy with subcortical cysts, benign familial macrocephaly, and macrocephaly with retardation and autism. *American Journal of Human Genetics* **88**(4), 422–32.

Markovic DS, Vinnakota K, van Rooijen N, Kiwit J, Synowitz M, Glass R, Kettenmann H. (2011). Minocycline reduces glioma expansion and invasion by attenuating microglial MT1-MMP expression. *Brain, Behavior, and Immunity* **25**(4), 624–8.

Matute C. (2011). Glutamate and ATP signalling in white matter pathology. *Journal of Anatomy* **219**(1), 53–64.

McAlpine D, Araki S. (1958). Minamata disease: an unusual neurological disorder caused by contaminated fish. *Lancet* **2**(7047), 629–31.

McFerrin MB, Sontheimer H. (2006). A role for ion channels in glioma cell invasion. *Neuron Glia Biology* **2**(1), 39–49.

McGeer PL, McGeer EG. (2008). Glial reactions in Parkinson's disease. *Movement Disorders* **23**(4), 474–83.

Mena MA, Garcia de Yebenes J. (2008). Glial cells as players in parkinsonism: the "good," the "bad," and the "mysterious" glia. *Neuroscientist* **14**(6), 544–60.

Mena MA, Casarejos MJ, Carazo A, Paino CL, Garcia de Yebenes J. (1996). *Glia* conditioned medium protects fetal rat midbrain neurones in culture from L-DOPA toxicity. *Neuroreport* **7**(2), 441–5.

Messing A, Brenner M, Feany MB, Nedergaard M, Goldman JE. (2012). Alexander disease. *Journal of Neuroscience* **32**(15), 5017–23.

Messing A, Daniels CM, Hagemann TL. (2010). Strategies for treatment in Alexander disease. *Neurotherapeutics* **7**(4), 507–15.

Meyer-Luehmann M, Spires-Jones TL, Prada C, Garcia-Alloza M, de Calignon A, Rozkalne A, Koenigsknecht-Talboo J, Holtzman DM, Bacskai BJ, Hyman BT. (2008). Rapid appearance and local toxicity of amyloid-beta plaques in a mouse model of Alzheimer's disease. *Nature* **451**(7179), 720–4.

Mosconi L, Pupi A, De Leon MJ. (2008). Brain glucose hypometabolism and oxidative stress in preclinical Alzheimer's disease. *Annals of The New York Academy Of Sciences* **1147**, 180–95.

Murray TJ. (2009). The history of multiple sclerosis: the changing frame of the disease over the centuries. *Journal of The Neurological Sciences* **277**(Suppl 1), S3–8.

Nagele RG, Wegiel J, Venkataraman V, Imaki H, Wang KC. (2004). Contribution of glial cells to the development of amyloid plaques in Alzheimer's disease. *Neurobiology of Aging* **25**(5), 663–74.

Nedergaard M, Cooper AJ, Goldman SA. (1995). Gap junctions are required for the propagation of spreading depression. *Journal of Neurobiology* **28**(4), 433–44.

Oberheim NA, Tian GF, Han X, Peng W, Takano T, Ransom B, Nedergaard M. (2008). Loss of astrocytic domain organization in the epileptic brain. *Journal of Neuroscience* **28**(13), 3264–76.

Oide T, Yoshida K, Kaneko K, Ohta M, Arima K. (2006). Iron overload and antioxidative role of perivascular astrocytes in aceruloplasminemia. *Neuropathology and Applied Neurobiology* **32**(2), 170–6.

Olabarria M, Noristani HN, Verkhratsky A, Rodriguez JJ. (2010). Concomitant astroglial atrophy and astrogliosis in a triple transgenic animal model of Alzheimer's disease. *Glia* **58**, 831–838.

Palop JJ, Mucke L. (2010). Amyloid-beta-induced neuronal dysfunction in Alzheimer's disease: from synapses toward neural networks. *Nature Neuroscience* **13**(7), 812–8.

Parkinson J. (1817). *An Essay on the Shaking Palsy* (also available in *Journal of Neuropsychiatry and Clinical Neurosciences* (2002), **14**, 223–226). London: Sherwood, Neely, and Jones.

Parpura V, Heneka MT, Montana V, Oliet SH, Schousboe A, Haydon PG, Stout RF, Jr., Spray DC, Reichenbach A, Pannicke T. *et al.* (2012). Glial cells in (patho)physiology. *Journal of Neurochemistry* **121**(1), 4–27.

Patel SC, Suresh S, Kumar U, Hu CY, Cooney A, Blanchette-Mackie EJ, Neufeld EB, Patel RC, Brady RO, Patel Y.C. *et al.* (1999). Localization of Niemann-Pick C1 protein in astrocytes: implications for neuronal degeneration in Niemann- Pick type C disease. *Proceedings of The National Academy Of Sciences Of The United States Of America* **96**(4), 1657 62.

Penfield W, Humphreys S. (1940). Epileptogenic lesions of the brain. A histologic study. *Archives of Neurology & Psychiatryy* **43**, 240–259.

Potts R, Leech RW. (2005). Thalamic dementia: an example of primary astroglial dystrophy of Seitelberger. *Clinical Neuropathology* **24**(6), 271–5.

Prust M, Wang J, Morizono H, Messing A, Brenner M, Gordon E, Hartka T, Sokohl A, Schiffmann R, Gordish-Dressman H. *et al.* (2011). GFAP mutations, age at onset, and clinical subtypes in Alexander disease. *Neurology* **77**(13), 1287–94.

Rajkowska G, Miguel-Hidalgo JJ. (2007). Gliogenesis and glial pathology in depression. *CNS & Neurological Disorders – Drug Targets* **6**(3), 219–33.

Rodriguez JJ, Verkhratsky A. (2011). Neuroglial roots of neurodegenerative diseases? *Molecular Neurobiology* **43**(2), 87–96.

Rodriguez JJ, Olabarria M, Chvatal A, Verkhratsky A. (2009). Astroglia in dementia and Alzheimer's disease. *Cell Death & Differentiation* **16**(3), 378–85.

Rodriguez JJ, Witton J, Olabarria M, Noristani HN, Verkhratsky A. (2010). Increase in the density of resting microglia precedes neuritic plaque formation and microglial activation in a transgenic model of Alzheimer's disease. *Cell Death and Disease* **1**, e1.

Rosenbaum AI, Maxfield FR. (2011). Niemann-Pick type C disease: molecular mechanisms and potential therapeutic approaches. *Journal of Neurochemistry* **116**(5), 789–95.

Rossi D, Volterra A. (2009). Astrocytic dysfunction: Insights on the role in neurodegeneration. *Brain Research Bulletin* **80**, 224–232.

Rossi D, Brambilla L, Valori CF, Roncoroni C, Crugnola A, Yokota T, Bredesen DE, Volterra A. (2008). Focal degeneration of astrocytes in amyotrophic lateral sclerosis. *Cell Death & Differentiation* **15**(11), 1691–700.

Rossi DJ, Brady JD, Mohr C. (2007). Astrocyte metabolism and signaling during brain ischemia. *Nature Neuroscience* **10**(11), 1377–86.

Rossner S, Lange-Dohna C, Zeitschel U, Perez-Polo JR. (2005). Alzheimer's disease beta-secretase BACE1 is not a neuron-specific enzyme. *Journal of Neurochemistry* **92**(2), 226–34.

Saadoun S, Papadopoulos MC. (2010). Aquaporin-4 in brain and spinal cord oedema. *Neuroscience* **168**(4), 1036–46.

Satoh J, Tabunoki H, Ishida T, Yagishita S, Jinnai K, Futamura N, Kobayashi M, Toyoshima I, Yoshioka T, Enomoto K. *et al.* (2011). Immunohistochemical characterization of microglia in Nasu-Hakola disease brains. *Neuropathology* **31**(4), 363–75.

Segal D, Koschnick JR, Slegers LH, Hof PR. (2007). Oligodendrocyte pathophysiology: a new view of schizophrenia. *International Journal of Neuropsychopharmacology* **10**(4), 503–11.

Seidel JL, Shuttleworth CW. (2011). Contribution of astrocyte glycogen stores to progression of spreading depression and related events in hippocampal slices. *Neuroscience* **192**, 295–303.

Seifert G, Steinhauser C. (2011). Neuron-astrocyte signaling and epilepsy. *Experimental Neurology*.

Seifert G, Carmignoto G, Steinhauser C. (2010). Astrocyte dysfunction in epilepsy. *Brain Research Reviews* **63**(1–2), 212–21.

Simard JM, Kent TA, Chen M, Tarasov KV, Gerzanich V. (2007). Brain oedema in focal ischaemia: molecular pathophysiology and theoretical implications. *The Lancet Neurology* **6**(3), 258–68.

Solito E, Sastre M. (2012). Microglia function in Alzheimer's disease. *Frontiers in Pharmacology* **3**, 14.

Sontheimer H. (2003). Malignant gliomas: perverting glutamate and ion homeostasis for selective advantage. *Trends In Neurosciences* **26**(10), 543–9.

Steinhauser C, Seifert G, Bedner P. (2012). Astrocyte dysfunction in temporal lobe epilepsy: K(+) channels and gap junction coupling. *Glia* **60**(8), 1192–1202.

Streit WJ. (2010). Microglial activation and neuroinflammation in Alzheimer's disease: a critical examination of recent history. *Frontiers in Aging Neuroscience* **2**, 22.

Streit WJ, Braak H, Xue QS, Bechmann I. (2009). Dystrophic (senescent) rather than activated microglial cells are associated with tau pathology and likely precede neurodegeneration in Alzheimer's disease. *Acta Neuropathologica* **118**(4), 475–85.

Strokin M, Seburn KL, Cox GA, Martens KA, Reiser G. (2012). Severe disturbance in the $Ca^{2+}$ signaling in astrocytes from mouse models of human infantile neuroaxonal dystrophy with mutated Pla2g6. *Human Molecular Genetics* **21**(12), 2807–14.

Struys-Ponsar C, Guillard O, van den Bosch de Aguilar P. (2000). Effects of aluminum exposure on glutamate metabolism: a possible explanation for its toxicity. *Experimental Neurology* **163**(1), 157–64.

Suarez-Fernandez MB, Soldado AB, Sanz-Medel A, Vega JA, Novelli A, Fernandez-Sanchez MT. (1999). Aluminum-induced degeneration of astrocytes occurs via apoptosis and results in neuronal death. *Brain Research* **835**(2), 125–36.

Sugaya E, Takato M, Noda Y. (1975). neuronal and glial activity during spreading depression in cerebral cortex of cat. *Journal of Neurophysiology* **38**(4), 822–41.

Takano T, Oberheim N, Cotrina ML, Nedergaard M. (2009). Astrocytes and ischemic injury. *Stroke* **40**(3 Suppl), S8–12.

Takeda M, Takahashi M, Matsumoto S. (2009). Contribution of the activation of satellite glia in sensory ganglia to pathological pain. *Neuroscience and Biobehavioral Reviews* **33**(6), 784–92.

Terry RD. (2000). Cell death or synaptic loss in Alzheimer disease. *Journal of Neuropathology and Experimental Neurology* **59**(12), 1118–9.

Tetreault NA, Hakeem AY, Jiang S, Williams BA, Allman E, Wold BJ, Allman JM. (2012). Microglia in the Cerebral Cortex in Autism. *Journal of Autism and Developmental Disorders*.

Thompson KA, McArthur JC, Wesselingh SL. (2001). Correlation between neurological progression and astrocyte apoptosis in HIV-associated dementia. *Annals of Neurology* **49**(6), 745–52.

Thornton IL, Rizzo JF, Cestari DM. (2011). Neuromyelitis optica: a review. *Seminars in Ophthalmology* **26**(4–5), 337–41.

Tian GF, Azmi H, Takano T, Xu Q, Peng W, Lin J, Oberheim N, Lou N, Wang X, Zielke H.R. *et al.* (2005). An astrocytic basis of epilepsy. *Nature Medicine* **11**(9), 973–81.

Tsuda M, Inoue K, Salter MW. (2005). Neuropathic pain and spinal microglia: a big problem from molecules in "small" glia. *Trends In Neurosciences* **28**(2), 101–7.

Turner BJ, Talbot K. (2008). Transgenics, toxicity and therapeutics in rodent models of mutant SOD1-mediated familial ALS. *Progress In Neurobiology* **85**(1), 94–134.

Turner MR, Cagnin A, Turkheimer FE, Miller CCJ, Shaw CE. (2004). Evidence of widespread cerebral microglial activation in amyotrophic lateral sclerosis: an [C-11](R)-PK11195 positron emission tomography study 1. *Neurobiology of Disease* **15**(3), 601–609.

van Caulaert C, Deviller C. (1932). Ammoniémie expérimentale après ingestion de chlorure d'ammonium chez l'homme à l'état normal et pathologique. *Compt Rend Soc Biol (Paris)* **111**, 50–52.

van der Knaap MS, Pronk JC, Scheper GC. (2006). Vanishing white matter disease. *The Lancet Neurology* **5**(5), 413–23.

Vangeison G, Rempe DA. (2009). The Janus-faced effects of hypoxia on astrocyte function. *Neuroscientist* **15**(6), 579–88.

Verkhratsky A, Olabarria M, Noristani HN, Yeh CY, Rodriguez JJ. (2010). Astrocytes in Alzheimer's disease. *Neurotherapeutics* **7**(4), 399–412.

Verkhratsky A, Sofroniew MV, Messing A, Delancrolle NC, Rempe D, Rodriguez JJ, Nedergaard M. (2012). Neurological diseases as primary gliopathies: a reassessment of neurocentrism. *ASN Neuro* **4**(3).

Wernicke C. (1881–1883). *Lehrbuch der Gehirnkrankheiten für Aerzte und Studirende.* Kassel und Berlin: Theodor Fischer.

Westphal M, Lamszus K. (2011). The neurobiology of gliomas: from cell biology to the development of therapeutic approaches. *Nature Reviews Neuroscience* **12**(9), 495–508.

Wharton SB, O'Callaghan JP, Savva GM, Nicoll JA, Matthews F, Simpson JE, Forster G, Shaw PJ, Brayne C, Ince PG. (2009). Population variation in glial fibrillary acidic protein levels in brain ageing: relationship to Alzheimer-type pathology and dementia. *Dementia and Geriatric Cognitive Disorders* **27**(5), 465–73.

Wright G, Soper R, Brooks HF, Stadlbauer V, Vairappan B, Davies NA, Andreola F, Hodges S, Moss RF, Davies D.C. *et al.* (2010). Role of aquaporin-4 in the development of brain oedema in liver failure. *Journal of Hepatology* **53**(1), 91–7.

Wyss-Coray T, Rogers J. (2012). Inflammation in Alzheimer disease-a brief review of the basic science and clinical literature. *Cold Spring Harbor Perspectives in Medicine* **2**(1), a006346.

Yamanaka K, Chun SJ, Boillee S, Fujimori-Tonou N, Yamashita H, Gutmann DH, Takahashi R, Misawa H, Cleveland DW. (2008). Astrocytes as determinants of disease progression in inherited amyotrophic lateral sclerosis. *Nature Neuroscience* **11**(3), 251–3.

Yeh CY, Vadhwana B, Verkhratsky A, Rodriguez JJ. (2012). Early astrocytic atrophy in the entorhinal cortex of a triple transgenic animal model of Alzheimer's disease. *ASN Neuro* **3**(5), 271–9.

Yenari MA, Kauppinen TM, Swanson RA. (2010). Microglial activation in stroke: therapeutic targets. *Neurotherapeutics* **7**(4), 378–91.

Yin Z, Milatovic D, Aschner JL, Syversen T, Rocha JB, Souza DO, Sidoryk M, Albrecht J, Aschner M. (2007). Methylmercury induces oxidative injury, alterations in permeability and glutamine transport in cultured astrocytes. *Brain Research* **1131**(1), 1–10.

Yoshida T, Sasaki M, Yoshida M, Namekawa M, Okamoto Y, Tsujino S, Sasayama H, Mizuta I, Nakagawa M. (2011). Nationwide survey of Alexander disease in Japan and proposed new guidelines for diagnosis. *Journal of Neurology* **258**(11), 1998–2008.

Zhao Y, Rempe DA. (2010). Targeting astrocytes for stroke therapy. *Neurotherapeutics* **7**(4), 439–51.

# Author Index

*Glial Physiology and Pathophysiology*, First Edition. Alexei Verkhratsky and Arthur Butt.
© 2013 John Wiley & Sons, Ltd. Published 2013 by John Wiley & Sons, Ltd.

# Subject Index